The Human Complement System in Health and Disease

The Human Complement System in Health and Disease

edited by

John E. Volanakis
University of Alabama at Birmingham
Birmingham, Alabama

Michael M. Frank
Duke University Medical Center
Durham, North Carolina

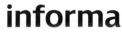
informa
healthcare

New York   London

Informa Healthcare USA, Inc.
52 Vanderbilt Avenue
New York, NY 10017

International Standard Book Number-10: 0-8247-9898-8 (Hardcover)
International Standard Book Number-13: 978-0-8247-9898-7 (Hardcover)

Library of Congress Cataloging-in-Publication Data

The human complement system in health and disease / edited by John E. Volanakis, Michael M. Frank
   p. cm.
     Includes bibliographical references and index.
  ISBN-13: 978-0-8247-9898-7
  ISBN-10: 0-8247-9898-8
  1. Complement (Immunology) 2. Immunopathology. I. Volanakis, John E. II. Frank, Michael M.
  [DNLM: 1.Complement--physiology. 2. Antigen-Antibody Complex--physiology. 3. Immune Complex Diseases--immunology. QW 680 H918 1998]

QR185.8.C6H86 1998
616.07'99--dc21
                                             97-46702

Visit the Informa Web site at
www.informa.com

and the Informa Healthcare Web site at
www.informahealthcare.com

Preface

It is now widely accepted that the activities of the complement system not only protect against invading pathogens, but also contribute to the regulation of other biological systems, specifically adaptive immunity. It is also recognized that deficiency, aberration, or exaggeration of these activities can lead to disease. Much of the knowledge on the molecular architecture, structure, cell biology, and pathophysiology of human complement has been gained only in recent years. It is becoming clear that complement studies are of importance in fields where they traditionally have not been considered central (e.g. transplantation). Complement research has been highly successful in applying a variety of technologies derived from biochemistry, molecular biology, immunology, cell biology, genetics, and pathology to the analysis of the components and intricate reactions of this highly complex system. The resulting information is scattered throughout original articles and reviews in many journals, and no single source exists that brings together current knowledge of the basic science and clinical aspects of complement. The goal of this volume is to fill this void.

The book consists of three sections. The first starts with a brief historical introduction and an overview of complement activation and includes detailed descriptions of the structure of human complement genes and proteins. Available information on the structure and chemical nature of ligand binding sites of complement proteins and of catalytic centers of enzymes is also included, and the section concludes with a chapter on the phylogeny of the system. The second section deals with the physiological functions and biology of complement. The emphasis is on new and potentially important findings that have not been adequately presented elsewhere. Older literature is also reviewed for the sake of completeness. The final section describes the relationship between complement and human diseases, where there now exists a body of information. Diseases resulting both from deficiency states and from excessive or inappropriate activation are discussed, as well as novel approaches to therapeutic manipulation of the complement system.

The 44 authors who wrote the 28 chapters of the book have produced much of the data they describe and most of them are recognized authorities in their respective subjects. We feel a sense of gratitude to all the contributors for their efforts, and for their willingness to integrate our comments and suggestions into the revised manuscripts. One of us (JEV) wishes to thank the Alexander von Humboldt Foundation for support during preparation of the book. Special appreciation is extended to Paula Kiley and Jeanette Clayton for competent secretarial assistance. It is our pleasure to thank Janet Sachs of Marcel Dekker, Inc., for her patience and efficiency.

John E. Volanakis
Michael M. Frank

Contents

Contributors

Joseph M. Ahearn   Department of Medicine, University of Pittsburgh School of Medicine, Pittsburgh, Pennsylvania

Gérard J. Arlaud   Laboratory of Molecular Enzymology, Institute for Structural Biology, Jean-Pierre Ebel, Grenoble, France

John P. Atkinson   Division of Rheumatology, Department of Internal Medicine, Washington University School of Medicine, St. Louis, Missouri

Milan Basta   Neuromuscular Disease Section, National Institute of Neurological Disorders and Stroke, National Institutes of Health, Bethesda, Maryland

Melvin Berger   Department of Pediatrics, Case Western Reserve University School of Medicine, and Rainbow Babies and Childrens Hospital, Cleveland, Ohio

Michael C. Carroll   Department of Pathology, Harvard Medical School, Boston, Massachusetts

Harvey R. Colten   Department of Pediatrics, Northwestern University Medical School, Chicago, Illinois

Neil R. Cooper   Department of Immunology, The Scripps Research Institute, La Jolla, California

Marinos C. Dalakas   Neuromuscular Disease Section, National Institute of Neurological Disorders and Stroke, National Institutes of Health, Bethesda, Maryland

Kevin A. Davies   Rheumatology Unit, Department of Medicine, Royal Postgraduate Medical School, Hammersmith Hospital, London, England

Alvin E. Davis III   Department of Pediatrics, Children's Hospital Research Foundation, University of Cincinnati College of Medicine, Cincinnati, Ohio

Peter Densen   Division of Infectious Diseases, Department of Internal Medicine, University of Iowa College of Medicine, Iowa City, Iowa

Julia A. Ember   Department of Immunology, The Scripps Research Institute, La Jolla, California

Douglas T. Fearon   Department of Medicine, University of Cambridge, Cambridge, England

Michael M. Frank   Department of Pediatrics, Duke University Medical Center, Durham, North Carolina

Gérard Garnier   Division of Allergy/Pulmonary Medicine, Department of Pediatrics, Washington University School of Medicine, St. Louis, Missouri

Tony E. Hugli   Department of Immunology, The Scripps Research Institute, La Jolla, California

Mark A. Jagels   Department of Immunology, The Scripps Research Institute, La Jolla, California

John D. Lambris   Department of Pathology and Laboratory Medicine, University of Pennsylvania, Philadelphia, Pennsylvania

Thomas J. Lawley   School of Medicine, Emory University, Atlanta, Georgia

M. Kathryn Liszewski   Division of Rheumatology, Department of Internal Medicine, Washington University School of Medicine, St. Louis, Missouri

Michael Loos   Institute of Medical Microbiology and Hygiene, Johannes Gutenberg-University, Mainz, Germany

Carolyn Mold   Department of Molecular Genetics and Microbiology, University of New Mexico Health Science Center, Albuquerque, New Mexico

Florin Niculescu   Department of Pathology, University of Maryland at Baltimore, School of Medicine, Baltimore, Maryland

Masaru Nonaka   Department of Biochemistry, Nagoya City University Medical School, Nagoya, Japan

Teresa J. Oglesby   Division of Rheumatology, Department of Internal Medicine, Washington University School of Medicine, St. Louis, Missouri

Franz Petry   Institute of Medical Microbiology and Hygiene, Johannes Gutenberg-University, Mainz, Germany

Jeffrey L. Platt   Departments of Surgery, Pediatrics and Immunology, Duke University Medical Center, Durham, North Carolina

Mnason E. Plumb   Department of Chemistry and Biochemistry, and the School of Medicine, University of South Carolina, Columbia, South Carolina

Ariella M. Rosengard   Department of Pathology, Johns Hopkins University School of Medicine, Baltimore, Maryland

Kenneth B. M. Reid   MRC Immunochemistry Unit, Department of Biochemistry, Oxford University, Oxford, England

Wendell F. Rosse   Department of Medicine and Immunology, Duke University Medical Center, Durham, North Carolina

Horea Rus   Department of Pathology, University of Maryland at Baltimore, School of Medicine, Baltimore, Maryland

Soheyla Saadi   Department of Surgery, Duke University Medical Center, Durham, North Carolina

Arvind Sahu   Department of Pathology and Laboratory Medicine, University of Pennsylvania, Philadelphia, Pennsylvania

Alan D. Schreiber   Department of Medicine, University of Pennsylvania School of Medicine, Philadelphia, Pennsylvania

Moon L. Shin   Department of Pathology, University of Maryland at Baltimore, School of Medicine, Baltimore, Maryland

James M. Sodetz   Department of Chemistry and Biochemistry, and the School of Medicine, University of South Carolina, Columbia, South Carolina

John E. Volanakis   Division of Clinical Immunology and Rheumatology, Department of Medicine, University of Alabama at Birmingham, Birmingham, Alabama

Eric Wagner   Departments of Surgery and Pediatrics, Duke University Medical Center, Durham, North Carolina

Mark J. Walport   Department of Medicine, Royal Postgraduate Medical School, Hammersmith Hospital, London, England

Clark West   Department of Pediatrics, University of Cincinnati College of Medicine, and Children's Hospital Medical Center, Cincinnati, Ohio

Rick A. Wetsel   Immunology Research Center, Institute of Molecular Medicine, University of Texas Health Science Center, Houston, Texas

Kim B. Yancey   Dermatology Branch, National Cancer Institute, National Institutes of Health, Bethesda, Maryland

1

Introduction and Historical Notes

MICHAEL M. FRANK
Duke University Medical Center, Durham, North Carolina

This volume reviews much of our understanding of complement chemistry, biology, and function in physiological systems. Much has been learned in the 100 years since the discovery of complement, but many of those who work in the field believe that our understanding is just beginning.

The development of our knowledge of the complement system parallels the history of immunology and its origins in the field of microbiology. Observations made in the latter half of the 19th century clarified the role of microbes in the causation of human illness. Vaccination had been known since the late 18th century and immunization appeared to be a likely method of protecting against infectious disease. The concept of antimicrobials had not yet been developed, but it was clear that individuals exposed to attenuated microorganisms were often immune to that organism. It was natural to ask the question, "What was responsible for that protection?" The work of Ehrlich, Metschnikoff, and a large number of others had led to an understanding that antibody and cells were important in such protection. There was controversy as to which of these provided the most important element of host defense.

As early as 1874, Traube and Gscheidlen had shown that microorganisms injected into the circulation were rapidly destroyed and the bloodstream maintained its sterility (1). The concept of bloodstream clearance of organisms was developed by these investigators and others. By 1884, Grohmann had noted that cell free serum in vitro was capable of killing microorganisms (2). Nuttall (1888) likewise inoculated defribinated blood with bacteria. He showed that outside of the body serum retained its bactericidal activity, although the activity was lost after a period of storage and the activity was heat labile (3). Buchner (1889) is generally credited with the first expression of the humoral theory of immunity: that a principle in fresh blood that he termed "alexin" (protective substance) was capable of killing bacteria. He thought that the alexin acted as an enzyme in destroying the bacteria, but he did not differentiate antibody from alexin (4). It is interesting that Baumgartner presented the theory, not taken seriously, that alexin damaged the membrane of the organism, causing an osmotic death (5).

In 1894 Pfeiffer began a series of experiments that revolutionized our understanding of the bactericidal action of serum (6). He reported that injection of cholera vibrios (called spirilla) into the peritoneum of immunized guinea pigs led to rapid dissolution of the organisms that could not be observed when injected into normal animals. In normals the organisms multiplied and killed the animal, but serum from an immunized animal, if injected into the normal, conferred protection. Heated serum also conferred protection, although it had lost all alexin activity. It was quickly shown by Bordet and Metschnikoff (7,8) that these phenomena could be duplicated in vitro and Bordet reported that cells were not required for the bactericidal effect. Bordet extended the concept of alexin by clearly identifying the heat-stable, specific antibody that recognized the antigen and the heat-labile, nonspecific activity present in all normal serum that had no activity by itself, but was lytic in the presence of antibody. Bordet also noted that a similar set of phenomena governed the lysis of red blood cells and introduced the concept of sensitization of the cells by immune sera (9). He noted that sensitized cells were lysed by fresh serum and realized that this represented the release of hemoglobin and the formation of erythrocyte ghosts that could be recovered from the reaction mixture. Others made the same observations independently. Bordet received the Nobel Prize for these observations.

Ehrlich and Morganroth extended these studies and presented the now-famous side chain theory as an explanation (10). They believed that immune cells had, on the surface, specific receptors that recognize antigen. On further immunization with antigen, more of these specific receptors were formed and were shed from the cells to circulate in the blood. They had a specific antigen-recognition site (haptophore group) that bound to antigen. They also had a specific complement-binding site (complementophore group) and activated complement after they had bound to antigen. Ehrlich conceived of complement acting like a bacterial toxin to damage the cells. He introduced the term *complement* to emphasize the fact that the fresh serum factor "complemented" the specific receptors, which he termed amboceptor, to emphasize the two types of recognition sites on the antibody molecule.

There was much confusion over the fact that complement appeared more or less lytic in different systems and the complement from different species differed in ability to lyse various targets. Ehrlich believed that each specific amboceptor had its own complement and Bordet believed that there was one type of complement. As early as 1909 Muir observed that complement of a species tended to be ineffective at lysing the cells of that species (11). Nevertheless, by 1910 it was known that alexin or complement activity was due to specific antibody and immunologically nonspecific protein factors. The concept that antibody promoted the killing of these organisms was established and the first studies of complement chemistry were yielding results.

In the early years of the 1900s, the first attempts at protein chemistry revealed that complement was not a single substance but consisted of multiple proteins. Buchner separated serum into water-soluble pseudoglobulin and insoluble euglobulin. He showed that the pseudoglobulin and euglobulin fractions no longer had bactericidal activity (12). Ferrata confirmed that neither pseudoglobulin nor euglobulin fractions of serum contained hemolytic activity (13). When these fractions were mixed together, complement activity was restored. It was possible to examine the action of these fractions sequentially and classify serum fractions into midpiece, which reacted with antibody; and end-piece, which reacted after midpiece to complete the lytic reaction.

Ehrlich's laboratory focused on the lysis of sheep erythrocytes sensitized with rabbit antibody in the presence of guinea pig serum. The reason for choosing this strange mixture of reagents is apparent. The laboratory had noted empirically that sheep erythrocytes were exquisitely sensitive to lysis by rabbit antisheep erythrocyte antibody and complement. We now know that sheep erythrocytes have on their surface a lipopolysaccharide antigen, the Forssman antigen, to which rabbits make large amounts of IgM and IgG hemolytic antibody. Sheep erythrocytes differ from those of most other species in that they are smaller, more spherical, and are remarkably sensitive to lyse by antibody and complement. The hemolytic titer of fresh guinea pig serum, as reflected in the ability to lyse antibody-sensitized sheep erythrocytes, is higher than that of most other species. Thus, it was possible using reagents easily available in the laboratory at the turn of the century, to develop a highly sensitive system for analyzing complement.

Brand, examining red cell lysis, recognized that complement action could be defined by a series of cellular intermediates important in hemolysis (14). By 1919 it was believed that complement consisted of at least three factors. This belief depended upon the earlier observation in 1903 by Flexner and Noguchi that cobra venom could destroy complement activity (15). Both midpiece and endpiece contained factors that could restore this activity. By 1913 Weil had prepared an erythrocyte, antibody, midpiece, intermediate that could be hemolyzed by the addition of heated serum (16). This finding was confirmed by Nathan who showed that as these cells were lysed, the third component was consumed (17). Ueno, in 1938, working in isolation in Japan, described a cellular intermediate product consisting of erythrocyte, antibody, C1, C4, and endpiece (18). His experiments established the order of the complement cascade. As early as 1914, Coca reported what was then called the third component of complement was capable of combining with yeast, and that yeast could be used to remove the third component from serum (19). This early work by Coca allowed for the later work in the 1950s by Pillemer that led to the discovery of the alternative pathway (20).

Investigators at that time were interested primarily in how human beings protect themselves from infection. In retrospect, it is clear that the system chosen for study consisting of sheep erythrocytes, rabbit antibody and guinea pig serum differed considerably from the systems they were interested in understanding. However, the assumption was made that discoveries in this model system would be immediately applicable to the systems of particular interest. It was much easier to study the lysis of sheep erythrocytes, since at the end of the reaction time the cells could be sedimented and the hemoglobin in the supernatant easily determined. If one studied the lysis of bacteria, one had to perform colony counts at the end of the reaction mixture to determine whether the bacteria were killed, which is a much more laborious procedure. Therefore, they missed the existence of a second or alternative pathway. Moreover, investigators focused on what bound to the sheep erythrocyte or bacterium, neglecting what was left behind in the supernate. They missed the important fact that such peptides left behind following complement activation have important inflammatory properties.

The serum fraction termed midpiece contained a protein that could interact with erythrocyte-bound hemolytic antibody. This protein was termed C1. In 1926, Gordon et al. reported the existence of the fourth component of complement, showing that ammonia destroyed a heat-stable factor in serum that was distinct from the third component (21). By the late 1950s, it was believed that there were four components of complement, and in the late 1950s, Manfred Mayer's group (Rapp) developed a mathematical model of complement action that suggested that the last-acting component, termed C3, might actually be a complex of two, three, or perhaps more components (22).

Nelson, et al., using laborious hemolytic assays and techniques of simple column chromatography, reported the existence of at least six separate factors that together made up C3. Müller-Eberhard and his colleagues, using more sophisticated techniques for protein isolation, began the arduous task of separating these proteins and characterizing them individually (23,24). During these early days, our understanding of complement paralleled our understanding of other physiological systems. The initial experiments were physiological, using the newly developed techniques of bacteriology. As early biochemical methods became available for the separation of proteins, these were applied to complement serum proteins and the proteins were laboriously separated. Mathematical models were applied in the 1950s to analyze the protein reactions and to clarify the steps in the sequence. With the advent of modern molecular biology, the focus turned to sequencing the proteins and determining their chromosomal localization and their structure.

Dourmashkin and Humphrey in the 1960s, using electron microscopy, first demonstrated the complement lesions in red cells. Ultimately, this finding confirmed the prediction of Mayer and his colleagues that complement caused a hole or donut in the cell surface, thereby destabilizing its osmotic equilibrium and inducing lysis.

The history of our knowledge of the alternative pathway is also fascinating. In 1954, Pillemer and his colleagues reported the results of a startling series of experiments (20). In studying the ability of a baker's yeast fraction, zymosan, to interact with serum, they noted that this insoluble polysaccharide interacted with the late-acting complement components without appearing to utilize the earlier components. The zymosan appeared to interact with a previously undescribed serum protein they termed properdin. Properdin-mediated C3 activation occurred in the absence of antibody, but did require the presence of a series of cofactors, termed properdin factor A and properdin factor B. Factor A was ammonia and hydrazine sensitive and heat stable. Factor B was stable to ammonia, but heat labile. Pillemer believed that these properdin factors were different from the previously described components of the classical complement pathway.

Pillemer found that at a temperature of 17°C properdin could interact with zymosan without consuming complement. The mixture of zymosan and serum could be centrifuged, leading to properdin-depleted serum in which complement was no longer activated by zymosan. Properdin could be eluted from zymosan, reintroduced into the serum and now at 37° zymosan could activate the complement. Thus, Pillemer believed that he had discovered a new complement pathway, not requiring antibody, but requiring properdin and the late-acting components of complement.

It was possible to study the ability of various microorganisms to be damaged by serum in which properdin had been removed by absorption. A series of papers followed that suggested that there were a wide variety of microorganisms whose destruction depended on the so-called properdin pathway. These included bacteria, viruses such as Newcastle disease virus, and even erythrocytes from patients with the disease paroxysmal nocturnal hemoglobinuria. Properdin was thought to play an important role in nonspecific immunity against infection.

In 1958, Nelson suggested a second interpretation of the data (25). He suggested that properdin was IgM antibody to zymosan. The antibody was required for zymosan to interact with complement. If the IgM antibody to zymosan was removed by absorption, zymosan would no longer interact with complement. If the antibody was restored, the interaction would again take place. The only additional concept needed was that a wide variety of organisms might have antigens on their surface that interacted with the polysaccharides important in the antigenicity of zymosan. Thus, the absorption might remove an IgM antibody that cross-reacted with a variety of microbial antigens and that was required for complement activation. The argument seemed compelling, since IgM was only then being identified and the properdin theory went into eclipse for over a decade. Several of Pillemer's students, including Pensky and Lepow continued to follow up Pillemer's original observations, identifying properdin as a protein and showing that it was unique and not identical to IgM.

The later history of the alternative pathway followed other rather disparate paths. In 1963, Schur and Becker suggested that F(ab)$'_2$ fragments of rabbit antibody in the form of antigen antibody complexes could fix or activate complement (26). Since C1 binding requires the Fc fragment of antibody, this was a surprising observation. Moreover, the F(ab)$'_2$ antigen antibody complexes could not fix all of the complement. The investigators came to the conclusion that there were two types of complement. One type could be absorbed with F(ab)$'_2$-containing fragments. The other only interacted with complement containing undigested antibody. This work did not receive wide recognition.

By the end of the 1960s, it was shown that guinea pig IgG antibodies, γ1, and γ2 could be separated and that γ2 antibodies behaved as expected, fixing or activating all of the components of complement after interacting with antigen. γ1 Antibodies also activated or fixed complement components when immune complexes were formed, however, only the late-acting components appeared to be activated and the early components were spared (27).

At about that time, Gewurz and colleagues noted that bacterial endotoxins consumed the late-acting components of complement, but appeared to spare the early components (28). This occurred even in agammaglobulinemic serum with no detectable antibody. The problem with these studies was that no one knew whether the observed variability reflected differences in antibody function, assay variability, or the presence of confounding regulatory molecules. Shortly thereafter, however, a strain of guinea pigs was developed totally lacking the early acting component of the classical pathway C4 (29). The serum of these guinea pigs had no ability to lyse sheep erythrocytes because of the failure of classical pathway activity. However, antigen–antibody complexes could activate the late-acting components in this serum. Thus, there was now no question that there was an alternative pathway of complement activation.

With many lines of evidence in multiple laboratories suggesting the presence of an alternative pathway of complement activation, there was a resurgence of interest in Pillemer's earlier observations. The laboratory of Müller-Eberhard turned to the analysis of an old observation (30). There is a protein in the venom of cobras capable of activating complement. Studies suggested that C1, C4, and C2 of the classical pathway were spared by cobra venom factor, but C3 and the later components were activated and destroyed. Further analysis suggested that cofactors were required and the cofactors had the same properties as those originally described by Pillemer, co-factor A, and co-factor B. Extensive analysis in several laboratories ultimately showed that cobra venom protein is a cobra analog of human C3b. It binds to factor B of the alternative pathway and in the presence of magnesium ion, factor D of the alternative pathway cleaves the factor B to form a C3 convertase. The search then began for the cobra venom protein analog in human serum. Ultimately it was found that hydrolyzed C3 in the presence of factors B and D formed a C3 convertase. The convertase was stabilized by properdin. Native C3 did not form the convertase, but only C3 with a hydrolyzed thioester that had undergone a conformational change or C3b itself served this function. Thus, the original hypothesis of Pillemer was confirmed.

The studies of the late 1970s and 1980s involved not finding new complement proteins. These in general had been discovered earlier. Now the emphasis was on characterizing the proteins and in defining regulatory steps in the complement cascade. An astonishing number of regulatory proteins were discovered and the reasons for their presence became clear. There are relatively few individuals missing any of the complement proteins, but complement is frequently involved in the causation of human disease. In these cases, it is almost always true that the complement is functioning in a physiologically normal fashion, but it is damaging host tissues rather than damaging invading microorganisms or foreign cells. The many regulatory molecules control activation in the host in attempts to regulate possible damage to host tissue. These regulatory proteins are discussed in detail later in this book. The 1970s and 1980s focused on defining these regulatory molecules, their mechanism of action, whether they were free in plasma or on cell surfaces, and how they functioned. Moreover, the critical role of complement in controlling cell function became a focus of study.

From the turn of the century it was known that bacteria injected in the bloodstream might be found in phagocytic cells and also might be found bound to surface of cellular elements in the bloodstream. Exudates containing phagocytic cells were more lytic for bacteria than serum or plasma. In severe cases of hemolytic anemia, it was noted that erythrocytes might be bound to the surface of monocytes or neutrophils or might be present in phagocytic cells. Nelson and his colleagues extended these studies in the 1950s to develop the concept of immune adherence, the coating of a particle by opsonic complement fragments that mediate adherence to phagocytic cells (31). Specific receptors for these complement fragments were identified and ultimately Fearon and colleagues isolated the first of these CR1, CD35 (32). Specific receptors for C4b, C3b, iC3b, C3dg, C1q, C5a, C3a, and others were found over the subsequent decades (33). Their importance in the biological activity of complement was established and the focus now is on determining how they trigger alterations in cellular function. Their importance in the removal of immune complexes from the circulation and in the phagocytosis of opsonized particles has become apparent. Their function during the induction phase of the immune response is just starting to become clear. The stage is set for a far more detailed understanding of the role of normal complement function in human disease. Part of the reason that his area has proceeded slowly has been the absence of patients in large numbers missing these complement factors and the limited study of immune function in these rare individuals. Individuals missing almost all of the complement proteins have been described. Often these people have autoimmune disease or a propensity for severe infection, particularly with *Neisseria* organisms. However, the numbers of individuals have been few and the animal models of complement deficiency that are available for use in their stead are quite limited.

In the 1920s, a guinea pig strain lacking C3 was reported by Hyde et al. (34). At that time, it was not known that C3 consisted of multiple proteins. The strain was lost over the years and we do not know which specific late component was missing in these guinea pigs. The development of C4-deficient guinea pigs missing classical pathway activity and C5-deficient mice, missing the activity of one of the later components, made study of these portions of the complement cascade easier. C6-deficient rabbits were described, but these animals were difficult to breed and available in small numbers and the number of studies performed with them was quite limited. C6-deficient rats, C3-deficient dogs, and factor H-deficient pigs have been described, but these animals are not yet generally available (35).

With the advent of modern molecular biology, it is possible to develop "knock-out" mice with specific gene defects preventing the synthesis of a specific protein. Given the fact that the chromosomal localization and DNA sequence of each of the complement proteins and regulators has been described, it is expected that such mouse models will become far more common. Much of modern cellular immunology depends on mouse models. These animals can be used in numbers and there is a large body of experimental data examining their immune response in a variety of settings convenient for study. It happens that the complement system in mice is particularly difficult to deal with since the proteins are labile, present in small amounts, and there is often an incompatibility between the mouse proteins, and the proteins available for study: human and guinea pig proteins. Complement protein purification traditionally relies on the availability of large amounts of plasma to simplify isolation. The difficulty working with mice made it particularly difficult to integrate the work developing in complement laboratories with the burgeoning literature in cellular immunology. It is now clear that those difficulties are of the past and further integration will come rapidly.

With our current understanding of molecules on cells and in plasma, their genes, their mechanism of action, their structure, and their function, we now see the birth of a new era in complement chemistry and biology where a further sophisticated understanding of physiology and disease will be forthcoming.

REFERENCES

1. Traube M, Gscheideln. Über Faeulniss und den Widerstand der lebenden Organismen gegen dieselbe. Zweiundfuenfzigster Jahres Bericht der Schlesischen Gesellschaft für vaterlaendische Cultur 1874; 179.
2. Grohmann W. Über die Einwirkung des zellenfreien Blutplasma auf einige pflanzliche Microorganismen (schimmel, spross, pathogene und nichtpathogene Spaltpilze). Dorpat: C. Mattiesen, 1884; 34.
3. Nuttall G. Experimente über die bacterienfeindlichen Einfluesse des thierischen Körpers. Z Hyg Infektionskr 1888; 4:353.
4. Buchner H. Über die bakterientödtende Wirkung des zellfreien Blutserums. Zbl Bakt (Naturwiss) 1889; 5:817, 6:1.
5. Baumgartner. Gehrbuch der pathogenen mikroorg. Hirzél, Leipzig. 1911. Quoted in Zinsser H. Infection and Resistance, New York: Macmillan, 1923:154.
6. Pfeiffer R, Issaeff R. Über die specifische Bedeutung der Choleraimmunität. Z Hyg Infektionskr 1894; 17:355.
7. Bordet J. Sur l'agglutination et la dissolution des globules rouges par le sérum d'animaux injecties de sang defibriné. Ann Inst Pasteur (Paris) 1898; 12:688.
8. Metschnikoff E. Sur la lutte des cellules de l'organisme contre l'invasion des microbes. Ann Inst Pasteur (Paris) 1887; 1:321.
9. Bordet J. Résumé of immunity In: Studies in Immunity. New York: J. Wiley and Sons, 1909.
10. Ehrlich P. Studies in Immunity. New York: J. Wiley and Sons, 1906.
11. Muir R. On the relationships between the complement and the immune bodies of different animals. J Pathol Bacteriol 1911; 16:523.
12. Buchner H. Über die nähere Natur der bakterientödtenden Substanz in Blutserum. Zbl Bakt (Naturwiss). 1889; 6:561.
13. Ferrata A. Die Unwirksamkeit der komplexen Hämolysine in salzfreien Lösungen und ihre Ursache. Berlin Klin Wochenschr 1907; 44:366.
14. Brand E. Über das Verhalten der Komplemente bei des Dialyse. Berlin Klin Wochenschr 1907; 44:1075.
15. Flexner S, Noguchi H. Snake venom in relation to haemolysis, bacteriolysis, and toxicity. J Exp Med 1903; 6:277.
16. Weil E. Über die Wirkungsweise des Komplements bei der Haemolyse. Biochem Z 1913; 48:347.
17. Nathan E. Über die Beziehungen der Komponenten des Komplements zu den ambozeptorbeladenen Blutköperchen. Z. Immunitaetsforsch 1914; 21:259.

18. Ueno S. Studien über die Komponenten des Komplementes. I and II. 1938; 7:201, 225.
19. Coca AF. A study of the anticomplementary action of yeast of certain bacteria and of cobra venom. Z Immunitaetsforsch 1914; 21:604.
20. Pillemer L, Blum L, Lepow IH, Ross OA, Todd EW, Wardlaw AC. The properdin system and immunity. I. Demonstration and isolation of a new serum protein, properdin, and its role in immune phenomena. Science 1954; 120:279–285.
21. Gordon J, Whitehead HR, Wormall A. The action of ammonia on complement. The fourth component. J Biochem 1926; 20:1028.
22. Rapp HJ. Mechanism of immune hemolysis: recognition of two steps in the conversion of $EAC'_{1,4,2}$ to E^*. Science 1958; 127:234.
23. Nelson RA, Jensen J, Gigli I, Tamura N. Methods for the separation, purification and measurement of nine components of hemolytic complement in guinea pig serum. Immunochemistry 1966; 3:111.
24. Muller-Eberhard HJ. Complement. Annu Rev Biochem 1975; 44:697–724.
25. Nelson RA. An alternative mechanism for the properdin system. J Exp Med 1968; 108:515–535.
26. Schur PH, Becker EL. Pepsin digestion of rabbit and sheep antibodies. The effect on complement fixation. J Exp Med 1963; 118:891–904.
27. Sandberg AL, Osler AG. Dual pathways of complement interaction with guinea pig immunoglobulins. J Immunol 1971; 107:1268–1273.
28. Gewurz H, Shin HS, Mergenhagen SE. Interactions of the complement system with endotoxic lipopolysaccharide: consumption of each of the six terminal complement components. J Exp Med 1968; 128:1049–1057.
29. Ellman L, Green I, Frank MM. Genetically controlled total deficiency of the fourth component of complement in the guinea pig. Science 1970; 170:74–75.
30. Gotze O, Muller-Eberhard HJ. The C3 activation system: an alternate pathway of complement activation. J Exp Med 1971; 134:90s–108s.
31. Nelson RA. The immune-adherence phenomenon. A hypothetical role of erythrocytes in defence against bacteria and viruses. Proc R Soc Med 1956; 49:55.
32. Fearon DT. Identification of the membrane glycoprotein that is the C3b receptor of the human erythrocyte, polymorphonuclear leukocyte, B lymphocyte and monocyte. J Exp Med 1980; 152:20.
33. Frank MM. Complement system. In: Frank MM, Austen KF, Claman HN, Unanue ER, eds. Samter's Immunologic Diseases, 5th Ed. Vol. I. Boston: Little, Brown, 1994; 489–500.
34. Hyde RR. Complement-deficient guinea-pig serum. J Immun 1923; 8:167.
35. Frank MM. Animal models for complement deficiencies. J Clin Immunol 1995; 15(6):113S–121S.

2

Overview of the Complement System

JOHN E. VOLANAKIS

University of Alabama at Birmingham, Birmingham, Alabama

I. INTRODUCTION

A century after its initial description as a heat-labile factor "complementing" the bacterio-lytic activity of antibodies (1–5), complement is widely recognized as a major multicompo-nent host-defense system. It comprises an ever-increasing number of proteins partitioned between the plasma and the cell membranes of blood and other cells (6). Following activation by bacterial or other pathogens, complement proteins generate fragments and protein complexes that mediate acute inflammatory reactions, clearance of foreign cells and molecules, and killing of pathogenic microorganisms. Most of these activities are mediated through the recruitment and/or activation of phagocytes, platelets, mast cells, and endothelial cells. Cell activation is effected either by binding of complement proteins or protein fragments to specific receptors or by insertion of protein complexes into cell membranes. The latter mechanism is also utilized to kill bacterial and other susceptible cells. In addition, it has been clearly established that complement activation products play a significant role in the regulation of adaptive immune responses. For example, optimal antibody responses to T-cell-dependent antigens require signals initiated by engagement of complement receptors on B cells.

A number of observations indicate that in addition to these well-recognized functions, complement can also elicit diverse responses from a variety of other cells and tissues. Such responses are not necessarily directly related to host defense. Early indications for such wider effects were provided by biosynthetic studies on complement proteins. As anticipated on the basis of earlier data (7–9), these extensive investigations demonstrated that hepatocytes are the main source of blood complement proteins, while macrophages and fibroblasts are responsible for local synthesis at tissue sites (see Chap. 10). These studies also revealed some unexpected sources of complement proteins. For example, astrocytes synthesize in vitro most complement proteins (10–12). Adipocytes are the main source of blood factor D (13) and also synthesize and secrete several other complement proteins (14). Rat endometrial epithelial cells secrete large amounts of C3 in response to estrogen (15). Human endometrium also secretes C3 and factor B (16).

A second line of evidence for a wider role of complement developed from studies on the expression of complement regulatory and receptor proteins. For example, complement-regulatory proteins are widely distributed throughout the female and male reproductive tracts, including oocytes and spermatozoa (17,18). Astrocytes also express complement

9

regulatory proteins (19,20) and receptors (21). The distribution of receptors for C3a and C5a, the two most active complement "anaphylatoxins," is of particular interest. Apart from inflammatory cells of myeloid origin, both receptors are widely distributed in human tissues, including lung, spleen, placenta, and throughout the brain (22). C5a receptor has been also demonstrated on hepatocytes, smooth muscle, endothelial cells, and astrocytes (23).

Some unexpected functions elicited by anaphylatoxins binding to their receptors have already been described. C3a-desArg was shown to stimulate triglyceride synthesis in human skin fibroblasts and adipocytes, probably through a PKC-mediated pathway (24) and C5a was shown to induce acute-phase protein genes in hepatocytes (25).

Other previously unrecognized complement functions are mediated by the large protein complexes formed during complement activation by the successive interaction of C5b, C6, C7, C8, and C9. The final complex, usually referred to as membrane attack complex (MAC) has traditionally been linked to complement-mediated cell lysis and death. However, as discussed in Chapters 13 and 15 of this volume, sublytic concentrations of the MAC have multiple additional effects on diverse cells, including expression of procoagulant activity by platelets and endothelial cells (26,27), secretion of interleukin 1 (IL-1) leading to autocrine activation of endothelial cells (28), and transduction of signals leading to activation of heterotrimeric G proteins and of the protein kinases ERK1 and JNK (29,30). More recent data have also shown that homologous MAC provides a mechanism for the export from cells of polypeptides devoid of signal sequences (31,32). Thus, the MAC could serve as a route for the release and perhaps also uptake of autocrine, paracrine, and/or endocrine signals (32). Therefore, it appears that the complement system is considerably more pleiotropic than generally recognized. As we enter a new century of complement research, it seems probable that additional evidence supporting the pleiotropic nature of complement will emerge, leading to a more complete understanding of the biology and pathophysiology of this complex protein system.

II. COMPLEMENT PROTEINS

A. General Features

About 35 proteins are presently known to participate in the complement system (Table 1). In their native state these proteins are either soluble in plasma or associated with cell membranes. Complement proteins can be categorized by function as those participating in the activation sequences, those regulating the activation and activities of the system, and those serving as cellular receptors for complement proteins or their fragments. Proteins participating in complement activation function as proteolytic enzymes, enzyme cofactors, or enzyme substrates, some of which are precursors of biologically active fragments. Regulatory proteins inhibit enzymes, thus ensuring that the extent of complement activation is proportional to the amount and duration of presence of complement activators. They also inactivate bioactive peptides and prevent complement activation on the surface of autologous cells, thus protecting the host's tissues from the harmful potential of complement activation. Some complement proteins overlap these functional categories. Also certain of these proteins have additional functions unrelated to the complement system.

B. Nomenclature

Nomenclature for proteins participating in complement activation follows two conventions (33,34). Eleven proteins originally described as components of the classical pathway are

Table 1 Proteins of the Complement System

Prevalent Form in Native State	Functional Group[a]		
	Activation Sequences	Regulatory	Receptors
Serum soluble	C1q, MBL	C1INH	
	C1r, C1s, MASP, D	C4bp, H, I, P	
	C2, B	C3a/C5a INA	
	C3, C4, C5	S protein, SP 40/40	
	C6, C7, C8, C9		
Membrane associated[b]		CR1	C1qR
		DAF, MCP	C3aR, C5aR
		HRF, CD59	CR1, CR2
			CR3, CR4

[a]Established symbols have been used for most complement proteins. In addition, the following generally accepted abbreviations have been used: INH, inhibitor, C4bp, C4b-binding protein; INA, inactivator; R, receptor (e.g., CR1, complement receptor type 1); MBL, mannose-binding lectin; MASP, MBL-associated serine protease; DAF, decay-accelerating factor; MCP, membrane cofactor protein; HRF, homologous restriction factor.
[b]CD numbers of membrane-associated proteins: CR1, CD35; CR2, CD21; CR3, CD18/CD11b; CR4, CD18/CD11c; C5aR, CD88; DAF, CD55; MCP, CD46

designated by the capital letter C and a number from 1 to 9. C1 is a Ca^{2+}-dependent complex of three distinct proteins termed C1q, C1r, and C1s. Two proteins participating in the activation of the alternative pathway are referred to as factors and are symbolized by capital letters (i.e., factor B and factor D). Proteins of the recently described lectin pathway are designated by their abbreviated trivial names (i.e., MBL for mannan-binding lectin [originally termed mannan-binding protein or MBP] and MASP for MBL-associated serine protease). A bar over a complement protein symbol (e.g., C1s) indicates an active serine protease. Proteolytic cleavage fragments are symbolized by lower case letters, as in C2a and C2b, and inactive proteins or protein fragments by the letter i (e.g. C3i, C2ai).

Some regulatory proteins, initially described as part of the alternative pathway, are termed factors and designated by capital letters, as in factor H and factor I. Other regulatory proteins are designated by trivial descriptive names and symbolized by their initials, as in DAF for decay-accelerating factor. Membrane-associated regulatory proteins have been assigned CD numbers (Table 1). Four of the complement receptors are symbolized by the letters CR for complement receptor and a number from 1 to 4. The remaining receptors are denoted by the symbol of the protein or protein fragment they bind followed by the capital letter R (e.g., C1qR, C5aR). Most complement receptors have been assigned CD numbers.

Polypeptide chains of native complement proteins are designated by Greek lower case letters (i.e., α, β, and γ) except for the C1q chains, which are termed A, B, and C. Nomenclature of complement protein modules follows the recommendations of an International Workshop held in 1994 in Margretetorp, Sweden (35).

C. Structure

Individual complement proteins or groups of proteins are structurally similar to members of various other protein families, indicating that the evolutionary origins of the complement system are diverse. For some complement proteins primary structure similarity to other proteins extends over their entire length. However, most complement proteins have a modular structure and sequence similarity with other proteins only involves short stretches of amino acids, organized in protein modules or domains. Complement proteins C3, C4, and C5, C1INH, and the C3a and C5a receptors are examples of the former group, while the majority of the remaining complement proteins belong to the latter group.

C3, C4, and C5 are described in detail in Chapter 5 of this volume. The three proteins are structurally similar to each other and belong to the same protein family as a_2-macroglobulin (36), an evolutionary ancient enzyme inhibitor (37). A unique structural characteristic of this group of blood proteins, which, however, is not shared by C5, is the presence of a thiolester bond, which on proteolytic cleavage/activation becomes exposed and thus extremely susceptible to nucleophilic attack (38,39). The metastable thiolester then reacts with $-NH_2$ or $-OH$ groups on cellular or protein surfaces to form amide or ester bonds, respectively, or is hydrolyzed (40,41). Covalent attachment of C4 and C3 to the surface of complement activators through this mechanism is essential to their function. Other examples of nonmodular complement proteins structurally similar to members of other protein families are provided by C1INH, which is a member of the serine protease inhibitor or serpin superfamily (42) and also by the C5a-receptor and C3a-receptor, both of which belong to the family of seven-membrane-domain, G protein-coupled receptors (22,43).

Most other complement proteins consist of either identical repeating modules or, more often, of different modules or domains derived from apparently unrelated protein families. This modular structure indicates that multiple exon shuffling and/or gene duplication events marked the evolution of the complement system (44,45). Groups of functionally related complement proteins have similar overall modular structures. Three major groups of modular complement proteins, the complement enzymes, the cytolytic proteins, and the regulatory and receptor proteins (Fig. 1) are discussed briefly below.

The seven complement enzymes, factor D, C1r, C1s, MASP, factor B, C2, and factor I, are discussed in detail in Chapter 4 of this volume. They are responsible, either directly or indirectly, for the production of biologically active complement fragments and complexes. They have in common a catalytic domain comprising about 230 amino acids, which is structurally similar to that found in all members of the large chymotrypsin-like subfamily of serine proteases (46,47). With the exception of factor D (48), complement enzymes have additional protein modules derived from various gene superfamilies. These modules are apparently involved in protein-protein interactions, endowing these proteases with their extremely restricted substrate specificity. MASP (49), C1r (50,51), and C1s (52,53) have identical modular structures. Each of these three enzymes contains two noncontiguous CUB modules at its NH_2-terminal region. CUB modules consist of approximately 110 amino acids folded in an antiparallel β-barrell; they are also found in several extracellular proteins participating in developmental processes (54). Each of these three proteases also has an epidermal growth factor (EGF)-like and two complement control protein (CCP) modules. EGF-like modules consist of about 40 amino acids, including 6 disulfide-linked cysteines and are folded into two antiparallel two-stranded β sheets (55,56). EGF-like modules in single or often multiple copies are also present in cellular receptors and a wide variety of other proteins of diverse function. CCP modules, also termed short consensus repeats (SCR) (57), constitute the main or exclusive building blocks of several complement regulatory or receptor proteins (58,59). They are also found in several noncomplement proteins, such as the IL-2 receptor and $β_2$-glycoprotein I (60).

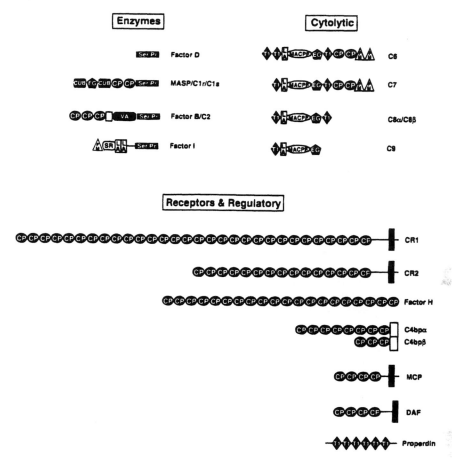

Figure 1 Modular structure of major groups of complement proteins. SerPr, serine protease domain. Protein module designation: CP, complement control protein (CCP); CUB, first found in C1r, C1s, *u*EGF, *b*one morphogenetic protein; EG, epidermal growth factor (EGF)-like; FM, factor I/membrane attack complex proteins C6/7 (FIMAC); LA, low-density lipoprotein-receptor class A, (LDLRA); MACPF, membrane attack complex (MAC) proteins/perforin; SR, scavenger receptor cysteine-rich (SRCR); T1, thrombospondin type-1 (TSP1); VA, von Willebrand factor type A (VWFA). (Adapted from Ref. 35).

CCP modules consist of about 60 amino acids and include 4 invariant disulfide-linked cysteines. They are folded in a series of β-strands that surround a hydrophobic core (61,62).

C2 (63,64) and factor B (65,66) have identical modular structures. In addition to the serine protease domain each contains three CCP modules at the NH$_2$-terminus followed by a von Willebrand factor type A (VWFA) module (67,68). VWFA modules are also present in extracellular matrix proteins and in integrins (69). They consist of about 200 amino acid residues arranged in a typical α/β open sheet or "Rossmann" fold (70,71).

Factor I has a unique structure, containing four modules of three different types in its NH$_2$-terminal half (72,73). A factor I/MAC proteins C6/C7 (FIMAC) module is followed by a scavenger receptor cysteine-rich (SRCR) and two tandem low-density lipoprotein receptor class A (LDLRA) modules. FIMAC modules contain about 70 residues and are characterized by an unusually high number, (ten) of disulfide-bridged cysteines (74). Their tertiary structure remains unknown. SRCR modules are found in several cell-surface proteins, including receptors (75). They consist of about 100 residues including 6 highly conserved disulfide-linked cysteines (75). LDLRA modules are found in several receptors and complement proteins (76). Each LDLRA module contains about 40 amino acid residues, including 6 disulfide-linked cysteines and a cluster of conserved acidic residues. The tertiary structure of LDLRA modules has not been reported, but consensus structure predictions combined with spectroscopy indicate a high β-sheet content (77).

The five polypeptide chains, C6 (74,78), C7(79), C8α (80), C8β (81), and C9 (82), which interact with C5b and with each other to form the MAC, have very similar modular structures (Fig. 1). The structure and function of these proteins is described in detail in Chapter 6 of this volume. They all share a common structural domain, termed membrane attack protein/perforin (MACPF) domain. As indicated by its designation, MACPF is also present in perforin, the cytolytic polypeptide of cytolytic T cells (83). The MACPF domain is about 340 amino acid residues long and can be subdivided into two regions, an NH$_2$-terminal one shared by all cytolytic complement proteins and a COOH-terminal one that is also present in perforin. All complement cytolytic proteins also contain two thrombospondin type-1 (TSP1) modules, except for C6 and C9, which contain three and one TSP1 modules, respectively. TSP1 modules, initially described in the cell adhesion protein thrombospondin (84), constitute the main structural element of the regulatory complement protein properdin (85) and are also found in malarial proteins (86). They consist of about 60 residues and contain six highly conserved cysteines, apparently forming disulfide bridges. Fourier transform infrared spectroscopy combined with secondary structural predictions has indicated that TSP1 modules are composed of β-sheets and an unusually high percentage of β-turns (87). Each of the five cytolytic proteins also contains one LDLRA and one EGF-like module. In addition, C6 and C7 contain two CCP and two FIMAC modules each. It seems likely that the protein modules found in the cytolytic polypeptides mediate protein–protein interactions, which are necessary for the stepwise assembly of the MAC.

Two important complement receptors, complement receptor type I (CR1) (57,88) and complement receptor type II (CR2) (89,90), and four regulatory proteins, DAF (91,92), membrane cofactor protein (MCP) (93), C4b-binding protein (C4bp) (94,95), and factor H (96,97), consist almost entirely of tandemly repeated CCP modules. Their number varies from 3 for the β-chain of C4bp to 30 for the most common allele of CR1 (Fig. 1). CCP modules are therefore responsible for the structural features of these proteins. They apparently also provide a suitable framework for binding sites for fragments of C3 and C4. Such binding sites usually extend over two or three contiguous CCP modules, most often at the NH$_2$-terminal end of these proteins (98,99). Complement regulatory and receptor proteins are discussed in Chapters 7 and 8, respectively, of this volume.

III. COMPLEMENT ACTIVATION

A. Overview

Activation is necessary for expression of biological activities by the complement system. Despite the participation of multiple structurally and functionally diverse proteins, complement activation is characterized by remarkable operational simplicity. This can best be illustrated in the context of prevalent ideas about the evolution of the system. It has been proposed (45,100) that the ancestral complement system consisted of a thiolester-containing, C3-like molecule and a phagocytic receptor recognizing its activated form. Cleavage/activation of this C3-like molecule, perhaps by a bacterial protease, would result in its covalent attachment to the bacterial surface through a transacylation reaction of the thiolester bond. Interaction of C3 with its receptor would then result in phagocytosis of the bacterial cell. Evolution of the system probably proceeded through the emergence of intrinsic complement C3-cleaving enzymes and the acquisition of additional functions by C3, which obviously maintained its central position in the system. Indeed, C3 is the most abundant complement protein in blood (130 mg/dl) and its proteolytic fragments not only express multiple biological activities but also are necessary for the assembly of several key enzymes of the activation sequences (101).

Duplication of the ancestral C3-like gene produced C4, which mostly participates in the complement activation sequences and C5, which produces fragments expressing important biological activities, including chemotaxis and cytolysis of bacterial cells. It should be noted that this is a hypothetical sequence of evolution of C3, C4, and C5. Evidence either supporting (102) or refuting (103, 104) this proposal has been presented. Nevertheless, it is clear that the most important biological activities of complement are derived from C3 and C5. Therefore, the majority of all other complement proteins appear to have evolved under pressures to ensure efficient and controlled production and utilization of the many biologically active fragments derived from C3 and from its structurally similar protein C5. In parallel, additional proteins evolved to control complement enzymes and to protect host tissues from potential complement-induced damage.

In humans and other mammals complement activation is initiated by a variety of pathogens and foreign molecules recognized either directly by complement proteins or indirectly through recognition molecules from other host defense systems, such as antibodies. Activation proceeds through two main phases. The first phase starts with recognition of the activator and proceeds through a series of highly specialized protein–protein interactions and proteolytic cleavages, which culminate in the assembly of bimolecular proteases, termed C3-convertases. Depending on the nature of the complement activator, one or two of the three available pathways, termed classical, lectin, and alternative, are predominantly activated to yield C3-convertases (Fig. 2). Activation pathways utilize different proteins to recognize pathogens and form C3-convertases. All C3-convertases however, cleave the same single peptide bond in C3, generating the same two active fragments: C3a, a small peptide, and C3b, a large 2-chain fragment.

The second or effector phase of complement activation proceeds through two pathways. The first consists of successive proteolytic cleavages of C3b attached to the surface of complement activators and results in the generation of several fragments with distinct biological activities. The second or cytolytic effector pathway is initiated by the formation of a C5-convertase and concludes with the assembly of the large potentially cytolytic MAC.

B. Assembly of C3 Convertases

1. Classical Pathway

The most extensively investigated mechanism for the assembly of a C3 convertase in the classical pathway of complement activation is the one initiated by antibodies of the IgG or IgM class in complex with their specific antigens (Fig. 3). Activation of this pathway is also triggered by the evolutionary ancient C-reactive protein (CRP) (105) in complex with one of its ligands, (106,107). Many pathogens, including gram-negative bacteria

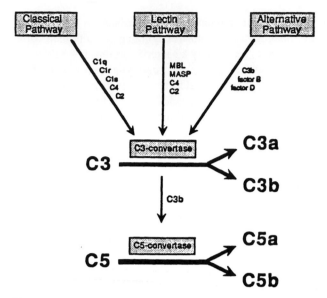

Figure 2 Complement-activation pathways.

(108,109) and various viruses (110,111), can also initiate formation of a C3 convertase in this pathway in the absence of specific antibodies. The demonstration that antibodies are not the only activators of the classical pathway has challenged the traditional belief that this pathway emerged at the same time as adaptive immune responses.

All classical pathway activators are recognized by C1q, which normally circulates in blood as a Ca^{2+}-dependent complex with two molecules each of the serine protease zymogens C1r and C1s (112,113). C1q is discussed in detail Chapter 3 of this volume. It has an unusually complex structure, consisting of six globular domains connected to a central region by collagen triple-helical strands (114,115). An activator-binding site is located in each of the six globular heads (116). In the case of immune complexes, C1q binding sites recognize the Cγ2 domains of IgG1, 2, or 3 (117,118) or the Cμ3 domain

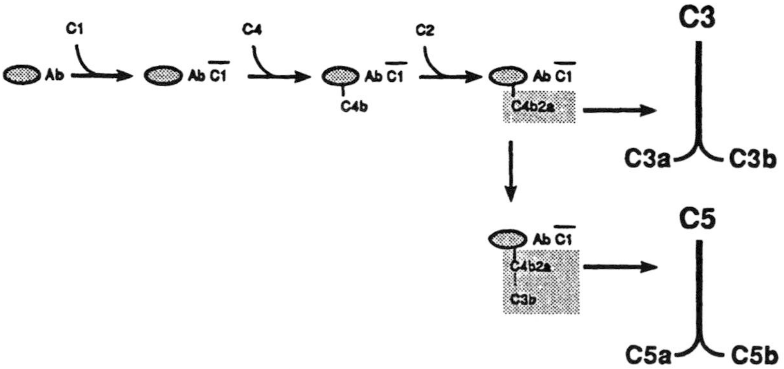

Figure 3 Assembly of complement convertases in the classical pathway of complement activation. Ab, antibody of IgG or IgM class. ⬤ Antigenic cell or protein.

(119,120) of IgM antibodies. In CRP, the C1q-binding site is located on the plane of the pentamer opposite to that containing the phosphocholine-binding site (121,122). Engagement of two or more of its activator binding sites is believed to induce a conformational change in C1q (123) that causes the autoactivation of C1r (124) from a single-chain zymogen to a disulfide-linked two-chain active protease designated $\overline{\text{C1r}}$. Next, $\overline{\text{C1r}}$ cleaves a single peptide bond in zymogen C1s to form the two-chain active protease $\overline{\text{C1s}}$ (124,125). $\overline{\text{C1s}}$ then cleaves the single Arg^{737}–Ala^{738} peptide bond on the α chain of C4, generating two fragments, a small peptide termed C4a released in the fluid-phase, and a large three-chain fragment called C4b that may become covalently attached to the surface of the activator (Fig. 3). Attachment of C4b is accomplished through a transacylation reaction involving the thiolester bond, which becomes metastable following the $\overline{\text{C1s}}$-catalyzed cleavage of C4. Of the two isotypes of C4, C4A preferentially reacts with -NH_2 groups to form amide bonds, whereas C4B preferentially reacts with -OH groups to form ester bonds (126,127). The latter reaction is much faster than the former and proceeds through the formation of an acyl intermediate involving the side-chain of His^{1106} (128). Attachment of C4b to the activator surface through either reaction is relatively inefficient, with the majority of mestastable C4b being hydrolyzed and remaining in the fluid phase. This fluid-phase C4b has no known function.

Following the covalent binding of C4b to the activating principle, C2 forms a Mg^{2+}-dependent complex with C4b. If C4b is attached at the appropriate distance from the site of its generation, bound C2 is cleaved by $\overline{\text{C1s}}$ at the Arg^{223}–Lys^{224} peptide bond, generating two fragments. The smaller one, C2b, is released in the fluid phase, while the larger, C2a, remains bound to C4b to form the bimolecular complex, $\overline{\text{C4b2a}}$, which is the C3 convertase of the classical pathway (129,130). The catalytic center of this protease resides in the serine protease domain of C2a. However, proteolytic activity against C3 is only expressed in the context of the bimolecular complex.

Several mechanisms discussed in Chapter 7 of this volume ensure that the extent of classical pathway activation is proportional to the amount and persistence of its activator. As discussed in Chapter 21, C1INH regulates the activity of $\overline{\text{C1}}$, forming tight stoichiometric complexes with both $\overline{\text{C1r}}$ and $\overline{\text{C1s}}$. This results in their removal from the activated C1 complex in the form of C1INH–$\overline{\text{C1r}}$–$\overline{\text{C1s}}$–C1INH tetramers (131,132). Removal of $\overline{\text{C1r}}$ and $\overline{\text{C1s}}$ leaves C1q alone bound to the complement activator. Such activator-bound C1q can then bind to its receptor, C1qRp (133), and enhance phagocytosis of the particle onto which it is attached (134). C1INH also prevents autoactivation of C1 in blood as well as activation by weak activators (135,136), probably by binding to activated C1r, thus preventing activation of C1s and subsequent proteins. Additional control of the classical pathway is exercised at the level of the C3-convertase. The $\overline{\text{C4b2a}}$ complex has a short half-life of about 1–5 min, after which it decays as a result of dissociation of C2a in an inactive form (137) The serum protein C4bp binds to C4b accelerating the decay/dissociation of the assembled convertase and preventing the formation of new one (138). C4bp also acts as a cofactor for the serine protease, factor I, which cleaves C4b into fragments, which cannot participate in the formation of C3 convertase (139). If a C3-convertase is formed on the surface of a host cell, cell-membrane associated DAF accelerates its dissociation/decay (140) and MCP, another host cell surface protein, serves as factor I cofactor for the cleavage/inactivation of C4b (141,142).

2. Lectin Pathway

A novel antibody- and C1-independent pathway leading to assembly of $\overline{\text{C4b2a}}$, C3 convertase was described recently (Fig. 4) (143,144). This pathway utilizes, mannan-binding

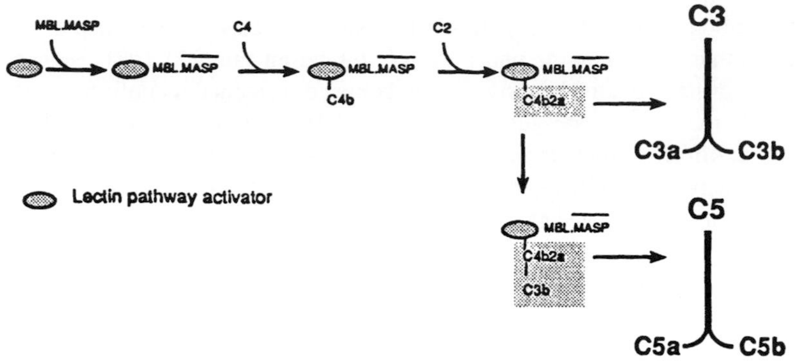

Figure 4 Assembly of complement convertases in the lectin pathway of complement activation. ⬭ Lectin pathway activator.

lectin (MBL) to recognize bacterial pathogens expressing terminal mannose or N-acetylglucosamine on their surface. Blood levels of MBL are genetically determined and increase during acute-phase reactions (145). MBL is structurally similar to C1q, consisting of four to six C-lectin domains connected to a central region by triple-helical collagen stems (146). MBL circulates in blood in complex with the zymogen form of the serine protease MASP, which has the same modular structure as C1r and C1s (49,147). Preliminary evidence for the presence of an additional MASP in the complex has been presented (148). Thus, the MBL-MASP complex is structurally similar to C1. Also, it appears that the two protein complexes are similar functionally. Binding of MBL to carbohydrate structures on pathogens results in activation of the single-chain zymogen MASP to an active two-chain serine protease, which in turn sequentially cleaves C4 and C2, resulting in the formation of pathogen-bound $\overline{C4b2a}$, C3 convertase (143,144). Expression of C3-convertase activity by the complex implies that MASP has identical peptide bond specificity as $\overline{C1s}$. Activated MASP can also cleave C3, suggesting that the activated MBL-MASP complex may be able to bypass C4 and C2 and also serve as a C3-convertase (149). It should be noted that a similar bypass pathway has been described for C1 (150,151). However, at this point the physiological significance of either of these "bypass" pathways remains unknown.

Similarly to $\overline{C1r}/\overline{C1s}$, activated MASP is inhibited by C1INH (152), which probably regulates the lectin activation pathway in a manner similar to the classical pathway.

3. Alternative Pathway

Assembly of a C3-convertase in the alternative pathway is initiated by a variety of cellular surfaces, including those of various pathogenic bacteria, parasites, viruses, virally infected cells, and fungi (153). Antibodies can also activate this pathway, but usually are not required. The first step in the formation of the C3-convertase is the covalent attachment of mestastable C3b to the surface of the activator (Fig. 5). Similarly to C4b, attachment of C3b is accomplished through a transacylation reaction between the carbonyl group of the metastable thiolester and either -NH$_2$ or -OH groups of protein or carbohydrate moeities on the activator surface (40,154). Since the half-life of mestastable C3b is very short, its

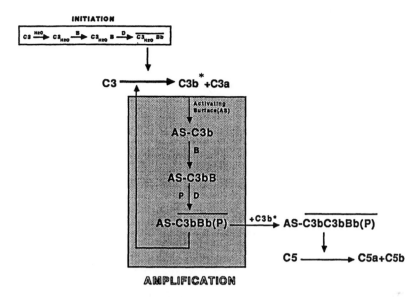

Figure 5 Assembly of the initiation and amplification convertases in the alternative pathway of complement activation. C3b*, metastable C3b.

availability in blood indicates the need for its continuous generation, irrespective of the presence of an activator. Indeed, low-level cleavage of C3, generating metastable C3b, seems to occur continuously under physiological conditions (155) and is apparently catalyzed by the so-called "initiation C3-convertase." Formation of this convertase depends on the slow spontaneous hydrolysis of the thiolester bond of C3, which occurs at an estimated rate of 0.2–0.4% of the C3 plasma pool/h (156). C3 with a hydrolyzed thiolester bond, termed $C3_{H_2O}$, is conformationally different from native C3 (157). A main functional characteristic of $C3_{H_2O}$ is its ability to form a Mg^{2+}-dependent complex with factor B. Within the context of this complex, factor B becomes susceptible to proteolytic attack by factor D, which catalyzes the hydrolysis of the single Arg^{234}–Lys^{235} peptide bond generating two fragments, Ba and Bb. Ba, the smaller fragment, is released in the fluid-phase while Bb remains bound to form $C3_{H_2O}Bb$, the initiation C3-convertase (156).

The series of reactions starting with the hydrolysis of the thiolester bond of C3 and concluding with the cleavage of C3 into C3a and C3b by the initiation C3-convertase are considered to occur continuously at slow rates. Thus, a supply of newly generated metastable C3b is always available in blood. Under normal conditions, (i.e., in the absence of an activating principle) the initiation C3-convertase and the products of its catalytic action, C3a and C3b, are efficiently inactivated by regulatory proteins and, therefore, do not have any pathophysiologic effects. Specifically, the $C3_{H_2O}Bb$ convertase has a short half-life, dissociating into $C3_{H_2O}$ and inactive Bb. This decay/dissociation is accelerated by factor H, which also acts as a cofactor for the factor I-catalyzed cleavage of $C3_{H_2O}$ into a form unable to form new initiation convertase. C3a is inactivated by anaphylatoxin inactivator, a serine carboxypeptidase N, which removes the COOH-terminal Arg residue, eliminating anaphylatoxin activity. Fluid-phase C3b binds to factor H, thus becoming susceptible to cleavage by factor I. Therefore, under physiological conditions the alternative pathway is activated continuously, but the rate of activation is kept very low by powerful regulatory mechanisms.

The balance between activation and control shifts dramatically in favor of activation when an alternative pathway activator gains access into blood or other fluids containing complement proteins. Metastable C3b binds covalently to the activator and the chemical nature of the activator surface favors binding of factor B, which forms a Mg^{2+}-dependent complex with C3b. Formation of this complex is thought to cause a conformational change in factor B, which can induce the enzymatically active conformation of factor D. Factor D then cleaves factor B into Ba and Bb, with Bb remaining bound to C3b. The resulting $\overline{C3bBb}$ complex has C3-convertase activity but is relatively ineffective because of its short half-life (158). The catalytic center of the C3-convertase resides in the serine protease domain of Bb, but proteolytic activity against C3 is expressed only in the context of the bimolecular complex. The $\overline{C3bBb}$ complex is bound by properdin (P), which extends its half-life from 1–2 min to approximately 18 min (159). The P-stabilized convertase catalyzes the hydrolysis of many C3 molecules to C3a and metastable C3b. Many of the metastable C3b molecules are hydrolyzed and remain in the fluid-phase, where they are subject to inactivation by the action of factors H and I. However, a substantial percentage of the generated metastable C3b covalently binds to the surface of the activator around the initial C3b molecule and initiates the formation of additional C3-convertase complexes, thus amplifying local production of C3a and metastable C3b. For this reason, the P-stabilized alternative pathway C3-convertase assembled on the surface of an activator is usually referred to as "amplification C3-convertase."

Metastable C3b, generated by any of the C3-convertases, cannot discriminate between nucleophilic groups on the surface of activators and nonactivators of the alternative pathway. Thus, C3b can become covalently attached to virtually any cell or protein surface in the immediate vicinity of its generation. However, C3b attached to the surface of a nonactivator of the alternative pathway, such as a cell or protein of the host, cannot initiate the assembly of an amplification C3-convertase, because the chemical composition of the surface endows it with a 100-fold higher affinity for factor H than factor B (160). As mentioned, factor H bound to C3b serves as a cofactor for factor I, which cleaves C3b, preventing the formation of a convertase. By comparison, C3b attached on an alternative pathway activator has about equal affinity for factors B and H. Because the concentration of factor H in blood (3.2 μM) is higher than that of factor B (2.2 μM), the initial burst of amplified complement activation occurring on the surface of an alternative pathway activator is eventually controlled by the action of factors H and I. This is indicated by the finding that the majority of C3 on the surface of the activator is in the form of factor I-cleaved C3b, termed C3bi (161). Thus, although adequate for the elimination of a foreign cell or molecule, alternative pathway activation is limited in time by the regulatory proteins.

A biochemical feature determining whether a cell surface can function as an alternative pathway activator is the relative amount of sialic acid present in membrane-associated glycoproteins and glycolipids. The presence of sialic acid on a cell surface increases the affinity of C3b for factor H, which prevents formation of C3-convertase (162,163). In addition to sialic acid, several membrane-associated proteins prevent the formation of an amplification C3-convertase on the surface of blood and other host cells. DAF and CR1 bind C3b, preventing the binding of factor B or dissociating C3b-bound Bb. MCP and CR1 serve as cofactors for factor I-catalyzed cleavage of C3b to C3bi, which cannot form a C3-convertase.

C. Effector Pathways

1. C3b Activation Pathway

Complement activation on the surface of an activator results in the covalent attachment of a large number of C3b molecules clustered around the initial C3-convertase. Such C3b molecules mediate several important biological activities. For example, as discussed in Chapter 20 of this volume, C3b binding to CR1 receptors on erythrocytes provides the main mechanism for the clearance of antigen–antibody complexes from blood. Also, as discussed in Chapter 12, recognition of bacterial cell-attached C3b by CR1 on phagocytic cells significantly contributes to the phagocytosis of bacteria. In addition, activator-attached C3b molecules serve as precursors for several smaller fragments with distinct and important functions. These smaller C3 fragments are produced mainly by the proteolytic action of factor I, which is active only in the context of complexes of C3b or its fragments with appropriate cofactor proteins. Unlike C3b, its proteolytic fragments cannot participate in the formation of alternative pathway C3-convertase. Accordingly, cleavage of C3b is usually referred to as "C3b-inactivation" and factor I is termed "C3b-inactivator." In the case of clustered C3b fragments attached to the surface of complement activators, this terminology is misleading, because the factor I-produced proteolytic fragments are recognized by specific receptors on effector cells and mediate important biological activities. On the other hand, cleavage by factor I of the sparse C3b molecules attached on the surface of host cells or of fluid-phase C3b does constitute inactivation as it prevents amplified complement activation, and host tissue injury. C3b proteolytic fragments on host cell surfaces cannot activate effector cells expressing specific receptors because of their low density.

Initially, factor I cleaves two neighboring peptide bonds on the α chain of C3b, resulting in the release of a small peptide, C3f, and the generation of C3bi, which remains attached to the activator surface (Fig. 6) (164). Both of these proteolytic cleavages require as cofactor, factor H, CR1, or MCP, which form bimolecular complexes with C3b, thus inducing the proteolytically active conformation of factor I. C3bi serves as ligand for two integrin-type receptors, CR3 (CD18/CD11b) and CR4 (p150/95; CD18/CD11c). Engagement of CR3 and probably also CR4 promotes the phagocytosis of cells carrying attached C3bi molecules. Factor I cleaves an additional peptide bond on the α chain of iC3b (164). This cleavage requires CR1 as cofactor (165) and results in the release into the fluid-phase of a large fragment, termed C3c, consisting of 3 polypeptide chains. The remaining fragment of the α chain of C3, termed C3dg remains attached to the activator surface. Factor H can also serve as cofactor for the proteolysis of C3bi by factor I, but is inefficient compared to CR1 (166,167). C3dg is the principal physiological ligand for CR2 and its binding to this receptor on B cells lowers the threshold for B-cell activation and enhances production of antibodies to T-cell dependent antigens (168–170).

Additional C3b fragments are produced by the action of other proteolytic enzymes, but their production in vivo and physiological significance has not been well established. Kallikrein can cleave C3bi at sites NH_2-terminal to that cleaved by factor I, generating a nonapeptide and a fragment, C3dK, slightly larger than C3dg. C3dK has been reported to express immunoregulatory activity (171), while the nonapeptide produces leukocytosis by mobilizing white blood cells from the bone marrow (172). Trypsin and possibly also other serine proteases can cleave C3dg into two smaller peptides, C3g, released in the fluid-phase, and C3d, which remains attached to the activator and like C3dg can serve as a ligand for CR2. Finally, a small fragment, C3e, split off C3b by proteolytic cleavage

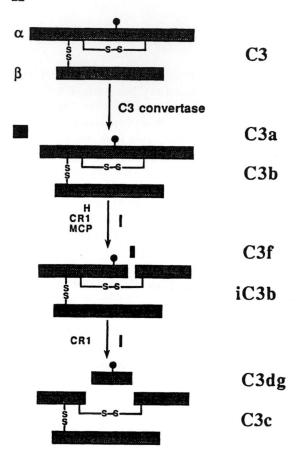

Figure 6 Schematic representation of the C3b activation pathway. The approximate position of the thiolester bond is indicated by the solid circle.

has also been reported to mobilize white blood cells from the bone marrow causing leukocytosis (173).

2. Cytolytic Pathway

Metastable C3b, generated by the action of a C3-convertase, can also react with nucleophiles on the noncatalytic subunits, C4b or C3b, of C3-convertases. Formation of the trimolecular complexes, $\overline{\text{C4b2a3b}}$ (174,175) or $(\overline{\text{C3b}})_2\overline{\text{Bb}}$ (176), through this mechanism results in loss of C3-convertase activity and acquisition of C5-cleaving or C5-convertase activity. Despite the change in substrate specificity, the catalytic center of the C5-convertases is the same as that of the parent C3-convertases, (i.e., it resides in the serine protease domain of C2a or Bb, respectively). The proteolytic activity of both C5-convertases is restricted to hydrolysis of the single Arg^{733}–Leu^{734} bond on the α chain of C5. Thus, cleavage of C5 by either C5-convertase generates the same two fragments: C5a and C5b. C5a is a small peptide expressing anaphylatoxin and chemotaxin activity (see Chap. 11), while C5b is a large two-chain fragment that initiates the assembly of the MAC (see Chap. 6). Formation of the MAC begins with the binding of C6 to a labile binding site of C5b and continues with the sequential binding of single molecules of C7 and C8 and of 6–12 molecules of C9. During these sequential reactions, hydrophobic domains of the participating proteins become exposed on the surface of the complex. Assembly of the MAC on the surface of a biological membrane favors interactions of these hydrophobic domains with the fatty acid chains of the phospholipid in the bilayer.

The complex becomes gradually inserted into the lipid bilayer and eventually forms a transmembrane channel. As discussed in Chapters 6, 13, 15, and 23, insertion of the MAC into cellular membranes can elicit cell functions or can lead to killing of susceptible cells. Formation and membrane insertion of the MAC are regulated by several proteins. The serum S-protein, also termed vitronectin, binds to the assembling complex at the C5b67 stage, inhibiting binding of C8 and precluding insertion into the lipid bilayer (177). Another serum protein, SP40,40 also binds to the C5b67 complex inhibiting its interaction with cell membranes (178). A cell membrane-associated protein, CD59, also termed HRF20, protectin, and MIRL, inhibits the formation of the MAC on cells of the host. CD59 binds to the complex at the C5b678 step, inhibiting binding and polymerization of C9 (179–181). CD59 exhibits species specificity in its action. Another membrane-associated MAC inhibitory protein termed homologous restriction factor (HRF) has been described (182), but its primary structure has not been reported. HRF seems to act in a manner similar to CD59.

IV. CONCLUDING REMARKS

Complement is a highly evolved, complex system of proteins. It constitutes a major element of host defenses and it functions in both innate and adaptive immunity. The system appears to be pleiotropic with newly described activities falling outside host defense.

Activation of the complement system proceeds through enzymatic amplification steps and is tightly regulated by specific proteins, which not only limit the extent of activation but also protect host cells from potential complement-mediated injury. However, as discussed in subsequent chapters of this volume, under conditions of misguided, excessive, or uncontrolled activation, complement protein products contribute to the pathogenesis of human disease. A better understanding of the system seems necessary to develop effective pharmacological control of complement activation in human disease.

REFERENCES

1. Nuttal G. Experimente über die bakterienfeindlichen einflüsse des thierischen körpers. Z Hyg Infenktionskr 1888; 4:353–394.
2. Buchner, H. Ueber die bakterientötende wirkung des zellenfreien blutserums. Zentralbl Bakteriol 1889; 5:817–823.
3. Pfeiffer R, Issaeff R. Ueber die spezifische bedeutung der choleraimmunität. Z Hyg Infektionskr 1894; 17:355–400.
4. Bordet J. Sur l' agglutination et la dissolution des globules rouges par le serum d'animaux injectés de sang defibriné. Ann Inst Pasteur 1898; 12:688–695.
5. Ehrlich P, Morgenroth J. Zur theorie der lysenwirkung. Berlin Klin Wochenschr 1899; 36:6–9.
6. Müller-Eberhard HJ. Molecular organization and function of the complement system. Annu Rev Biochem 1988; 57:321–347.
7. Ehrlich P, Morgenroth J. Ueber hemolysine. Berlin Klin Wochenschr 1900; 37:453–458.

8. Alper CA, Johnson AM, Birtch AG, Moore RD. Human C3: evidence for the liver as the primary site of synthesis. Science 1969; 163:286–280.

9. Stecher VJ, Thorbecke GJ. Sites of synthesis of serum proteins. I. Serum proteins produced by macrophages in vitro. J Immunol 1967; 99:643–652.

10. Barnum SR, Ishii Y, Agrawal A, Volanakis JE. Production and interferon-γ-mediated regulation of complement component C2 and factors B and D by the astroglioma cell line U105-MG. Biochem J 1992; 287:595–601.

11. Gasque P, Julen N, Ischenko AM, Picot C, Mauger C, Chauzy C, Ripoche J, Fontaine M. Expression of complement components of the alternative pathway by glioma cell lines. J Immunol 1992; 149:1381–1387.

12. Gasque P, Ischenko A, Legoedec J, Mauger C, Schouft M-T, Fontaine M. Expression of the complement classical pathway by human glioma in culture. A model for complement expression by nerve cells. J Biol Chem 1993; 268:25068–25074.

13. White RT, Damm D, Hancock N, Rosen BS, Lowell BB, Usher P, Flier JS, Spiegelman BM. Human adipsin is identical to complement factor D and is expressed at high levels in adipose tissue. J Biol Chem 1992; 267:9210–9213.

14. Choy LN, Rosen BS, Spiegelman BM. Adipsin and an endogenous pathway of complement from adipose cells. J Biol Chem 1992; 267:12736–12741.

15. Brown EO, Sundstrom SA, Komm BS, Yi Z, Teuscher C, Lyttle CR. Progesterone regulation of estradiol-induced rat uterine secretory protein, complement C3. Biol Reprod 1990; 42:713–719.

16. Hasty LA, Lambris JD, Lessey BA, Pruksananonda K, Lyttle CR. Hormonal regulation of complement components and receptors throughout the menstrual cycle. Am J Obstet Gynecol 1994; 170:168–175.

17. Fenichel P, Donzeau M, Cervoni F, Menezo Y, Hsi BL. Expression of complement regulatory proteins on human eggs and preimplantation embryos. Am J Reprod Immunol 1995; 33:155–164.

18. Simpson KL, Holmes CH. Differential expression of complement regulatory proteins decay-accelerating factor (CD55), membrane cofactor protein (CD46) and CD59 during human spermatogenesis. Immunology 1994; 81:452–461.

19. Yang C, Jones JL, Barnum SR. Expression of decay-accelerating factor (CD55), membrane cofactor protein (CD46) and CD59 in the human astroglioma cell line, D54-MG, and primary rat astrocytes. J Neuroimmunol 1993; 47:123–132.

20. Gasque P, Fontaine M, Morgan BP. Complement expression in human brain. Biosynthesis of terminal pathway components and regulators in human glial cells and cell lines. J Immunol 1995; 154:4726–4733.

21. Gasque P, Chan P, Mauger C, Schouft M-T, Singhrao S, Dierich MP, Morgan BP, Fontaine M. Identification and characterization of complement C3 receptors on human astrocytes. J Immunol 1996; 156:2247–2255.

22. Ames RS, Li Y, Sarau HM, Nuthulaganti P, Foley JJ, Ellis C, Zeng Z, Su K, Jurewicz AJ, Hertzberg RP, Bergsma DJ, Kumar C. Molecular cloning and characterization of the human anaphylatoxin C3a receptor. J Biol Chem 1996; 271:20231–20234.

23. Gasque P, Chan P, Fontaine M, Ischenko A, Lamacz M, Götze O, Morgan BP. Identification and characterization of the complement C5a anaphylatoxin receptor on human astrocytes. J Immunol 1995; 155:4882–4889.

24. Baldo A, Sniderman AD, St-Luce S, Avramoglu RK, Maslowska M, Hoang B, Monge JC, Bell A, Mulay S, Cianflone K. The adipsin–acylation stimulating protein system and regulation of intracellular triglyceride synthesis. J Clin Invest 1993; 92:1543–1547.

25. McCoy R, Haviland DL, Molmenti EP, Ziambaras T, Wetsel RA, Perlmutter DH. N-formylpeptide and complement C5a receptors are expressed in liver cells and mediate hepatic acute phase gene regulation. J Exp Med 1995; 182:207–217.

26. Sims PJ, Wiedmer T. Induction of cellular procoagulant activity by the membrane attack complex of complement. Semin Cell Biol 1995; 6:275–282.

27. Hamilton KK, Hattori R, Esmon CT, Sims PJ. Complement proteins C5b-9 induce vesiculation of the endothelial plasma membrane and expose catalytic surface for assembly of the prothrombinase enzyme complex. J Biol Chem 1990; 265:3809–3814.

28. Saadi S, Holzknecht RA, Patte CP, Stern DM, Platt JL. Complement-mediated regulation of tissue factor activity in endothelium. J Exp Med 1995; 182:1807–1814.

29. Niculescu F, Rus H, Shin S, Lang T, Shin ML. Generation of diacylglycerol and ceramide during homologous complement activation. J Immunol 1993; 150:214–224.

30. Niculescu F, Rus H, Shin ML. Receptor-independent activation of guanine nucleotide-binding regulatory proteins by terminal complement complexes. J Biol Chem 1994; 269:4417–4423.

31. Benzaquen LR, Nicholson-Weller A, Halperin JA. Terminal complement proteins C5b-9 release basic fibroblast growth factor and platelet-derived growth factor from endothelial cells. J Exp Med 1994; 179:985–992.

32. Acosta JA, Benzaquen LR, Goldstein DJ, Tosteson MT, Halperin JA. The transient pore formed by homologous terminal complement complexes functions as a bidirectional route for the transport of autocrine and paracrine signals across human cell membranes. Mol Med 1996; 2:755–765.

33. World Health Organization. Nomenclature of complement. Bull WHO 1968; 39:935–938.

34. IUIS-WHO Nomenclature Committee. Nomenclature of the alternative activating pathway of complement. J Immunol 1981; 127:1261–1262.

35. Bork P, Bairoch A. Extracellular protein modules. Trends Biochem Sci 1995; 20:Suppl: March C03.

36. Sottrup-Jensen L, Stepanik TM, Kristensen T, Lønblad PB, Jones CM, Wierzbicki DM, Magnusson S, Domdey H, Wetsel RA, Lundwall A, Tack BF, Fey GH. Common evolutionary origin of α_2-macroglobulin and complement components C3 and C4. Proc Natl Acad Sci USA 1985; 82:9–13.

37. Quigley JP, Armstrong PB. A homologue of $\alpha 2$ macroglobulin purified from the hemolymph of the horseshoe crab *Limulus polyphemus*. J Biol Chem 1985; 260:12715–12719.

38. Tack BF, Harrison RA, Janatova J, Thomas ML, Prahl JW. Evidence for presence of an internal thiolester bond in third component of human complement. Proc Natl Acad Sci USA 1980; 77:5764–5768.

39. Isenman DE, Cooper NR. The structure and function of the third component of human complement-I. The nature and extent of conformational changes accompanying C3 activation. Mol Immunology 1981; 18:331–339.

40. Law SK, Lichtenberg NA, Levine RP. Evidence for an ester linkage between the labile binding site of C3b and receptive surfaces. J Immunol 1979; 123:1388–1394.

41. Law SK, Lichtenberg NA, Levine RP. Covalent binding and hemolytic activity of complement proteins. Proc Natl Acad Sci USA 1980; 77:7194–7198.

42. Bock SC, Skriver K, Nielsen E, Thøgersen HC, Wiman B, Donaldson VH, Eddy RL, Marrinan J, Radziejewska E, Huber R, Shows TB, Magnusson S. Human C1̄ inhibitor: primary structure, cDNA cloning, and chromosomal localization. Biochemistry 1986; 25:4292–4301.

43. Gerard NP, Gerard C. The chemotactic receptor for human C5a anaphylatoxin. Nature 1991; 349:614–617.

44. Doolittle RF. The genealogy of some recently evolved vertebrate proteins. Trends Biochem Sci 1985; 10:233–237.

45. Dodds AW, Day AJ. The phylogeny and evolution of the complement system. In: Whaley K, Loos M, Weiler JM, eds. Complement in Health and Disease, 2nd ed. Dordrecht: Kluwer, 1993:39–88.

46. Greer J. Comparative modeling methods: application to the family of the mammalian serine proteases. Proteins Struct Funct Genet 1990; 7:317–334.

47. Perona JJ, Craik CS. Structural basis of substrate specificity in the serine proteases. Protein Sci 1995; 4:337–360.
48. Volanakis JE, Narayana SVL. Complement factor D: a novel serine protease. Protein Sci 1996; 5:553–564.
49. Takayama Y, Takada F, Takahashi A, Kawakami M. A 100-kDa protein in the C4-activating component of Ra-reactive factor is a new serine protease having module organization similar to C1r and C1s. J Immunol 1994; 152:2308–2316.
50. Journet A, Tosi M. Cloning and sequencing of full-length cDNA encoding the precursor of human complement component C1r. Biochem J 1986; 240:783–787.
51. Gagnon J, Arlaud GJ. Primary structure of the A chain of human complement-classical-pathway enzyme C1r. *N*-terminal sequences and alignment of autolytic fragments and CNBr-cleavage peptides. Biochem J 1985; 225:135–142.
52. Tosi M, Duponchel C, Meo T, Julier C. Complete cDNA sequence of human complement C1s and close physical linkage of the homologous genes C1s and C1r. Biochemistry 1987; 26:8516–8524.
53. Mackinnon CM, Carter PE, Smyth SJ, Dunbar B, Fothergill JE. Molecular cloning of cDNA for human complement component C1s. The complete amino acid sequence. Eur J Biochem 1987; 169:547–553.
54. Bork P, Beckmann G. The CUB domain. A widespread module in developmentally regulated proteins. J Mol Biol 1993; 231:539–545.
55. Campbell ID, Bork P. Epidermal growth factor-like modules. Curr Opin Cell Biol 1993; 3:385–392.
56. Rao Z, Handford P, Mayhew M, Knott V, Brownlee GG, Stuart D. The structure of a Ca^{2+}-binding epidermal growth factor-like domain: its role in protein-protein interactions. Cell 1995; 82:131–141.
57. Klickstein LB, Wong WW, Smith JA, Weis JH, Wilson JG, Fearon DT. Human C3b/C4b receptor (CR1). Demonstration of long homologous repeating domains that are composed of the short consensus repeats characteristic of C3/C4 binding proteins. J Exp Med 1987; 165:1095–1112.
58. Kristensen T, D'Eustachio P, Ogata RT, Chung LP, Reid KBM, Tack BF. The superfamily of C3b/C4b-binding proteins. Fed Proc 1987; 46:2463–2469.
59. Holers VM, Cole JL, Lublin DM, Seya T, Atkinson JP. Human C3b- and C4b-regulatory proteins: a new multi-gene family. Immunol Today 1985; 6:188–191.
60. Reid KBM, Day AJ. Structure–function relationships of the complement components. Immunol Today 1989; 10:177–180.
61. Norman DG, Barlow PN, Baron M, Day AJ, Sim RB, Campbell ID. Three-dimensional structure of a complement control protein module in solution. J Mol Biol 1991; 219:717–725.
62. Barlow PN, Norman DG, Steinkasserer A, Horne TJ, Pearce J, Driscoll PC, Sim RB, Campbell ID. Solution structure of the fifth repeat of factor H: a second example of the complement control protein module. Biochemistry 1992; 31:3626–3634.
63. Bentley DR. Primary structure of human complement component C2: homology to two unrelated protein families. Biochem J 1986; 239:339–345.
64. Horiuchi T, Macon KJ, Kidd VJ, Volanakis JE. cDNA cloning and expression of human complement component C2. J Immunol 1989; 142:2105–2111.
65. Mole JE, Anderson JK, Davison EA, Woods DE. Complete primary structure for the zymogen of human complement factor B. J Biol Chem 1984; 259:3407–3412.
66. Horiuchi T, Kim S, Matsumoto M, Watanabe I, Fujita S, Volanakis JE. Human complement factor B: cDNA cloning, nucleotide sequencing, phenotypic conversion by site-directed mutagenesis and expression. Mol Immunol 1993; 30:1587–1592.
67. Sadler JE. von Willebrand factor. J Biol Chem 1991; 266:22777–22780.
68. Perkins SJ, Smith KF, Williams SC, Haris PI, Chapman D, Sim RB. The secondary structure of the von Willebrand factor type A domain in factor B of human complement by Fourier transform infrared spectroscopy. J Mol Biol 1994; 238:104–119.

69. Colombatti A, Bonaldo P. The superfamily of proteins with von Willebrand factor type A-like domains: one theme common to components of extracellular matrix, hemostasis, cellular adhesion, and defense mechanisms. Blood 1991; 77:2305–2315.

70. Lee J-O, Rieu P, Arnaout MA, Liddington R. Crystal structure of the A domain from the α subunit of integrin CR3 (CD11b/CD18). Cell 1995; 80:631–638.

71. Qu A, Leahy DJ. Crystal structure of the I-domain from the CD11a/CD18 (LFA-1, $\alpha_L\beta2$) integrin. Proc Natl Acad Sci USA 1995; 92:10277–10281.

72. Goldberger G, Bruns GAP, Rits M, Edge MD, Kwiatkowski DJ. Human complement factor I: analysis of cDNA-derived primary structure and assignment of its gene to chromosome 4. J Biol Chem 1987; 262:10065–10071.

73. Catterall CF, Lyons A, Sim RB, Day AJ, Harris TJR. Characterization of the primary amino acid sequence of human complement control protein Factor I from an analysis of cDNA clones. Biochem J 1987; 242:849–856.

74. Haefliger J-A, Tschopp J, Vial N, Jenne DE. Complete primary structure and functional characterization of the sixth component of the human complement system. Identification of the C5b-binding domain in complement C6. J Biol Chem 1989; 264:18041–18051.

75. Freeman M, Ashkenas J, Rees DJG, Kingsley DM, Copeland NG, Jenkins NA, Krieger M. An ancient, highly conserved family of cysteine-rich protein domains revealed by cloning type I and type II murine macrophage scavenger receptors. Proc Natl Acad Sci USA 1990; 87:8810–8814.

76. Südhof TC, Goldstein JL, Brown MS, Russell DW. The LDL receptor gene: a mosaic of exons shared with different proteins. Science 1985; 228:815–822.

77. Ullman CG, Haris PI, Smith KF, Sim RB, Emery VC, Perkins SJ. β-Sheet secondary structure of an LDL receptor domain from complement factor I by consensus structure predictions and spectroscopy. FEBS Letters 1995; 371:199–203.

78. DiScipio RG, Hugli TE. The molecular architecture of human complement component C6. J Biol Chem 1989; 264:16197–16206.

79. DiScipio RG, Chakravarti DN, Müller-Eberhard HJ, Fey GH. The structure of human complement component C7 and the C5b-7 complex. J Biol Chem 1988; 263:549–560.

80. Rao AG, Howard OMZ, Ng SC, Whitehead AS, Colten HR, Sodetz JM. Complementary DNA and derived amino acid sequence of the α subunit of human complement protein C8: evidence for the existence of a separate α subunit messenger RNA. Biochemistry 1987; 26:3556–3564.

81. Howard OMZ, Rao AG, Sodetz JM. Complementary DNA and derived amino acid sequence of the β subunit of human complement protein C8: identification of a close structural and ancestral relationship to the α subunit and C9. Biochemistry 1987; 26:3565–3570.

82. DiScipio RG, Gehring MR, Podack ER, Kan CC, Hugli TE, Fey GH. Nucleotide sequence of cDNA and derived amino acid sequence of human complement component C9. Proc Natl Acad Sci USA 1984; 81:7298–7302.

83. Liu C-C, Walsh CM, Young JD-E. Perforin: structure and function. Immunol Today 1995; 16:194–201.

84. Lawler J, Hynes RO. The structure of human thrombospondin, an adhesive glycoprotein with multiple calcium-binding sites and homologies with several different proteins. J Cell Biol 1986; 103:1635–1648.

85. Goundis D, Reid KBM. Properdin, the terminal complement components, thrombospondin and the circumsporozoite protein of malaria parasites contain similar sequence motifs. Nature 1988; 335:82–85.

86. Robson KJH, Hall JRS, Jennings MW, Harris TJR, Marsh K, Newbold CI, Tate VE, Weatherall DJ. A highly conserved amino-acid sequence in thrombospondin, properdin and in proteins from sporozoites and blood stages of a human malaria parasite. Nature 1988; 335:79–82.

87. Perkins SJ, Nealis AS, Haris PI, Chapman D, Goundis D, Reid KBM. Secondary structure in properdin of the complement cascade and related proteins: a study by Fourier transform infrared spectroscopy. Biochemistry 1989; 28:7176–7182.

88. Klickstein LB, Bartow TJ, Miletic V, Rabson LD, Smith JA, Fearon DT. Identification of distinct C3b and C4b recognition sites in the human C3b/C4b receptor (CR1, CD35) by deletion mutagenesis. J Exp Med 1988; 168:1699–1717.

89. Moore MD, Cooper NR, Tack BF, Nemerow GR. Molecular cloning of the cDNA encoding the Epstein-Barr virus/C3d receptor (complement receptor type 2) of human B lymphocytes. Proc Natl Acad Sci USA 1987; 84:9194–9198.

90. Weis JJ, Toothaker LE, Smith JA, Weis JH, Fearon DT. Structure of the human B lymphocyte receptor for C3d and the Epstein-Barr virus and relatedness to other members of the family of C3/C4 binding proteins. J Exp Med 1988; 167:1047–1066.

91. Medof ME, Lublin DM, Holers VM, Ayers DJ, Getty RR, Leykam JF, Atkinson JP, Tykocinski ML. Cloning and characterization of cDNAs encoding the complete sequence of decay-accelerating factor of human complement. Proc Natl Acad Sci USA 1987; 84:2007–2011.

92. Caras IW, Davitz MA, Rhee L, Weddell G, Martin DW, Jr., Nussenzweig V. Cloning of decay-accelerating factor suggests novel use of splicing to generate two proteins. Nature 1987; 325:545–549.

93. Lublin DM, Liszewski MK, Post TW, Arce MA, LeBeau MM, Rebentisch MB, Lemons RS, Seya T, Atkinson JP. Molecular cloning and chromosomal localization of human membrane cofactor protein (MCP). J Exp Med 1988; 168:181–194.

94. Chung LP, Bentley DR, Reid KBM. Molecular cloning and characterization of the cDNA coding for C4b-binding protein, a regulatory protein of the classical pathway of the human complement system. Biochem J 1985; 230:133–141.

95. Hillarp A, Dahlbäck B. Cloning of cDNA coding for the β chain of human complement component C4b-binding protein: sequence homology with the α chain. Proc Natl Acad Sci USA 1990; 87:1183–1187.

96. Kristensen T, Wetsel RA, Tack BF. Structural analysis of human complement protein H: homology with C4b binding protein, β_2-glycoprotein I, and the Ba fragment of B. J Immunol 1986; 136:3407–3411.

97. Ripoche J, Day AJ, Harris TJR, Sim RB. The complete amino acid sequence of human complement factor H. Biochem J 1988; 249:593–602.

98. Ahearn JM, Fearon DT. Structure and function of the complement receptors, CR1 (CD35) and CR2 (CD21). Adv Immunol 1989; 46:183–219.

99. Liszewski MK, Farries TC, Lublin DM, Rooney IA, Atkinson JP. Control of the complement system. Adv Immunol 1996; 61:201–283.

100. Lachmann PJ. An evolutionary view of the complement system. Behring Inst Mitt 1979; 63:25–37.

101. Volanakis JE. Participation of C3 and its ligands in complement activation. Curr Top Microbiol Immunol 1990; 153:1–21.

102. Nonaka M, Takahashi M. Complete complementary DNA sequence of the third component of complement of lamprey: implication for the evolution of thioester containing proteins. J Immunol 1992; 148:3290–3295.

103. Mavroidis M, Sunyer JO, Lambris JD. Isolation, primary structure, and evolution of the third component of chicken complement and evidence for a new member of the α_2-macroglobulin family. J Immunol 1995; 154:2164–2174.

104. Hughes AL. Phylogeny of the C3/C4/C5 complement-component gene family indicates that C5 diverged first. Mol Biol Evol 1994; 11:417–425.

105. Agrawal A, Kilpatrick JM, Volanakis JE. Structure and function of human C-reactive protein. In: Mackiewicz A, Kushner I, Baumann H, eds. Acute Phase Proteins: Molecular Biology, Biochemistry and Clinical Applications. Boca Raton: CRC Press, 1993; 79–92.

106. Kaplan MH, Volanakis JE. Interaction of C-reactive protein complexes with the complement system. I. Consumption of human complement associated with the reaction of C-reactive protein with pneumococcal C-polysaccharide and with the choline phosphatides, lecithin and sphingomyelin. J Immunol 1974; 112:2135–2147.

107. Claus DR, Siegel J, Petras K, Skor D, Osmand AP, Gewurz H. Complement activation by interaction of polyanions and polycations. III. Complement activation by interaction of multiple polyanions and polycations in the presence of C-reactive protein. J Immunol 1977; 118:83–87.

108. Clas F, Loos M. Antibody-independent binding of the first component of complement (C1) and its subcomponent C1q to the S and R forms of *Salmonella minnesota*. Infect Immun 1981; 31:1138–1144.

109. Loos M. Antibody-independent activation of C1, the first component of complement. Ann Immunol (Inst Pasteur) 1982; 133C:165–179.

110. Cooper NR, Jensen FC, Welsh RM, Jr., Oldstone MBA. Lysis of RNA tumor viruses by human serum: direct antibody-independent triggering of the classical complement pathway. J Exp Med 1976; 144:970–984.

111. Ebenbichler CF, Thielens NM, Vornhagen R, Marschang P, Arlaud GJ, Dierich MP. Human immunodeficiency virus type 1 activates the classical pathway of complement by direct C1 binding through specific sites in the transmembrane glycoprotein gp[41]. J Exp Med 1991; 174:1417–1424.

112. Strang CJ, Siegel RC, Phillips ML, Poon PH, Schumaker VN. Ultrastructure of the first component of human complement: electron microscopy of the crosslinked complex. Proc Natl Acad Sci USA 1982; 79:586–590.

113. Arlaud GJ, Colomb MG, Gagnon J. A functional model of the human C1 complex. Immunol Today 1987; 8:106–111.

114. Shelton E, Yonemasu K, Stroud RM. Ultrastructure of the human complement component C1q. Proc Natl Acad Sci USA 1972; 69:65–68.

115. Reid KBM, Porter RR. Subunit composition and structure of subcomponent C1q of the first component of human complement. Biochem J 1976; 155:19–23.

116. Hughes-Jones NC, Gardner B. Reaction between the isolated globular subunits of the complement component C1q and IgG-complexes. Mol Immunol 1979; 16:697–701.

117. Burton DR. Immunoglobulin G: functional sites. Mol Immunol 1985; 22:161–206.

118. Duncan AR, Winter G. The binding site for C1q on IgG. Nature 1988; 332:738–740.

119. Painter RH. The binding of C1q to immunoglobulins. Behring Inst Mitt 1993; 93:131–137.

120. Arya S, Chen F, Spycher S, Isenman DE, Shulman MJ, Painter RH. Mapping of amino acid residues in the Cµ3 domain of mouse IgM important in macromolecular assembly and complement-dependent cytolysis. J Immunol 1994; 152:1206–1212.

121. Agrawal A, Volanakis JE. Probing the C1q-binding site on human C-reactive protein by site-directed mutagenesis. J Immunol 1994; 152:5404–5410.

122. Shrive AK, Cheetham GMT, Holden D, Myles DAA, Turnell WG, Volanakis JE, Pepys MB, Bloomer AC, Greenhough TJ. Three dimensional structure of human C-reactive protein. Nature Struct Biol 1996; 3:346–354.

123. Golan MD, Burger R, Loos M. Conformational changes in C1q after binding to immune complexes: detection of neoantigens with monoclonal antibodies. J Immunol 1982; 129:445–447.

124. Dodds AW, Sim RB, Porter RR, Kerr MA. Activation of the first component of human complement (C1) by antibody–antigen aggregates. Biochem J 1978; 175:383–390.

125. Schumaker VN, Hanson DC, Kilchherr E, Phillips ML, Poon PH. A molecular mechanism for the activation of the first component of complement by immune complexes. Mol Immunol 1986; 23:557–565.

126. Isenman DE, Young JR. The molecular basis for the difference in immune hemolysis activity of the Chido and Rodgers isotypes of human complement component C4. J Immunol 1984; 132:3019–3027.

127. Carroll MC, Fathallah DM, Bergamaschini L, Alicot EM, Isenman DE. Substitution of a single amino acid (aspartic acid for histidine) converts the functional activity of human complement C4B to C4A. Proc Natl Acad Sci USA 1990; 87:6868–6872.

128. Dodds AW, Ren X-D, Willis AC, Law SKA. The reaction mechanism of the internal thioester in the human complement component C4. Nature 1996; 379:177–179.

129. Stroud RM, Austen KF, Mayer MM. Catalysis of C'2 Fixation by C'1a: Reaction kinetics, competitive inhibition by TAMe, and transferase hypothesis of the enzymatic action of C'1a on C'2, one of its natural substrates. Immunochemistry 1965; 2:219–234.

130. Kerr MA. The human complement system: assembly of the classical pathway C3 convertase. Biochem J 1980; 189:173–181.

131. Ziccardi RJ, Cooper NR. Active disassembly of the first complement component, C1, by C1 inactivator. J Immunol 1979; 123:788–792.

132. Sim RB, Arlaud GJ, Colomb MG. C1̄ inhibitor-dependent dissociation of human complement component C1̄ bound to immune complexes. Biochem J 1979; 179:449–457.

133. Nepomuceno RR, Henschen-Edman AH, Burgess WH, Tenner AJ. cDNA cloning and primary structure analysis of C1qRp, the human C1q/MBL/SPA receptor that mediates enhanced phagocytosis in vitro. Immunity 1997; 6:119–129.

134. Guan E, Robinson SL, Goodman EB, Tenner AJ. Cell-surface protein identified on phagocytic cells modulates the C1q-mediated enhancement of phagocytosis. J Immunol 1994; 152:4005–4016.

135. Ziccardi RJ. A new role for C1-inhibitor in homeostasis: control of activation of the first component of human complement. J Immunol 1982; 128:2505–2508.

136. Tseng Y, Poon PH, Zavodszky P, Schumaker VN. Spontaneous activation of serum C1 in vitro. Role of C1̄ inhibitor. J Immunol 1991; 147:1884–1890.

137. Stroud RM, Mayer MM, Miller JA, McKenzie AT. C'2a^d, an inactive derivative of C'2 released during decay of EAC'42a. Immunochemistry 1966; 3:163–176.

138. Gigli I, Fujita T, Nussenzweig V. Modulation of the classical pathway C3 convertase by plasma proteins C4 binding protein and C3b inactivator. Proc Natl Acad Sci USA 1979; 76:6596–6600.

139. Fujita T, Gigli I, Nussenzweig V. Human C4-binding protein. II. Role in proteolysis of C4b by C3b-inactivator. J Exp Med 1978; 148:1044–1051.

140. Medof ME, Kinoshita T, Nussenzweig V. Inhibition of complement activation on the surface of cells after incorporation of decay-accelerating factor (DAF) into their membranes. J Exp Med 1984; 160:1558–1578.

141. Seya T, Turner JR, Atkinson JP. Purification and characterization of a membrane protein (gp45–70) that is a cofactor for cleavage of C3b and C4b. J Exp Med 1986; 163:837–855.

142. Oglesby TJ, Allen CJ, Liszewski MK, White DJG, Atkinson JP. Membrane cofactor protein (CD46) protects cells from complement-mediated attack by an intrinsic mechanism. J Exp Med 1992; 175:1547–1551.

143. Matsushita M, Fujita T. Activation of the classical complement pathway by mannose-binding protein in association with a novel C1s-like serine protease. J Exp Med 1992; 176:1497–1502.

144. Ji Y-H, Fujita T, Hatsuse H, Takahashi A, Matsushita M, Kawakami M. Activation of the C4 and C2 components of complement by a proteinase in serum bactericidal factor, Ra reactive factor. J Immunol 1993; 150:571–578.

145. Turner MW. Mannose-binding lectin: the pluripotent molecule of the innate immune system. Immunol Today 1996; 17:532–540.

146. Taylor ME, Brickell PM, Craig RK, Summerfield JA. Structure and evolutionary origin of the gene encoding a human serum mannose-binding protein. Biochem J 1989; 262:763–771.

147. Sato T, Endo Y, Matsushita M, Fujita T. Molecular characterization of a novel serine protease involved in activation of the complement system by mannose-binding protein. Int Immunol 1994; 6:665–669.

148. Vorup-Jensen T, Stover C, Poulsen K, et al. Cloning of cDNA encoding a human MASP-like protein (MASP-2). Mol Immunol 1996; 33:81 (abstract).

149. Matsushita M, Fujita T. Cleavage of the third component of complement by mannose-binding protein-associated serine protease (MASP) with subsequent complement activation. Immunobiology 1995; 194:443–448.

150. May JE, Frank MM. A new complement-mediated cytolytic mechanism—the C1-bypass activation pathway. Proc Natl Acad Sci USA 1973; 70:649–652.

151. May JE, Frank MM. Hemolysis of sheep erythrocytes in guinea pig serum deficient in the fourth component of complement. II. Evidence for involvement of C1 and components of the alternate complement pathway. J Immunol 1973; 111:1668–1676.

152. Matsushita M, Fujita T. Inhibition of mannose-binding protein-associated serine protease (MASP) by C1 inhibitor (C1 INH). Mol Immunol 1996; 33:44 (abstract).

153. Pangburn MK, Müller-Eberhard HJ. The alternative pathway of complement. Semin Immunopathol 1984; 7:163–192.

154. Law SKA, Minich TM, Levine RP. Binding reaction between the third human complement protein and small molecules. Biochemistry 1981; 20:7457–7463.

155. Nicol AE, Lachmann PJ. The alternative pathway of complement activation. The role of C3 and its inactivator (KAF). Immunology 1973; 24:259–275.

156. Pangburn MK, Schreiber RD, Müller-Eberhard HJ. Formation of the initial C3-convertase of the alternative complement pathway. Acquisition of C3b-like activities by spontaneous hydrolysis of the putative thioester in native C3. J Exp Med 1981; 154:856–867.

157. Isenman DE, Kells DI, Cooper NR, Müller-Eberhard HJ, Panbgurn MK. Nucleophilic modification of human complement protein C3 correlation of conformational changes with acquisition of C3b-like functional properties. Biochemistry 1981; 20:4458–4467.

158. Brade V, Lee GD, Nicholson A, Shin HS, Mayer MM. The reaction of zymosan with the properdin system in normal and C4-deficient guinea pig serum. Demonstration of C3- and C5-cleaving multi-unit enzymes, both containing factor B, and acceleration of their formation by the classical complement pathway. J Immunol 1973; 111:1389–1400.

159. Fearon DT, Austen KF. Properdin: binding to C3b and stabilization of the C3b-dependent C3 convertase. J Exp Med 1975; 142:856–863.

160. Fearon DT, Austen KF. Activation of the alternative complement pathway due to resistance of zymosan-bound amplification convertase to endogenous regulatory mechanisms. Proc Natl Acad Sci USA 1977; 74:1683–1687.

161. Law SK, Fearon DT, Levine RP. Action of the C3b-inactivator on cell-bound C3b. J Immunol 1979; 122:759–765.

162. Fearon DT. Regulation by membrane sialic acid of β1H-dependent decay-dissociation of amplification C3 convertase of the alternative complement pathway. Proc Natl Acad Sci USA 1978; 75:1971–1975.

163. Kazatchkine MD, Fearon DT, Austen KF. Human alternative complement pathway: membrane-associated sialic acid regulates the competition between B and β1H for cell-bound C3b. J Immunol 1979; 122:75–81.

164. Davis AE, III, Harrison RA. Structural characterization of factor I mediated cleavage of the third component of complement. Biochemistry 1982; 21:5745–5749.

165. Medof ME, Iida K, Mold C, Nussenzweig V. Unique role of the complement receptor CR$_1$ in the degradation of C3b associated with immune complexes. J Exp Med 1982; 156:1739–1754.

166. Ross GD, Lambris JD, Cain JA, Newman SL. Generation of three different fragments of bound C3 with purified factor I or serum. I. Requirements for factor H *vs* CR$_1$ cofactor activity. J Immunol 1982; 129:2051–2060.

167. Sahn A, Isaacs S, Lambris JD. Modulation of complement by recombinant vaccinia virus complement control protein. Mol Immunol 1996; 33:61 (abstract).

168. Carter RH, Spycher MO, Ng YC, Hoffman R, Fearon DT. Synergistic interaction between complement receptor type 2 and membrane IgM on B lymphocytes. J Immunol 1988; 141:457–463.

169. Croix DA, Ahearn JM, Rosengard AM, Han S, Kelsoe G, Ma M, Carroll MC. Antibody response to a T-dependent antigen requires B cell expression of complement receptors. J Exp Med 1996; 183:1857–1864.

170. Dempsey PW, Allison MED, Akkaraju S, Goodnow CC, Fearon DT. C3d of complement as a molecular adjuvant: bridging innate and acquired immunity. Science 1996; 271:348–350.

171. Thoman ML, Meuth JL, Morgan EL, Weigle WO, Hugli TE. C3d-K a kallikrein cleavage fragment of iC3b is a potent inhibitor of cellular proliferation. J Immunol 1984; 133:2629–2633.

172. Hoeprich PD, Jr, Dalinden CA, Lachmann PJ, Davis AE, III, Hugli TE: A synthetic nonapeptide corresponding to the NH_2-terminal sequence of C3d-k causes leukocytosis in rabbits. J Biol Chem 1985; 260:2597–2600.

173. Rother K. Leukocyte mobilizing factor: a new biologic activity derived from the third component of complement. Eur J Immunol 1972; 2:550–558.

174. Takata Y, Kinoshita T, Kozono H, Takeda J, Tanaka E, Hong K, Inoue K. Covalent association of C3b with C4b within C5 convertase of the classical complement pathway. J Exp Med 1987; 165:1494–1507.

175. Kozono H, Kinoshita T, Kim YU, Takata-Kozono Y, Tsunasawa S, Sakiyama F, Takeda J, Hong K, Inoue K. Localization of the covalent C3b-binding site on C4b within the complement classical pathway C5 convertase, C4b2a3b. J Biol Chem 1990; 265:14444–14449.

176. Kinoshita T, Takata Y, Kozono H, Takeda J, Hong K, Inoue K. C5 convertase of the alternative complement pathway: covalent linkage between two C3b molecules within the trimolecular complex enzyme. J Immunol 1988; 141:3895–3901.

177. Podack ER, Müller-Eberhard HJ. Isolation of human S-protein, an inhibitor of the membrane attack complex of complement. J Biol Chem 1979; 254:9908–9914.

178. Hamilton KK, Zhao J, Sims PJ. Interaction between apolipoproteins A-I and A-II and the membrane attack complex of complement: affinity of the apoproteins for polymeric C9. J Biol Chem 1993; 268:3632–3638.

179. Davies A, Simmons DL, Hale G, Harrison RA, Tighe H, Lachmann PJ, Waldmann H. CD59, an LY-6-Like protein expressed in human lymphoid cells, regulates the action of the complement membrane attack complex on homologous cells. J Exp Med 1989; 170:637–654.

180. Holguin MH, Fredrick LR, Bernshaw NJ, Wilcox LA, Parker CJ. Isolation and characterization of a membrane protein from normal human erythrocytes that inhibits reactive lysis of the erythrocytes of paroxysmal nocturnal hemoglobinuria. J Clin Invest 1989; 84:7–17.

181. Hüsler T, Lockert DH, Kaufman KM, Sodetz JM, Sims PJ. Chimeras of human complement C9 reveal the site recognized by complement regulatory protein CD59. J Biol Chem 1995; 270:3483–3486.

182. Zalman LS, Wood LM, Müller-Eberhard HJ. Isolation of a human erythrocyte membrane protein capable of inhibiting expression of homologous complement transmembrane channels. Proc Natl Acad Sci USA 1986; 83:6975–6979.

3

C1q and Mannose-Binding Lectin

KENNETH B. M. REID
Oxford University, Oxford, England

I. GENE STRUCTURES

A. Human C1q

The genes encoding the A, B, and C chains of human C1q are located within the region 1p34.1–1p36.3 on the short arm of chromosome 1 (1) (Table 1). They are tandemly arranged 5′ to 3′ in the order A–C–B on a 24 kb stretch of DNA, with each gene being approximately 3 kb long and each containing (2) a single intron of approximately 1.2 kb. The first exon, in each of the A-, B-, and C-chain genes, encodes the leader sequence, a short (2–5 residues) N-terminal region and approximately half the total length of collagen-like Gly–Xaa–Yaa repeating triplet sequence found in each chain. There are 84 residues of collagen-like sequence in each chain but interruptions to the continuity of the coding of the Gly-Xaa-Yaa repeating triplet sequence are seen in the A and C chains close to the beginning of the second exon. The second exon in each of the three genes encodes the remaining half of collagen-like Gly–Xaa–Yaa repeating triplet sequence along with the approximately 135 residues that make up the C1q–C-terminal module. Mutations leading to C1q deficiency have been found in all three chains and are recessive in nature. The number of individuals for which the molecular basis of C1q deficiency has been established is now seven and in each case the cause of the defect has been shown to be

Table 1 Chromosomal Location of Human Genes Coding for Proteins with Globular and Collagenous Domains

Name	Gene symbol	Chromosome location
C1qA-chain	C1QA	1p34.1–p36.3
C1qB-chain	C1QB	1p34.1–p36.3
C1qC-chain	C1QC	1p34.1–p36.3
Collagen VIII α-2 polypeptide	COL8A2	1p34.3–p32.3
Mannose-binding lectin	MBL	10q21
Lung surfactant protein A (SP-A)	SFTP1	10q22–q23
Lung surfactant protein D (SP-D)	SFTP4	10q22–q23
Collagen XIII α-1 polypeptide	COL13A1	10q22

due to a point mutation or single nucleotide deletion (Table 2). Several of the mutations causing C1q deficiency create a novel restriction site, or delete a normal restriction site, which has allowed rapid screening of groups of patients with systemic lupus erythematosus (SLE) for evidence of the same mutation. For example, the G to T mutation within the codon for amino acid 186 in the A chain (3) (Table 2) deletes a PvuII restriction site in exon 2 of the A chain. The G to A mutation within the codon for amino acid 6 of the C chain (3) (Table 2) creates a novel SfcI restriction site in exon 1 of the C chain (Table 2). However, when 158 DNA samples from patients with SLE were screened for these mutations, none were found (4). Analysis of DNA from 50 SLE patients for the loss of a Taq1 restriction site introduced by the C to T mutation within the codon 150 of the B chain (Table 2) showed no evidence for the defective mutation (5). There are no reports of extensive screening for the presence of polymorphic sites within the genes encoding all three chains of C1q in normal individuals. To date, only one polymorphism, detected with the restriction enzyme PstI, has been found in the B chain gene and this was the result of screening the DNA from 50 healthy individuals using 12 common restriction enzymes and cDNA probes from the A- and B-chain clones (5).

B. Human Mannose-Binding Lectin*

The human Mannose-binding lectin (MBL) gene has been localized to the 10q11.2-q21 region of chromosome 10 by Southern blot analysis of human/rodent somatic cell hybrids and *in situ* hybridization of metaphase spreads, using a cDNA probe (6) (Table 1). Analysis and sequencing of cosmid and lambda clones has shown that the 7 kb-long gene encoding human MBL contains four exons that each correspond to distinct regions of the protein structure (7). Exon 1 encodes the signal peptide, the cysteine-containing N-terminal region and seven Gly-Xaa-Yaa triplets of the collagen-like region; exon 2 encodes the remaining 12 Gly-Xaa-Yaa triplets of the collagen-like region; exon 3 encodes the α-helical neck region and exon 4 encodes the carbohydrate recognition domain (CRD) and the 3', nontranslated region of the mRNA. The 5' region of the MBL gene contains features which are characteristic of acute phase proteins (7). These regions are apparently active since modest (1.5 to 3 times) increases in the serum MBL levels have been reported in patients who had undergone surgery and also in individuals who suffered from malarial attacks (8). Basal serum levels of MBL are controlled by gene variants within the promotor, and also the structural, regions of the gene (9,10). There are four structural variants described for the MBL gene that have been defined by Garred and co-workers as A, B, C, and D alleles, where A represents the wild type and B, C, and D define point mutations within codons 54, 57, and 52, respectively, which are clustered within a short segment

---

* This protein is usually called "mannan-binding protein" or "mannose-binding protein" in the recent literature. Both of these names abbreviate to MBP, but the use of the names "mannan-binding lectin" or "mannose-binding lectin," which both abbreviate to MBL (the official gene symbol for the gene, on human chromosome 10, which encodes the protein) are perhaps preferable since the abbreviation MBP is already used for myelin basic protein (and is the official gene symbol for that protein) and MBP is also used for the major basic protein of eosinophils. However, to date, there is no official IVIS recommended nomenclature ruling in favor of using the name mannose-binding lectin and the abbreviation MBL for the description of this protein at the protein and gene levels.

Table 2 Mutations Causing C1q Deficiency Have been Identified Within the Genes of All Three Chains of C1q

C1q chain	Mutation	Result of mutation	Number of patients identified	References
Patients in whom no C1q function, or antigenicity, was dectected in plasma				
A	C→T within codon for amino acid 186	Codon for Gln_{186}→premature stop codon	2	3,4
B	C→T within codon for amino acid 150	Codon for Arg_{150}→premature stop codon	1	5
C	C→T within codon for amino acid 41	Codon for Arg_{41}→premature stop codon	1	4
C	Deletion of C nucleotide within codon for amino acid 43	Change in reading frame from residue 43 gives stop codon at position 108	1	4
Patients in whom C1q antigenicity, but no C1q function, was detected in plasma				
C	G→A within codon for amino acid 6	Gly→Arg at position 6	2	3,4

of exon 1 and which each result in single amino acid substitutions within the collagen-like region of the MBL polypeptide chains (Table 3). These substitutions therefore completely disrupt the ability to form collagen-like triple helical structures by the MBL polypeptide chains of individuals who are homozygous for the B, C, or D alleles and greatly reduce the formation of triple-helical structure in heterozygous individuals. The B, C, and D alleles are therefore one cause of complete deficiency or low levels of serum MBL (9). However, mutations in the promotor region (Table 3) also regulate MBL levels and therefore individuals homozygous for the wild type A allele can still display very low levels of serum MBL (10).

II. POLYPEPTIDE CHAIN AND SUBUNIT STRUCTURES

A. Human C1q

The human C1q molecule (460 kDa) is composed of 18 polypeptide chains (6A, 6B, and 6C) that are similar in length and amino acid sequence. Analysis of the complete amino acid sequences of each of the three types of chain, as derived from protein, cDNA, and genomic sequencing, shows that the A-chain (223 residues long), B-chain (226 residues long), and C-chain (217-residues long) each have a short (3–9 residues) N-terminal region (containing a half-cystine residue involved in interchain disulfide bond formation), followed by a collagen-like sequence of approximately 81 residues and a C-terminal globular region of approximately 135 residues (2,11). The only interchain disulfide bridges in human C1q are located between the half-cystine residues at positions A-4 and B-4, in the A- and B-chains, and between the half-cystine residues at position C-4 in pairs of C-chains. This interchain disulfide bonding yields 6A-B dimer subunits and 3C-C dimer

Table 3   Serum Levels of MBL are Influenced by Allelic Variations Seen Within Both the Promotor and Structural Coding Regions of the Gene

Variants within the promotor region

Genotype	Position of polymorphic site	Cause of polymorphism
H/L	−550	G→C transition
YX	−220	G→C transition

Variants differing by one nucleotide within the region covered by codons 52–57 that encode part of the collagen-like sequence

Allele	Position of polymorphic site		
	Codon 52	Codon 54	Codon 57
A	CGT	GCC	GCA
(wild type)	Arg	Gly	Gly
B	CGT	G<u>A</u>C	GGA
	Arg	<u>Asp</u>	Gly
C	CGT	<u>GCC</u>	GA<u>A</u>
	Arg	Gly	<u>Glu</u>
D	<u>T</u>GT	GCC	<u>GGA</u>
	<u>Cys</u>	Gly	Gly

subunits (Fig. 1a). It is proposed that the collagen-like sequences in the A- and B-chains of an A-B subunit form a triple-helical collagen-like structure with the equivalent sequence in one of the C-chains present in a C-C subunit. This would give rise to 'structural units', composed of two A-B subunits and one C-C subunit, which are held together by both covalent (the C-C disulfide bond), and noncovalent (the two triple helical regions), bonds (Fig. 1a). Three of these structural units are then considered to associate, via strong noncovalent bonds in the fibril-like central portion, to yield the hexameric C1q molecule (12).

Approximately 60% of the proline and lysine residues within the collagen-like regions of the A-, B-, and C-chains are hydroxylated as summarized in Sellar et al.[2] to yield 4-hyroxyproline and hydroxylysine, respectively. There is no hydroxylation of these residues seen within the globular, approximately 135-residues-long, non-collagen-like C-terminal regions of C1q which are defined as "complement C1q carboxy-terminal" modules abbreviated to "C1q" modules (13).

Overall comparison of the amino acid sequences of the three chains of C1q with each other shows that the leader sequences, of 22–28 residues, do not show any significant degree of identity apart from a leucine-rich core seen in the B- and C-chains (2). The hydrophobic leader peptides are cleaved at an alanine (B- and C-chains), or threonine (A chain), residue at position -1 to yield the mature chains. Comparison of the mature chains shows that there are four conserved cysteines in each chain (at positions 4, 135, 154, and 171, as per the B chain numbering). The cysteines at position 4 are involved in the interchain disulfide bridges yielding the A–B and C–C subunits, and it is proposed that the cysteines at positions 135 and 154 form an intrachain disulfide bond in each of the chains while the cysteine at position 171, in each chain, is present as a free thiol group. The alignment and comparison of the collagen-like amino acid sequences of the chains of human C1q shows little similarity, apart from the conservation of glycine over the Gly-Xaa-Yaa repeating triplet sequences, with only three proline residues (at positions 17, 59 and 67) and one glutamic acid residue (at position 34) being conserved in all three chains. The conserved glutamic residue, within these Gly–Xaa–Yaa triplets, is located immediately preceding the region where the triple-helix, formed from the three C1q chains, appears to "bend" when viewed in the electron microscope (14,15) (Fig. 1a). In the A-chain a threonine residue is inserted between two Gly–Xaa–Yaa triplets at position A-39, and in the C-chain an alanine residue is substituted for a glycine residue at position C-36 while the B-chain does not have an interruption but does have an "extra" Gly–Xaa–Yaa triplet over this region compared to the A- and C-chains. Molecular modeling can place all the Gly–Xaa–Yaa triplets in human C1q in an almost perfect triple helix with the helix appearing to bend over the region of the interruptions in the A- and C-chains (16).

On comparison of the C-terminal regions of the three chains of C1q (immediately after the collagen-like region, from residue 90 onwards as based on the B-chain numbering), approximately 27% of the residues are completely conserved. These include three cysteines and a large number of hydrophobic and neutral residues, which seem likely to be the framework residues which form the scaffold of the 135-residues long C1q C-terminal module and to import on it its largely β-sheet structure, as has been predicted from Fourier-transform infrared spectroscopy and analysis of the sequence (17). Modules of the same type as the C1q C-terminal module are also found in a variety of noncomplement proteins that include the C-terminal regions of the human type VIII (18) and type X collagens (19), precerebellin (20), the chipmunk hibernation proteins (21), the human endothelial cell protein designated "multimerin" (22), a serum protein Acrp-30 that is

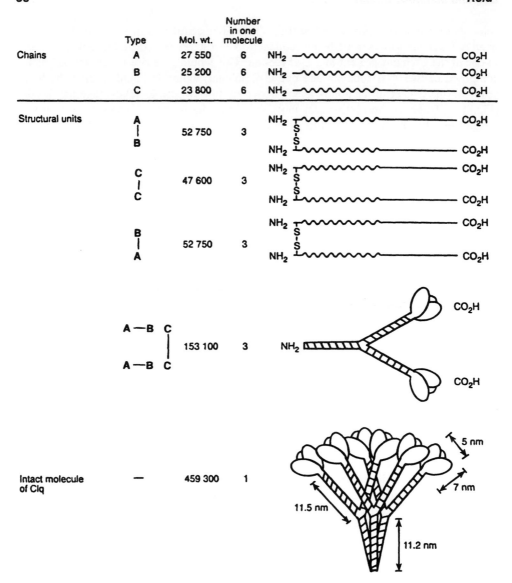

Chains	Type	Mol. wt.	Number in one molecule
	A	27 550	6
	B	25 200	6
	C	23 800	6

Structural units			
A–B		52 750	3
C–C		47 600	3
B–A		52 750	3
A—B C / A—B C		153 100	3

| Intact molecule of C1q | — | 459 300 | 1 |

Figure 1a   A molecular model of C1q. ∿∿∿∿ and ⊐⊐⊐⊐⊐⊐ denote collagen-like amino acid sequence and triple-helical structure, respectively. The molecule consists of 18 chains with the N-terminal portions of the A, B, or C chains having collagen-like sequences that adopt a triple-helical structure. Each of the six globular "heads" contains one each of the C-terminal portions (or domains) of the A, B, and C chains, thus each head is shown as a composite of three domains. The A and B chains are disulfide bonded at the N-terminal region. The C chain is disulfide bonded to the C chain of another monomeric ABC subunit. Three dimeric subunits are held by noncovalent forces to give the hexameric structure of an intact molecule of C1q. The C1r- and C1s-binding sites are located in the collagen regions, whereas the binding sites for the Fc regions of IgG or IgM are in the globular heads.

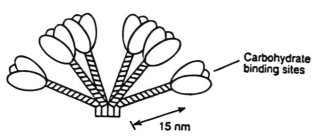

Figure 1b A side view of the hexameric form of human serum MBP. ⲛⲧⲧⲧⲧⲧⲧⲛ denotes triple-helical structure. In contrast to C1q, the three chains in each monomeric subunit are identical. Each head of MBP contains three C-type lectin domains.

secreted from mouse adipocytes (23) and the sunfish inner-ear specific structural protein (24). In several of these proteins the chains containing these C1q-like carboxyterminal modules appear likely to form a homotrimeric structure (as in type X collagen, multimerin, Acrp-30 and possibly precerebellin and the inner-ear-specific protein). However, in the other proteins a heterotrimeric structure is probably formed (as in C1q and the hibernation protein, which both have three types of chain, and the type VIII collagen, which has two α1 and one α2 chains). The C1q molecule is the only one of these proteins for which, to date, a function has been ascribed to the module (i.e., binding to the Fc regions of antibody IgM and IgG on the formation of immune complexes involving these types of antibodies).

B. Human Mannose-Binding Lectin

Human serum MBL is composed of oligomers of one type of polypeptide chain (227 residues long) with a molecular mass of approximately 32 kDa. Three of these identical chains associate to form a 96 kDa subunit which is considered to form a range of oligomers, from dimers (2 × 96kDa) to hexamers (6 × 96kDa) (Fig. 1b). The derived amino acid sequence of human MBL (7) shows that it has an N-terminal region (of 21 residues) that contains three cysteines, which are involved in the formation of interchain disulfide bonds within and between trimeric subunits. The repeating Gly–Xaa–Yaa triplet region (of 59 residues), which follows the N-terminal region, forms a triple helical collagen-like structure with the repeating triplet regions from two other chains. Immediately C-terminal to the collagen-like sequence there is a stretch of 34 amino acids, known as the neck region, that forms a three-stranded α-helical-coiled coil when associated with the equivalent regions in two other chains. The 113 residues, located at the C-terminal end of each chain of MBL, form an independently folded C-type lectin carbohydrate recognition domain (CRD). The MBL polypeptide chains trimerize via a triple-helical collagen-like region, formed from the 59 residues of Gly–Xaa–Yaa in each chain, and also via the α-helical-coiled coil section located between the triple helical region and the C-type lectin CRDs. Each trimeric subunit of MBL, formed from three identical MBL polypeptide chains, therefore contains a cluster of three C-type lectin CRDs at its C-terminal end (as has been shown by x-ray crystallography [25]). Dimers to hexamers of this subunit yield the spectrum of MBL oligomers seen in serum (26). The hexameric form of MBL is shown in Figure 1b.

There is no information yet available concerning the precise bond arrangement in MBL, with respect to interchain bonds between trimeric 96 kDa subunits. It has been suggested from studies involving sucrose density gradient analysis followed by sodium dodecyl sulfate–polyacrylamide gel electropheresis (SDS-PAGE) analysis, that dimers, trimers, and tetramers of the 96 kDa subunits account for approximately 75% of the serum MBL (26). This is consistent with another study, utilizing gel-filtration followed by SDS-PAGE analysis, indicating that human MBL was composed of mainly trimers, tetramers, and pentamers (27) and also the finding of a range of dimers, trimers, tetramers, pentamers, and hexamers by electron microscopy (28).

III. INTERACTIONS WITH OTHER PROTEINS

A. Enzymes Associated with C1q and MBL

1. Interaction of Human C1q with Enzymes C1r and C1s

The C1 complex is composed of one molecule of C1q and two molecules of proenzyme C1r and two molecules of proenzyme C1s. C1q acts as the recognition unit of the C1 complex, by binding to the Fc regions of antibody IgG, or IgM, in immune complexes. The C1r and C1s act as a catalytic unit in the form of a calcium-dependent $C1r_2 C1s_2$ tetramer, which, after activation of the proenzyme forms, brings about classical pathway activation of components C4 and C2. The proenzyme forms of C1r and C1 are both single-chain polypeptides of approximately 83 kDa. They appear to have an almost rodlike shape when the purified C1s–C1r–C1r–C1s tetramer is viewed in the electron microscope (i.e., with the $C1r^2$ dimer at the core of the tetramer[29,30]). Both C1r and C1s are seen as two globular domains connected by an elongated structure, with the larger of the globular domains containing the catalytic site in activated C1r and C1s. A model of the C1 complex has been proposed (31) in which the C1s–C1r–C1r–C1s tetramer adopts a distorted figure eight structure with the smaller globular "interaction" domains located outside the collagen-like strands of C1q while the globular catalytic domains remain closely associated within the collagen-like strands. This model is in agreement with the observations that the large collagen-like fragment of C1q (the C1q "stalks" that can be prepared by limited proteolysis with pepsin) can interact with the $C1r_2$–$C1s_2$ complex (32) and that these stalks behave as an inhibitor of the reconstruction of C1 complex activity from mixtures of C1q and $C1s_2 C1s_2$ (33).

2. Interaction of Human MBL with the MBL-Associated
Serine Proteases MASP-1 and MASP-2

Kawasaki and co-workers established in 1987 that MBL was involved in activation of complement through the classical pathway (34). It then became clear that MBL was identical to the carbohydrate-recognition portion of the serum Ra-reactive factor, which recognized and bound to the Ra polysaccharides of various strains of *Salmonella typhimurium* and *Escherichia coli*. The Ra-reactive factor was known to provide antibody-independent defense against a range of pathogenic organisms by activating the classical pathway of complement. It is now recognized that, after the trimeric C-type lectin domain clusters present in MBL have bound to carbohydrate structures on the surface of pathogens, one or more of the MASP proenzymes associated with the MBL become activated. This then leads to the activation of C4 and C2 in a similar manner to their activation by C1s via the activated C1 complex (35,36). Two MBL-associated serine proteases designated as

MASPs have been characterized. The initial MASP described is also called P100(37) and in this chapter it will be defined as MASP-1. The MASP-1 has a similar overall domain organization to that of C1r and C1s(37, 38): a polypeptide chain of approximately 83 kDa with the following domains: an N-terminal C1r/C1s-like module (CUB module) followed by an epidermal growth factor module (EGF) then another CUB module, two complement control protein (CCP) module, and finally a C-terminal serine protease domain. It is not known which portion of the MBL the MASP-1 proenzyme interacts, but by analogy with the $C1q$-$C1r_2$ $C1s_2$ interaction it appears likely that MASP-1 will be bound to the collagen-like regions of MBL in the form of a dimer. It has been reported that MASP-1, once activated, can, in turn, activate C4, C2, and C3 (34–36,39,40). However, another enzyme that co-purifies with MBL and MASP-1 has been characterized and shown by sequence analysis and function to be closely related to MASP-1, C1r, and C1s (41). This novel protease has been named MASP-2 in view of the fact it associates with MBL and was shown under certain conditions to cleave C4, whereas, under the same conditions, the MASP-1 was unable to cleave C4 (41). It has therefore been postulated that there may be an MBL–MASP-1–MASP-2 complex analogous in overall organization and function to the $C1q$–$C1r_2$–$C1s_2$ complex (41), with MASP-1 and MASP-2 fulfilling C1r-like and C1s-like roles, respectively. Much more research is required before this view is accepted since it has not been conclusively shown that there is a MBL–MASP-1–MASP-2 complex; if proenzyme MASP-1 can autoactivate in the same manner as C1r; if MASP-1 can activate proenzyme MASP-2; or if the preparations of MASP-1 used in the earlier studies did, in fact, contain MASP-2. At present it can be concluded that there are two closely related MASP proenzymes and that both are found in MBL preparations and appear likely to interact with MBL via the collagenous portions of the MBL molecule.

B. Proteins, Glycoproteins, and Carbohydrates That Are Recognized by and Bring About Activation of the C1 Complex and MBL–MASP-1/MASP-2 Complex

1. Interaction of Human C1 with IgG and IgM and Other Protein Activators

It is generally accepted that the globular "heads" of C1q contain binding sites for the Fc regions of IgG (42,43) and also for the Fc regions of IgM, although this has not been formally demonstrated in the case of IgM. Human C1q shows only weak binding to the Fc regions of nonaggregated IgG whereas, upon the presentation of multiple, closely-spaced Fc regions, as are found in immune complexes, the strength of the binding of the hexameric C1q to antibody IgG increases dramatically. The different subclasses of human IgG vary in their ability to bind C1q and activate complement, with IgG1 and IgG3 being the most active, IgG2 less active, and Ig4 inactive. Since a single molecule of antibody IgM contains multiple (five or six) Fc regions it is considered that binding of C1q takes place by exposure of the Fc regions on the binding of IgM Fab regions to multiple antigenic sites. The C1q binds to the $C\gamma2$ domain of IgG and the $C\mu3$ domain of IgM and the interactions in both cases appear to be primarily ionic. The three charged residues Glu-318, Lys-320, and Lys-322 in the $C\gamma2$ domain have been implicated in the binding of C1q to IgG, as judged by a site-directed mutagenesis study of a mouse Ig2b antihapten hybridoma antibody (44). The Glu–X–Lys–X–Lys sequence motif is conserved in all the IgG subclasses in humans and mice and therefore it is surprising that the human IgG4 subclass shows no binding, thus it is possible that access of the C1q heads to the $C\gamma2$

regions of IgG4 is sterically hindered by the Fab regions. The charged residues Asp-417, Glu-418, and His-420 in the $C\mu3$ region of IgM are considered to be involved in binding the C1q heads (45,46) and Asp-356 has also been implicated. It is therefore probable that charged residues, such as lysine, arginine, and histidine, in the globular head sequences of C1q are involved in Fc–C1q interactions. There is support for this view from a number of studies involving chemical modification of charged residues within C1q (as reviewed by Painter [46] and Smith et al. [17]). Each globular head of C1q is composed of the C-terminal halves (3×136 residues) of one A-, one B-, and one C-chain. It is not known if each of these C-terminal globular regions is an independently folding module (with the A-, B-, and C-chain C-terminal regions having distinct binding properties) or whether the different binding functions of C1q are dependent upon a combined globular structure that relies on contributions from all three chains. Expression of the human B-chain C-terminal region (residues B-90 to B-226) in *E. coli* has allowed the assessment of monomeric, dimeric, and highly aggregated forms of this region for the ability to bind to IgG and IgM. The results indicated that there was preferential binding of the dimeric, or aggregated, forms of the B-chain C-terminal region to IgG rather than IgM (47). This is consistent with the view that each head of C1q may be composed of three independently folded modules, each of which have different binding functions.

Many of the nonimmunoglobulin activators, which are considered to interact with C1q and bring about activation of C1r and C1s within the C1 complex, appear to interact with the collagen-like regions of C1q rather than the globular heads. These activators include nucleic acids, lipids, polysaccharides, polyanionic molecules, and microbial extracts, as well as several proteins (48). Two proteins, C-reactive protein (CRP) and serum amyloid protein (SAP) have been shown to interact specifically with C1q and bring about C1 activation. CRP is composed of five identical, noncovalently-linked, nonglycosylated subunits each of 24 kDa, and its three-dimensional structure has recently been determined (49). It binds in a Ca^{2+}-dependent manner to phosphocholine present in the cell walls of *Streptococcus pneumoniae*. This interaction with pneumococcal C-polysaccharide results in strong activation of the classical pathway of complement (50). It has been proposed that there are two binding sites on the A-chain of C1q with which CRP can interact to bring about activation of the C1 complex (51). One site is located completely within the collagen-like region (residues A14–26) while the other is located at the junction bridging the collagen-like and globular regions (residues A76–92). Since CRP is an acute-phase protein, its serum levels can rise more than 100-fold during infection. Its ability to interact with *Streptococcus pneumoniae* and activate complement is important at early stages of infection prior to the production of anticapsular antibodies (52) SAP, which is structurally homologous to CRP but behaves as a lectin that can bind tightly to various carbohydrates (53), can also bind to the collagen-like region C1q and activate the classical pathway in a manner analogous to that shown for CRP (54) and β-amyloid peptides, which also show this property of C1 activation (55). However, the finding that endotoxin also appears to activate the classical complement pathway via residues 14–26 of the C1q A-chain (48) does indicate that perhaps there may not be a high degree of specificity of interaction between C1q and these various proteins (CRP, SAP, β amyloid) via the 14–26 site in the A-chain. As well as endotoxin a variety of other extracts from bacteria, viruses, parasites, and mammalian cells have been found to bring about antibody-independent activation of C1 (reviewed by Gerwurz et al. [48]). These include the outer membrane proteins from bacteria and certain viral proteins, such as pI5E of the Moloney leukemia virus (56) and the gp41 fragment of gp160 of human immunovirus (HIV)-1. The site of C1q that recognizes gp41 is considered to lie within the globular head regions of C1q (57).

2. Interaction of Human MBL with Carbohydrate Structures That Results in Activation of the Classical Pathway

MBL has been shown to interact, via its carbohydrate-binding properties, with the cell surfaces, or purified fractions from cell surfaces, of a wide range of organisms. These include pathogenic strains of gram-negative and gram-positive bacteria, yeasts, viruses, mycobacteria, parasites, and protozoa (as summarized by Epstein et al. [58]). None of the cell surface targets for MBL on these organisms have been fully characterized but they are presumed to be mainly glycoproteins and glycolipids bearing appropriate mannose, GlcNAc, fucose, and glucose residues at the nonreducing ends of their carbohydrate structures, which allows their recognition by MBL.

One human serum glycoprotein has been shown to be recognized by MBL. It is the agalactosyl form of IgG, known as IgG-GO. The interaction of MBL with aggregated IgG-GO (which would mimic immune complexes composed of IgG–GO) results in activation of the classical pathway of complement (59). The absence of galactose at the reducing ends of the complex carbohydrate structure seen in the Fc region of IgG allows recognition of the exposed reducing sugar residue by MBL. Since IgG-GO levels are raised in conditions such as rheumatoid arthritis, the ability of MBL to activate one of the major routes of inflammation in this fashion may be of clinical significance.

C. Cell-Surface Proteins That Interact with, and Are Considered to Act as Receptors for, C1q and MBL

1. Interaction of C1q with Cell-Surface Proteins

C1q is considered to be able to interact with cell surfaces via both its collagen-like regions and its globular head regions. However, the acceptance, as true cell-surface molecules, of some of the putative C1q-receptors that have been described, is controversial. This being the case, this section on C1q–C1q receptor interaction sites has been mainly restricted to a brief description of two possible sites on the collagen-like region of the C1q molecule that may serve as primary sites of interaction between C1q and the putative receptors. Three molecules have been characterized and designated as cell-surface receptors with an affinity for the collagen-like region of C1q. They are cC1q R (60,61), C1qRp (62,63), and $C1qR_{O_2^-}$ (64). The cC1q R molecule is found in a wide range of cells and appears to be calreticulin or a very closely-related isoform of calreticulin (65). As well as interacting with C1q, the calreticulin-like cC1qR binds to the collectins MBL, SP-A conglutinin, and Collectin-43 (66,67). The C1q Rp is a 126 kDa, heavily glycosylated, cell-surface membrane protein, found on monocytes and macrophages, which has been shown to enhance phagocytosis mediated via C1q, MBL, or SP-A (62,63). The $C1qR_{O_2^-}$ is a receptor present on neutrophils that triggers superoxide production on binding the collagen-like region of C1q (68) and does not appear to interact with MBL or SP-A These three putative receptors are considered to bind to either of two distinct sites on the collagen-like region of C1q. The first site has been located (69) just prior to the bend region of the collagen triple helix where a cluster of charged amino acids is seen (over residues 18–32 in all three chains, using the B-chain numbering). This site is considered to be utilized when C1q interacts with cells via the molecule considered to be a variant of calreticulin and designated cC1q-R. The cC1q-R molecule has also been shown to bind to the collectins SP-A, MBP, and conglutinin via highly charged sections, located immediately N-terminal to the bend regions, in the collagen-like triple helices present in human SP-A (residues 29–43) and human MBP (residues 35–49) (69). Bovine conglutinin also has a highly charged section within the N-terminal of its collagen-like triple helical region (residues 32–46) that is considered to be the receptor binding site, since a truncated form of conglutinin, lacking the N-terminal 55 residues, shows no binding to the cC1q-R (69). The phagocytosis-enhancing receptor C1q Rp (62,63) may also bind to the same highly charged sections, located just prior to the bend in the triple helical regions, present in C1q, SP-A, and MBP (62,63).

A second binding site on the collagen-like region of C1q, which involves the interaction of C1q with neutrophil cell-surface molecules and stimulation of neutrophil superoxide production (i.e., binding of C1q to $C1qR_{O_2^-}$), has been localized (70). By means of limited proteolysis of the collagen-like fragment of C1q it was shown that the neutrophil receptor for this region interacts with the collagen-helix of C1q in the area of amino acid residues 38–60 of either A- or C-chain (i.e., located just C-terminal to the bend region in the C1q of collagen-like triple helix). More recent studies suggest that the sequence Gly–X–Hyl–Gly–Gln–Hyl–Gly–Glu within the C-chain may constitute an important part of the receptor binding site (70), especially since the same peptide sequence is also found in the macrophage scavenger receptor system (except that the lysines are not hydroxylated in the macrophage scavenger receptor) where it has been shown to be involved in ligand binding and uptake.

REFERENCES

1. Sellar GC, Cockburn D, Reid KBM. Localization of the gene cluster encoding the A, B and C chains of human C1q to 1p34.1–1p36.3. Immunogenetics 1992; 35:214–216.
2. Sellar GC, Blake DJ, Reid KBM. Characterization and organization of the genes encoding the A-, B- and C-chains of human complement subcomponent C1q: the complete derived amino acid sequence of human C1q. Biochem J 1991; 274:481–490.
3. Petry F, Le DT, Kirschfink M, Loos M. Non-sense and missense mutations in the structural genes of complement component C1qA and C chains are linked with two different types of complete selective C1q deficiencies. J Immunol 1995; 155:4734–4738.
4. Slingsby JH, Topaloglu R, Norsworthy PJ, Pearce GJ, Vaishnaw AK, Bakkaloglu A, Morley B, Walport MJ. Molecular basis of C1q deficiency in four patients. Mol Immunol 1996; 33 Suppl 1:70.
5. McAdam RA, Goundis D, Reid KBM. A homozygous point mutation results in a stop codon in the C1q B-chain of a C1q-deficient individual. Immunogenetics 1988; 27:259–264.
6. Sastry K, Herman GA, Day L, Deignan E, Bruns G, Morton CC, Ezekowitz RA. The human mannose-binding protein gene. Exon structure reveals its evolutionary relationship to a human pulmonary surfactant gene and localization to chromosome 10. J Exp Med 1989; 170:1175–1189.
7. Taylor ME, Brickell PM, Craig RK, Summerfield JA. Structure and evolutionary origin of the gene encoding a human serum mannose-binding protein. Biochem J 1989; 262:763–771.
8. Thiel S, Holmskov U, Hviid L, Laursen SB, Jensenius JC. The concentration of the C-type lectin mannan-binding protein, in human plasma increases during an acute phase response. Clin Exp Immunol 1992; 90:31–35.
9. Madsen HO, Garred P, Kurtzhals JAL, Lamm LU, Ryder LP, Thiel S, Svejgaard A. A new frequent allele is the missing link in the structural polymorphism of the human mannan-binding protein. Immunogenetics 1994; 40:37–44.

10. Madsen HO, Garred P, Kurtzhals JAL, Lamm LU, Ryder LP, Svejgaard A. Interplay between promotor and structural gene variants control basal serum level of mannan-binding protein. J Immunol 1995; 155:3013–3020.

11. Reid KBM. Proteins involved in the activation and control of the two pathways of human complement. Biochem Soc Trans 1983; 11:1–12.

12. Reid KBM, Porter RR. Subunit composition and structure of subcomponent C1q of the first component of human complement. Biochem J 1976; 155:19–23.

13. Doolittle R. The multiplicity of domains in proteins. Annu Rev Biochem 1995; 64:287–314.

14. Knobel HR, Villiger W, Isliker H. Chemical analysis and electron microscopy studies of human C1q prepared by different methods. Eur J Immunol 1975; 5:78–82.

15. Brodsky-Doyle B, Leonard KR, Reid KBM. Circular-dichroism and electron-microscopy studies of human subcomponent C1q before and after limited proteolysis by pepsin. Biochem J 1976; 159:279–286.

16. Kilchherr E, Hofmann H, Steigemann W, Engel J. A Structural model of the collagen-like region of C1q comprising the kink region and the fibre-like packing of the six triple helices. J Mol Biol 1985; 186:403–415.

17. Smith KF, Haris PI, Chapman D, Reid KBM, Perkins SJ. β-Sheet secondary structure of the trimeric globular domain of C1q of complement and collagen types VIII and X by Fourier-transform infrared spectroscopy and averaged structure predictions. Biochem J 1994; 301:249–256.

18. Yamaguchi N, Benya PD, van der Rest M, Nimomiya Y. The cloning and sequencing of α1 (VIII) collagen cDNAs demonstrate that the type VIII collagen is a short chain collagen and contains triple helical and carboxyl-terminal non-triple-helical domains similar to those of type X collagen. J Biol Chem 1989; 264:16022–16029.

19. Ninomiya Y, Gordon M, van der Rest M, Schmid T, Linsenmayer T, Olsen BR. The developmentally regulated type X collagen gene contains a long open reading frame without introns. J Biol Chem 1986; 261:5041–5050.

20. Urade Y, Oberdick J, Molinar-Rode R, Morgan JI. Precerebellin is a cerebellum specific with similarity to the globular domains of complement C1q B chain. Proc Natl Acad Sci USA 1991; 88:1069–1073.

21. Takamatsu N, Ohba KI, Kondo J, Shiba T. Hibernation-associated gene regulation of plasma proteins with a collagen-like domain in mammalian hibernators. Mol Cell Biol 1993; 13:1516–1521.

22. Hayward CPM, Hassell JA, Denomme GA, Rachubinski RA, Brown C, Kelton JG. The cDNA sequence of human endothelial cell multimerin. A unique protein with RGDs, coiled-coil and epidermal growth factor-like domains and a carboxyl terminus similar to the globular domain of component C1q and collagens type VIII and X. J Biol Chem 1995; 270:18246–18251.

23. Scherer PE, Williams S, Fogliano M, Baldini G, Lodish HF. A novel serum protein similar to C1q, produced exclusively in adipocytes. J Biol Chem 1995; 270:26746–26749.

24. Davis JG, Oberholtzer JC, Burns FR, Greene MI. Molecular cloning and characterization of an inner ear-specific structural protein. Science 1995; 267:1031–1034.

25. Sherrif S, Chang CY, Ezekowitz RAB. Human mannose-binding protein carbohydrate recognition domain trimerizes through a triple α-helical coiled-coil. Struct Biol 1994; 1:789–794.

26. Lipscombe RJ, Sumiya M, Summerfield JA, Turner MW. Distinct physiochemical characteristics of human mannose binding protein expressed by individuals of differing genotype. Immunology 1995; 85:660–667.

27. Yokota Y, Arai T, Kawasaki T. Oligomeric structures required for complement activation of serum mannan-binding proteins. J Biochem 1995; 117:414–419.

28. Lu J, Thiel S, Wiedemann H, Timpl R, Reid KBM. Binding of the pentamer/hexamer forms of mannan-binding protein to zymosan activates the proenzyme C1r$_2$ C1s$_2$ complex, of the classical pathway of complement, without involvement of C1q. J Immunol 1990; 144:2287–2294.

29. Tschopp J, Villiger W, Fuchs H, Kilchherr E, Engel J. Assembly of subcomponents C1r and C1s of the first component of complement: electron microscopic and ultracentrifuge studies. Proc Natl Acad Sci USA 1980; 77:7014–7018.

30. Strang CJ, Siegel RC, Phillips ML, Poon PH, Schumaker VN. Ultrastructure of the first component of human complement: electron-microscopy of the crosslinked complex. Proc Natl Acad Sci USA 1982; 79:586–590.

31. Arlaud GJ, Colomb MG, Gagnon J. A functional model of the human C1 complex. Immunol Today 1987; 8:106–111.

32. Siegel RC, Schumaker VN. Measurement of the association constants of the complexes formed between intact C1q or pepsin treated C1q stalks and the unactivated or activated C1r2 C1s2 tetramers. Mol Immunol 1983; 20:53–66.

33. Reid KBM, Sim RB, Faiers AP. Inhibition of the reconstitution of the haemolytic activity of the first component of human complement by a pepsin-derived fragment of subcomponent C1q. Biochem J 1977; 161:239–245.

34. Ikeda K, Sannoh T, Kawasaki N, Kawasaki T, Yamashina I. Serum lectin with known structure activates complement through the classical pathway. J Biol Chem 1987; 262:7451–7454.

35. Matsushita M, Fujita T. Activation of the classical complement pathway by mannose-binding protein in association with a novel C1s-like serine protease. J Exp Med 1992; 176:1497–1502.

36. Ji YH, Fujita T, Hatsuse H, Takahashi A, Matsushita M, Kawakami M. Activation of the C4 and C2 components of complement by a proteinase in serum bactericidal factor, Ra reactive factor. J Immunol 1993; 150:571–578.

37. Takayama Y, Takada F, Takahashi A, Kawakami M. A 100-kDa protein in the C4-activating component of Ra-reactive factor is a new serine protease having module organization similar to C1r and C1s. J Immunol 1994; 152:2308–2316.

38. Sato T, Endo Y, Matsushita M, Fujita T. Molecular characterisation of a novel serine protease involved in activation of the complement system by mannose-binding protein. Int Immunol 1994; 6:665–669.

39. Ogata RT, Low PJ, Kawakami M. Substrate specificities of the protease of mouse serum Ra-reactive factor. J Immunol 1995; 154:2351–2357.

40. Matsushita M, Fujita T. Cleavage of the third component of complement (C3) by mannose-binding protein associated serine protease (MASP) with subsequent complement activation. Immunobiol 1995; 194:443–448.

41. Vorup-Jensen T, Stover C, Poulsen K, Laursen SB, Eggleton P, Reid KBM, Willis AC, Schwaeble W, Lu J, Holmskov U, Jensenius JC, Thiel S. Cloning of cDNA encoding a human MASP-like protein (MASP-2). Mol Immunol 1996; 33 Suppl 1:81.

42. Paques EP, Huber R, Preiss H, Wright JK. Isolation of the globular region of the subcomponent C1q of the C1 component of complement. Hoppe-Seylers Z Physiol Chem 1979; 360:177–183.

43. Hughes-Jones NC, Gardener B. Reaction between the isolated globular subunits of the complement component C1q and IgG-complexes. Mol Immunol 1979; 16:697–701.

44. Duncan AR, Winter G. The binding site for C1q on IgG. Nature 1988; 332:738–740.

45. Perkins SJ, Nealis AS, Sutton BJ, Feinstein A. The solution structure of human and mouse immunoglobulin M by synchrotron X-ray scattering and molecular graphics modelling: a possible mechanism for complement activation. J Mol Biol 1991; 221:1345–1366.

46. Painter RH. The binding of C1q to immunoglobulins. Behring Inst Mitt 1993; 93:131–137.

47. Kishore U, Leigh LEA, Willis AC, Eggleton P, Reid KBM. Production and characterization of a recombinant form of the C-terminal globular region of the B-chain of C1q. Mol Immunol 1996; 33 Suppl 1:88.

48. Gewurz H, Ying SC, Jiang H, Lint TE. Non-immune activation of the classical pathway of complement. Behring Inst Mitt 1993; 93:138–147.

49. Shrive AK, Cheetam GMT, Holden D, Myles DAA, Tumell WG, Volanakis JE, Pepys MB, Bloomer AC, Greenhough TJ. Three-dimensional structure of human C-reactive protein. Nature Struct Biol 1996; 3:346–353.

50. Volanakis JE. Complement activation by C-reactive protein complexes. Ann NY Acad Sci 1982; 389:235–249.

51. Jiang H, Robey FA, Gewurz H. Localisation of sites through which C-reactive protein binds and activates complement to residues 14–26 and 76–92 of the human C1q A-chain. J Exp Med 1992; 175:1374–1379.

52. Yother J, Volanakis JE, Briles DE. Human C-reactive protein is protective against fatal *Streptococcus pneumoniae* infection in mice. J Immunol 1982; 128:2374–2376.

53. Hind CRK, Collins PM, Baltz ML, Pepys MB. Human serum amyloid P component, a circulating lectin with specificity for the cyclic 4,6-pyruvate acetal of galactose. Biochem J 1985; 25:107–111.

54. Ying SC, Gewurz AT, Jiang H, Gewurz H. Human serum amyloid P component oligomers bind and activate the classical pathway complement pathway via residues 14–26 and 76–92 of the collagen-like region of C1q. J Immunol 1993; 150:169–176.

55. Jiang H, Burdick D, Glabe CG, Cotman CW, Tenner AJ. β-Amyloid activates complement by binding to a specific region of the collagen-like domain of the C1q A-chain. J Immunol 1994; 152:5050–5059

56. Bartholomew RM, Esser AF, Müller-Eberhard HJ. Lysis of oncoma viruses by human serum. Isolation of the viral complement (C1) receptor and identification as p15E. J Exp Med 1978; 147:844–853.

57. Thielens NM, Bally IM, Ebenbichler CF, Dierich MP, Arlaud GJ. Further characterization of the interaction between the C1q subcomponent of human C1 and the transmembrane envelope glycoprotein gp41 of HIV-1. J Immunol 1993; 151:6583–6590.

58. Epstein J, Eichbaum Q, Sheriff S, Ezekowitz RAB. The collectins in innate immunity. Curr Opin Immunol 1996; 8:29–35.

59. Malhotra R, Wormald MR, Rudd PM, Fischer PB, Dwek RA, Sim RB. Glycosylation changes of IgG associated with rheumatoid arthritis can activate complement via the mannose-binding protein. Nature Med 1995; 1:237–243.

60. Ghebrehiwet B, Silvestri L, McDevitt C. Identification of the Raji cell membrane-derived C1q inhibitor as a receptor for human C1q. Purification and immunochemical characterization. J Exp Med 1984; 160:1375–1389.

61. Ghebrehiwet B. Functions associated with the C1q receptor. Behring Inst Mitt 1989; 84:204–215.

62. Tenner AJ, Robinson SL, Ezekowitz RAB. Mannose binding protein (MBP) enhances mononuclear phagocyte function via a receptor that contains the 126000 Mr component of the C1q receptor. Immunity 1995; 3:485–493.

63. Ruiz S, Tenner AJ. C1q and pulmonary surfactant protein A (SPA) trigger enhanced phagocytic capacity with identical kinetics and via the same 126,000 Mr cell surface "C1q receptor." Mol Immunol 1996; 33 Supplement 1:65.

64. Ruiz S, Henschen-Edman AH, Tenner AJ. Localization of the site on the complement component C1q required for the stimulation of neutrophil superoxide production. J Biol Chem 1995; 270:30627–30634.

65. Lu J, Sim RB. Collectins and collectin receptors. In: Erdei A, ed. New Aspects of Complement Structure and Function. Austin, TX: R.G. Landes Company, 1994:85–106.

66. Malhotra R, Thiel S, Reid KBM, Sim RB. Human leukocyte C1q receptor binds other soluble proteins with collagen domains. J Exp Med 1990; 172:955–959.

67. Malhotra R, Haurum J, Thiel S, Sim RB. Interaction of C1q receptor with lung surfactant protein A. Eur J Immunol 1992; 22:1437–1445.

68. Goodman EB, Tenner AJ. Signal transduction mechanisms of C1q-mediated superoxide production. Evidence for the involvement of temporally distinct staurosporine-insensitive and sensitive pathways. J Immunol 1992; 148:3920–3928.

69. Malhotra R, Laursen SB, Willis AC, Sim RB. Localization of the receptor-binding site in the collectin family of proteins. Biochem J 1993; 293:15–19.
70. Ruiz S, Henschen-Edman AH, Tenner AJ. Identification of a region of the C1q C-chain that is critical for the stimulation of neutrophil superoxide production by C1q. Mol Immunol 1996; 33 Suppl 1:38.

4

Complement Enzymes

JOHN E. VOLANAKIS
University of Alabama at Birmingham, Birmingham, Alabama

GÉRARD J. ARLAUD
Institute for Structural Biology, Jean-Pierre Ebel, Grenoble, France

Complement activation and the associated production of biologically active protein fragments is effected by a group of seven proteolytic enzymes, factor D (EC 3–4–21–46), C1r (EC 3–4–21–41), C1s (EC 3–4–21–42), MASP, factor B (EC 3–4–21–47), C2, and factor I (EC 3–4–21–45), all of which are serine proteases (SPs). On the basis of their primary structure, complement SPs belong to the chymotrypsin family and, on the basis of their specificity for Arg residues, to the trypsin subfamily. Members of the chymotrypsin family of SPs are ubiquitous and are involved in a wide range of biological processes, which in addition to complement activation include blood coagulation, kinin production, fibrinolysis, fertilization, digestion, and probably also cell differentiation (1,2). After a short overview of shared structural and functional features of SPs, this chapter will describe the genomic organization, structure, function, and structural correlates of function of the complement SPs.

I. OVERVIEW OF STRUCTURE AND FUNCTION OF SERINE PROTEASES

The high-resolution crystal structures of several chymotrypsin-like SPs have been reported (3–6). All have very similar structural folds, consisting of two antiparallel β-barrel type domains. Each barrel contains six β-strands that have the same topology in all enzymes. Because all chymotrypsin-like SPs, including the complement ones, have conserved in their primary sequence certain critical structural elements, it is generally assumed that they also have conserved the chymotrypsin structural fold.

   Four features essential for catalysis have been conserved in the structure of SPs: a catalytic triad, a substrate specificity pocket, a nonspecific binding site for the P_1–P_3 residues of the substrate, and an oxyanion-binding hole (7). The importance of the catalytic triad residues, Asp^{102}, His^{57}, and Ser^{195} (chymotrypsinogen numbering has been used for all SP domains throughout this paper to facilitate comparisons) for efficient substrate hydrolysis was established many years ago (8–10). However, the original proposal that the three residues participate in a charge-relay system (10) has not been supported by more recent studies (11–13). It is currently believed that substrate hydrolysis is effected by nucleophilic attack on the carbonyl carbon of the scissile bond by the Ser^{195} hydroxyl oxygen; His^{57} serves as a general base catalyst, increasing the nucleophilicity of Ser^{195}; Asp^{102} is necessary for maintaining the proper tautomer of His^{57} in the ground state and for stabilizing the developing positive charge of His^{57} during the transition state (14). The topology of the catalytic triad residues relative to each other is crucial for their synergistic action and is invariable in all chymotrypsin-like SPs of known structure. All complement enzymes have conserved the three catalytic residues and the surrounding highly conserved regions (Fig. 1). Therefore, they should be expected to employ the typical SP catalytic mechanism. Functional support for this proposal is provided by the fact that all complement enzymes are inhibited by diisopropylfluorophosphate. However, the catalytic triad of factor D, the only complement enzyme of known three-dimensional structure (15), displays considerable plasticity, such that in its "resting-state" the enzyme has an apparently nonfunctional catalytic triad.

The three-dimensional structure of the substrate specificity pocket of chymotrypsin-like SPs is highly conserved, despite differences in substrate specificity among them. In γ-chymotrypsin the pocket has three walls formed by residues 189–195, 214–220, and 225–228 (16), which are similar to the corresponding residues of trypsin (Fig. 1). The difference in substrate specificity between the two enzymes is attributed mainly to residue 189, which is located at the bottom of the specificity pocket. The presence of an Asp at this position endows trypsin with specificity for positively charged Arg and Lys residues, while in chymotrypsin the preference for bulky aromatics is largely defined by Ser-189. With the exception of factor B and C2, complement SPs have an Asp at position 189, which is consistent with their specificity for Arg peptide bonds (Table 1). An unexpected finding is that C2 has a Ser and factor B an Asn residue at the 189 position, although both cleave Arg bonds. However, both enzymes have an Asp at position 187, which could conceivably be located within the pocket and serve to bind the guanidinium side chain of the P_1* Arg residue of the substrate.

Additional structural elements, particularly the conformation of the invariable Gly^{216} as well as distant surface loops that contribute to the geometry of the specificity pocket without binding the substrate (17,18), play crucial roles in substrate specificity and catalysis. Comparative analyses of crystal structures of chymotrypsin, trypsin, and chymotrypsin-like trypsin mutants have indicated that the main chain conformation of Gly^{216} is a crucial structural determinant for the correct orientation of the scissile bond of the substrate (19). In turn, accurate positioning of the scissile bond relative to the oxyanion hole and the Ser^{195}, His^{57} dyad is a major kinetic determinant of substrate specificity. In all SPs analyzed, Gly^{216} forms two antiparallel β-strand H-bonds with the P_3 residue of the substrate. The H-bonds formed in trypsin and chymotrypsin are different and are believed to act as specificity determinants (19). It would be of interest to analyze the effect on substrate specificity of the presumed H-bonds between Gly^{216} of complement SPs and the corresponding P_3 residues.

Despite their overall structural similarity to typical pancreatic SPs, complement enzymes have unique features that allow them to carry out their highly specialized functions. With the exception of factor D, complement enzymes have additional domains,

---

* The nomenclature for the individual amino acid residues (P_1, P_2, etc.) of a substrate and the corresponding subsites (S_1, S_2, etc.) of the enzyme is that of Schechter and Berger (36).

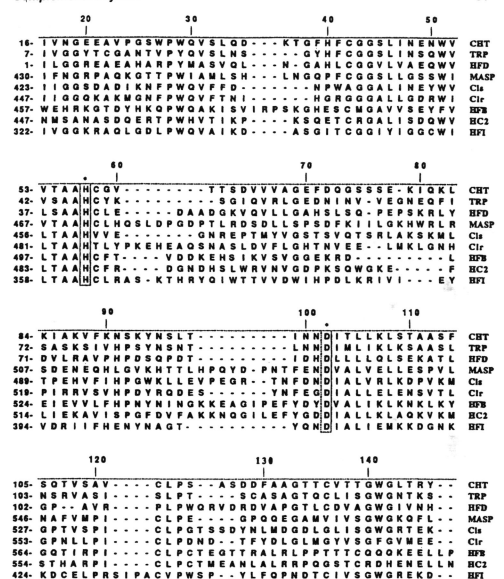

Figure 1a Amino acid sequence alignment of typical pancreatic serine proteases and complement serine protease domains. The catalytic triad residues His[57], Asp[102], and Ser[195] are boxed. Residues forming the walls of the primary specificity pocket in γ-chymotrypsin are shaded. Numbers at the top are for residues of the chymotrypsinogen sequence and numbers on the left are for the amino acid sequence of each intact protein. CHT, bovine chymotrypsin; TRP, bovine trypsin; HFD, human factor D; MASP, MBL-associated serine protease; HFB, human factor B, HC2, human C2, HFI, human factor I.

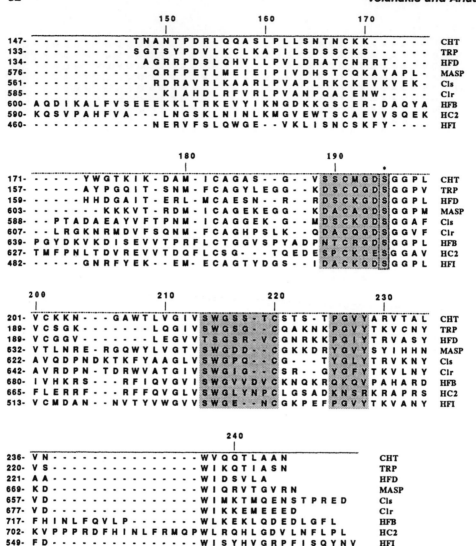

Figure 1b Amino acid sequence alignment of typical pancreatic serine proteases and complement serine protease domains. The catalytic triad residues His[57], Asp[102], and Ser[195] are boxed. Residues forming the walls of the primary specificity pocket in γ-chymotrypsin are shaded. Numbers at the top are for residues of the chymotrypsinogen sequence and numbers on the left are for the amino acid sequence of each intact protein. CHT, bovine chymotrypsin; TRP, bovine trypsin; HFD, human factor D; MASP, MBL-associated serine protease; HFB, human factor B, HC2, human C2, HFI, human factor I.

Table 1 Complement Enzymes: Natural Substrates and Cleavage Sites

Zymogen	Active Enzyme	Cofactor(s)	Substrate	Cleavage Sites[a]								
				P_5	-P_4	-P_3	-P_2	-P_1	-P_1'	-P_2'	-P_3'	-P_4'
C1r	C1r		C1r	^{442}Glu	-Gln	-Arg	-Gln	-Arg	-Ile	-Ile	-Gly	-Gly
C1r	C1r̄		C1s	^{418}Glu	-Glu	-Lys	-Gln	-Arg	-Ile	-Ile	-Gly	-Gly
C1r	C1r̄		C1r	^{275}Ser	-Gly	-Asp	-Ser	-Arg	-Gly	-Trp	-Lys	-Leu
				^{207}Ile	-Arg	-Val	-Glu	-Arg	-Gly	-Leu	-Thr	-Leu
?	?		MASP[b]	^{425}Lys	-Leu	-Met	-Ala	-Arg	-Ile	-Phe	-Asn	-Gly
C1s	C1s̄		⎡C4⎤[c]	^{733}Ala	-Gly	-Leu	-Gln	-Arg	-Ala	-Leu	-Glu	-Ile
MASP	MASP		⎣C2⎦	^{219}Glu	-Ser	-Leu	-Gly	-Arg	-Lys	-Ile	-Gln	-Ile
D	D	C3b	B	^{230}Glu	-Gln	-Gln	-Lys	-Arg	-Lys	-Ile	-Val	-Leu
B	C3bBb		C3⎤	^{722}Leu	-Gly	-Leu	-Ala	-Arg	-Ser	-Asn	-Leu	-Asp
C2	C4b2a		C3⎦									
B	(C3b)₂Bb		C5⎤	^{729}Met	-Gln	-Leu	-Gly	-Arg	-Leu	-His	-Met	-Lys
C2	C4b3b2a		C5⎦									
I	I	H, MCP, CR1	C3b	^{1772}Gln	-Leu	-Pro	-Ser	-Arg	-Ser	-Val	-Lys	-Ile
				^{1294}Ala	-Ser	-Leu	-Leu	-Arg	-Ser	-Glu	-Glu	-Thr
		CR1	iC3b	^{928}Glu	-Arg	-Leu	-Gly	-Arg	-Glu	-Gly	-Val	-Gln
		C4bp, MCP, CR1	C4b	^{933}Asp	-His	-Arg	-Gly	-Arg	-Thr	-Leu	-Glu	-Ile
				^{1313}Ser	-Ser	-Thr	-Gly	-Arg	-Asn	-Gly	-Phe	-Lys

[a]The nomenclature for the individual amino acid residues (P1, P2, ... P1', P2', etc.) of the substrate is that introduced by Schechter and Berger (36).
[b]The enzyme that cleaves and activates MASP has not been identified.
[c]C1s and MASP cleave identical peptide bonds in C4 and C2.

which contain protein modules also present in functionally unrelated proteins. In MASP, C1r, C1s, and factor I the SP domain occupies the smaller of two, disulfide-linked polypeptide chains. In the former three enzymes the two-chain structure arises from cleavage of a peptide bond of the single polypeptide chain zymogen form during complement activation. Factor I apparently has no circulating zymogen form and cleavage of its single-chain biosynthetic precursor probably occurs intracellularly before secretion. Conversion of pro-factor D to factor D also takes place intracellularly by cleavage of a single peptide bond, which results in the release of a small activation peptide. Factor B and C2 lack the highly conserved and functionally important N-terminal sequence of SPs. Instead, following activation their SP domains remain attached to a von Willebrand factor type A (VWFA) module. These and additional unique structural properties endow complement SPs with their extremely restricted substrate specificity, which is necessary for their function and reflected in their low reactivity with synthetic substrates and active site inhibitors.

II. FACTOR D

Factor D is the least abundant and smallest complement protein, consisting only of a SP domain. The location and structure of the factor D gene have not been reported. The enzyme catalyzes the cleavage of C3b-bound factor B leading to the formation of the alternative pathway C3-convertase. It differs from other SPs in blood in that it apparently requires neither enzymatic cleavage for expression of proteolytic activity nor inactivation by a serpin-type inhibitor for its control. Instead, transition of factor D from the catalytically inactive to the active state seems to be effected by fully reversible conformational changes. An initial understanding of the structural correlates of these unusual features has emerged from recent structural and mutational studies (reviewed in ref. 20).

A. Protein Structure and Function

1. Primary and Tertiary Structure

The almost complete primary structure of factor D was initially determined at the protein level (21,22). Subsequently, the complete amino acid sequence was deduced from the nucleotide sequence of cDNA clones (23). The single polypeptide chain of the mature protein consists of 228 amino acid residues with a calculated Mr of 24,376. There are no potential *N*-glycosylation sites and no carbohydrate is present in the purified protein (24). The primary sequence shows 33–35% residue identity with pancreatic bovine trypsin, bovine chymotrypsin A, porcine elastase, and human neutrophil elastase (20). Alignment of the factor D sequence with that of 35 other mammalian SPs (6) demonstrated that the majority of the invariable and conserved residues of the superfamily have been retained in factor D. In addition, four disulfide bridges that are highly conserved among SPs are also present in factor D (15). They form between half-cystine residues 42 and 58 ("histidine loop"), 168 and 182 ("methionine loop"), 191 and 220 ("bridge between primary and secondary substrate binding sites"), and 136 and 201 ("B-C chain bridge") (Fig. 2).

In addition to the mature polypeptide chain, the factor D cDNA encodes a putative leader peptide followed by seven residues, AAPPRGR, that could represent an activation peptide. However, factor D purified from serum or urine lacks an activation peptide, its N-terminal sequence, ILGG-, corresponding to the highly conserved one of active SPs of the chymotrypsin family (25,26). The discrepancy was solved by the demonstration that expression of factor D cDNA in insect cells, by using baculovirus, resulted in secretion of DFP-resistant, proteolytically inactive factor D, consisting of two molecular forms with respective activation peptides AAPPRGR and APPRGR (27). Catalytic amounts of trypsin converted recombinant, pro-factor D to its enzymatically active form, which exhibited the same N-terminus and proteolytic activity as native factor D. No autoactivation of the zymogen was observed and no activation by a serum enzyme could be demonstrated (27).

Figure 2 Schematic representation of the structures of human complement serine proteases. The structure shown for MASP is that of the first species discovered in human (89). The relative positions of the disulfide bridges, carbohydrates, and of the amino acid residues of the catalytic triad are represented on scale. For most structures, the disulfide bridges have been drawn on the basis of homologies with other proteins or protein modules of known structure. The disulfide bridge pattern of factor I cannot be deduced from available information. The two letter module nomenclature is that recommended by Bork and Bairoch. Unlabeled portions represent connecting segments. N represents the Asn residues known to undergo posttranslational hydroxylation in C1r and C1s. (α,γ), fragments generated by limited proteolysis. (♦), potential Asn-linked glycosylation sites. Arrows indicate peptide bonds cleaved on activation.

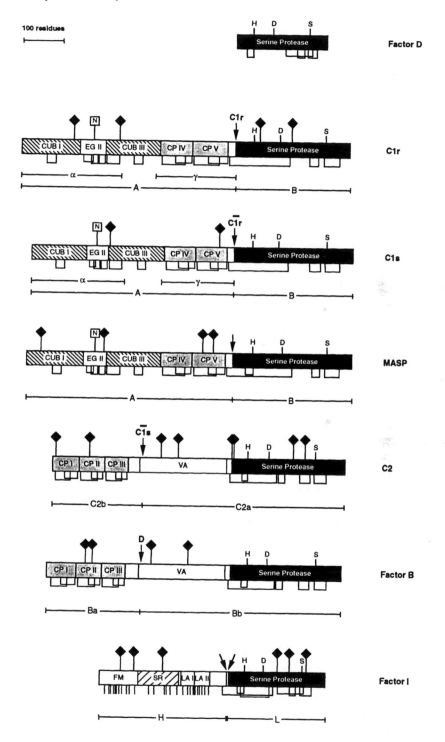

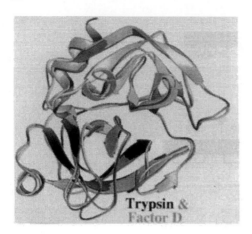

Figure 3 Superposition of the main-chain structures of factor D (gray) and trypsin (black). The models were generated using the ribbons program (Carson M, Bugg CE. J Mol Graph 1986;4:121–122).

Furthermore, expression of the same factor D cDNA in COS or CHO cells resulted in secretion of active enzyme (28). Taken together these data support the proposal (25,26) that the activation peptide of pro-factor D is cleaved off within the secretory pathway of mammalian cells by a trypsin-like maturase or convertase (29), which is not present in insect cells. This is unlike other mammalian SPs and similar to many prohormones and other proproteins (30).

The crystal structure of factor D was solved by using a combination of multiple isomorphous replacement and molecular replacement methods (15). Two molecules, A and B, related by a noncrystallographic twofold axis are present in the triclinic unit cell. They are similar to each other, but display distinct orientations of the side chains of residues in their active centers. As expected from the conserved SP primary structure, both molecules of factor D have the characteristic chymotrypsin structural fold (Fig. 3). The only major differences in backbone structure occur in surface loops connecting secondary structural elements. Despite its typical SP three-dimensional structure, factor D displays unique conformations of key catalytic and substrate-binding residues. These atypical structural elements include residues of the catalytic triad, the substrate specificity pocket, and the nonspecific substrate-binding site of factor D.

Available crystal structures of several SPs have demonstrated that in the chymotrypsin family the geometric relations of the side chains of the three residues of the catalytic triad, Asp^{102}, His^{57}, and Ser^{195} are invariable and crucial for catalysis (7). Nevertheless, in factor D the canonical orientation of the side chains of the catalytic triad residues has not been conserved (Fig. 4). In molecule A, the carboxyl of Asp^{102} is pointed away from His^{57} and is freely accessible to the solvent, while the geometry of the His^{57}-Ser^{195} dyad is identical to that of trypsin. In molecule B, the imidazole of His^{57} is oriented away from Ser^{195}, having assumed the energetically favored *trans* conformation. The space filled in trypsin by the side chain of His^{57} is occupied in molecule B by Ser^{215}. In molecule A, Ser^{215} is within the specificity pocket forming an H-bond with Arg^{218}. If we assume that forms A and B are alternative conformations, residues Thr^{214} and Gly^{216} appear to act as hinges allowing Ser^{215} to swing in and out of the specificity pocket, forcing His^{57} to

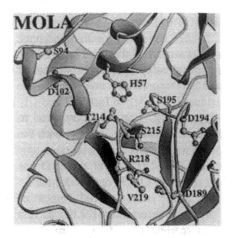

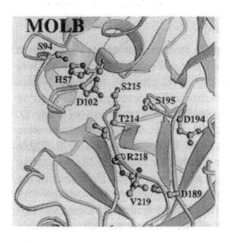

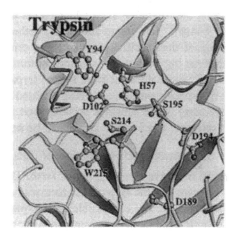

Figure 4 Active centers of molecules A (MOLA) and B (MOLB) of factor D and (C) of trypsin. Models were generated using the ribbons program. The side chains of residues of the catalytic triad and of the primary specificity pocket are shown. Coordinates for bovine trypsin (1ptc) were obtained from the Brookhaven Protein Data Bank.

assume a *cis* or *trans* conformation, respectively. Neither of these two orientations of the catalytic triad residues would allow expression of catalytic activity, indicating the need for a realignment via a conformational change.

Factor D cleaves only the Arg[233]–Lys[234] bond of its natural substrate factor B (Table 1). Therefore, like all complement enzymes it belongs to the trypsin subfamily of chymotrypsin-like SPs, which as a rule have an aspartate at position 189 in the bottom of the specificity pocket. Extensive studies (31–33) have established that the presence of a negative charge at the base of the pocket is essential for catalysis by trypsin. Factor D also has an Asp at position 189 (Figs. 1 and 4), but in both molecules A and B Asp[189] forms a salt bridge with Arg[218]. This salt link probably restricts access of the side chain of the P$_1$ Arg[233] of factor B to the negative charge of Asp[189]. Again, a reorientation seems necessary for optimal substrate binding and catalysis.

Superposition of the specificity pockets of factor D and trypsin (34) reveals that two of the walls formed by residues 189–195 and 225–228 have very similar backbone conformations in the two enzymes. However, the conformation of the third wall of the pocket of factor D, formed by residues 214–220, is considerably different from that of trypsin. Residues 214 and 215 of factor D are Thr and Ser, respectively, compared to the highly conserved Ser and Trp in trypsin (Fig. 1). Residue 218 is Arg in factor D and Gly in trypsin and Val^{219} of factor D is missing from trypsin (Fig. 1 and 4). Compared to trypsin, the loop 214–219 of factor D is substantially raised toward the solvent with the Arg^{218}-Asp^{189} salt bridge acting as a tether. This positioning results in considerable narrowing of the specificity pocket. The orientation of the 214–219 loop of factor D has additional implications for substrate binding, because it results in a backbone conformation of Gly^{216} quite different from that of trypsin. As noted, Gly^{216} is an essential element of the nonspecific substrate-binding site and a crucial structural determinant for the correct positioning of the substrate scissile bond. Thus, again a reorientation of key elements of the substrate binding site appears to be necessary for efficient catalysis by factor D.

2. Expression and Regulation of Catalytic Activity

Results of active site mapping of factor D with peptide thioester substrates (35) support the concept that the atypical conformation of key catalytic and substrate-binding residues of factor D are not compatible with expression of high-level catalytic activity. A series of peptide thioesters, containing an Arg at the P$_1$ position and various groups and amino acids at P$_2$, P$_3$, and P$_4$, were used to investigate the specificity and reactivity of factor D. Of 12 dipeptides tested only three containing Arg, Val, or Lys in the P$_2$ position were hydrolyzed at measurable rates. Lys is also present at the P$_2$ position of factor B (Table 1). More recently Z-Lys-SBzl was also shown to be cleaved by factor D (28), indicating that, like trypsin, the P$_1$ site is reactive with both Arg and Lys residues. Extension of the peptide thioesters to include Gln at the P$_3$ and P$_4$ positions, which are also occupied by Gln in factor B, resulted in complete loss of reactivity. Thus, neither Bz-Gln–Lys-Arg-SBzl nor Bz-Gln-Gln-Lys-Arg-SBzl was hydrolyzed at measurable rates. Also, tripeptide thioesters containing four other amino acids at P$_3$ (Gly, Glu, Lys, Phe) did not react with factor D. In addition to this high degree of specificity, factor D exhibited an extremely low reactivity with peptide thioesters. Compared to C1s (37), its functional homologue in the classical pathway, the reactivity (k_{cat}/K_m) of factor D was two to three orders of magnitude lower. Compared to trypsin, factor D was as much as 3×10^3 less efficient in hydrolyzing thioesters. The reactivity of factor D with isocoumarins substituted with basic groups was similarly low (38). These compounds are very effective inhibitors of trypsin-like enzymes (39). Their mechanism of action involves the initial formation of an acyl enzyme. By comparison to C1s, the inhibitory rates of factor D by its best inhibitor were three orders of magnitude lower. The inhibitory rates obtained with the best inhibitors of trypsin and coagulation SPs (39) were five orders of magnitude higher than those measured for factor D.

The low reactivity of factor D with synthetic substrates and active site inhibitors is consistent with the atypical three-dimensional structure of its active center and supports the notion of an inactive conformation of resting-state factor D. Mutational analyses have identified structural determinants responsible for the unique conformation of the active center and the low esterolytic activity of factor D. Replacement of three residues, Ser^{94}, Thr^{214}, and Ser^{215} with Tyr, Ser, and Trp, respectively, which are found in the corresponding positions of trypsin, resulted in a mutant enzyme with about 20-fold higher k_{cat}/K_m for hydrolysis of Z-Lys-SBzl (40). The increased reactivity could be accounted for by an increase in k_{cat} and could be directly attributed to a reorientation of the side chains of the catalytic triad residues, as demonstrated by the high-resolution crystal structure of the S94Y/T214S/S215W factor D.

Mutational replacement of all residues lining the specificity pocket of factor D with those present in trypsin did not result in increased esterolytic activity (28,34). This suggested that structural elements outside the pocket are important determinants of substrate specificity and reactivity. A similar conclusion had been arrived at previously in studies on the substrate specificity of chymotrypsin (31). It was subsequently shown that in addition to the binding pocket residues, surface loops connecting the walls of the pocket have a major effect on substrate specificity, although they do not directly come in contact with the substrate (17,18). Substituting one of these loops of factor D with the corresponding one of trypsin had no major effect on esterolytic activity. However, combining this mutation with the specificity pocket mutations resulted in markedly increase reactivity with k_{cat}/K_m of two orders of magnitude higher than wild-type factor D (34).

In conclusion, the mutational studies identified structural elements responsible for the unique active center conformation and low reactivity with synthetic substrates of resting-state factor D. They include unique residues lining the specificity pocket (Lys[192], Thr[214], Ser[215], Arg[218], and Val[219]), residues forming the surface loop 184–188 (Glu[184], Ser[185], Asn[186], Arg[187], Arg[188]), and Ser[94]. Results of esterolytic assays indicate that these residues act synergistically.

In sharp contrast to its low esterolytic activity, the proteolytic activity of factor D during activation of the alternative pathway is comparable to that of other complement enzymes. Factor D is the limiting enzyme in the activation sequence of the alternative pathway (25), but this is due to its low concentration in blood, which is maintained by a very fast (60% per hour) catabolic rate (41,42). At 9–10 times physiological serum concentrations the enzyme becomes nonlimiting (25). The pronounced difference between the rates of hydrolysis of small synthetic esters and C3b-bound factor B can be explained adequately by the proposal (20) that the C3bB complex induces the conformational changes necessary for the realignment of the atypical active center residues of factor D. These changes probably are, at least in part, similar to those induced by the mutations discussed above. Native factor B and small peptide esters cannot induce these conformational changes probably because they cannot form crucial contacts with the enzyme. A corollary to this hypothesis is that, following cleavage of C3b-bound factor B, the active center of factor D reverts to its resting-state inactive conformation. This mechanism and the inability of factor D to cleave uncomplexed factor B provide for the regulation of its proteolytic activity. Thus, the need for a circulating profactor D and an activating enzyme and also for a serpin-type inhibitor are obviated.

III. C1r AND C1s

A. Gene Organization

The genes encoding human C1r and C1s have been assigned to chromosome 12, and further located by *in situ* hybridization analysis on the short arm of the chromosome, in region p13 (43). The C1r and C1s genes are arranged in a tail-to-tail orientation, and lie in close proximity, with a distance between their 3' ends of about 9.5 kb (44). This unusual disposition raises the possibility of the occurrence in this short intergenic region of regulatory elements shared by both genes, providing a plausible explanation for the observation that almost all hereditary deficiencies of C1r and C1s reported so far are of the combined type (45). The exon–intron structure of the human C1s gene has been mapped by electron microscopy of genomic DNA-cDNA hybrids, indicating that the protein is encoded by 12 exons (46). Sequence analysis reveals that, at variance with other SPs (47), the entire SP domain of C1s, including a short N-terminal segment encompassing the proteolytic activation site by C1r, is encoded by a single uninterrupted exon. This unusual feature is also shared by C1r (48) and by haptoglobin, a member of the SP family that lacks proteolytic activity (46). Other striking similarities between C1r, C1s, and haptoglobin, both at the gene and protein level, support the notion that these three proteins define a specific branch in the evolution of the SP family.

B. Protein Structure and Function

1. Modular Structure of C1r and C1s

The complete primary structures of human C1r (49–52) and C1s (53–56) have been elucidated from either protein or DNA sequencing. The two proteins are very similar with respect to overall structural organization. Proenzyme C1r and C1s are single-chain glycoproteins containing 688 and 673 amino acids, respectively, and each is split upon activation, through cleavage of a single Arg-Ile bond, into two polypeptide chains A and B linked by a single disulfide bridge (Table 1, Fig. 2). Twelve additional disulfide bridges are present in C1r and C1s (10 in each A chain and 2 in each B chain). The complete disulfide bridge pattern of C1s has been determined (57) but only some of the bonds have been formally identified in C1r (58).

The N-terminal A chains (446 and 422 amino acids in C1r and C1s, respectively) share the same type of modular structure, each comprising five modules, including two pairs of internal repeats (I/III and IV/V), and a single copy of module II (Fig. 2). The N-terminal and central modules I and III belong to the CUB type, initially recognized in C1r/C1s, the sea urchin protein Uegf, and the human bone morphogenetic protein-1 (59), and subsequently identified in an increasing number of other extracellular proteins, mostly known to be involved in developmental processes. Four cysteine residues forming two disulfide bridges (Cys1–Cys2; Cys3–Cys4) are conserved in all CUB modules, except for the N-terminal modules I of C1r and C1s, which only contain the Cys3–Cys4 disulfide bond. Although no three-dimensional structure of a CUB module has been reported yet, secondary structure predictions suggest that this approximately 110 amino acid residue domain has an antiparallel β-barrel fold comparable to that observed in the immunoglobulin-like module (59).

Modules II contain approximately 50 amino acids and belong to the family of epidermal growth factor (EGF)-like modules, which are often found in multiple copies and in association with different other modules, within extracellular or membrane-bound proteins usually involved in blood coagulation, fibrinolysis, neural development, and cell adhesion (60). In addition to six conserved cysteine residues forming three disulfide bonds (Cys1-Cys3; Cys2-Cys4; Cys5-Cys6), the EGF modules of C1r and C1s contain the consensus pattern Asp/Asn, Asp/Asn, Gln/Glu, Asp*/Asn*, Tyr/Phe (where * indicates a β-hydroxylated residue) characteristic of a subset of EGF-like modules shown to participate in calcium binding. Similar EGF-like modules have been identified in various vitamin K-dependent plasma proteins and in fibrillin (61). The EGF module of C1r contains, at position 150, an *erythro*-β-hydroxyasparagine (62), whereas the corresponding asparagine residue of C1s (position 134) is only partially (about 50%) hydroxylated (63). Indeed, this posttranslational modification is probably not directly involved in calcium binding, since recombinant C1s expressed in the baculovirus/insect cells system shows no detectable β-hydroxylation, but nevertheless retains its calcium-dependent interaction properties (64). An unusual feature of the EGF module of C1r compared to other known EGF modules, including that of C1s, is the large size of the loop between Cys1 and Cys3. This loop also contains the single polymorphic site (Ser/Leu) identified in C1r from both protein (52) and cDNA sequence analyses (50,51), providing a molecular basis for the occurrence of two common alleles at the C1r locus (65). A number of high-resolution structures of EGF modules have been determined, indicating that the main structural feature is the presence of two antiparallel two-stranded β-sheets (60). Preliminary analyses by nuclear magnetic resonance (NMR) spectroscopy of the EGF module of C1r produced by chemical synthesis indicate that it is folded in a comparable manner, but the large loop between Cys1 and Cys3 appears to be disordered (66).

Modules IV and V of C1r and C1s are tandem repeats of 60–70 amino acids that belong to the complement control protein (CCP) module type found, always in multiple copies, in several complement proteins as well as in proteins unrelated to the complement system (67). Like all other CCP modules, those in C1r and C1s contain four conserved cysteine residues forming two disulfide bridges (Cys1-Cys3; Cys2-Cys4), and exhibit a consensus sequence restricted to a few hydrophobic and neutral residues.

There is more sequence similarity between corresponding modules (IV or V) of C1r and C1s than between modules IV and V of either protein. The solution structures of three different CCP modules from human factor H have now been determined by NMR spectroscopy, indicating that they fold autonomously and share a common overall topology, consisting of a compact hydrophobic core wrapped in five β-strands, with the N- and C-termini located at opposite poles of the long axis of the molecule (68,69). Three-dimensional homology models of the CCP modules IV and V of C1r and C1s have been built on the basis of the structural coordinates of the factor H modules. Each module shows a typical five-β-stranded globular structure, with some modifications, mostly located in the C-terminal region of the modules and occurring at the surface (70,71). In both C1r and C1s, CCP module V is followed by a 15-residue intermediary segment homologous to the activation peptide of chymotrypsinogen, which in the proenzymes connects module V to the SP domain. Activation occurs through cleavage of the Arg-Ile bond between this segment and the SP, which remain covalently linked to each other by a disulfide bridge.

The C-terminal B chains (242 and 251 amino acids in C1r and C1s, respectively) are SP domains that belong to the chymotrypsin-like family. The three residues of the catalytic triad (His[57], Asp[102], and Ser[195] in chymotrypsinogen) are surrounded by conserved sequences, although with some exceptions (e. g., Pro[198] is substituted by Val and Ala in C1r and C1s, respectively; see Fig. 1). Both C1r and C1s have an Asp residue at the S_1 subsite, indicative of trypsin-like specificity, consistent with the fact that both proteases cleave arginyl bonds in their natural protein substrates (72). Thus, autoactivation of proenzyme C1r and subsequent activation of C1s by activated C1r both involve cleavage of Arg-Ile bonds. Also, active C1s cleaves a single Arg-Ala bond in C4, and a single Arg-Lys bond in C2 (Table 1). With respect to esterolytic activity, activated C1r cleaves with low catalytic efficiency a restricted number of synthetic ester substrates containing a P_1 Arg or Lys residue. In contrast, C1s is an efficient esterase and cleaves a wider range of substrates containing an Arg, Lys (37), or, unexpectedly, a Tyr residue at the P_1 position, suggesting that, in addition to the anionic S_1 subsite, its specificity pocket may involve a hydrophobic component (72). C1r and C1s contain two disulfide bridges conserved in other chymotrypsin-like SPs: the "methionine loop" and the disulfide bridge connecting the primary and secondary substrate binding sites. In contrast, both proteases lack the "histidine loop" disulfide bridge present in all other known mammalian SPs.

A three-dimensional model of the SP domain of C1s has been constructed using chymotrypsin as a template (70). Although the two proteases only exhibit 33% sequence identity, as much as 74% of their residues appear to be structurally conserved (i. e., superposable within a limit of 1.5 Å). Compared to chymotrypsin, the core of the C1s protease domain, including the catalytic triad, is highly conserved, whereas major differences occur at the surface. These include two insertions of seven and eight residues, forming extended loops at the entrance of the active site cleft (Fig. 5), three deletions also occurring within the same area, and a five-residue extension at the C-terminal α-helical end of the protease. Homology modeling of the SP domain of C1r (71) indicates that major modifications also occur in the vicinity of the active site cleft, suggesting that in both proteases these may be involved in substrate recognition. With respect to the activation of C1r and C1s, it should be emphasized that both three-dimensional models

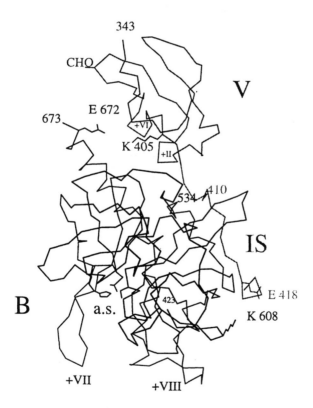

Figure 5   Three-dimensional Cα model of the C-terminal catalytic region of human C1s. V, CCP module V; IS, intermediary segment; B, serine protease domain. The side chains of the amino acids involved in ionic bonds (E672-K405, E418-K608), and of the active site amino acids, as well as the α carbons of Cys410 and Cys534 connecting the intermediary segment and the serine protease, are shown. The two extended loops at the entrance of the active site cleft are denoted +VII and +VIII. CHO, N-linked oligosaccharide. a.s., active site (from ref. 70).

are consistent with a mechanism involving formation of a salt bridge between the α-amino group of the N-terminal Ile of the SP domain and the carboxyl group of Asp[194], as this occurs in chymotrypsin.

The SP domain of C1s is not glycosylated, whereas that of C1r has two *N*-linked oligosaccharides, located in the regions following the His residue of the catalytic triad, and the Cys residue involved in the disulfide bridge connecting the SP to the A chain (Fig. 2). The N-terminal A chains of both proteases contain two *N*-linked oligosaccharides each, located in modules CUB I and III of C1r, and in modules CUB III and CCP V of C1s (Fig. 2). All of these oligosaccharides belong to the complex type, as judged from their contents in N-acetylglucosamine, mannose, galactose, and sialic acid. Detailed analysis performed on C1s has shown that the oligosaccharide linked to module III is biantennary and bisialylated, whereas that on module V is biantennary bisialylated, or triantennary trisialylated, or fucosylated triantennary trisialylated, in relative proportions 1:1:1 (73).

2. Protein–Protein Interactions

A fundamental feature of C1r and C1s is that during classical pathway activation they do not act as isolated proteases, but exert their catalytic activities within a calcium-dependent tetramer C1s-C1r-C1r-C1s, which binds to the nonenzymatic protein C1q to form the C1 complex (58). Both proteases are therefore involved in various protein–protein interactions, both within the C1s-C1r-C1r-C1s tetramer, and between the tetramer and C1q. It is well established that the structural determinants responsible for the calcium-dependent C1r-C1s interactions involved in the assembly of the C1s-C1r-C1r-C1s tetramer are located in the N-terminal regions of the A chain of each protein (74). Both regions exhibit characteristic low-temperature transitions (midpoints 32–37°C) that are abolished, or shifted to higher temperatures in the presence of calcium ions (75,76). With the use of limited proteolysis with trypsin under controlled conditions, fragments of about 200 amino acid residues corresponding to these regions of C1r and C1s have been obtained (77). These fragments (C1rα, C1sα) each comprise modules CUB I, EGF II, and the N-terminal disulfide loop of CUB III (Fig. 2). Each fragment contains one high-affinity calcium binding site, with Kds of 32–38 μM, comparable to those determined for the intact proteins. They also retain the ability to mediate calcium-dependent protein-protein interactions, as shown by the formation of C1rα-C1sα heterodimers, which bind 2 calcium atoms/mol, consistent with the fact that the C1s-C1r-C1r-C1s tetramer binds four calcium atoms/mol. Various studies performed on C1s (63,78) suggest that the structural determinants required for calcium binding and the calcium-dependent C1r-C1s interaction are contributed to by both the N-terminal CUB module I and the EGF module II. Strong support for this view is provided by the observation that the isolated EGF module of C1r produced by chemical synthesis binds calcium with an affinity about 300 times lower than that measured for fragment C1rα (66). Also, deletion of CUB module I from C1r impairs its calcium-dependent interaction properties (79). These data and current knowledge on other calcium-binding proteins involving EGF modules (61) are consistent with the hypothesis that the EGF modules of C1r and C1s, like all other known EGF modules of the same type, contribute most but not all of the necessary calcium ligands, with the N-terminal CUB modules providing one or more ligands to complete the coordination sphere of calcium. This would result in the formation of a calcium-dependent CUB-EGF association that probably constitutes the domain responsible for the C1r-C1s interactions within the C1s-C1r-C1r-C1s tetramer.

With respect to the assembly of the C1 complex, binding of C1s-C1r-C1r-C1s to C1q appears to be a complex process involving multiple sites contributed to by both C1r and C1s. Thus, proenzyme C1r alone binds weakly to C1q in the presence of calcium (80,81), and interaction between C1s-C1r-C1r-C1s and C1q is abolished by chemical modification of acidic amino acids of C1r (82). However, the C1r/C1q interaction is strengthened by fragment C1sα, as shown by the ability of the calcium-dependent C1sα-C1r-C1r-C1sα tetramer to form a stable and functional pseudo-C1 complex (81,83). Based on these and other available data, a likely hypothesis is that assembly of the C1 complex involves primarily a binding site in the calcium-binding α region of C1r, and that interaction with the corresponding C1sα region induces a conformational change that enhances its affinity for C1q (81). Although the structural determinants responsible for these interactions remain to be identified, it is very likely that the calcium-binding regions of C1r and C1s, particularly their N-terminal CUB-EGF modules, play a major role in the interaction between C1s-C1r-C1r-C1s and C1q, and therefore represent key elements of the architecture of macromolecular C1.

3. Catalytic Activities

Early experiments based on limited proteolytic cleavage of C1r and C1s allowed identification in each protease of regions responsible for catalytic activity (74). The corresponding fragments (γ-B), derived from the C-terminal part of each protease, originate from cleavage of peptide bonds located within a short sequence stretch at the C-terminal end of the CUB module III, and comprise CCP modules IV and V, the 15-residue intermediary segment, and the SP domain (Fig. 2). The γ-B fragment obtained by limited proteolysis of activated C1s with plasmin is monomeric and forms the outer portions of the C1s-C1r-C1r-C1s tetramer (74,84). Studies by differential scanning calorimetry are consistent with the presence in C1s γ-B of three independently folded domains, corresponding to CCP modules IV and V, and the SP domain (85). From a functional point of view, the C1s γ-B fragment fully retains the catalytic properties of native activated C1s, as shown by its ability to cleave both synthetic esters and the protein substrates C4 and C2.

In the case of C1r, autolytic cleavage of the active protease, as well as limited proteolysis by various extrinsic proteases of different specificities yield noncovalent (γ-B)₂ homodimers, which form the core of the C1r-C1r dimer and of the C1s-C1r-C1r-C1s tetramer (86). Again, as observed for C1s, the activated C1r (γ-B)₂ fragment retains the enzymic properties of intact C1r, as shown by its ability to cleave and activate proenzyme C1s. The proenzyme form of these (γ-B)₂ regions has also been obtained by limited proteolysis, and exhibits the same autoactivation properties as native C1r, including similar activation kinetics and identical inhibition patterns (i. e., inhibition by 4-nitrophenyl-4'-guanidinobenzoate and insensitivity to diisopropylfluorophosphate) (87). However, in contrast to C1r, activation of the (γ-B)₂ regions is totally insensitive to calcium ions, indicating that they contain the structural elements necessary for intramolecular activation, but probably lack a regulatory element associated with the N-terminal calcium-binding region of C1r. The latter hypothesis is consistent with the finding that deletion of the EGF module from C1r decreases the stability of the zymogen (79).

Recent studies based on the combined use of chemical cross-linking and homology modeling have provided insights into the structure of the catalytic regions of C1r and C1s (70,71). Three-dimensional models of the C-terminal part of these regions, comprising CCP module V, the intermediary segment, and the SP domain, have been constructed and indicate that, in both proteases, module V interacts with the SP on the side opposite to both the active site and the Arg-Ile bond cleaved on activation (Fig. 5). With respect to C1s, a likely role for module V could be a contribution to the correct positioning of protein substrates with respect to the active center, as indicated by previous data on the presence of a C4-binding site within the γ region of C1s (88). In both C1r and C1s, chemical cross-linking yielded no information with respect to the relative positioning of CCP modules IV and V, which is consistent with the NMR solution structure of a pair of CCP modules from factor H (69), showing that there exists a wide range of angles of twist of one module with respect to the other. If this feature applies to C1r and C1s, the module V/SP domain unit may be expected to rotate about the long axis of module V with respect to module IV. Such a rotation may be a key element of the activation mechanism of C1. It may allow the SP domain to C1r to switch from a "proenzyme" position allowing cleavage of one C1r monomer by the other to an "active" position allowing cleavage of C1s by activated C1r. Once activated, the SP domain of C1s may likewise be expected to move outside the C1 complex, thereby gaining access to its substrates C4 and C2 (70). With respect to the catalytic regions of C1r, cross-linking studies performed on the $(\gamma$-B$)_2$ fragment produced by autolytic cleavage of the active protease also provide evidence for mutual intermonomer interactions between the region preceding module IV of one monomer, and the SP domain of the other monomer (71,86). Based on this information, a three-dimensional model of the activated $(\gamma$-B$)_2$ dimer has recently been built, indicating that the monomers interact in a "head-to-tail" configuration, with their active sites facing opposite directions towards the outside of the dimer. This configuration likely corresponds to the active state of the dimer, since it allows access of the C1r active sites to the Arg-Ile activation sites in the C1s γ-B regions, proposed to interact with opposite sides of the C1r $(\gamma$-B$)_2$ dimer (58,84). In contrast, the proenzyme configuration of the dimer is expected to allow the activation site of each monomer to fit into the prosite of the other monomer, which implies that a dramatic conformational change must take place between the proenzyme and active states.

IV. MANNOSE-BINDING LECTIN-ASSOCIATED SERINE PROTEASE

A. Gene Organization

The gene encoding human MBL-associated serine protease (MASP) has been mapped by fluorescence *in situ* hybridization to the q27–q28 region of the long arm of chromosome 3 (89,90). This location is clearly different from those of the C1r and C1s genes. The exon–intron structure of the MASP gene has also been partially determined (48), indicating that, in contrast to C1r and C1s, the SP domain is encoded by at least six exons. Based on this information and other differences seen at the gene and protein level, it has been proposed that MASP belongs to a branch of the phylogenetic tree of human SPs that is distinct, and possibly more ancient, than that defined by C1r, C1s, and haptoglobin (48).

B. Protein Structure and Function

The primary structure of MASP (originally called P100) has been deduced from DNA sequencing in both human (89,91) and mouse (92,93). The proteins from the two species, each containing 680 amino acids, share more than 87% sequence identity and show no insertions or deletions with respect to each other. As in C1r and C1s, activation occurs through cleavage of a single Arg-Ile bond that splits the protein into two disulfide linked polypeptide chains of 429 and 251 amino acids. Also, both human and mouse MASPs exhibit the same type of modular structure as C1r and C1s (Fig. 2). Thus, the N-terminal chain of MASP contains the five modules and the short intermediary segment described in C1r and C1s and, in view of the location of the cysteine residues, very likely exhibits the same disulfide bridge pattern. The EGF-like module of MASP also contains the consensus pattern that characterizes calcium-binding EGF modules, including the Asn residue that undergoes β-hydroxylation in C1r and C1s. A particular feature of the N-terminal chain is the occurrence of four potential N-glycosylation sites, located at identical positions in both human and mouse MASPs, in the N-terminal CUB module, the EGF module, and the CCP module V. The presence of an N-linked oligosaccharide in the EGF module is unusual, since only O-linked oligosaccharides have been described in this type of module (60). The C-terminal SP domain of MASP belongs to the chymotrypsin-like family and, based on the presence of an Asp residue at position 189, is expected to have a trypsin-like specificity. Unlike C1r and C1s, MASP has conserved Pro[198] and the two cysteine residues forming the "histidine loop" disulfide bridge (Fig. 1). Sequence comparison of the whole proteins shows that human MASP exhibits 36% and 37% homology with human C1r and C1s, respectively, indicating no preferential relationship with either protein.

Although it was initially reported that MBL can bind and activate the proenzyme C1s-C1r-C1r-C1s tetramer (94), it seems now established that MBL is preferentially, if not exclusively, associated in serum with a SP component that includes MASP (95). The resulting MBL–MASP complex (also known as Ra-reactive factor) mediates the assembly of the C4b2a, C3-convertase of the classical pathway upon binding to mannose and N-acetylglucosamine residues on certain microorganisms, thereby providing an activation mechanism (the "lectin pathway") distinct from that mediated by C1. The single MASP species originally found associated with MBL in human serum can be dissociated from MBL in the presence of EDTA and exhibits C1s-like proteolytic activity, as shown by its ability to cleave C4 and C2 (95). Further studies have provided evidence that, in contrast with C1s, human MASP also cleaves C3 (96), a property that is shared by murine MASP (97). Based on the above findings, it was assumed until recently that, in contrast to C1q, MBL is associated with a single MASP species that would exhibit both the C1r autoactivating ability and the C1s proteolytic activity (95). This scheme should be reconsidered in light of the recent identification in human serum of another MBL-associated SP termed MASP-2, showing the same modular structure as C1r, C1s, and the originally discovered MASP (98). It has been postulated that MASP-2 is a further component of the MBL-MASP complex, which may have a C1-like composition (Chapter 3). Obviously, further studies will be necessary to get a clear picture of the assembly and activation of this newly discovered complex protease that may play an important role in innate immunity.

V. FACTOR B AND C2

Factor B and C2 provide the catalytic subunits of the C3 and C5 convertases in the alternative and classical pathway, respectively. They are structurally and functionally similar single-chain glycoproteins, that probably represent gene duplication products.

A. Gene Organization

The single genes encoding human factor B (*Bf*) and C2 are located in the class III region of the major histocompatibility complex on chromosome 6 (99). The 5' end of the *C2* gene lies approximately 600 kb centromeric of the 5' end of the HLA-B gene (100,101). *Bf* lies centromeric to the *C2* gene and has the same transcriptional orientation. The cap site of *Bf* is located only 421 bp downstream of the poly(A) signal of *C2* (102). This proximity is compensated for by the presence of a termination sequence or polymerase II "pause" site, which contains a GGGGGA direct repeat and is located 44 bp downstream of the C2 poly(A) site (103). The nuclear factor MAZ binds to this site contributing to termination from the *C2* gene and ensuring unimpeded initiation from the *Bf* promoter (104).

The *C2* and *Bf* genes contain 18 exons each and have very similar exon/intron organizations (105,106). The main difference between the two genes is their size, being 18 kb for *C2* and 6 kb for *Bf*. The large size of some introns of the *C2* gene accounts for this difference. The largest intron of *C2* follows exon 3 and contains a human-specific (107) SINE-type retroposon, derived from the human endogenous retrovirus HERV-K10 (108). The *C2* retroposon, termed SINE-R.C2, is associated with a variable number of tandem repeats (VNTR) locus, which gives rise to a multiallelic RFLP of the *C2* gene (109). Several dimorphic RFLPs have also been described for the *C2* gene, while *Bf* is considerably less polymorphic (110).

B. Protein Structure and Function

1. Modular Structure of Factor B and C2

The complete primary structures of factor B (111,112) and C2 (113,114) have been determined from protein and/or cDNA sequencing. Factor B consists of 739 residues with a calculated M_r of 83,000 and C2 of 732 residues with M_r of 81,000. The two polypeptides exhibit 39% amino acid residue identity. Factor B contains four sites for potential *N*-linked glycosylation, while C2 contains eight sites (Fig. 2) The carbohydrate content of the two proteins, 8.6 and 15.9% for factor B and C2, respectively, indicates that all sites are occupied by oligosaccharides (24). The difference in glycosylation probably accounts for the difference in molecular mass between the two mature proteins (factor B, 90 kDa; C2, 102 kDa).

Factor B and C2 have similar modular structures, consisting of, from the N-terminus, three CCP modules, short connecting segments, single VWFA modules, short connecting segments, and SP domains (Fig. 2). Transmission electron micrographs of factor B and C2 have shown three-lobed structures for both proteins (115,116). In the assembled C3-convertases, Bb and C2a were visualized as two-lobed structures bound to C3b and C4b, respectively, through a single lobe (115). Apparently, the third lobe of each intact protein corresponds to the N-terminal fragment, Ba and C2b, which is cleaved off by the action of factor D and C1s, respectively. In addition to the three CCP modules and the connecting segment of their parent proteins, Ba and C2b also contain the seven N-terminal residues of the VWFA module.

The three CCP modules of factor B and C2 extend from the N-terminus to residue 195 and 186, respectively. They are encoded by single exons and consist of 58–74 residues each. They have maintained the conserved residues of the CCP modules superfamily and should be expected to have the typical β-sheet sandwich structure (68,69) discussed above for C1s and C1r. The CCP/VWFA connecting segments contain 32 residues in factor B and 30 in C2. They are encoded by exons 5, which in addition encode the 2–3 N-terminal residues of the VWFA modules. It is of interest that the S189F mutation within the connecting region of C2 causes type II C2 deficiency, characterized by a block in C2 secretion (117). It is of further interest that another mutation, G444R, which also causes type II C2 deficiency, is within the VWFA/SP connecting segment (117). It thus appears that the two connecting segments of C2 play a role in the overall folding and/or conformation of the polypeptide.

The VWFA modules of C2 and factor B extend between residues 217 and 432 and 228 and 443, respectively. They are encoded by exons 6–10 of their respective genes. They are structurally similar to modules present in three copies in von Willebrand factor and in 1–12 copies in a wide range of proteins. WVFA modules consist of about 200 residues and are present in collagen types VI, VII, XII, and XIV, cartilage matrix protein, and other extracellular matrix proteins, as well as in the α subunits of certain heterodimeric integrins, including LFA-1 (CD11a/CD18), CR3 (CD11b/CD18), CR4 (CD11c/CD18), VLA1, and VLA2 (118,119). All of these proteins are involved in cell–cell, cell–matrix, or matrix–matrix interactions and their VWFA modules are believed to mediate ligand binding. Single free Cys residues and two N-linked potential glycosylation sites are present in the VWFA modules of factor B and C2, although at different positions (Fig. 2).

Recently the high-resolution crystal structures of the VWFA modules of the α chains of CR3 (CD11b; 120) and LFA-1 (CD11a; 121) were reported. The two structures are essentially identical and conform to the classical α/β open sheet or "Rossmann" fold. Both consist of a β-sheet core formed by five parallel and one short antiparallel β strands. This central sheet is surrounded on both faces by seven amphipathic α-helices. Single Mg^{2+} or Mn^{2+} binding sites were located in CR3 and LFA-1, respectively on the surface of the module at the top of the β sheet. Residues whose side chains coordinate the divalent cation either directly or through H-bonds to coordinating water molecules are completely conserved in all cation-binding VWFA modules. They have been called the MIDAS (metal ion-dependent adhesion site) motif. The motif consists of a Asp–Xxx–Ser–Xxx–Ser sequence, where Xxx can be any amino acid, and Thr and Asp residues from other parts of the polypeptide chain (120). The crystal structure reveals that the sixth coordinating site of the cation is "available," suggesting a direct role of this site in ligand binding. The MIDAS motif has been maintained in factor B and C2, both of which require Mg^{2+} for ligand binding. The putative Mg^{2+}-coordinating residues of factor B are ASp^{251}, Ser^{253}, Ser^{255}, Thr^{328}, and Asp^{364} and those of C2 Asp^{240}, Ser^{242}, Ser^{244}, Thr^{315}, and Asp^{356}. Homology modeling of the factor B VWFA module, based of the CR3 crystal coordinates indicated that the overall structural folds of the two modules are quite similar (122). A number of differences were noted, but mainly involved the length of surface loops connecting secondary structural elements.

The SP domains of factor B and C2 extend from residues 457 and 447, respectively, to the C-terminus. They are encoded by exons 11–18 of their respective genes. Exons 11 also encode short connecting segments of 13 and 14 residues in factor B and C2, respectively, and exons 18 also encode 3' untranslated segments. The SP domains have conserved the main structural elements of the superfamily, including the catalytic triad and substrate-binding sites residues, except for the already mentioned absence of Asp^{189} of other trypsin-like enzymes (Fig. 1). Alignment of the factor B and C2 sequences with those of nine SPs of known high-resolution crystal structure suggested that they have also maintained the chymotrypsin structural fold (123). However, factor B and C2 exhibit several differences from typical SPs, which probably subserve their highly specialized functions. One of their major unique features is the absence of the highly conserved N-terminal sequence, which is generated during zymogen activation (Fig. 1). In other SPs the positively-charged α-N-terminus folds into the interior of the protein and forms a salt bridge with the negatively charged carboxyl group of Asp^{194}. This molecular movement is accompanied by a rearrangement of the specificity pocket and expression of catalytic activity (124). In factor B and C2, cleavage leading to zymogen activation occurs at a distant site from the SP domain, which remains attached to the VWFA module. Thus, assumption of the active conformation must be achieved through a different mechanism. Additional major differences from canonical SPs include 12–13 residue insertions following residues 146 and 170 (Fig. 1). Comparison to SPs of known crystal structure indicates that both insertions are probably located at the protein surface and therefore they should not disturb the core-β-sheet structure (123).

Comparison to typical SPs indicates that factor B and C2 have maintained three of the highly conserved disulfide bridges. They form between half cystine residues 42 and 58, 168 and 182, and 191 and 220 (Figs. 1, 2).

Two additional disulfide bridges are present. The first between Cys122 and the Cys corresponding to position 3 of chymotrypsinogen apparently forms between the SP domain and the VWFA/SP linking segment. It is homologous to the disulfide linking the A and B chains of C1r, C1s, and MASP and the heavy and light chains of factor I (Fig. 2). The final disulfide bridge between Cys125 and Cys139 appears to be unique to factor B and C2 and probably requires a structural rearrangement of the molecule to be formed (123). The factor B SP domain has no *N*-linked glycosylation sites, whereas that of C2 has 4. Two of them occur at residues 16 and 20 (i. e., in the region forming the N-terminus salt-bridge with Asp^{194} in other SPs, again indicating a different conformation of this region of C2).

2. Topology of Ligand-Binding Sites

Models for the assembly of C3 convertases have proposed that initial binding of factor B or C2 to activator-attached C3b or C4b, respectively, is mediated by two low-affinity sites, one on Ba or C2b and the other on the VWFA modules (116,125–127). Mg^{2+} apparently acts as an allosteric effector of the latter site (128). Cleavage of factor B or C2 by factor D or C1s, respectively, induces a transient conformational change in this site, resulting in increased binding avidity for C3b or C4b, sequestration of Mg^{2+}, and expression of proteolytic activity for C3.

Initial evidence for the presence of a C4b-binding site on C2b was provided by the demonstration of a C4b2b complex (129,130). In addition, it was shown (131) that purified C2b accelerated the dissociation of the C4b2a complex. Further evidence for a C4b-binding site was subsequently provided by the demonstration that anti-C2b mAbs inhibited binding of C2 to C4b (126). Using a panel of C2/factor B chimeras, in which intact or partial CCP modules of factor B were substituted for the corresponding ones of C2, it was shown that the epitope of the inhibitory mAbs is located on the second CCP of C2 (132). Functional analysis of the chimeras indicated that all three CCP modules of C2 contribute to the C4b-binding site. Evidence that Ba contains a C3b-binding site was also provided by the demonstration (116) that an mAb recognizing an epitope on the 2nd CCP (132) inhibited binding of factor B to C3b. In addition, it was shown that Ba could inhibit the formation of the C3bB complex and that it could be cross-linked to C3b in a metal-ion-independent fashion (125). More recently a panel of factor B CCP mutants was used to identify C3b binding sites on Ba (133). Two sites, one on the carboxyl end of the 2nd CCP and the other in the first intercysteine region of the 3rd CCP were shown to contribute to C3b-B binding.

Indirect evidence for the presence of a C4b-binding site on the VWFA module of C2 was initially provided by studies on the oxidation of C2 by I_2, which results in increased binding avidity of C2a for C4b (134). The effect of I_2 was directly attributed to oxidation of the free thiol of Cys^{241} at the N-terminal region of VWFA (135). Site-directed mutagenesis studies of that region of C2 demonstrated that substitution of Leu or Ala for Asp^{240} or Ser^{244}, respectively, resulted in more than 100-fold decrease of C2 activity (136). Asp^{240} and Ser^{244} are two of the five invariable residues of the MIDAS, Mg^{2+} binding motif of C2 (120). Thus, these data directly implicated the putative Mg^{2+}-binding site of C2 in C4b-binding. With respect to the VWFA module of factor B, indirect evidence for the presence of a C3b-binding site was originally provided by the demonstration that the module contains the Mg^{2+}-binding site of factor B (137). It was subsequently shown that mutations of residues of the MIDAS motif led to almost complete loss of factor B activity (133). More recently, a series of chimeras were constructed by substituting surface loops surrounding the putative Mg^{2+}-binding site of the C2 VWFA for the corresponding ones of factor B (122). Functional analysis of the chimeras indicated that the loops connecting β strand A to α helix 1 and β strand D to α helix 5 define regions participating in C3b binding. The results also suggested that the former loop mediates the conformational regulation of the affinity of Bb for C3b.

3. Catalytic Activities

Full expression of the proteolytic activities of factor B and C2 only occurs in the context of the C3/C5 convertase complexes. A k_{cat}/K_m of 3.1×10^5 $s^{-1}M^{-1}$ was measured for cleavage of C3 by fluid-phase C3bBb, while the initiation convertase $C3_{H_2O}Bb$ was slightly less efficient with k_{cat}/K_m of 1.6×10^5 $s^{-1}M^{-1}$ (138). For the classical pathway C3-convertase, C4b2a, a K_m of $1.8 \times 10^{-6}M$ has been measured for C3 cleavage (139). This is in the same range as the K_m of $5.7 \times 10^{-6}M$ measured for C3bBb (138). Uncomplexed Bb retains about 1% of the proteolytic activity of its C3b-complexed counterpart (140). In addition, low level proteolytic activity has also been demonstrated for a 33 kDa fragment, containing the SP domain of factor B (141). Cleavage of C3 by this fragment is Mg^{2+}-independent but is enhanced by the presence of C3b (137).

Factor B and C2, as well as their fragments Bb and C2a, express esterolytic activity (139,142) and their active sites have been mapped with peptide thioester substrates (35). All synthetic substrates reactive with C2 contained the tripeptide sequences Leu-Ala-Arg or Leu-Gly-Arg, which correspond to the cleavage sites of C3 and C5, respectively (Table 1). Tetrapeptide thioesters were better substrates for C2 than either tri- or pentapeptides while dipeptides were not hydrolyzed. C2a was more reactive than C2 and it hydrolyzed the pentapeptide thioester Z-Leu-Gly-Leu-Ala-Arg-SBzl four times better than C2. The best substrate for factor B was the dipeptide Z-Lys-Arg-SBzl. Bb was about an order of magnitude more reactive than factor B and its best substrate was the tetrapeptide Z-Gly-Leu-Ala-Arg-SBzl. Overall, C3-like substrates were considerably more reactive than C5-like substrates. Using their best substrates, the k_{cat}/K_m values of C2, C2a, factor B, and Bb were 8.6×10^3, 1.2×10^4, 1.4×10^3, and 9.2×10^3 s^{-1} M^{-1}, respectively, as compared to 7.8×10^6 $s^{-1}M^{-1}$ measured for the hydrolysis of the most reactive thioester by trypsin.

VI. FACTOR I

Factor I cleaves three peptide bonds on the α' chain of C3b (143,144) and two bonds on the α' chain of C4b (145). Its action is limited to bimolecular complexes of C3b and C4b with the regulatory proteins factor H, C4b-binding protein, MCP, or CR1 (146). By its action factor I blocks the formation of the alternative pathway amplification C3 convertase and of both C5 convertases. It also generates important biological activities from C3b. Factor I shares with factor D the property of having neither a circulating structural zymogen nor an inhibitor in the blood. Thus, like factor D, its proteolytic activity must be regulated by unique mechanism(s).

A. Gene Organization

The gene encoding factor I (*IF*) is located on chromosome 4q25, telomeric of the EGF gene and centromeric of the IL2 gene (147). It contains 13 exons and spans 63 kb of DNA (148). *IF* is unusual in that the first exon is small, 86 bp, and it is followed by a large 36 kb intron. There is a close association between *IF* exons and structural modules of the protein (148).

B. Protein Structure and Function

The primary structure of factor I has been determined from partial amino acid sequences (149,150) and from nucleotide sequences of cDNA clones (151,152). The approximately 2.4 kb mRNA encodes a pre-pro-factor I polypeptide chain of 583 residues, which includes an 18-residue leader peptide. The mature protein in blood is composed of two, disulfide-linked, polypeptide chains, heavy and light, of 50 and 38 kDa, respectively. The light chain consists of an SP domain (Fig. 2). This structure is derived from the 565-residue pro-factor I polypeptide via intracellular proteolytic removal of four basic amino acids, Arg-Arg-Lys-Arg, linking the two chains. Similar intracellular processing, involving the proteolytic excision of basic tetrapeptides by cathepsin-like enzymes also converts pro-C3, pro-C4, and pro-C5 to the corresponding mature secreted proteins (153). In the case of factor I, the intracellular processing of the proprotein generates in the light chain a typical active SP N-terminal sequence (Fig. 1). It therefore corresponds to the cleavage of single peptide bonds that converts typical SP zymogens in blood to active two-polypeptide chain enzymes. Pro-factor I has never been identified in plasma, but it has been detected in biosynthetic studies using hepatoma cell lines and also under cell-free conditions (154). There are six potential *N*-glycosylation sites in mature factor I, three on each chain. On the basis of a carbohydrate content of 27% (154) and an approximate 23 kDa difference between the calculated size of the unglycosylated polypeptide and the one estimated for the mature protein, it would appear that all potential sites are glycosylated.

Like most other SPs in blood, factor I has a modular structure. It is of interest that among complement proteins, only components of the membrane attack complex share modules with factor I. Starting from the N-terminus, the heavy chain of factor I contains a factor I/membrane attack complex proteins C6/7 (FIMAC) module, a scavenger receptor Cys-rich (SRCR) module, and two low-density lipoprotein receptor class A (LDLRA) modules (Fig. 2). The FIMAC module consists of 70 residues, extending between positions 22 and 91 of the heavy chain and is encoded by exon 2. In addition to factor I, this module is only known to occur in C6 and C7. Both proteins have two FIMAC copies at their C-termini (155). The FIMAC module is characterized by a high number of conserved Cys (10), all of which are assumed to be disulfide-bridged (155). Its function is unknown, although it has been suggested that in C6 and C7 it participates in protein–protein interactions (156).

The SRCR module of factor I contains 103 residues starting at position 96 of the heavy chain. It is encoded by exons 3 and 4. This module also occurs in one to four copies in diverse secreted and cell-surface proteins, including the murine and bovine type I macrophage scavenger receptors, the CD5 and CD6 lymphocyte surface antigens, and the sea urchin speract receptor (157,158). SRCR is characterized by six highly conserved, disulfide-linked Cys and a number of other consensus residues, the distribution of which is reminiscent of the consensus sequence of the Ig module. The factor I SRCR module is missing the fifth conserved Cys, but it has a nonconserved Cys residue between Cys 2 and 3. Thus, like other SRCR modules the factor I one probably has three disulfide bridges.

The two LDLRA modules extend between residues 199 and 237, and 238 and 277, and are encoded by exons 5 and 6, respectively. LDLRA modules were first described in the LDL receptor (159) and in C9 (160,161). They are found as groups of modules in LDLR and related surface receptors and in single copies in the complement polypeptides, C6, C7, C8α, C8β, and C9. The module is characterized by six conserved Cys and a cluster of acidic residues, which is particularly conserved in the sequence Asp–Cys–Xxx–Asp-Gly-Ser-Asp-Glu that occurs near the C-terminal end of the module. The conserved negatively charged residues of the LDL receptor are thought to bind to closely spaced positively charged residues of apoprotein E, a high-affinity ligand for the receptor. By using a combination of secondary structure predictions and Fourier transform infrared spectroscopy, it was shown that the LDLRA module of factor I contains mostly turns and loops with a small amount of β-sheet stabilized by the disulfide bridges (162). It was suggested that the clustered acidic residues are located on an exposed surface loop.

The SP domain of factor I spans the entire length of the L chain between residues 322 and 565 of profactor I (159). It is encoded by exons 9–13 of the *IF* gene, which have an organization similar to that of trypsin (148). Factor I has conserved most of the invariable amino acids of SPs, including the residues of the catalytic triad, the Asp[189] residue in the bottom of the specificity pocket, and the conserved residues of the nonspecific substrate-binding site (Fig. 1). Overall, it exhibits the highest sequence similarity with tissue plasminogen activator (41% identical residues) and plasma kallikrein (37%) and among complement SPs with factor D (28%) (152). Alignment of factor I with SP of known crystal structure (123) has indicated that it has probably conserved the chymotrypsin fold. A small insertion and a small deletion occur at the protein surface, but should not be expected to disturb the core β-sheet structure (123). The factor I SP domain has 11 Cys residues, eight of which correspond to conserved disulfides. In addition Cys[122] apparently forms a bridge with Cys[309] of the heavy chain. This disulfide is homologous to bridges linking the A and B chains of C1r, C1s, and MASP (Fig. 2). Another disulfide bridge unique to factor I probably forms between Cys[50] and Cys[117]. Three potential *N*-linked glycosylation sites are present in the SP domain of factor I. They are all expected to be occupied by oligosaccharides (152) and are located in loop regions probably exposed to the solvent (123).

Factor I shares several properties with factor D. No structural zymogen and no inhibitor has been identified in blood for either enzyme. Both enzymes cleave their natural substrates only in the context of bimolecular complexes with cofactor proteins. Factor D is a poor esterase and no reactive substrate was identified for factor I among 50 peptide thioesters examined (38). This is unique among secreted SPs, all of which have been shown to hydrolyze thioester substrates. Finally, compared to other SPs (39), the rates of inhibition of both enzymes by substituted isocoumarins were very low (38). These structural and functional similarities have led to the suggestion that the proteolytic activities of both enzymes are regulated by similar mechanisms. The structural evidence supporting a reversible substrate-induced conformation of factor D, associated with expression of proteolytic activity was reviewed in II.B above. A similar mechanism seems possible for factor I, although no structural evidence exists for an inactive, "resting-state" conformation of its active center. It is, however relevant that diisopropylfluorophosphate, a mechanism-based inhibitor of all SPs, binds to and inactivates factor I only in the presence of C3b (163). This finding provides indirect evidence for a C3b-induced realignment of the catalytic center of factor I.

REFERENCES

1. Stroud RM. A family of protein-cutting proteins. Sci Am 1974; 231:74–88.
2. Smith CL, DeLotto R. Ventralizing signal determined by protease activation in *Drosophila* embryogenesis. Nature 1994; 368:548–551.
3. Birktoft JJ, Blow DM. Structure of crystalline α-chymotrypsin. V. The atomic structure of tosyl-α-chymotrypsin at 2 Å resolution. J Mol Biol 1972; 68:187–240.
4. Fehlhammer H, Bode W, Huber R. Crystal structure of bovine trypsinogen at 1.8 Å resolution. II. Crystallographic refinement, refined crystal structure, and comparison with bovine trypsin. J Mol Biol 1977; 111:414–438.
5. Sawyer L, Shotton DM, Campbell JW, et al. The atomic structure of crystalline porcine pancreatic elastase at 2.5 Å resolution. Comparisons with the structure of α-chymotrypsin. J Mol Biol 1978; 118:137–208.
6. Greer J. Comparative modeling methods: application to the family of the mammalian serine proteases. Proteins Struct Funct Genet 1990; 7:317–334.
7. Perona JJ, Craik CS. Structural basis of substrate specificity in the serine proteases. Protein Sci 1995; 4:337–360.
8. Dixon GH, Go S, Neurath H. Peptides combined with ^{14}C-diisopropyl phosphoryl following degradation of ^{14}C-DIP-trypsin with α-chymotrypsin. Biochim Biophys Acta 1956; 19:193–195.
9. Shaw E, Mares-Guia M, Cohen W. Evidence for an active-center histidine in trypsin through use of a specific reagent, 1-chloro-3-tosylamido-7-amino-2-heptanone, the chloromethyl ketone derived from N$^{\alpha}$-tosyl-L-lysine. Biochemistry 1965; 4:2219–2224.
10. Blow DM, Birktoft JJ, Hartley BS. Role of a buried acid group in the mechanism of action of chymotrypsin. Nature 1969; 221:337–340.
11. Bachovchin WW, Roberts JD. Nitrogen-15 nuclear magnetic resonance spectroscopy. The state of histidine in the catalytic triad of α-lytic protease. Implications for the charge-relay mechanism of peptide-bond cleavage by serine proteases. J Am Chem Soc 1978; 100:8041–8047.
12. Kossiakoff AA, Spencer SA. Direct determination of the protonation states of aspartic acid-102 and histidine-57 in the tetrahedral intermediate of the serine proteases: neutron structure of trypsin. Biochemistry 1981; 20:6462–6474.
13. Warshel A, Naray-Szabo G, Sussman F, Hwang JK. How do serine proteases really work? Biochemistry 1989; 28:3629–3637.
14. Craik CS, Roczniak S, Largman C, Rutter WJ. The catalytic role of the active site aspartic acid in serine proteases. Science 1987; 237:909–913.

15. Narayana SVL, Carson M, El-Kabbani O, et al. Structure of human factor D, a complement system protein at 2.0 Å resolution. J Mol Biol 1994; 235:695–708.

16. Cohen GH, Silverton EW, Davies DR. Refined crystal structure of γ-chymotrypsin at 1.9 Å resolution. Comparison with other pancreatic serine proteases. J Mol Biol 1981; 148:449–479.

17. Hedstrom L, Szilágyi L, Rutter WJ. Converting trypsin to chymotrypsin: the role of surface loops. Science 1992; 255:1249–1253.

18. Hedstrom L, Perona JJ, Rutter WJ. Converting trypsin to chymotrypsin: residue 172 is a substrate specificity determinant. Biochemistry 1994; 33:8757–8763.

19. Perona JJ, Hedstrom L, Rutter WJ, Fletterick RJ. Structural origins of substrate discrimination in trypsin and chymotrypsin. Biochemistry 1995; 34:1489–1499.

20. Volanakis JE, Narayana SVL. Complement factor D, a novel serine protease. Protein Sci 1996; 5:553–564.

21. Johnson DMA, Gagnon J, Reid KBM. Amino acid sequence of human factor D of the complement system. Similarity in sequence between factor D and proteases of non-plasma origin. FEBS Lett 1984; 166:347–351.

22. Niemann MA, Bhown AS, Bennett JC, Volanakis JE. Amino acid sequence of human factor D of the alternative complement pathway. Biochemistry 1984; 23:2482–2486.

23. White RT, Damm D, Hancock N, et al. Human adipsin is identical to complement factor D and is expressed at high levels in adipose tissue. J Biol Chem 1992; 267:9210–9213.

24. Tomana M, Niemann M, Garner C, Volanakis JE. Carbohydrate composition of the second, third, and fifth components and factors B and D of human complement. Mol Immunol 1985; 22:107–111.

25. Lesavre PH, Müller-Eberhard HJ. Mechanism of action of factor D of the alternative complement pathway. J Exp Med 1978; 148:1498–1509.

26. Volanakis JE, Bhown AS, Bennett JC, Mole JE. Partial amino acid sequence of human factor D: Homology with serine proteases. Proc Natl Acad Sci USA 1980; 77:1116–1119.

27. Yamauchi Y, Stevens JW, Macon KJ, Volanakis JE. Recombinant and native zymogen forms of human complement factor D. J Immunol 1994; 152:3645–3653.

28. Kim S, Narayana SVL, Volanakis JE. Mutational analysis of the substrate binding site of human complement factor D. Biochemistry 1994; 33:14393–14399.

29. Vernet T, Tessier DC, Richardson C, et al. Secretion of functional papain precursor from insect cells. Requirement for N-glycosylation of the pro-region. J Biol Chem 1990; 265:16661–16666.

30. Steiner DF, Smeekens SP, Ohagi S, Chan SJ. The new enzymology of precursor processing endoproteases. J Biol Chem 1992; 267:23435–23438.

31. Gráf L, Jancsó A, Szilágyi L, et al. Electrostatic complementarity within the substrate binding pocket of trypsin. Proc Natl Acad Sci USA 1988; 85:4961–4965.

32. Evnin LB, Vásquez JR, Craik CS. Substrate specificity of trypsin investigated by using a genetic selection. Proc Natl Acad Sci USA 1990; 87:6659–6663.

33. Perona JJ, Hedstrom L, Wagner R, Rutter WJ, Craik CS, Fletterick RJ. Exogenous acetate reconstitutes the enzymatic activity of Asp189Ser trypsin. Biochemistry 1994; 33:3252–3259.

34. Kim S, Narayana SVL, Volanakis JE. Catalytic role of a surface loop of the complement serine protease factor D. J Immunol 1995; 154:6073–6079.

35. Kam C-M, McRae BJ, Harper JW, Niemann MA, Volanakis JE, Powers JC. Human complement proteins D, C2, and B. Active site mapping with peptide thioester substrates. J Biol Chem 1987; 262:3444–3451.

36. Schechter I, Berger A. On the size of the active site in proteases. I. Papain. Biochem Biophys Res Commun 1967; 27:157–162.

37. McRae BJ, Lin T-Y, Powers JC. Mapping the substrate binding site of human C$\overline{1}$r and C$\overline{1}$s with peptide thioesters: development of new sensitive substrates. J Biol Chem 1981; 256:12362–12366.

38. Kam C-M, Oglesby TJ, Pangburn MK, Volanakis JE, Powers JC. Substituted isocoumarins as inhibitors of complement serine proteases. J Immunol 1992; 149:163–168.

39. Kam C-M, Fujikawa K, Powers JC. Mechanism-based isocoumarin inhibitors for trypsin and blood coagulation serine proteases: new anticoagulants. Biochemistry 1988; 27:2547–2557.

40. Kim S, Narayana SVL, Volanakis JE. Crystal structure of a complement factor D mutant expressing enhanced catalytic activity. J Biol Chem 1995; 270:24399–24405.

41. Volanakis JE, Barnum SR, Giddens M, Galla JH. Renal filtration and catabolism of complement protein D. N Engl J Med 1985; 312:395–399.

42. Pascual M, Steiger G, Estreicher J, Macon K, Volanakis JE, Schifferli JA. Metabolism of complement factor D in renal failure. Kidney Int 1988; 34:529–536.

43. Van Cong N, Tosi M, Gross MS, et al. Assignment of the complement serine protease genes C1r and C1s to chromosome 12 region 12p13. Hum Gen 1988; 78:363–368.

44. Kusumoto H, Hirosawa S, Salier JP, Hagen FS, Kurachi K. Human genes for complement components C1r and C1s in a close tail-to-tail arrangement. Proc Natl Acad Sci USA 1988; 85:7307–7311.

45. Loos M, Heinz HP. Complement deficiencies 1. The first component: C1q, C1r, C1s. Prog Allergy 1986; 39:212–231.

46. Tosi M, Duponchel C, Meo T. Complement genes C1r and C1s feature an intronless serine protease domain closely related to haptoglobin. J Mol Biol 1989; 208:709–714.

47. Rogers J. Exon shuffling and intron insertion in serine protease genes. Nature 1985; 315:458–459.

48. Endo Y, Sato T, Matsushita M, Fujita T. Exon structure of the gene encoding the human mannose-binding protein-associated serine protease light chain: Comparison with complement C1r and C1s genes. Int Immunol 1996; 8:1355–1358.

49. Arlaud GJ, Gagnon J. Complete amino acid sequence of the catalytic chain of human complement subcomponent C1r. Biochemistry 1983; 22:1758–1764.

50. Leytus SP, Kurachi K, Sakariassen KS, Davie EW. Nucleotide sequence of the cDNA coding for human complement C1r. Biochemistry 1986; 25:4855–4863.

51. Journet A, Tosi M. Cloning and sequencing of full-length cDNA encoding the precursor of human complement component C1r. Biochem J 1986; 240:783–787.

52. Arlaud GJ, Willis AC, Gagnon J. Complete amino acid sequence of the A chain of human complement-classical-pathway enzyme C1̄r. Biochem J 1987; 241:711–720.

53. Carter PE, Dunbar B, Fothergill JE. The serine proteinase chain of human complement component C1s. Biochem J 1983; 215:565–571.

54. Spycher SE, Nick H, Rickli EE. Human complement component C1̄s. Partial sequence determination of the heavy chain and identification of the peptide bond cleaved during activation. Eur J Biochem 1986; 156:49–57.

55. Mackinnon CM, Carter PE, Smyth SJ, Dunbar B, Fothergill JE. Molecular cloning of cDNA for human complement component C1s. The complete amino acid sequence. Eur J Biochem 1987; 169:547–553.

56. Tosi M, Duponchel C, Meo T, Julier C. Complete cDNA sequence of human complement C1s and close physical linkage of the homologous genes C1s and C1r. Biochemistry 1987; 26:8516–8524.

57. Hess D, Schaller J, Rickli EE. Identification of the disulfide bonds in human complement C1s. Biochemistry 1991; 30:2827–2833.

58. Arlaud GJ, Colomb MG, Gagnon J. A functional model of the human C1 complex. Immunol Today 1987; 8:106–111.

59. Bork P, Beckmann G. The CUB domain. A widespread module in developmentally regulated proteins. J Mol Biol 1993; 231:539–545.

60. Campbell ID, Bork P. Epidermal growth factor-like modules. Curr Opin Cell Biol 1993; 3:385–392.

61. Rao Z, Hanford P, Mayhew M, Knott V, Brownlee GG, Stuart D. The structure of a Ca²⁺-binding epidermal growth factor-like domain: its role in protein–protein interactions. Cell 1995; 82:131–141.

62. Arlaud GJ, van Dorsselaer A, Bell M, Mancini A, Aude C, Gagnon J. Identification of erythro-β-hydroxyasparagine in the EGF-like domain of human C1r. FEBS Lett 1987; 222:129–134.

63. Thielens NM, van Dorsselaer A, Gagnon J, Arlaud GJ. Chemical and functional characterization of a fragment of C1̄s containing the epidermal growth factor homology region. Biochemistry 1990; 29:3570–3578.

64. Luo C, Thielens NM, Gagnon J, et al. Recombinant human complement subcomponent C1s lacking β-hydroxyasparagine, sialic acid, and one of its two carbohydrate chains still reassembles with C1q and C1r to form a functional C1 complex. Biochemistry 1992; 31:4254–4262.

65. Kamboh MI, Ferrell RE. Genetic studies of low abundance human plasma proteins. III. Polymorphism of the C1r subcomponent of the first complement component. Am J Hum Genet 1986; 39:826–831.

66. Hernandez JF, Bersch B, Pétillot Y, Gagnon J, Arlaud GJ. Chemical synthesis and characterization of the EGF-like module of human C1r. Mol Immunol 1996; 33:18 (abstract).

67. Reid KBM, Bentley DR, Campbell RD, et al. Complement system proteins which interact with C3b or C4b. A superfamily of structurally related proteins. Immunol Today 1986; 7:230–234.

68. Norman DG, Barlow PN, Baron M, Day AJ, Sim RB, Campbell ID. Three-dimensional structure of a complement control protein module in solution. J Mol Biol 1991; 219:717–725.

69. Barlow PN, Steinkasserer A, Norman DG, et al. Solution structure of a pair of complement modules by nuclear magnetic resonance. J Mol Biol 1993; 232:268–284.

70. Rossi V, Gaboriaud C, Lacroix M, et al. Structure of the catalytic region of human complement protease C1s: study by chemical cross-linking and three-dimensional homology modeling. Biochemistry 1995; 34:7311–7321.

71. Lacroix M, Rossi V, Gaboriaud C, et al. Structure of the catalytic regions of human C1r. Study by chemical cross-linking and 3-D homology modeling. Mol Immunol 1996; 33:19 (abstract).

72. Arlaud GJ, Thielens NM. Human complement serine proteases C1r and C1s and their proenzymes. Methods Enzymol 1993; 223:61–82.

73. Pétillot Y, Thibault P, Thielens NM, et al. Analysis of the *N*-linked oligosaccharides of human C1s using electrospray ionisation mass spectrometry. FEBS Lett 1995; 358:323–328.

74. Villiers CL, Arlaud GJ, Colomb MG. Domain structure and associated functions of subcomponents C1r and C1s of the first component of human complement. Proc Natl Acad Sci USA 1985; 82:4477–4481.

75. Busby TF, Ingham KC. Calcium-sensitive thermal transitions and domain structure of human complement subcomponent C1r. Biochemistry 1987; 26:5564–5571.

76. Busby TF, Ingham KC. Domain structure, stability, and interactions of human complement C1s: characterization of a derivative lacking most of the B chain. Biochemistry 1988; 27:6127–6135.

77. Thielens NM, Aude CA, Lacroix MB, Gagnon J, Arlaud GJ. Ca²⁺ binding properties and Ca²⁺-dependent interactions of the isolated NH₂-terminal α fragments of human complement proteases C1̄r and C1̄s. J Biol Chem 1990; 265:14469–14475.

78. Illy C, Thielens NM, Gagnon J, Arlaud GJ. Effect of lactoperoxidase-catalyzed iodination on the calcium-dependent interactions of human C1s. Location of the iodination sites. Biochemistry 1991; 30:7135–7141.

79. Cseh S, Gal P, Sarvari M, et al. Functional effects of domain deletions in a multidomain serine protease, C1r. Mol Immunol 1996; 33:351–359.

80. Lakatos S. Subunit interactions in the first component of complement, C1. Biochem Biophys Res Commun 1987; 149:378–384.

81. Thielens NM, Illy C, Bally IM, Arlaud GJ. Activation of human complement serine-proteinase C1r is down-regulated by a calcium-dependent intramolecular control that is released in the C1 complex through a signal transmitted by C1q. Biochem J 1994; 301:509–516.

82. Illy C, Thielens NM, Arlaud GJ. Chemical characterization and location of ionic interactions involved in the assembly of the C1 complex of human complement. J Protein Chem 1993; 12:771–781.

83. Busby TF, Ingham KC. NH$_2$-terminal calcium-binding domain of human complement $\overline{\text{C1s}}$ mediates the interaction of $\overline{\text{C1r}}$ with C1q. Biochemistry 1990; 29:4613–4618.

84. Weiss V, Fauser C, Engel J. Functional model of subcomponent C1 of human complement. J Mol Biol 1986; 189:573–581.

85. Medved LV, Busby TF, Ingham KC. Calorimetric investigation of the domain structure of human complement $\overline{\text{C1s}}$: reversible unfolding of the short consensus repeat units. Biochemistry 1989; 28:5408–5414.

86. Arlaud GJ, Gagnon J, Villiers CL, Colomb MG. Molecular characterization of the catalytic domains of human complement serine protease C1r. Biochemistry 1986; 25:5177–5182.

87. Lacroix MB, Aude CA, Arlaud GJ, Colomb MG. Isolation and functional characterization of the proenzyme form of the catalytic domains of human $\overline{\text{C1r}}$. Biochem J 1989; 257:885–891.

88. Matsumoto M, Nagaki K, Kitamura H, Kuramitsu S, Nagasawa S, Seya T. Probing the C4-binding site on C1s with monoclonal antibodies. Evidence for a C4/C4b-binding site on the gamma domain. J Immunol 1989; 142:2743–2750.

89. Sato T, Endo Y, Matsushita M, Fujita T. Molecular characterization of a novel serine protease involved in activation of the complement system by mannose-binding protein. Int Immunol 1994; 6:665–669.

90. Takada F, Seki N, Matsuda YI, Takayama Y, Kawakami M. Localization of the genes for the 100-kDa complement-activating components of Ra-reactive factor (CRARF and *crrarf*) to human 3q27-q28 and mouse 16B2-B3. Genomics 1995; 25:757–759.

91. Takada F, Takayama Y, Hatsuse H, Kawakami M. A new member of the C1s family of complement proteins found in a bactericidal factor, Ra-reactive factor, in human serum. Biochem Biophys Res Commun 1993; 196:1003–1009.

92. Takahashi A, Takayama Y, Hatsuse H, Kawakami M. Presence of a serine protease in the complement-activating component of the complement-dependent bactericidal factor, RaRF, in mouse serum. Biochem Biophys Res Commun 1993; 190:681–687.

93. Takayama Y, Takada F, Takahashi A, Kawakami M. A 100-kDa protein in the C4-activating component of Ra-reactive factor is a new serine protease having module organization similar to C1r and C1s. J Immunol 1994; 152:2308–2316.

94. Lu J, Thiel S, Wiedemann H, Timpl R, Reid KBM. Binding of the pentamer/hexamer forms of mannan-binding protein to zymosan activates the proenzyme C1r$_2$-C1s$_2$ complex of the classical pathway of complement, without involvement of C1q. J Immunol 1990; 144:2287–2294.

95. Matsushita M, Fujita T. Activation of the classical complement pathway by mannose-binding protein in association with a novel C1s-like serine protease. J Exp Med 1992; 176:1497–1502.

96. Matsushita M, Fujita T. Cleavage of the third component of complement by mannose-binding protein-associated serine protease (MASP) with subsequent complement activation. Immunobiology 1995; 194:443–448.

97. Ogata RT, Low PJ, Kawakami M. Substrate specificities of the protease of mouse serum Ra-reactive factor. J Immunol 1995; 154:2351–2357.

98. Vorup-Jensen T, Stover C, Poulsen K, et al. Cloning of cDNA encoding a human MASP-like protein (MASP-2). Mol Immunol 1996; 33:81 (abstract).

99. Carroll MC, Campbell RD, Bentley DR, Porter RR. A molecular map of the human major histocompatibility complex class III region linking complement genes C4, C2, and factor B. Nature 1984; 307:237–241.

100. Dunham I, Sargent CA, Trowsdale J, Campbell RD. Molecular mapping of the human major histocompatibility complex by pulsed-field gel electrophoresis. Proc Natl Acad Sci USA 1987; 84:7237–7241.

101. Carroll MC, Katzman P, Alicot EM, et al. Linkage map of the human major histocompatibility complex including the tumor necrosis factor genes. Proc Natl Acad Sci USA 1987; 84:8535–8539.

102. Wu L-C, Morley BJ, Campbell RD. Cell-specific expression of the human complement protein factor B gene: evidence for the role of two distinct 5'-flanking elements. Cell 1987; 48:331–342.

103. Ashfield R, Enriquez-Harris P, Proudfoot NJ. Transcriptional termination between the closely linked human complement genes C2 and factor B: common termination factor for C2 and c-myc? EMBO J 1991; 10:4197–4207.

104. Bossone SA, Asselin C, Patel AJ, Marcu KB. MAZ, a zinc finger protein, binds to cMYC and *C2* gene sequences regulating transcriptional initiation and termination. Proc Natl Acad Sci USA 1992; 89:7452–7456.

105. Ishii Y, Zhu Z-B, Macon KJ, Volanakis JE. Structure of the human C2 gene. J Immunol 1993; 151:170–174.

106. Campbell RD, Bentley DR. The structure and genetics of the C2 and factor B genes. Immunol Rev 1985; 87:19–37.

107. Zhu Z-B, Jian B, Volanakis JE. Ancestry of SINE-R.C2, a human-specific retroposon. Hum Genet 1994; 93:545–551.

108. Zhu Z-B, Hsieh SL, Bentley DR, Campbell RD, Volanakis JE. A variable number of tandem repeats (VNTR) locus within the human complement C2 gene is associated with a retroposon derived from a human endogenous retrovirus. J Exp Med 1992; 175:1783–1787.

109. Zhu Z-B, Volanakis JE. Allelic associations of multiple restriction fragment length polymorphisms of the gene encoding complement protein C2. Am J Hum Genet 1990; 46:956–962.

110. Cross SJ, Edwards JH, Bentley DR, Campbell RD. DNA polymorphism of the *C2* and factor B genes. Detection of a restriction fragment length polymorphism which subdivides haplotypes carrying the *C2C* and factor B *F* alleles. Immunogenetics 1985; 21:39–48.

111. Mole JE, Anderson JK, Davison EA, Woods DE. Complete primary structure for the zymogen of human complement factor B. J Biol Chem 1984; 259:3407–3412.

112. Horiuchi T, Kim S, Matsumoto M, Watanabe I, Fujita S, Volanakis JE. Human complement factor B: cDNA cloning, nucleotide sequencing, phenotypic conversion by site-directed mutagenesis, and expression. Mol Immunol 1993; 30:1587–1592.

113. Bentley DR. Primary structure of human complement component C2: homology to two unrelated protein families. Biochem J 1986; 239:339–345.

114. Horiuchi T, Macon KJ, Kidd VJ, Volanakis JE. cDNA cloning and expression of human complement component C2. J Immunol 1989; 142:2105–2111.

115. Smith CA, Vogel C-W, Muller-Eberhard HJ. MHC class III products: an electron microscopic study of the C3 convertases of human complement. J Exp Med 1984; 159:324–329.

116. Ueda A, Kearney JF, Roux KH, Volanakis JE. Probing functional sites on complement protein B with monoclonal antibodies. J Immunol 1987; 138:1143–1149.

117. Wetsel RA, Kulics J, Lokki M-L, et al. Type II human complement C2 deficiency. Allele-specific amino acid substitutions (Ser[189] → Phe; Gly[444] → Arg) cause impaired C2 secretion. J Biol Chem 1996; 271:5824–5831.

118. Colombatti A, Bonaldo P. The superfamily of proteins with von Willebrand factor type A-like domains: one theme common to components of extracellular matrix, hemostasis, cellular adhesion, and defense mechanisms. Blood 1991; 77:2305–2315.

119. Perkins SJ, Smith KF, Williams SC, Haris PI, Chapman D, Sim RB. The secondary structure of the von Willebrand factor type A domain in factor B of human complement by Fourier transform infrared spectroscopy. J Mol Biol 1994; 238:104–119.

120. Lee J-O, Rieu P, Arnaout MA, Liddington R. Crystal structure of the A domain from the α subunit of integrin CR3 (CD11b/CD18). Cell 1995; 80:631–638.

121. Qu A, Leahy DJ. Crystal structure of the I-domain from the CD11a/CD18 (LFA-1, $\alpha_L\beta2$) integrin. Proc Natl Acad Sci USA 1995; 92:10277–10281.

122. Tuckwell DS, Xu Y, Newham P, Humphries MJ, Volanakis JE. Surface loops adjacent to the putative cation-binding site of the complement factor B von Willebrand factor type-A module determine C3b binding specificity. Biochemistry 1997; 36:6605–6613.

123. Perkins SJ, Smith KF. Identity of the putative serine–proteinase fold in proteins of the complement system with nine relevant crystal structures. Biochem J 1993; 295:109–114.

124. Stroud RM, Krieger M, Koeppe II RE, Kossiakoff AA, Chambers JL. Structure-function relationships in the serine proteases. In: Reich, Rifkin, Shaw, eds. Proteases and Biological Control. New York: Cold Spring Harbor Laboratory, 1975:13–32.

125. Pryzdial ELG, Isenman DE. Alternative complement pathway activation fragment Ba binds to C3b. Evidence that formation of the factor B-C3b complex involves two discrete points of contact. J Biol Chem 1987; 262:1519–1525.

126. Oglesby TJ, Accavitti MA, Volanakis JE. Evidence for a C4b binding site on the C2b domain of C2. J Immunol 1988; 141:926–931.

127. Volanakis JE. Participation of C3 and its ligands in complement activation. Curr Top Microbiol Immunol 1990; 153:1–21.

128. Fishelson Z, Pangburn MK, Muller-Eberhard HJ. C3 convertase of the alternative complement pathway. Demonstration of an active, stable C3b, Bb (Ni) complex. J Biol Chem 1983; 258:7411–7415.

129. Nagasawa S. Stroud RM. Cleavage of C2 by C1 into the antigenically distinct fragments C2a and C2b: demonstration of binding of C2b to C4. Proc Natl Acad Sci USA 1977; 74:2998–3001.

130. Kerr MA. The human complement system. Assembly of the classical pathway C3 convertase. Biochem J 1980; 189:173–181.

131. Nagasawa S, Kobayashi C, Maki-Suzuki T, Yamashita N, Koyama J. Purification and characterization of the C3 convertase of the classical pathway of human complement system by size exclusion high-performance liquid chromatography. J Biochem 1985; 97:493–499.

132. Xu Y, Volanakis JE. Contribution of the complement control protein modules of C2 in C4b-binding assessed by analysis of C2/factor B chimeras. J Immunol 1997; 158:5958–5965.

133. Hourcade DE, Wagner LM, Oglesby TJ. Analysis of the short consensus repeats of human complement factor B by site-directed mutagenesis. J Biol Chem 1995; 270:19716–19722.

134. Polley MJ, Müller-Eberhard HJ. Enhancement of the hemolytic activity of the second component of human complement by oxidation. J Exp Med 1967; 126:1013–1025.

135. Parkes C, Gagnon J, Kerr MA. The reaction of iodine and thiol-blocking reagents with human complement components C2 and factor B. Biochem J 1983; 213:201–209.

136. Horiuchi T, Macon KJ, Engler JA, Volanakis JE. Site-directed mutagenesis of the region around CYS-241 of complement component C2: Evidence for a C4b-binding site. J Immunol 1991; 147:584–589.

137. Sánchez-Corral P, Antón LC, Alcolea JM, Marqués G, Sánchez A, Vivanco F. Proteolytic activity of the different fragments of factor B on the third component of complement (C3): involvement of the N-terminal domain of Bb in magnesium binding. Mol Immunol 1990; 27:891–900.

138. Pangburn M, Müller-Eberhard HJ. The C3 convertase of the alternative pathway of human complement. Enzymic properties of the bimolecular proteinase. Biochem J 1986; 235:723–730.

139. Cooper NR. Enzymatic activity of the second component of complement. Biochemistry 1975; 14:4245–4251.

140. Fishelson Z, Müller-Eberhard HJ. Residual hemolytic and proteolytic activity expressed by Bb after decay-dissociation of C3b,Bb. J Immunol 1984; 132:1425–1429.

141. Lambris JD, Müller-Eberhard HJ. Isolation and characterization of a 33,000-Dalton fragment of complement factor B with catalytic and C3b binding activity. J Biol Chem 1984; 259:12685–12690.

142. Ikari N, Hitomi Y, Ninobe M, Fujii S. Studies on esterolytic activity of alternative complement component factor B. Biochim Biophys Acta 1983; 742:318–323.

143. Davis AE, III, Harrison RA. Structural characterization of factor I mediated cleavage of the third component of complement. Biochemistry 1982; 21:5745–5749.

144. Medof ME, Iida K, Mold C, Nussenzweig V. Unique role of the complement receptor CR1 in the degradation of C3b associated with immune complexes. J Exp Med 1982; 156:1739–1754.

145. Fujita T, Gigli I, Nussenzweig V. Human C4-binding protein. II. Role in proteolysis of C4b by C3b-inactivator. J Exp Med 1978; 148:1044–1051.

146. Seya T, Nakamura K, Masaki T, Ichihara-Itoh C, Matsumoto M, Nagasawa S. Human factor H and C4b-binding protein serve as factor I-cofactors both encompassing inactivation of C3b and C4b. Mol Immunol 1995; 32:355–360.

147. Shiang R, Murray JC, Morton CC, et al. Mapping of the human complement factor I gene to 4q25. Genomics 1989; 4:82–86.

148. Vyse TJ, Bates GP, Walport MJ, Morley BJ. The organization of the human complement factor I gene (IF): a member of the serine protease gene family. Genomics 1994; 24:90–98.

149. Davis AE. The C3b inactivator of the human complement system: homology with serine proteases. FEBS Lett 1981; 134:147–150.

150. Yuan J-m, Hsiung L-m, Gagnon J. CNBr cleavage of the light chain of human complement Factor I and alignment of the fragments. Biochem J 1986; 233:339–345.

151. Catterall CF, Lyons A, Sim RB, Day AJ, Harris TJR. Characterization of the primary amino acid sequence of human complement control protein Factor I from an analysis of cDNA clones. Biochem J 1987; 242:849–856.

152. Goldberger G, Bruns GAP, Rits M, Edge MD, Kwiatkowski DJ. Human complement factor I: Analysis of cDNA-derived primary structure and assignment of its gene to chromosome 4. J Biol Chem 1987; 262:10065–10071.

153. Barnum SR, Fey G, Tack BF. Biosynthesis and genetics of C3. Curr Top Microbiol Immunol 1989; 153:23–43.

154. Goldberger G, Arnaout MA, Aden D, Kay R, Rites M, Colten HR. Biosynthesis and postsynthetic processing of human C3b/C4b inactivator (Factor I) in three hepatoma cell lines. J Biol Chem 1984; 259:6492–6497.

155. Haefliger J-A, Tschopp J, Vial N, Jenne DE. Complete primary structure and functional characterization of the sixth component of the human complement system. Identification of the C5b-binding domain in complement C6. J Biol Chem 1989; 264:18041–18051.

156. DiScipio RG. Formation and structure of the C5b-7 complex of the lytic pathway of complement. J Biol Chem 1992; 267:17087–17094.

157. Freeman M, Ashkenas J, Rees DJG, et al. An ancient, highly conserved family of cysteine-rich protein domains revealed by cloning type I and type II murine macrophage scavenger receptors. Proc Natl Acad Sci USA 1990; 87:8810–8814.

158. Aruffo A, Melnick MB, Linsley PS, Seed B. The lymphocyte glycoprotein CD6 contains a repeated domain structure characteristic of a new family of cell surface and secreted proteins. J Exp Med 1991; 174:949–952.

159. Südhof TC, Goldstein JL, Brown MS, Russell DW. The LDL receptor gene: a mosaic of exons shared with different proteins. Science 1985; 228:815–822.

160. DiScipio RG, Gehring MR, Podack ER, Kan CC, Hugli TE, Fey GH. Nucleotide sequence of cDNA and derived amino acid sequence of human complement component C9. Proc Natl Acad Sci USA 1984; 81:7298–7302.

161. Stanley KK, Kocher h-P, Luzio JP, Jackson P, Tschopp J, Dickson J. The sequence and topology of human complement component C9. EMBO J 1985; 4:375–382.

162. Ullman CG, Haris PI, Smith KF, Sim RB, Emery VC, Perkins SJ. β-Sheet secondary structure of an LDL receptor domain from complement factor I by consensus structure predictions and spectroscopy. FEBS Lett 1995; 371:199–203.

163. Nilsson-Ekdahl K, Nilsson UR, Nilsson B. Inhibition of factor I by diisopropylfluorophosphate. Evidence of conformational changes in factor I induced by C3b and additional studies on the specificity of factor I. J Immunol 1990; 144:4269–4274.

5

The Chemistry and Biology of C3, C4, and C5

JOHN D. LAMBRIS and ARVIND SAHU
University of Pennsylvania, Philadelphia, Pennsylvania

RICK A. WETSEL
University of Texas Health Science Center, Houston, Texas

I. INTRODUCTION

The complement proteins C3, C4, and C5 are structural homologues and their interactions are paramount for complement activation. All three proteins are members of the α_2-macroglobulin superfamily (1). A comparison of their primary sequences and interactions with other protein suggests that they are more related to each other than to any other known protein. Structurally they are similar in size ($\sim$200 kDa), subunit structure (α-β in C3 and C5 and α-β-γ in C4), order of chains and arginine linker in the biosynthetic precursor, presence of internal thioester bond (not in C5), and probably even in disulfide linkages. All three proteins are proteolytically cleaved during complement activation to produce C3a, C4a, and C5a anaphylatoxins and both C3 and C4 are further cleaved by factor I in the presence of different cofactors to generate essentially similar products. Moreover, solution scattering studies also depict them as similar two-domain structures (2–4).

Presence of C3 activity has been reported in different animal species including invertebrates (5). The phylogenetic analysis of C3 from different species was instrumental in delineating the structural elements involved in its different functions and also led to one of the most interesting findings. Trout, a tetraploid fish possesses four different forms of C3, suggesting that during the tetraploidization event the C3 locus was duplicated and each locus was probably diverged and duplicated to generate four different C3 proteins (6). Thus, from these findings one could speculated that C4 and C5 are also the result of similar genome duplication events, in which genes were duplicated from C3 or a common ancestor, and evolved to C4 and C5. However, this has to have happened before the emergence of salmonids since trout have a functional C5 molecule. In fact, at the DNA level a C3/C4/C5-like protein has recently been identified in sea urchin (7). Purification and functional analysis of this protein may lead to the identification of such an ancestor molecule. In this chapter we focus our discussion on the structure of human C3, C4, and C5, both at protein and gene levels. Emphasis has been given to the interactions of these proteins with other complement proteins.

II. COMPLEMENT COMPONENT C3

A. Structure and Chemical Characterization

Human C3 is a key complement protein that helps organize the classical as well as the alternative pathway of complement activation. It is the most abundant complement component in serum (1–2 mg/ml) and has been characterized as a glycoprotein comprised of a 115 kDa α-chain linked to a 75 kDa β-chain by a single disulfide bond and noncovalent forces (Fig. 1). The primary structure, deduced from the cDNA sequence (8), consists of 1663 amino acids, including a 22 amino acid signal peptide. A complete disulfide bridge pattern has been determined for C3 (9,10): four linkages were found in C3a and a single bridge was determined in the β-chain as well as the C3d portion of the α-chain. The N- and C-terminal regions of the α-chain were found to be connected with each other with a disulfide linkage. It is interesting that six linkages are clustered in the 46 kDa C-terminal peptide of the α-chain. Molecular modeling of C3, based on data derived from x-ray scattering studies, depicts it as a two-domain structure with a flat ellipsoid associated with a smaller flat domain. These two domains move closer together following proteolytic activation of C3 and removal of C3a (2). Methylamine-treated C3 and C3b have been crystallized (11), although, data could be collected only at 7.7 Å resolution. Nevertheless, recent study on the α-2 macroglobulin (12) suggests that even data collected at low resolution (~10 Å) should allow one to determine the domain arrangement of the molecule. Carbohydrate analysis revealed that human C3 possesses two N-linked carbohydrate moieties, positioned at residues 63 of the β-chain ($Man_5GlcNac_2 + Man_6GlcNac_2$) and 917 of the α-chain ($Man_8GlcNac_2 + Man_9GlcNac_2$), which together account for 1.5% of the molecular weight of C3 (13,14).

One of the important characteristics of C3 is its ability to bind covalently to acceptor molecules on cell surfaces (15) via ester or amide linkages (16). In most biological systems the majority of C3b is linked via an ester bond, indicating a strong preference for the hydroxylated targets. This feature has been attributed to the thioester bond present within the C3d region of C3, which is sensitive to nucleophilic attack. The thioester bond is the product of an intramolecular transacylation between the thiol group of cysteine and the γ-amide group of the glutamine within the C3 sequence Gly-Cys[988]–Gly-Glu-Gln[991]-Asn (17). This thioester moiety is also found in two other plasma proteins, namely C4 and α_2-macroglobulin. In native C3, the thioester bond appears to be protected within a hydrophobic pocket and is exposed in the C3b fragment upon cleavage of C3 by C3 convertases. Thus, the transiently exposed thioester bond (half life ~100μs) can then participate in a transacylation reaction with nucleophilic groups present on cell surfaces, complex carbohydrates, or immune complexes (17–21). Until recently, attachment of C3b to different acceptors has been considered as a nonspecific reaction. However, recent studies clearly demonstrate that C3b displays a high degree of specificity in reacting with targets such as carbohydrates, C3b, C4b, and IgG (18,19,22,23) and that this specificity plays an important factor in complement activation (18.) In human IgG[1] and C4b, Thr[144] and Ser[1213], respectively, were identified as the major if not the only sites with which C3b reacts (19,22). These findings demonstrate the selection of a single residue out of several hundred potential hydroxyl and amino group-containing targets on these two proteins. Thus, the belief that metastable C3b reacts randomly or nonspecifically is not correct. The deposition of C3b to surface structures is necessary to initiate the formation of the membrane attack complex (MAC), the phagocytosis of foreign particles, and the enhancement of effector cell–target cell contact.

B. Activation and Degradation

Cleavage of C3 between residues 726 and 727 (Arg-Ser) by either the classical (C4b,2a) or the alternative (C3b,Bb) pathway C3 convertases leads to the generation of C3b (185

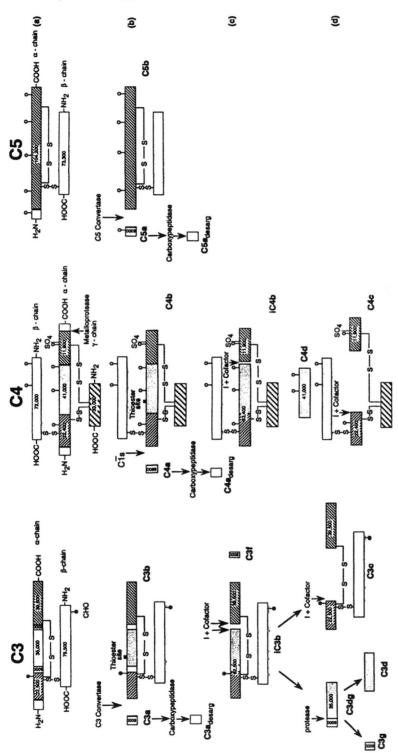

Figure 1 Activation and degradation of C3, C4, and C5. The cleavage sites are indicated by arrows. The locations of *N*-linked carbohydrate sites in C3 and potential *N*-linked carbohydrate sites on C4 and C5 are indicated with closed and open balloons respectively. The molecular weights of polypeptides are calculated on the basis of their deduced amino acid sequences. Only disulfide bridges that are relevant to the degradation pattern are shown. (a) Native Molecule, cleavage by C1s, C3-convertase or C5-convertase generate anaphylatoxin. (b) Cleavage by factor I in the presence of cofactors CR1, H, MCP (for C3b) and CR1, MCP, C4Bp (for C4b). (c&d), Further cleavage by factor I in the presence of a cofactor CR1, H (for i C3b) and CR1, C4bp (for i C4b) generates C3c and C3dg or C4c and C4d, respectively.

kDa) and C3a (9 kDa). In contrast to native C3, C3b expresses multiple binding sites for other complement components, including C5, properdin (P), factors H, B, and I, C4-binding protein (C4bp), CR1 (C3b-receptor), and the membrane cofactor protein (MCP) (24). Binding of these proteins to C3b leads either to amplification of the C3 convertase (by B and P in the presence of factor D) and initiation of the assembly of the MAC, or to the inactivation of C3b (by factor I) (25). Whether amplification or inactivation occurs depends on the nature of the surface to which C3b is attached.

The inactivation of C3b by factor I, an event by which complement activation is downregulated, proceeds in three steps (26,27) and requires one of several cofactor molecules (MCP, CR1, or H). The cleavage of the α'-chain of C3b first between residues 1281–1282 (Arg-Ser) and then between residues 1298–1299 (Arg-Ser) (Fig. 1) of C3 liberates the C3f fragment (Mr 2,000) and yields iC3b (28–30). A third factor I cleavage site, with CR1, or factor H serving as cofactors (28,29,31) has been reported to exist at residues 932–933 (Arg-Glu) of the α-chain of C3, generating the C3c and C3dg fragments (30). Our recent laboratory data on cofactor activity of CR1, factor H, and MCP suggest that the first cleavage can occur in the presence of any of the three cofactors, the second cleavage requires the presence of CR1, factor H, or MCP, but the third cleavage occurs preferentially in the presence of CR1. The cofactor activity of factor H for the third site was minimal, required buffers of low ionic strength, and was observed only after extensive incubation (27,32).

Previous study of Nilsson-Ekdahl et al. (33) suggested that factor I cleavage generates three different C3dg-like fragments with N-termini corresponding to residues 933 (cleavage between Arg-Glu), 939 (cleavage between Lys-Glu), and 919, 924, or 930 (cleavage between Lys-Thr, Arg-Thr or Arg-Leu). From the above cleavages and those occurring in C4 (34), it appears that factor I preferentially cleaves Arg/Lys-X bonds, but that this specificity is restricted by the required presence of one of several cofactor molecules (factor H, C4bp, CR1, or MCP). The cleavages by factor I in the region between residues 918–940 have been debated so far. The presence of sequences His-Thr, His-Leu, and Gln-Gly, at the proposed factor I cleavage site in rabbit, mouse, and rat C3, respectively, (35–37) supported the hypothesis that some of the observed cleavages may be mediated by enzyme(s) other than factor I. However, a recent study by Farries et al. (38) using site-directed mutagenesis of the P1 arginine residues of human C3b showed that replacement of both Arg[1281] and Arg[1298] by Gln although significantly reduced the factor I-mediated cleavages allowed for slow cleavage between residues 1281–1282, indicating that factor I possesses a broader specificity than previously anticipated.

C. Biosynthesis, Gene Structure, and Deficiencies

C3 is synthesized as single chain pre-pro molecule with the α- and β-chains linked by a tetra-arginine sequence, which is removed by a furin-like enzyme (39) during posttranslational modification. Following translocation through the endoplasmic reticulum to the Golgi, N-linked high-mannose type carbohydrate moieties are attached at residues 917 of the α-chain and 63 of the β-chain (Fig. 1) (13,14). The vast majority (more than 90%) of C3 biosynthesis occurs in the liver (40), but synthesis at numerous other sites (reviewed in (41)) may be involved in localized inflammatory processes. C3 expression is regulated by cytokines such as interferon (IFN), interleukin-1 (IL-1), and tumor necrosis factor (TNF) (41). Regulation of C3 synthesis appears to be tissue-specific, as in the cases of estrogen regulation in the uterus (42) or vitamin D regulation in osteoblasts (43).

The 41 kb gene for human C3 has been localized to chromosome 19 (44). Of the 41 exons (ranging in size from 52 to 213 bases) contained in the gene, 16 encode the β chain, and 25 the α chain (45,46). Each of the major binding sites in the α chain of C3 appear to be encoded by single exons (reviewed in [41]). It is interesting to note that the highly conserved thioester domain is encoded by class 1-1 exons, the type most commonly reshuffled and duplicated (47). Coding regions of C4 and C5 also contain approximately 40 exons and the exons flanking the thioester site in C4 are similar to those of C3.

In humans, two major C3 protein polymorphisms have been identified, based on the agarose gel electrophoretic mobility of the allotypes (48). The C3 slow (C3S) and C3 fast (C3F) variants exhibit very similar specific hemolytic activities (49) and have been described in many populations; C3S is the more common allotype with a frequency of 0.79, 0.95, 0.97, and 0.99 in White, African-American, South American Indian, and Asian populations, respectively.

Since 1972, inherited C3 deficiency has been described in 16 families representing a variety of ethnic and national origins (50). Inherited C3 deficiencies are characterized by a heightened susceptibility to bacterial infections that lead to purulent lesions. In addition several C3-deficient patients have shown impaired chemotactic activity, sluggish response of neutrophils to infectious agents, and development of immune complex disease, specifically, systemic lupus erythematosus, and membrane proliferative glomerulonephritis (51). Although the antibody response to routine immunizations is normal, an impaired switch from IgM to IgG was observed in two C3 deficient patients immunized with limited doses of the T-dependent antigen, bacteriophage φX174 (52,52A). A similar defective antibody response was observed in C3-deficient guinea pigs (51) and dogs (53). These findings and those made using pharmacologically C3-depleted animals suggest that C3 may play an important role in the generation of a normal immune response (reviewed in [50,51]).

Recently, the molecular genetic basis of C3 deficiency has been examined in five unrelated kindred. Collectively these studies have demonstrated that C3 deficiency is caused by numerous molecular genetic defects. Two of the C3-deficient kindred contain point mutations at 5'-donor splice sites in the C3 gene; one of these is a 5'-donor splice site mutation in intron 18 of the C3 gene described in an English male. This mutation causes a cryptic 5'-splice site in exon 18 that is used during RNA processing generating a 61-nucleotide deletion in the C3 RNA. This deletion results in a shift in the reading frame of the C3 transcript and a premature stop in translation (54). The other splice site mutation has been described in the C3-deficient gene of a Taiwanese aborinigal (Atayal tribe) female (55); a 5'-donor splice site mutation in intron 10 causes exon 10 to be skipped during RNA processing, resulting in the generation of a premature stop codon. The third family carries an 800-bp deletion in the C3 gene that includes exons 22 and 23 and is the cause of inherited C3 deficiency in the Afrikaaner population of South Africa (56). A missense mutation in exon 13 was discovered recently in a fourth family that results in a critical amino acid substitution in the C3 β-chain (Asp^{549} to Asn). This Asn^{549} substitution causes impaired secretion of the intracellular C3 protein (57). The exact molecular genetic defect in a fifth kindred is yet to be delineated; however, fibroblast skin cells indicate that C3 protein deficiency in this Laotian family results from reduced levels of C3 specific mRNA (58).

III. COMPLEMENT COMPONENT C4

A. Structure and Chemical Characterization

The fourth component of complement (C4) plays a central role in activation of the classical pathway. In humans, C4 exists in two functional isoforms, as a transcription product of two separate genes. It is a plasma glycoprotein (0.64 mg/ml) of 200 kDa of which 7% is carbohydrate and contains three polypeptide chains: α (95 kDa), β (75 kDa) and γ (33 kDa) (59,60). The N-terminal region of the α-chain is linked by disulfide bonds to both the β- and the γ-chains, whereas the C-terminal region of the α-chain is linked only to the γ-chain (Fig. 1) (61). Analogous to C3 and C5, C4 is also synthesized as a single polypeptide chain (pro-C4), which is glycosylated (62) before being processed by a plasmin-like protease (63), sulfated (64), and secreted as a multichain protein. The order of the three subunits in pro-C4 molecule is β-α-γ (65). After secretion, the protein is further processed in the plasma by the removal of a small C-terminal fragment of the α-chain by a metalloprotease (66). The half-time required for processing and secretion of C4 was determined to be ~60–90 min (67), which is comparable to that required by C3 and C5 (68,69). The primary structure of C4 has been derived from a cDNA sequence encoded by a 5.5-kb mature mRNA and contains 1722 amino acids (65). Currently the three-dimensional structure of C4 is not known, however electron microscopic studies (70) and x-ray and neutron scattering (3) depict it as a multidomain structure.

Like C3 and α-2 macroglobulin, C4 contains an internal thioester bond as a result of posttranslational modification that links the sulfhydryl group of Cys^{991} to the carbonyl group of Gln^{994} with release of ammonia (71). This bond is located in the C4d region of the C4 molecule. It has been shown that formation of this bond is entirely spontaneous and does not involve any enzymes or high-energy metabolites (72). During activation of the classical pathway, proteolytic cleavage of native C4 by C1s produces a low-molecular-weight anaphylatoxic peptide C4a (8.8 kDa) and a major cleavage fragment C4b (191 kDa) that contains a short lived, highly reactive thioester bond. The activated thioester of C4b reacts with hydroxyl or amino groups of the receptive surface to form ester or amide bonds, which is required for subsequent steps in complement activation. Isotypes of C4 differ in their reactivity, C4A shows strong reactivity with amino groups while C4B displays preference for hydroxyl groups (73,74). If one disregards polymorphic variations, both isotypes of C4 are identical in sequence except for four amino acid residues located 107 residues C-terminal to the thioester site. C4A contains Pro-Cys-Pro-Val-Leu-Asp, whereas C4B contains Leu-Ser-Pro-Val-Ile-His and the structural basis for this specificity has been allocated to histidine at position 1106 (75). Recently, a mechanism for the binding of C4A and C4B has been proposed (76). It is suggested that if the key residue at position 1106 is nonnucleophilic (Asp, as in C4A) the activated thioester reacts directly with the nucleophilic groups present on the acceptor molecule. Thus in C4A the reaction with more nucleophilic amino groups is predominant and hydrolysis is slower. However, if the residue at position 1106 is nucleophilic (His, as in C4B), it reacts with the thioester and forms an acyl-intermediate. The released thiol then serves as a base to catalyze the transfer of the acyl group to hydroxyl- and amino-nucleophiles. It is important to mention here that the four amino acid residues responsible for isotypic variation and other four substitutions at the C4d region of C4 (residues 1054, 1157, 1188, and 1191) are responsible for generating the two Rodgers and six Chido serological determinants (77,78).

B. Activation and Degradation

The conversion of C4 to C4b by C1s (cleavage between residues 737 and 738) initiates a series of conformational changes in the molecule and exposes antigenic sites (79) as well as binding sites for various proteins. Structural studies found that C4 activation leads to decrease in the surface hydrophobicity and changes in the backbone conformation (80). The newly formed C4b encompasses binding sites for various complement proteins such as C2, C3, C5, C4bp, CR1, and MCP. The binding of C2, C3, and C5 leads to the activation of the pathway, while that of C4bp, CR1, and MCP shut off the activation process. Binding of C2 to C4b in the presence of magnesium ions followed by the cleavage of C2 by C1s results in formation of the C3 convertase C4b,2a (81,82). This complex then cleaves C3 and cleaved molecules bind covalently to C4b to form a C5 convertase C4b,2a,3b; a major fraction of C3b gets hydrolyzed with water. The covalent binding site of C3 on C4b was determined to be Ser^{1217} (22). It has been proposed, although not conclusively demonstrated, that in this trimolecular complex both C3b and C4b participate in C5 binding (83). Site-directed mutagenesis of the C4 β-chain residue arginine 458 to tryptophan, which occurs naturally in the hemolytically inactive A6 allotype of C4, abolished the ability of the molecule to participate as C5 binding subunit of the convertase (84). Binding of C4bp, CR1, and MCP to C4b allows the cleavage of C4b by factor I into functionally inactive species C4c and C4d (34,85–87). The factor I-mediated cleavages have been reported to be located at residues 937–938 (Arg-Thr) and 1318–1319 (Arg-Asn) of the α'-chain of the C4b (numbering according to (65)).

C. Biosynthesis, Gene Structures, and Deficiencies

C4 is primarily synthesized in the liver. However, like most complement components, it is also synthesized in various other extrahepatic tissues including kidney, lung, spleen, brain, and mammary glands (88). It has been reported that acute inflammatory response, tissue injury, and treatment with interferon-γ results in a two- to three-fold increase in C4 synthesis (89). Expression of C4 appears to be tissue specific (reviewed in [90]). Much interest has been focused on the regulation of C4 expression, since deficiency of C4 leads to repeated bacterial infections, systemic or discoid lupus erythematosus, immune complex diseases, and is sometimes fatal (91). Recent study with C3- and C4-deficient mice suggests that deficiency of either protein results in increased susceptibility to lethal group B streptococcal infection (92).

The genes encoding C4A and C4B are located within the major histocompatibility complex (MHC) class III region on the short arm of chromosome 6 (93). This region also contains genes encoding tumor necrosis factor α and β (94,95), heat shock proteins HSP 70 (96), C2, factor B, and adrenal steroid 21-hydroxylase genes P450c21A and B (93). The duplication of the C4/P450c21 gene cluster has been thought to occur before mammalian speciation; mice (97) and cattle (98) also have duplicated genes for C4 and P450c21. Both *C4* genes are arranged in tandem loci that are ~10 kb apart. The *C4A* gene is about

22 kb long, but the *C4B* gene is either 22 kb or 16 kb long. The difference in size is due to the presence of a single large intron located about 2.5 kb from the 5' end of the gene. The genes for P450c21 A and B are located downstream of each C4 gene. The complete structure of both C4 genes has been determined in humans (99,100). The C4A gene consists of 41 exons, which encode a transcript for precursor protein of 1744 amino acid residues. It is interesting that some unique features of C4 like the α-γ chain junction, the tyrosine sulfation sites, and the postsecretory metalloprotease cleavage site are encoded by a single exon (exon 33) (99). Human C4 genes A and B are highly polymorphic. To date at least 40 alleles for each gene have been reported. These include null alleles (C4A Q0 and C4B Q0), which are responsible for the absence of C4A and C4B protein in the serum. Although most of these are due to gene deletion, about 40% are due to nonexpression of unaltered genes (101,102). It is possible that this variation in expression of C4 may be due to polymorphism in regulatory elements. Recent studies demonstrated that the area of transcriptional activity for C4 in the hepatocyte cell line (HepG2) occurs ~500 base pairs 5' to the C4A and C4B transcriptional start sites. However, this region is identical in different C4 allotypes as well as MHC haplotypes including HLA B57, C4A6, C4B1, DR7; thus variation in expression of C4 cannot be explained at the transcriptional level (103).

IV. COMPLEMENT COMPONENT C5

A. Structure and Chemical Characterization

C5 (190,000 M_r) is contained in human serum at a concentration of approximately 0.075 mg/ml and can be highly purified by several procedures (104–106). C5 is comprised of two polypeptide chains, α and β, with approximate molecular weights of 115,000 and 75,000, respectively (Fig. 1) (107,108). Biosynthesized as a single-chain promolecule, C5 is enzymatically cleaved into its two-chain structure during processing and secretion. After cleavage, the two chains are held together by at least one disulfide bond as well as noncovalent forces (109–111).

Primary amino acid structures of human and murine C5 were obtained from cDNA sequencing data (112–115). The deduced amino acid sequence of precursor human pre- pro-C5 is 1676 amino acids, which includes an 18 amino acid signal peptide, and an arginine rich linker sequence (RPRR) located between the amino-terminal β-chain and the carboxy-terminal α-chain. The signal and linker peptides are processed from the promolecule during secretion, yielding the mature, native two chain structure. The β- and α-chains of mature C5 are comprised of 655 and 999 amino acids, respectively. The mass of C5 is composed of approximately 3.0% carbohydrate (116,117). Galactose (0.3%), mannose (0.6%), N-acetylglucosamine (1.5%), and N-acetylneuraminate (0.6%) have been detected in C5 (116). One oligosaccharide moiety, of approximately 3000 M_r, has been localized in human C5. This complex is attached to the asparagine at residue 64 in the C5 α-chain and is comprised of mannose, galactose, glucosamine, and sialic acid. In addition, there are four possible asparagine-linked carbohydrate moieties in the C5 α-chain.

There are 29 cysteine residues in the primary structure of human C5, of which all but one are thought to be involved in disulfide linkages. This free cysteine residue is located at position 27 in the C5 α-chain. Only three of the cysteine residues are in the C5 β-chain. Extensive detailed disulfide mapping studies have not been done for human

C5 as have been done for C3 (see above and [118,119]). However, it is likely that a single disulfide bond links the C5 α- and β-chains, since the β cysteine residues are identically positioned in the C3 and C5 molecules.

Circular dichroism studies indicate that the native C5 molecule is 17% alpha helix and 20% beta sheet (117). Electron microscopy, neutron and x-ray scattering, and physical chemical studies have indicated that C5 exhibits an asymmetrical two-domain shape with a sedimentation coefficient of 7.9 S (4,117).

B. Activation and Degradation

C5 is cleaved during activation of either complement pathway into C5a and C5b fragments (Fig. 1). The convertase enzymes responsible for C5 activation, C4b,2a,3b and (C3b)$_2$,Bb,P for the classical (120–122) and alternative (123) pathways, respectively, activate C5 by cleavage at a site (arginyl-leucyl, pos 74–75) in the α-chain. After activation, the 11,200 M$_r$ peptide (C5a) derived from the amino-terminus of the α-chain is released into the surrounding. C5a shares the same anaphylatoxin properties exhibited by C3a, but is 100 times more potent, on a molar basis, in eliciting the responses. In addition to its anaphylatoxic properties, C5a stimulates directed migration of neutrophils (124,125) eosinophils (126), basophils (127), and monocytes (128,129). The C5a peptide is regulated by the plasma enzyme carboxypeptidase N (E.C.3.4.12.7) that removes the carboxy-terminal arginine from C5a forming the C5a des Arg derivative (130). On a molar basis, human C5a des Arg expresses only 1% as much anaphylactic activity (131) and 1.0% as much PMN chemotactic activity as does undigested C5a (132,133). The restricted C5a des Arg anaphylatoxin activity can be enhanced by a serum-derived "cochemotaxin" (134,135) or by removal of the oligosaccharide moiety (131,136).

A number of physiologically relevant proteolytic enzymes cleave C5 to express C5a-like biological activities. For example, trypsin (125,137,138) α-thrombin (139), elastase (140), and cathepsin G (141) modify C5 to express neutrophil chemotactic and lysosomal enzyme-releasing activities. It was initially assumed that these enzymes cleaved the C5a peptide from the parent molecule (142,143). One report documented that the C5a fragment was released after limited trypsin digestion (144). However, four independent laboratories have determined that the actual site of initial trypsin cleavage is interior into the C5 α-chain producing 25,000 and 90,000 M$_r$ fragments that remain disulfide-bound to the parent molecule (107,108,145–147). In fact, it is now well documented that the first three trypsin cleavage events do not release C5 fragments (145–147). It is interesting that the trypsin-modified C5 molecule, which has the same molecular weight as native C5, elicits neutrophil responses such as chemotactic migration and lysosomal enzyme release (146). The mechanism by which trypsin-modified C5 mediates the C5a-like activities is presently not known.

C. Biosynthesis, Gene Structure, and Deficiencies

With the use of a panel of hamster–human somatic cell hybrids, the human C5 gene was mapped to chromosome 9 (112). *In situ* chromosomal hybridization studies employing metaphase cells localized the gene to bands 9q32–34 (112). Two genes that have been localized to the same region are spectrin and the Abelson murine leukemia viral oncogene homologue (148–151). The mouse C5 gene has been mapped to chromosome 2 (152). By employing overlapping genomic cosmid clones, both the murine and human C5 genes have been fully characterized (153,154). The human C5 gene is approximately 79 Kb in length and contains 41 exons. Comparison of the C5 gene with the homologous family members C3 and C4 reveal that all three genes share striking similarities in organization and exon size, although C3 (41 kb), and C4 (20 kb) are smaller because they have shorter introns.

Human C5 is present in plasma at a concentration of 0.075 mg/ml (155), most of which is thought to be synthesized in hepatocytes (156), but additional synthesis of hemolytically active C5 has been demonstrated in lung, spleen, and fetal intestine (157). Biosynthetic labeling and immunoprecipitation studies have suggested that human mono-cytes (158–161), macrophages (160,162), and type II alveolar epithelial cells (163) synthe-size C5. Regulated expression of C5 has not been explored in depth. In one study, histamine was demonstrated to inhibit the synthesis of functionally and immunochemically detectable C5 in peritoneal murine macrophages (164). The effect appeared to be mediated by histamine type 2 receptors and resulted in decreased synthesis of pro-C5.

Several C5-deficient families have been reported (165–173) from different ethnic backgrounds and from different geographic regions. Sera from homozygous C5-deficient individuals lack bactericidal activity and have severely impaired ability to induce chemo-taxis (166,168,170) Consequently, all C5-deficient individuals display a propensity for severe recurrent infections, particularly to neisserial species, including meningitis and extragenital gonorrhea (165,168,169,171–174). In addition, one individual with complete C5 protein deficiency has systemic lupus erythematosus, but it is not clear if this is directly related to her C5 deficiency (165). The molecular genetic basis of human C5 deficiency has been examined only recently (175). In the study of three C5-deficient African–American families it was determined that C5 deficiency is caused by several molecular genetic defects, C5 deficiency in the African–American population can be explained in part by two distinct nonsense mutations in exons 1 and 36 compound heterozygosity exists in all of the reported African-American C5–deficient families, and none of the C5-deficient white families contains the exon 1 and exon 36 mutations.

The molecular basis of C5 deficiency has been studied extensively in the mouse. Approximately 40% of commercially available inbred mice strains are C5 deficient (176,177). All C5-deficient mouse strains examined contain a two basepair deletion in exon 7 of the C5 structural gene, accounting for the C5 protein deficiency (114)

Polymorphisms of C5 have been examined only cursorily. A protein polymorphism of C5 has been reported in populations of the South Pacific region (178). A phenylalanine to serine amino acid substitution has been observed at residue 500 of the β-chain from cDNA sequencing studies (115).

V. INTERACTION OF C3, C4, AND C5 WITH RECEPTORS AND CELL-ASSOCIATED REGULATORY PROTEIN

The cleavage fragments, both soluble and/or surface bound, generated during complement activation have the potential to bind specifically to several cell surface receptors, known as CR1, CR2, CR3, CR4, CR5, and C3a-, C4a- and C5a- receptor. These ligand–receptor interactions lead to various biological responses (Table 1, for detailed reviews see also [179–183]).

A. C3a, C4a, and C5a Anaphylatoxin Receptors

In vitro and in vivo studies have shown that one of the major biological consequences of complement activation is the generation of three small cationic peptides C3a, C4a, and C5a, collectively referred to as complement anaphylatoxins. All three peptides are 74–77 amino acids in length and are derived from the amino terminus of the parent molecule's α-chain. All three peptides mediate many biological phenomena that occur during an inflammatory response, including smooth muscle contraction, histamine release from mast cells, vasodilation, and increased vascular permeability. In addition, one of the peptides, C5a, is a potent chemoattractant for neutrophils and other leukocytes. The complement anaphylatoxin peptides exert their effects by binding to G protein-coupled receptors on specific target cells, resulting in receptor phosphorylation and activation of pertinent intracellular signal transduction pathways. The cloning of the cDNA encoding the C3a and C5a receptors has recently been accomplished demonstrating that each receptor is a member of the superfamily of rhodopsin-type receptors, containing seven transmembrane loops (184–186). Numerous laboratories have generated deletion, site-directed, and chimeric C5a receptor cDNA mutants, as well as sequence-specific antisera, in attempts to localize structural elements that bind the C5a ligand (reviewed in 183). Taken together, the data from these laboratories have demonstrated that the ligand-binding site of the C5a receptor is complex and consists of at least two physically separable binding domains. One binds the C5a amino terminus (amino acids 1–20) and disulfide-linked core (amino acids 21–61), while the second binds the C5a carboxy-terminal end (amino acids 62–74). Similar mutational analyses have not yet been done for the C3a-receptor.

Until recently, expression of the complement anaphylatoxin receptors was thought to be limited primarily to peripheral blood leukocytes, including neutrophils, eosinophils, monocytes, and macrophages, as well as the differentiated myeloid cell lines U937 and HL-60. This belief was established from a wealth of functional and binding data generated during the past two decades, which examined the effects of C5a on peripheral blood cells (187). Cloning of the C3a and C5a receptors has now made it possible to generate antisense probes and antireceptor antisera that have been used recently to examine the cellular expression of the C3a and C5a receptors in detail. These studies have yielded very surprising results. For example, *in situ* hybridization, flow cytometry, and immunohistochemistry have demonstrated that several non-myeloid-derived tissue cells express the C5a receptor. These cells include liver parenchymal cells, lung vascular smooth muscle and endothelial cells, bronchial and alveolar epithelial cells (188), as well as astrocytes isolated from adult spinal cords (189). Comparative studies with the C3a receptor are currently underway and also indicate that the C3a receptor is expressed by many different cell types of nonmyeloid origin. These data suggest that the C5a anaphylatoxin mediates previously unrecognized functions by binding to nonmyeloid tissue cells that express the C5a receptor.

Based on the results of cross-desensitization of smooth muscle contraction by the three complement anaphylatoxins, it has been generally accepted that C3a and C4a bind to the identical receptor. However, recent investigations have suggested that there are two distinct receptors for C3a and C4a, at least on monocytes and macrophages. This conclusion was first drawn from studies that demonstrated that C4a, but not C3a, suppressed chemotac-

Table 1 C3, C4, and C5 Receptors and Binding Proteins

Protein	Specificity	Structure	Cell type(s)	Key features
Cell Surface Proteins				
CR1	C3b, C4b iC3b, C3c	4 allotypes 160 kDa 190 220	Erythrocytes, eosinophils, monocytes, macrophages, neutrophils, B and some T lymphocytes, glomerular podocytes, follicular dendritic cells, mast cells	Member of RCA, accelerates dissociation of CP and AP C3 convertases, cofactor for factor I, helps processing immune complexes, involved in phagocytosis
CR2	iC3b, C3dg EBV gp 350	140 kDa	B cells, T cells, follicular dendritic cells, Polymorphonuclear cells	Member of RCA Plays a role in immunoregulation
CR3	iC3b, C3dg	170 kDa α chain 95 kDa β chain	Polymorphonuclear cells, monocytes, natural killer cells, some B and T lymphocytes	Involved in phagocytosis of iC3b-coated particles, adhesion of neutrophils, cytotoxicity of cells bearing activated complement components, member of leukocyte integrins
CR4 (p150, 95)	iC3b	150 kDa α chain 95 kDa β chain	Monocytes, macrophages, NK and ADCC effector lymphocytes, neutrophils	Functions in cell adhesion
C3aR	C3a, C4a	95 kDa	Mast cells, neutrophils, basophils, monocytes, T lymphocytes, eosinophils	Depending on cell type, functions include chemotaxis, chemokinesis, cell aggregation and adhesion, release of lysosomal contents, may play a role in immunoregulation
C5aR	C5a	43 kDa	Neutrophils, eosinophils, monocytes, macrophages, liver parenchymal cells, lung vascular smooth muscle and endothelial cells, bronchial and alveolar epithelial cells, astrocytes	Depending on cell type functions include, directed chemotaxis, cell adhesion and aggregation,release of granular enzymes and histamine, augments the humoral and cellular responses

C3eR	C3dk, C3e	Not characterized	Neutrophils, monocytes	Lysosomal enzyme release, leukocytosis
DAF	C3b,Bb C4b, 2a	75 kDa	Erythrocytes, all leukocytes, platelets	Accelerates decay of CP and AP C3 convertases
MCP	C3b, iC3b C4b	45–70 kDa	Neutrophils, monocytes, platelets, reticulocytes, most lymphocytes, granulocytes, endothelial cells, epithelial cells, mesenchymal cells	Member of RCA, cofactor for factor I, does not accelerate decay of C3 convertases
Undefined	C3 (β chain)	Neutrophils, eosinophils	Eosinophil cytotoxicity inhibitor (275) Inhibitor of neutrophil adherence (275)	
Serum proteins				
Factor B	C3b, C3(H₂O)	93 kDa		Catalytic subunit of AP C3 convertase
Factor H	C3b, iC3b C3c, C3d	150 kDa		Accelerates the dissociation of AP C3 convertase cofactor for factor I
Factor I	C3b, iC3b	88 kDa		C4b/C3b inactivator
Properdin	C3b, C3c	55–220 kDa		Stabilizes AP C3 convertase
C4bp	C4b, C3b	460–540 kDa 70 kDa α chain 45 kDa β chain		Cofactor for factor I accelerates the decay of CP C3 convertase

Table 1 Continued

Protein	Specificity	Structure	Cell type(s)	Key features
Proteins of foreign origin				
gC-1	C3, C3b iC3b, C3c	120 kDa	HSV-1 infected cells	Accelerates the decay of AP C3 convertase, inhibits binding of properdin and C5 to C3
gC-2	C3, C3b iC3b, C3c	100 kDa	Cells transfected with gC-2 gene	Stabilizes AP C3 convertase Does not inhibit properdin and C5 binding to C3
Undefined	C3b, iC3b		EBV	Accelerates the decay of AP C3 convertase cofactor for factor I
VCP	C3b, C4b	35 kDa	Vaccinia	Accelerates the decay of CP and AP convertases cofactor for factor I
gp60/70 gp185	C3d iC3b	60–70 kDa 185 kDa	*Candida albicans*	Possibly involved in virulence by mediating adherence to mammalian cells
CMTp87–93	C3bBb	87–93 kDa	*Trypanosoma cruzi*	Accelerates the decay of AP and CP C3 convertases
gp160	C3b	160 kDa		Accelerates decay of AP C3 convertase
Undefined	C3b	Not characterized	*Schistosoma mansoni*	
Undefined [276]	C3b	Not characterized	*Babesia rhodhani*	

Other proteins

Conglutinin	iC3b	300 kDa		Physiological role unknown
Undefined [257]	C3	26 kDa		Inhibits C3 activation
Fibronectin [277]	C3c, C3d	250 kDa α chain 250 kDa β chain	Extracellular matrix	
Interleukin 2 [278]	C3b, C3c			Modulates proliferation of helper T cells
ProMBP [258]	C3dg	50–90 kDa	Eosinophilic leukocytes	
Laminin [279]	C3d	400 kDa α chain (2) 225 kDa β chains	Extracellular matrix	

CP, classic pathway; AP, alternative pathway; RAC, regulators of complement activation.

tic responses of monocytes (190,191). More convincing studies have recently showed that C4a failed to inhibit C3a binding to guinea-pig macrophages and C4a desensitized guinea-pig macrophages still responded to C3a-induced Ca^{2+} mobilization (192). Now that the C3a receptor has been cloned, this issue will soon be resolved.

B. C3b/C4b Receptor (CR1, CD35)

The complement receptor type one, CR1, is a 220 kDa protein containing 30 SCRs and is present on the cell surface of a wide variety of circulating cells (Table 1) exhibiting an unusual genetic polymorphism with four allotypes having molecular masses of 160 (C form), 190 (A), 220 (B), and 250 (D) kDa. CR1 serves as a receptor for C3b and C4b, and also for iC3b and C3c but with lower affinity. Dimeric C3b binds with a higher affinity than monovalent C3b, suggesting that multivalency of surface-bound C3b may be physiologically important in CR1-mediated functions. Previous studies shown that the CR1-binding site in C3 is localized within the 42 N-terminal amino acids of the α′-chain of C3b at residues 727–768 (Fig. 2) (193). Recently, utilizing chimeric C3 molecules, it has been found that CR1 binds to at least two sites on C3 and the major CR1 binding site are located within residues 727–768 (27). The binding site of CR1 on C4 has not yet been localized. The biological effects arising as a consequence of interaction of CR1 with either C3b or C4b are diverse. This interaction leads to the inhibition of complement activation, either by decay of the C3 convertase of both complement pathways or by acting as a cofactor for the factor I-mediated cleavage of C3b or C4b; the processing of immune complexes; the promotion of binding and phagocytosis of C3b- and C4b-coated particles by phagocytic cells (see chapter 12, this volume).

C. C3d/EBV Receptor (CR2, CD21)

Complement receptor type two, CR2, is a 140 kDa glycoprotein expressed on B cells, some T cells, and follicular dendritic cells (194–197). It binds to iC3b, C3dg, and C3d fragments of C3 (198), while a low-affinity binding has been reported for C3b (199). One of the binding sites in C3d has been localized to residues 1201–1214 (PGKQLYNVEAT-SYA) (Fig. 2) (200) and is similar to the sequence in a viral envelope protein (gp350) of Epstein-Barr virus (EBV) that mediates binding of EBV to CR2 (201,202). Participation of residues 1199–1210 in CR2 binding was also analyzed by others using a site-directed mutagenesis approach (203). In this study 8 of 11 residues of this region were mutated, either individually or in a group. Substitution of alanine at positions 1999–1200 (ED), 1203–1204 (KQ), or 1207–1208 (NV) had no effect on binding to CR2, whereas a triple mutant containing substitutions of all six residues, showed a 20% reduction in binding compare to the wild-type C3. These findings suggest that C3d residues other than 1201–1214 are also involved in CR2 binding; however they do not rule out the possible involvement of these residues in CR2 binding. We believe, based on the following data, that residues 1201–1214 and an additional site on C3d, which is yet to be identified, are involved in CR2 binding. First, a synthetic peptide corresponding to this region binds to Raji cells in a CR2-dependent manner (200,204). Second, the CR2-binding site in EBV gp350 is homologous to these residues and mutations in this region of intact EBV gp350 abolish the binding to CR2 (205). Third, a mutant-carrying substitution of six residues (ED, KQ, and NV) with alanine displayed 20% reduction in binding to CR2 (203). Two other sites sharing sequence homology with the CR2 binding site on C3d have been

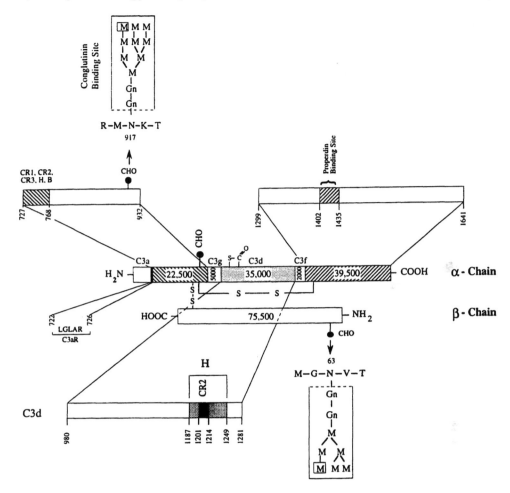

Figure 2 Schematic model of human C3 shows binding sites of different proteins. The molecule consists of an α- and a β-chain, linked by a disulfide bond. The N-linked high-mannose carbohydrates are located at residues 63 (β-chain) and 917 (α-chain) of C3. Binding sites for receptors (CR1, CR2, and CR3), regulatory proteins (H and P), and binding proteins (B and conglutinin) are shown. The numbering of amino acid residues is based on the sequence of human C3 deduced from the cDNA, starting at the N-terminus of the mature protein (8).

identified as residues 295–306 of the β-chain and 744–755 of the α-chain and peptides representing these segments have been found to bind to CR2 (204). The existence of multiple CR2 binding sites in C3 may play a role in CR2 mediated responses (see below).

CR2, in addition to being the receptor for C3d and EBV, also serves as a receptor for interferon α (INFα), an interaction thought to be involved in the antiproliferative effects of this cytokine on B cells (206). The binding site of interferon α for CR2 was localized to a segment of INFα-spanning residues 92–99. The sequence similarity of this region to the CR2 binding sites on C3d and gp350 led to the suggestion that it binds to the same region on CR2 as C3d and EBV (206). The amino acid sequence similarity, however, is low and further work is required to determine the relationship of the CR2-binding site on INFα to those on C3d and EBV.

CR2 has long been implicated in the regulation of B cell responses (see chapter 14, this volume). The valency of the ligand interacting with CR2 appears to be important to the outcome of the response. Thus, polyvalent C3d/C3dg enhances proliferation of activated B cells and this effect can be inhibited by monovalent C3d/C3dg (207,208). Polyvalent, but not monovalent C3dg, is capable of priming human B lymphocytes for anti-IgM induced proliferation, and polyvalent CR2-ligands increase the anti-IgM-induced B cell intracytoplasmic Ca^{2+} influx, whereas monovalent ligands have an opposite effect (209,210). B cell activation via CR2 has been associated with phosphorylation and increased expression of the receptor, as well as its translocation to the nucleus (211–213). CR2 has been shown to be associated with CD19 (214) and treatment of B cells with anti-CD19 antibodies leads to activation of both a protein tyrosine kinase and a phospholipase C (215). In addition to the CR2/CD19 complex, CR2 also associates with CR1, forming a complex that may assist B-cell activation by capturing and maintaining C3b/iC3b-containing antigens (216).

In relation to CR2-mediated responses, it is interesting to note the in vivo experiments in which it was found that either anti-CR2 antibodies or recombinant CR2-IgG1 molecules suppressed antibody responses to T-cell-dependent and independent antigens (217–219). Of utmost importance was the recent study of Dempsey et al. (220), which clearly showed that antigen coupled to C3d molecule(s) enhanced the antibody production to the coupled antigen; in other words, C3d can act as a "natural adjuvant." These data suggest that agents that inhibit the interaction of CR2 with its ligand(s) may be used as immunosuppressants.

D. iC3b Receptor (CR3, CD11b/CD18)

CR3 is a two-chain molecule with a 170 kDa α-chain and a 95 kDa β-chain that binds to iC3b in a divalent cation dependent manner and assists in opsonization and phagocytosis of foreign substances. Unlike CR1 and CR2, CR3 does not contain CCP modules, but is a member of a family of proteins with unique α-chains and noncovalently associated identical β-chain. These proteins are classified as the leukocyte integrins (221) and are characterized by the presence of the Arg-Gly-Asp (RGD) sequence within the ligand binding site. The presence of these residues (1393–1395) in human C3 led to the speculation that RGD (222) is involved in iC3b–CR3 interaction. Using synthetic peptides, the CR3-binding site within iC3b was localized to a 21 amino acid segment spanning residues 1361–1381 of C3 and containing an RGD sequence (222). The ability of *Xenopus* C3b/iC3b to bind to *Xenopus* macrophages (223) despite the absence of RGD sequence in *Xenopus* C3 (224) raised questions about the importance of this sequence in CR3 interaction (225). Experiments involving site-directed mutagenesis have confirmed the hypothesis that RGD is not involved in CR3 binding, and in addition showed that none of the residues within the segment 1361–1381 are involved in this binding (226). Further study demonstrated that the N-terminus of the α'-chain of C3b, which encompasses charged residues 730–731 (DE) and 736–737 (EE), are involved in this interaction (227). We and others have shown that a weak but specific interaction occurs between CR3 and C3d-coated erythrocytes (198,228). This suggests that although C3d may not be the only region involved in CR3 binding, it contributes to this interaction.

E. p150/95 (CR4, CD11c/CD18)

The p150/95 glycoprotein, also a member of the family of leukocyte integrins, is expressed on myeloid cells and on some activated lymphocytes (Table 1). It binds iC3b in a divalent cation-dependent manner (229,230). The binding of purified p150,95 to iC3b-coated erythrocytes is blocked by I-domain-specific mAb, indicating that the I-domain of the p150,95 α subunit mediates the binding. The physiological role of p150/95 is not yet clear but it appears to have similar properties to CR3.

F. Decay-Accelerating Factor (CD55) and Membrane Cofactor Protein (CD46)

The complement regulatory proteins, decay-accelerating factor (DAF), and membrane cofactor protein (MCP) are structurally similar and both protect host tissues from complement-mediated damage by downregulating complement activation (reviewed in ref. 231 see also chapter 7, this volume). DAF is a 75 kDa integral membrane glycoprotein with many oligosaccharide side chains, present on virtually all blood cells, where it inactivates convertases of both pathways. DAF becomes anchored to the cell membrane via a covalent linkage with a glycosyl-phosphatidyl inositol and may be involved in signal transduction. A soluble form of DAF is also present in plasma, urine, and other body fluids (232). DAF is differentiated from other complement regulatory proteins in that it does not serve as a cofactor for I. The amino acid sequence of DAF deduced from the cDNA depicts a protein composed of 4 CCP modules with a 24 amino acid terminal segment of markedly hydrophobic character, serving as a membrane anchor (231). MCP is a single-chain glycoprotein ranging in size from 45 to 70 kDa, depending on the degree of glycosylation (231). Present on the same cell types as DAF (except erythrocytes), MCP differs in that it serves as a cofactor for factor I mediated cleavage of C3b and C4b deposited on self-tissue, but does not accelerate decay of convertases. Four different isoforms were identified in humans (233,234). Study on the interaction of MCP with C3 showed that the first and second factor I-mediated cleavages of C3b can occur in its presence. However, unlike CR1 and factor H, it does not support the conversion of iC3b to C3c and C3d (27). This study also showed that the N-terminus of α′-chain of C3 (727–768) that is involved in the binding of factor H and CR1 is not involved in MCP binding (27). This conclusion was based on two experiments. First, the truncated inactivated C3 molecule devoid of residues 727–768 lost its ability to be cleaved by factor I with CR1 or factor H as cofactors, although no significant change was observed in the cofactor activity of MCP. Second was the absence of any effect of anti-C3[727–768] on the MCP cofactor activity. Whether MCP binds to a single or to a multiple binding sites of C3 is unclear at present.

VI. INTERACTION OF C3, C4 AND C5 WITH SOLUBLE COMPLEMENT PROTEINS

A. Factor I

Factor I is a 88 kDa serine protease that circulates in activated form. Among the different downregulators of complement activation at the C3 level, factor I is the only protein with enzymatic activity. It functions by inactivating C3b and C4b in the presence of different cofactor molecules (see above). The generated iC3b/C4c cannot participate in complement activation due to their inability to bind to factor B or C2, respectively. Although direct binding of factor I to C3b has not been shown, it was found that such interaction occurs and is necessary in order for factor I to expose its active site (33).

B. Factor B

Factor B is a single-chain 93 kDa serine protease serving as the catalytic subunit of the C3/C5 convertases in the alternative pathway. It contains five domains, three CCP modules at the N-terminus, a type A von Willebrand factor module (VWFA), and trypsin-like serine protease domain at the C-terminus. Binding of B to C3b involves multiple sites on the factor B molecule including the Ba and Bb fragments (235). One binding site for factor B was shown to be located in the NH2-terminus of the α'-chain of C3 (236,241), while another has been proposed to be located in a region spanning residues 933–942 of C3 (237). This proposal is supported by data showing that mAbs from both the C3c and C3d domains inhibit factor B binding to C3b (238,239). Taniguchi-Sidel and Isenman (227) have used site-directed mutagenesis to show that mutation of residues [736]EE and, to lesser extent, residues [730]DE to the isosteric amides diminishes significantly the binding and modulation of factor B, thus suggesting that these segments are involved in B binding to C3b. However, experiments showing that chimeric C3 molecules, in which residues [736]EE were substituted by DS or YMRSS, supported the cleavage of factor B by factor D suggested that residues other than [736]EE must also contribute to this interaction. Furthermore, deletion of residues 727–768 of C3 renders the molecule nonfunctional in terms of factor B cleavage, suggesting that this segment of C3 is somehow involved in factor B binding. In view of the finding that anti-CVF[728–771] reacted with the Hu/Tr and Hu/Xe chimeric C3 molecules (residues 727–768 of human C3 were replaced by the corresponding segment of trout or *Xenopus* C3, respectively) but not with the *Xenopus* or trout C3, it appears that the folding of the C3 molecule within the segment spanning residues 727–768 is influenced by residues outside this segment (27). Thus, additional data are needed to clarify if residues within 727–768 are directly or indirectly involved in factor B binding.

C. Factor H

Factor H is a single-chain serum glycoprotein composed of 20 CCP modules. It downregulates amplification of the alternative pathway by binding either to surface-bound or to fluid-phase C3b and accelerating the decay of the C3b,Bb convertase or acting as a cofactor for factor I. The factor H-binding site in C3 was found to be a discontinuous one, comprised of amino acids present in a segment spanning residues 1199–1274 of the C3 sequence, which also encompasses the CR2-binding site (240). Additional sites of interaction in C3 for H have been found within the CR1-binding site (241,27) and suggest that these two molecules share binding sites (both molecules are factor I cofactors). However, the findings that human CR1, but not H, bind to *Xenopus* iC3, and that H, but not CR1, interacts with Trout iC3 suggest that, although these three molecules recognize the same domains in human C3, their exact binding sites are different (242). The inability of human factor B to bind to either *Xenopus* or trout C3 (242) likewise suggests that its binding site on human C3b is different from that for H and CR1. Thus, the ability of H and CR1 to compete with B for binding to C3b may be due to an allosteric or steric effect and not to competition for the same binding site. Because CR1, factor B, and factor H appear to bind to distinct sites in C3, it was hypothesized that there may be multiple sites of interaction in C3 for these molecules and that some of these sites may be common for some of the molecules (27). Such a hypothesis would explain the ability of these molecules to compete for binding to C3b. In addition, it would also explain previous reports describing the following: that Abs from the C3c and C3d region inhibit binding of CR1, factor H, and factor B to C3b (236,238,243–245); that two sites exist in CR1 and factor B for binding to C3b (239); and that the extent of C3b binding to various ligands is higher than that of C3c and/or C3d (246).

D. C4 Binding Protein (C4bp)

C4bp is a serum protein that regulates the formation of the classical pathway C3 convertase by serving as a cofactor in the inactivation of C4b by factor I. It is expressed as a family of three isoforms (247,248). The major isoform contains seven α-chains (70 kDa) and one β-chain (45 kDa), which are linked by disulfide linkages to form a spiderlike structure. The two other isoforms are $\alpha 7\beta 0$ and $\alpha 6\beta 1$. C4bp, like its functional analogue in the alternative pathway, factor H, contains the consensus repeating units (CCP) found in other C3b-binding proteins (249). Although C4bp's principal role is in the classical pathway, it has been shown to bind C3b and serve as a cofactor for the factor I cleavage of C3b. However, approximately five times more C4bp than H is needed to cleave fluid phase C3b and C4bp showed no cofactor activity when C3b was surface bound. The physiological significance of C4bp participating in the alternative pathway is unknown.

E. Properdin

The plasma glycoprotein properdin is not required for activation, but allows rapid amplification of surface-bound C3b by stabilizing the C3b,Bb convertase. The localization of the properdin-binding site in C3b was greatly assisted by the phylogenetic analysis of C3. Originally, properdin was shown to bind both C3b and C3c (250) and subsequent studies placed the properdin binding site within residues 1385–1541 of C3 (251). Comparison of the amino acid sequences of human, mouse, and rabbit C3 (properdin-binding proteins) with those sequences from human and mouse C4, C5, and α_2-macroglobulin (homologous but non-properdin-binding proteins) identified a region, residues 1402–1435 of the human C3 sequence, that was conserved and therefore a possible candidate for the properdin-binding site. A synthetic peptide (C3$^{1402-1435}$) corresponding to this segment of C3 was shown to bind properdin, inhibit properdin binding to C3, and inhibit the activation of the alternative pathway by rabbit erythrocytes (252). These results showed conclusively that properdin stabilization of the C3 convertase is necessary for efficient amplification of the enzyme cascade during complement activation and is in agreement with studies on patients with properdin deficiency showing that properdin is essential for optimal complement activation (253).

VII. INTERACTION OF C3, C4, AND C5 WITH OTHER SOLUBLE PROTEINS

The lectin conglutinin is a 300 kDa collagen-like plasma protein that binds to iC3b in a Ca^{2+} dependent manner (254). The binding specificity of conglutinin is for terminal N-acetylglucosamine, mannose, and fucose residues (255). Although the physiological role of the iC3b–conglutinin interaction is not known, binding studies have identified the conglutinin-binding site on C3 as the carbohydrate moiety attached to Asn^{917} (256). Another protein that binds to C3 and inhibits C3 activation was isolated from a rabbit bronchoalveolar lavage (257). It runs as a 26 kDa protein on sodium dodecyl sulfate (SDS) polyacrylamide gels. Detailed characterization of this protein should enable us to find out if it is a cleaved fragment of complement receptor or a new protein. Recently it has been discovered that C3dg forms a complex with the proform of eosinophil major basic protein (proMBP) and angiotensinogen (258). The physiological importance of this finding is not clear at present.

VIII. INTERACTION OF C3, C4, AND C5 WITH BINDING PROTEINS OF FOREIGN ORIGIN

A variety of pathogens express C3-binding capabilities (Table 1), which, through different mechanisms, allow them to evade complement-mediated destruction (for review see 259, 260 and chapter 18, this volume). Members of the herpes family of viruses code for proteins that become expressed on the cell membrane of infected cells and act as receptors for C3b. Two types of herpes simplex virus (HSV-1 and HSV-2) produce homologous glycoproteins, (gC-1 and gC-2) that protect against complement-mediated neutralization (261–263). Decay-accelerating activity, specific for the convertase of the alternative pathway is expressed by gC-1, but not gC-2, which appears to stabilize this convertase (264). It was likewise found that gC-1, but not gC-2, can destabilize the C3 convertase by inhibiting the binding of properdin to C3b. In contrast to gC-2, gC-1 also blocks C5 binding to C3b (265,266). EBV is another herpes virus that experiences proteins that downregulate complement activation, but in contrast to HSV, EBV expresses both cofactor activity for factor I and decay-accelerating activity for the alternative pathway convertase (267). A complement-regulating protein has also been identified in vaccinia. Vaccinia virus complement control protein (VCP) is a major protein secreted by cells infected with vaccinia virus. It contains four CCP modules, which show homology to the C4-binding protein (268). Binding of VCP to C3b or C4b results in decay of the classical and alternative pathway C3 convertases, respectively (269). It also acts as a cofactor in the proteolytic inactivation of C4b and C3b by factor I. In contrast to factor H and CR1, which display cofactor activity in factor I-mediated cleavage of C3b resulting in cleavage of the α-chain between Arg^{1281}–Ser^{1282} (generating $iC3b_1$), Arg^{1298}–Ser^{1299} (generating $iC3b_2$) and Arg^{932}–Glu^{933} (generating C3c and C3dg), VCP displayed cofactor activity primarily for site 1, leading to generation of $iC3b_1$.

Several proteins expressed by the protozoan *Trypanosoma cruzi* inhibit complement activation by possessing decay-accelerating activity for both classical and alternative pathways (270), or only for the alternative pathway convertase (271). Molecules present on the pseudohyphae of the fungus, *Candida albicans* bind to iC3b and C3d fragments of C3 (272,273), although, in contrast to binding of other pathogens to C3 fragments, these molecules do not protect the organism from complement-mediated destruction but may play a role in virulence by mediating adherence to mammalian cells (274).

REFERENCES

1. Sottrup-Jensen L, Stepanik TM, Kristensen T, Lonbald PB, Jones CM, Wierzbicki DM, Magnusson S, Domdey H, Wetsel RA, Lundwall A. Common evolutionary origin of alpha

2-macroglobulin and complement components C3 and C4. Proc Natl Acad Sci USA 1985; 82:9–13.

2. Perkins SJ, Sim RB. Molecular modelling of human complement component C3 and its fragments by solution scattering. Eur J Biochem 1986; 157:155–168.

3. Perkins SJ, Nealis A, Sim RB. Molecular modeling of human complement C4 and its fragments by x-ray and neutron solution scattering. Biochemistry 1990; 29:1167–1175.

4. Perkins SJ, Smith KF, Nealis AS, Lachmann PJ, Harrison RA. Structural homologies of component C5 of human complement with components C3 and C4 by neutron scattering. Biochemistry 1990; 29:1175–1180.

5. Lambris JD, Mavroidis M, Sunyer JO. Phylogeny of third component of complement, C3. In: Erdei A, ed. New Aspects of Complement Structure and Function. Austin: R.G. Landes Co., 1994:15–34.

6. Sunyer JO, Zarkadis IK, Sahu A, Lambris JD. Multiple forms of complement C3 in trout that differ in binding to complement activators. Proc Natl Acad Sci USA 1996.

7. Smith LC, Chang L, Britten RJ, et al: Sea urchin genes experessed in activated coelomocytes are identified by expressed sequence tags. J Immunol 1996; 156:593–602.

8. De Bruijn MHL, Fey GH. Human complement component C3: cDNA coding sequence and derived primary structure. Proc Natl Acad Sci USA 1985; 82:708–712.

9. Huber R, Scholze H, Paques EP, Deisenhofer J. Crystal structure analysis and molecular model of human C3a anaphylatoxin. Hoppe-Seylers Z Physiol Chem 1980; 361:1389–1399.

10. Dolmer K, Sottrupjensen L. Disulfide bridges in human complement component C3b. FEBS Lett 1993; 315:85–90.

11. Dolmer K, Thirup S, Andersen GR, Sottrup-Jensen L, Nyborg J. Crystallization of human methylamine-treated complement C3 and C3b. Acta Cryst 1994; D50:786–789.

12. Andersen GR, Koch TJ, Dolmer K, Sottrup-Jensen L, Nyborg J. Low resolution x-ray structure of human methylamine-treated α_2-macroglobulin. J Biol Chem 1995; 270:25133–25141.

13. Hase S, Kikuchi N, Ikenaka T, Inoue K. Structures of sugar chains of the third component of human complement. J Biochem (Tokyo) 1985; 98:863–874.

14. Hirani S, Lambris JD, Muller-Eberhard HJ. Structural analysis of the asparagine-linked oligosaccharides of human complement component C3. Biochem J 1986; 233:613–616.

15. Müller-Eberhard HJ, Dalmasso AP, Calcott MA. The reaction mechanism of β1c-globulin (C'3) in immune hemolysis. J Exp Med 1966; 123:33–54.

16. Law SK, Lichtenberg NA, Levine RP. Evidence for an ester linkage between the labile binding site of C3b and receptive surfaces. J Immunol 1979; 123:1388

17. Levine RP, Dodds AW. The thiolester bond of C3. Curr Top Microbiol Immunol 1990; 153:73–82.

18. Sahu A, Kozel TR, Pangburn MK. Specificity of the thioester-containing reactive site of human C3 and its significance to complement activation. Biochem J 1994; 302:429–436.

19. Sahu A, Pangburn MK. Covalent attachment of human complement C3 to IgG: identification of the amino acid residue involved in ester linkage formation. J Biol Chem 1994; 269:28997–29002.

20. Sahu A, Pangburn MK. Tyrosine is a potential site for covalent attachment of activated commplement component C3. Mol Immunol 1995; 32:711–716.

21. Sahu A, Pangburn MK. Investigation of mechanism-based inhibitors of complement targeting the activated thioester of human C3. Biochem Pharmacol 1996; 51:797–804.

22. Kim YU, Carroll MC, Isenman DE, Nonaka M, Pramoonjago P, Takeda J, Inoue K, Kinoshita T. Covalent binding of C3b to C4b within the classical complement pathway C5 convertase: determination of amino acid residues involved in ester linkage formation. J Biol Chem 1992; 267:4171–4176.

23. Kinoshita T, Takata Y, Kozono H, Takeda J, Hong K, Inoue K. C5 convertase of the alternative complement pathway: covalent linkage between two C3b molecules within the trimolecular complex enzyme. J Immunol 1988; 141:3895–3901.

24. Lambris JD. The multifunctional role of C3, the third component of complement. Immunol Today 1988; 9:387–393.

25. Davis AEI, Harrison RA, Lachmann PJ. Physiologic inactivation of fluid phase C3b: isolation and structural analysis of C3c, C3d,g, ($\beta\alpha\beta_2$D), and C3g. J Immunol 1984; 132:1960–1966.

26. Lambris JD. Chemistry, biology and phylogeny of C3. Complt Profiles 1993; 1:16–45.

27. Lambris JD, Lao Z, Oglesby TJ, Atkinson JP, Hack E, Becherer JD. Dissection of CR1, factor H, MCP, and factor B binding and functional sites in third complement component. J Immunol 1996; 156:4821–4832.

28. Ross GD, Lambris JD, Cain JA, Newman SL. Generation of three different fragments of bound C3 with purified factor I or serum. I. Requirements for factor H vs CR1 cofactor activity. J Immunol 1982; 129:2051–2060.

29. Medicus RG, Melamed J, Arnaout MA. Role of human factor I and C3b receptor in the cleavage of surface-bound C3b. Eur J Immunol 1983; 13:465–470.

30. Davis AE III, Harrison RA. Structural characterization of factor I mediated cleavage of the third component of complement. Biochemistry 1982; 21:5745–5749.

31. Medof ME, Iida K, Mold C, Nussenzweig V. Unique role of the complement receptor CR1 in the degradation of C3b associated with immune complexes. J Exp Med 1982; 156:1739–1754.

32. Sahu A, Isaacs S, Lambris JD. Modulation of complement by recombinant vaccinia virus complement control protein (abst). Mol Immunol 1996; 33:61.

33. Ekdahl KN, Nilsson UR, Nilsson B. Inhibition of factor I by diisopropylfluorophosphate. Evidence of conformational changes in factor I induced by C3b and additional studies on the specificity of factor I. J Immunol 1990; 144:4269–4274.

34. Press EM, Gagnon J. Human complement component C4: structural studies on the fragments derived from C4b by cleavage with C3b inactivator. Biochem J 1981; 199:351–357.

35. Wetsel RA, Lundwall A, Davidson F, Gibson T, Tack BF, Fey GH. Structure of murine complement component C3. II. Nucleotide sequence of cloned complementary DNA coding for the alpha chain. J Biol Chem 1984; 259:13857–13862.

36. Kusano M, Choi NH, Tomita M, Yamamoto K, Migita S, Sekiya T, Nishimura S. Nucleotide sequence of cDNA and derived amino acid sequence of rabbit complement component C3 alpha-chain. Immunol Invest 1986; 15:365–378.

37. Misumi Y, Sohda M, Ikehara Y. Nucleotide and deduced amino acid sequence of rat complement C3. Nucleic Acids Res 1990; 18:365–378.

38. Farries TC, Napper CM, Harrison RA. Factor I-mediated conversion of C3b to iC3b, studied using mutagenesis of C3 (abstr). Mol Immunol 1996; 33:58.

39. Misumi Y, Oda K, Fujiwara T, Takami N, Tashiro K, Ikehara Y. Functional expression of furin demonstrating its intracellular localization and endoprotease activity for processing of proalbumin and complement pro-C3. J Biol Chem 1991; 266:16954–16959.

40. Alper CA, Johnson AM, Birtch AG, Moore FD. Human C′3: evidence for the liver as the primary site of synthesis. Science 1969; 163:286–288.

41. Barnum SR, Fey G, Tack BF. Biosynthesis and genetics of C3. Curr Top Microbiol Immunol 1990; 153:23–38.

42. Sundstrom SA, Komm BS, Ponce-de-Leon H, Yi Z, Teuscher C, Lyttle RC. Estrogen regulation of tissue-specific expression of complement C3. J Biol Chem 1989; 264(28):16941–16947.

43. Hong MH, Jin CH, Sato T, Ishimi Y, Abe E, Suda T. transcriptional regulation of the production of the third component of complement (C3) by 1alpha, 25-dihydroxyvitamin- D3 in mouse marrow-derived stromal cells (ST2) and primary osteoblastic cells. Endocrinology 1991; 129:2774–2779.

44. Whitehead AS, Solomon E, Chambers S, Bodmer WF, Povey S, Fey G. Assignment of the structural gene for the third component of complement to chromosome 19. Proc Natl Acad Sci USA 1982; 79:5021–5025.

45. Barnum SR, Amiguet P, Amiguet-Barret F, Fey G, Tack BF. Complete intron/exon organization of DNA encoding the chain of human C3. J Biol Chem 1989; 264:8471–8474.

46. Vik DP, Amiguet P, Moffat GJ, Fey M, Amiguetbarras F, Wetsel RA, Tack BF. Structural features of the human C3-gene: intron/exon organization, transcriptional start site, and promoter region sequence. Biochemistry 1991; 30:1080–1085.

47. Fong KY, Botto M, Walport MJ, So AK. Genomic organization of human complement component C3. Genomics 1990; 7:579–586.

48. Welch TR, Beischel LS, Witte DP. Differential expression of complement C3 and C4 in the human kidney. J Clin Invest 1993; 92:1451–1458.

49. Colten HR, Alper CA: Hemolytic efficiencies of genetic variants of human C3. J Immunol 1972; 1184–1187.

50. Singer L, Colten HR, Wetsel RA: Complement C3 deficiency: human, animal, and experimental models. In: Cruse JM, ed. Pathobiology. Basel: S. Karger AG, 1994:14–28.

51. Bitter-Suermann D, Burger R. C3 deficiencies. Curr Top Microbiol Immunol 1990; 153:223–233.

52. Ochs HD, Wedgwood RJ, Heller SR, Beatty PG. Complement, membrane glycoproteins, and complement receptors: their role in regulation of the immune response. Clin Immunol Immunopathol 1986; 40:94–104.

52A. Fischer MB, Ma M, Goerg S, Zhou X, Xia J, Finco O, Han S, Kelsoe G, Howard RG, Rothstein TL, Kremmer E, Rosen FS, Carroll MC. Regulation of the B cell response to T-dependent antigens by classical pathway complement. J Immunol 1996; 157:549–556.

53. O'Neil KM, Ochs HD, Heller SR, Cork LC, Morris JM, Winkelstein JA. Role of C3 in humoral immunity defective antibody production in C3-deficient dogs. J Immunol 1988; 140:1939–1945.

54. Botto M, Fong KY, So AK, Rudge A, Walport MJ. Molecular basis of hereditary C3 deficiency. J Clin Invest 1990; 86:1158–1163.

55. Huang JL, Lin CY. A hereditary C3 deficiency due to aberrant splicing of exon 10. Clin Immunol Immunopathol 1994; 73:267–273.

56. Botto M, Fong KY, So AK, Barlow R, Routier R, Morley BJ, Walport MJ. Homozygous hereditary C3 deficiency due to a partial gene deletion. Proc Natl Acad Sci USA 1992; 89:4957–4961.

57. Singer L, Whitehead WT, Akama H, Katz Y, Fishelson Z, Wetsel RA. Inherited human complement C3 deficiency. An amino acid substitution in the β-chain (ASP549 to ASN) impairs C3 secretion. J Biol Chem 1994; 269:28494–28499.

58. Singer L, Kramer J, Borzy MS, Wetsel RA. Inherited complement C3 deficiency: reduced C3 mRNA and protein levels in a Laotian kindred. Clin Immunol Immunopathol. In press.

59. Gigli I, von Zabern I, Porter RR. The isolation and structure of C4, the fourth component of human complement. Biochem J 1977; 165:439–446.

60. Schreiber RD, Muller-Eberhard HJ. Fourth component of human complement: description of a three chain structure. J Exp Med 1974; 140:1324–1335.

61. Seya T, Nagasawa S, Atkinson JP. Location of the interchain disulfide bonds of the fourth component of human complement (C4): evidence based on the liberation of fragments secondary to thiol-disulfide interchange reactions. J Immunol 1986; 136:4152–4156.

62. Chan AC, Atkinson JP. Oligosaccharide structure of human C4. J Immunol 1985; 134:1790–1798.

63. Goldberger G, Colten HR. Precursor complement protein (pro-C4) is converted in vitro to native C4 by plasmin. Nature 1980; 286:514–516.

64. Karp DR. Post-translational modificatin of the fourth component of complement. Sulfation of the alpha chain. J Biol Chem 1983; 258:12745–12748.

65. Belt KT, Carroll MC, Porter RR. The structural basis of the multiple forms of human complement component C4. Cell 1984; 36:907–914.

66. Chan AC, Mitchell KR, Munns TW, Karp DR, Atkinson JP. Identification and partial characterization of the secreted form of the fourth component of human complement. Evidence that it is different from major plasma form. Proc Natl Acad Sci USA 1983; 80:268–272.

67. Roos MH, Kornfeld S, Shreffler DC. Characterization of the oligosaccharide units of the fourth component of complement (Ss protein) synthesized by murine macrophages. J Immunol 1980; 124:2860–2861.

68. Morris KM, Aden DP, Knowles BB, Colten HR. Complement biosynthesis by the human hepatoma-derived cell line HepG2. J Clin Invest 1982; 70:906–913.

69. Morris KM, Goldberger G, Colten HR, Aden DP, Knowles BB. Biosynthesis and processing of a human presursor complement protein, pro-C3, in a hepatoma-derived cell line. Science 1982; 215:399–400.

70. Smith CA, Vogel CW, Müller-Eberhard HJ. MHC Class III products: an electron microscopic study of the C3 convertases of human complement. J Exp Med 1984; 159:324–329.

71. Janatova J, Tack BF. Fourth component of human complement: studies of an amine-sensitive site comprised of a thiol component. Biochemistry 1981; 20:2394–2402.

72. Pangburn MK. Spontaneous thioester bond formation in alpha 2-macroglobulin, C3 and C4. FEBS Lett 1992; 308:280–282.

73. Isenman DE, Young JR. The molecular basis for the difference in immune hemolysis activity of the Chido and Rodgers isotypes of human complement component C4. J Immunol 1984; 132:3019–3027.

74. Law SKA, Dodds AW, Porter RR. A comparison of the properties of two classes, C4A and C4B, of the human complement component C4. EMBO J 1984; 3:1819–1823.

75. Carroll MC, Fathallah DM, Bergamaschini L, Alicot EM, Isenman DE. Substitution of a single amino acid (aspartic acid for histidine) converts the functional activity of human complement C4B to C4A. Proc Natl Acad Sci USA 1990; 87:6868–6872.

76. Dodds AW, Ren XD, Willis AC, Law ASK. The reaction mechanism of the internal thioester in the human complement component C4. Nature 1996; 379:177–179.

77. Yu CY, Campbell RD, Porter RR. A structural model for the Rodgers and the Chido antigenic determinants and their correlation with the human complement C4A/C4B isotypes. Immunogenetics 1988; 27:399–405.

78. Giles CM. Antigenic determinants of human C4, Rodgers and Chido (abstr). Exp Clin Immunogenet 1988; 5:99–144.

79. Gorski JP, Muller-Eberhard HJ. Enhancement of C3 convertase activity by antibody to β-chain of C4. J Immunol 1980; 124:1523.

80. Isenman DE, Kells DIC. Conformational and functional changes in the fourth component of human complement produced by nucleophilic modification and by proteolysis with C1s. Biochemistry 1982; 21:1109–1117.

81. Kerr MA. The human complement system: assembly of the classical pathway C3 convertase. Biochem J 1980; 189:173–181.

82. Muller-Eberhard HJ, Polley MJ, Calcott RM. Formation and functional significance of a molecular complex derived from the second and the fourth component of human complement. J Exp Med 1967; 125:359–380.

83. Kinoshita T, Takata Y, Kozono H, Takeda J, Hong K, Inoue K. C5 convertase of the alternative complement pathway: covalent linkage between two C3b molecules within the trimolecular complex enzyme. J Immunol 1988; 141:3895–3901.

84. Ebanks RO, Isenman DE. Evidence for the involvement of arginine 462 and the flanking sequence of human C4 beta-chain in mediating C5 binding to the C4b subcomponent of the classical complement pathway C5 convertase. J Immunol 1995; 154:2808–2820.

85. von Zabern I, Bloom EL, Chu V, Gigli I. The fourth component of human complement treated with amines or chaotropes or frozen-thawed (C4b-Like C4): interaction with C4 binding protein and cleavage by C3b/C4b inactivator. J Immunol 1982; 128:1433–1438.

86. Kinoshita T, Medof ME, Hong K, Nussenzweig V. Membrane-bound C4b interacts endogenously with complement receptor CR1 of human red cells. J Exp Med 1986; 164:1377–1388.

87. Seya T, Turner JR, Atkinson JP. Purification and characterization of a membrane protein (gp45-70) that is a cofactor for cleavage of C3b and C4b. J Exp Med 1986; 163:837–855.

88. Cox J, Robins DM. Tissue-specific variation in C4 and C4-Spl gene regulation. Nucleic Acids Res 1988; 16:6857–6870.

89. Johansson BG, Kindmark CO, Trell EY, Wollheim FA. Sequencial changes of plasma proteins after myocardial infraction. Scand J Clin Lab Invest 1972; 27:117–126.

90. Colten HR. Tissue-specific regulation of inflammation. J Appl Physiol 1992; 72:1–7.

91. Passwell J, Schreiner GF, Nonaka M, Beuscher HU, Colten HR. Local extrahepatic expression of complement genes C3, factor B, C2, and C4 is increased in murine lupus nephritis. J Clin Invest 1988; 82:1676–1684.

92. Wessels MR, Butko P, Ma M, Warren HB, Lage AL, Carroll MC. Studies of group B streptococcal infection in mice deficient in complement component C3 or C4 demonstrate an essential role for complement in both innate and acquired immunity. Proc Natl Acad Sci USA 1995; 92:11490–11494.

93. Carroll MC, Campbell RD, Bentley DR, Porter RR. A molecular map of the human major histocompatibility complex class III region linking complement genes C4, C2 and factor B. Nature 1984; 307:237–241.

94. Dunham I, Sargent CA, Trowsdale J, Campbell RD. Molecular mapping of the human major histocompatibility complex by pulsed-field gel electrophoresis. Proc Natl Acad Sci USA 1987; 84:7237–7241.

95. Spies T, Morton CC, Nedospasov SA, Fiers W, Pious D, Strominger J. Genes for the tumor necrosis factor α and β are linked to the human major histocompatibility complex. Proc Natl Acad Sci USA 1986; 83:8699–8702.

96. Sargent CA, Dunham I, Trowsdale J, Campbell RD. Human major histocompatibility complex contains genes for the major heat shok protein HSP 70. Proc Natl Acad Sci USA 1989; 1968–1972.

97. Amor M, Tosi M, Duponchel C, Steinmetz M, Meo T. Liver cDNA probes disclose two cytochrome P450 genes duplicated in tandem with the complement C4 loci of the mouse H-2S region. Proc Natl Acad Sci USA 1985; 82:4453–4457.

98. Skow LE, Womack JE, Petresh JM, Miller WL. Synteny mapping of the genes for steroid 21-hydroxylase, alpha-A-crystallin, and class I bovine leucocyte (BoLA) in cattle. DNA 1988; 7:143–149.

99. Yu CY. The complete exon–intron structure of a human complement component C4A Gene: DNA sequences, polymorphism, and linkage to the 21-hydroxylase gene. J Immunol 1991; 146:1057–1066.

100. Ulgiati D, Townend DC, Christiansen FT, Dawkins RL, Abraham LJ. Complete sequence of the complement C4 gene from the HLA-A1, B8, C4AQO, C4B1, DR3 haplotype. Immunogenetics 1996; 43:250–252.

101. Schneider PM, Carroll MC, Alper CA, Rittner C, Whitehead AS, Yunis EJ, Colten HR. Polymorphism of human complement C4 and steroid 21-hydroxylase genes: restriction fragment length polymorphism revealing structural deletions, homoduplications, and size variants. J Clin Invest 1986; 78:650–657.

102. Barba G, Rittner C, Schneider PM. Genetic basis of human complement C4A deficiency: detection of a point mutation leading to nonexpression. J Clin Invest 1993; 91:1681–1686.

103. Vaishnaw AK, Hargreaves R, Campbell RD, Morley BJ, Walport MJ. DNase I hypersensitivity mapping and promoter polymorphism analysis of human C4. Immunogenetics 1995; 41:354–358.

104. Wetsel RA, Jones MA, Kolb WP. Immunoadsorbent affinity purification of the fifth component (C5) of human complement and development of a highly sensitive hemolytic assay. J Immunol Methods 1980; 35:319–335.

105. Kunkel SL, Kreutzer DL, Goralnick S, Ward PA. Purification of the third and fifth components of human complement: application of hydrophobic chromatography. J Immunol Methods 1980; 35:337–351.

106. Hammer CH, Wirtz GH, Renfer L, Gresham HD, Tack BF. Large scale isolation of functionally active components of the human complement system. J Biol Chem 1981; 256:3995–4006.

107. Nilsson UR, Mandle RJ, McConnell-Mapes JA: Human C3 and C5: subunit structure and modification by trypsin and C42-C423. J Immunol 1975; 114:815–822.

108. Tack BF, Morris SC, Prahl JW. Fifth component of human complement: purification from plasma and polypeptide chain structure. Biochemistry 1979; 18:1490–1497.

109. Minta JO, Ngan BY, Pang AS. Purification and characterization of a single chain precursor C3-protein (pro-C3) from normal human plasma. J Immunol 1979; 123:2415–2420.

110. Ooi YM, Colten HR. Biosynthesis and post-synthetic modification of a precursor (pro-C5) of the fifth component of mouse complement (C5). J Immunol 1979; 123:2494–2498.

111. Ooi YM, Harris DE, Edelson PJ, Colten HR. Post-translational control of complement (C5) production by resident and stimulated mouse macrophages. J Immunol 1980; 124:2077–2081

112. Wetsel RA, Lemons RS, Le Beau MM, Barnum SR, Noack D, Tack BF. Molecular analysis of human complement component C5: localization of the structural gene to chromosome 9. Biochemistry 1988; 27:1474–1482.

113. Wetsel RA, Ogata RT, Tack BF. Primary structure of the fifth component of murine complement. Biochemistry 1987; 26:737–743.

114. Wetsel RA, Fleischer DT, Haviland DL. Deficiency of the murine fifth complement component (C5). A 2-base pair gene deletion in a 5'-exon. J Biol Chem 1990; 265:2435–2440.

115. Haviland DL, Haviland JC, Fleischer DT, Hunt A, Wetsel RA. Complete cDNA sequence of human complement pro-C5. Evidence of truncated transcripts derived from a single copy gene. J Immunol 1991; 146:362–368.

116. Tomana M, Niemann M, Garner C, Volanakis JE. Carbohydrate composition of the second, third and fifth components and factors B and D of human complement. Mol Immunol 1985; 22:107–111.

117. DiScipio RG, Smith CA, Müller-Eberhard HJ, Hugli TE. The activation of human complement component C5 by a fluid phase C5 convertase. J Biol Chem 1983; 258:10629–10636.

118. Matsuda T, Seya T, Nagasawa S. Location of the inter-chain disulfide bonds of the third component of human complement. Biochem Biophys Res Commun 1985; 127:264–269.

119. Janatova J. Detection of disulphide bonds and localization of interchain linkages in the third (C3) and the fourth (C4) components of human complement. Biochem J 1986; 233:819–825.

120. Arroyave CM, Muller-Eberhard HJ. Interactions between human C5, C6, and C7 and their functional significance in complement-dependent cytolysis. J Immunol 1973; 111:536–545.

121. Goldlust MB, Shin HS, Hammer CH, Mayer MM. Studies of complement complex C5b,6 eluted from EAC-6: reaction of C5b,6 with EAC4b,3b and evidence on the role of C2a and C3b in the activation of C5. J Immunol 1974; 113:998–1007.

122. Thompson RA, Lachmann PJ. Reactive lysis: the complement-mediated lysis of unsensitized cells. I. The characterization of the indicator factor and its identification as C7. J Exp Med 1970; 131:629–641.

123. Schreiber RD, Pangburn MK, Lesavre PH, Müller-Eberhard HJ. Initiation of the alternative pathway of complement: recognition of activators by bound C3b and assembly of the entire pathway from six isolated proteins. Proc Natl Acad Sci USA 1978; 75:3948–3952.

124. Shin HS, Snyderman R, Friedman E, Mellors A, Mayer MM. Chemotactic and anaphylatoxic fragment cleaved from the fifth component of guinea pig complement. Science 1968; 162:361–363.

125. Ward PA, Newman LJ. A neutrophil chemotactic factor from human C'5. J Immunol 1969; 102:93–99.

126. Kay AB, Shin HS, Austen KF. Selective attraction of eosinophils and synergism between eosinophil chemotactic factor of anaphylaxis (ECF-A) and a fragment cleaved from the fifth component of complement (C5a). Immunology 1973; 24:969–976.

127. Lett-Brown MA, Boetcher DA, Leonard EJ. Chemotactic responses of normal human basophils to C5a and to lymphocyte-derived chemotactic factor. J Immunol 1976; 117:246–252.

128. Hausman MS, Snyderman R, Mergenhagen SE. Humoral mediators of chemotaxis of mononuclear leukocytes. J Infect Dis 1972; 125:595–602.

129. Snyderman R, Shin HS, Hausman MH. A chemotactic factor for mononuclear leukocytes. Proc Soc Exp Biol Med 1971; 138:387–390.

130. Goetzl EJ, Austen KF: Stimulation of neutrophil leucocyte aerobic glucose metabolism by purified chemotactic factors. J Clin Invest 1974; 53:591–599.

131. Gerard C, Hugli TE. Identification of classical anaphylatoxin as the des-Arg form of the C5a molecule: evidence of a modulator role for the oligosaccharide unit in human des-Arg74-C5a. Proc Natl Acad Sci USA 1981; 78:1833–1837.

132. Chenoweth DE, Hugli TE. Human C5a and C5a analogs as probes of the neutrophil C5a receptor. Mol Immunol 1980; 17:151–161.

133. Webster RO, Hong SR, Johnston RB Jr, Henson PM. Biological effects of the human complement fragments C5a and C5ades Arg on neutrophil function. Immunopharmacology 1980; 2:201–219.

134. Perez HD, Goldstein IM, Chernoff D, Webster RO, Henson PM. Chemotactic activity of C5ades Arg: evidence of a requirement for an anionic peptide 'helper factor' and inhibition by a cationic protein in serum from patients with systemic lupus erythematosus. Mol Immunol 1980; 17:163–169.

135. Perez HD, Goldstein IM, Webster RO, Henson PM. Enhancement of the chemotactic activity of human C5a des arg by an anionic polypeptide ("cochemotaxin") in normal human serum and plasma. J Immunol 1981; 126:800–804.

136. Gerard C, Chenoweth DE, Hugli TE. Response of human neutrophils to C5a: a role for the oligosaccharide moiety of human C5ades Arg-74 but not of C5a in biologic activity. J Immunol 1981; 127:1978–1982.

137. Goldstein IM, Hoffstein S, Gallin J, Weissmann G. Mechanisms of lysosomal enzyme release from human leukocytes: microtubule assembly and membrane fusion induced by a component of complement. Proc Natl Acad Sci USA 1973; 70:2916–2920.

138. Phan SH, Ward PA. Generation of biologic activity from the purified alpha-chain of C5. J Immunol 1979; 123:2735–2740.

139. Hugli TE. Complement factors and inflammation: effects of α-thrombin on components C3 and C5. In: Lundblad RL, Fenton JW, Mann KG, eds. Chemistry and Biology of Thrombin. Ann Arbor, MI: Ann Arbor Sciences, 1977:345–360.

140. Brozna JP, Senior RM, Kreutzer DL, Ward PA. Chemotactic factor inactivators of human granulocytes. J Clin Invest 1977; 60:1280–1288.

141. Ward PA, Kreutzer DL, Senior RM. The modulation of leukotaxis by neutral proteases and other factors from neutrophils. In: Havemann K, Janoff A, eds. Neutral Proteases of Human Polymorphonuclear Leukocytes. Baltimore, MD: Urban and Schwarzenberg, 1978:279–286.

142. Cochrane CG, Müller-Eberhard HJ. The derivation of two distinct anaphylatoxins activities from the third and fifth components of complement. J Exp Med 1968; 127:371–386.

143. Goldstein IM, Brai M, Osler AG, Weissmann G. Lysosomal enzyme release from human leukocytes: mediation by the alternate pathway of complement activation. J Immunol 1973; 111:33–37.

144. Minta JO, Man DP. Cleavage of human C5 by trypsin: characterization of the digestion products by gel electrophoresis. J Immunol 1977; 119:1597–1602.

145. Wetsel RA, Kolb WP. Complement-independent activation of the fifth component (C5) of human complement: limited trypsin digestion resulting in the expression of biological activity. J Immunol 1982; 128:2209–2216.

146. Wetsel RA, Kolb WP. Expression of C5a-like biological activities by the fifth component of human complement (C5) upon limited digestion with noncomplement enzymes without release of polypeptide fragments. J Exp Med 1983; 157:2029–2048.

147. Al Salihi A, Ripoche J, Fontaine M. Localization of a hydrophobic domain in human C5. Mol Immunol 1988; 25:367–377.

148. Groffen J, Stephenson JR, Heisterkamp N, Bartram C, de Klein AG, G. The human c-abl oncogene in the Philadelphia translocation. J Cell Physiol (Suppl) 1984; 3:179–191.

149. Jhanwar SC, Neel BG, Hayward WS, Chaganti RS. Localization of the cellular oncogenes ABL, SIS, and FES on human germ-line chromosomes. Cytogenet Cell Genet 1984; 38:73–75.

150. Westbrook CA, Le Beau MM, Diaz MO, Groffen J, Rowley JD. Chromosomal localization and characterization of c-abl in the t(6;9) of acute nonlymphocytic leukemia. Proc Natl Acad Sci USA 1985; 82:8742–8746.

151. Barton DE, Yang-feng TL, Leto T, Marchesi V, Francke U. NEAS encoding a non-erythroid α-spectrin is on chromosome 9, region q33-q34 and on mouse chromosome 2 (abstr). Cytogenet Cell Genet 1987; 46:578.

152. D'Eustachio P, Kristensen T, Wetsel RA, Riblet R, Taylor BA, Tack BF. Chromosomal location of the genes encoding complement components C5 and factor H in the mouse. J Immunol 1986; 137:3990–3995.

153. Haviland DL, Haviland JC, Fleischer DT, Wetsel RA. Structure of the murine fifth complement component (C5) gene. A large, highly interrupted gene with a variant donor splice site and organizational homology with the third and fourth complement component genes. J Biol Chem 1991; 266:11818–11825.

154. Carney DF, Haviland DL, Noack D, Wetsel RA, Vik DP, Tack BF. Structural aspects of the human C5 gene. Intron/exon organization, 5'-flanking region features, and characterization of two truncated cDNA clones. J Biol Chem 1991; 266:18786–18791.

155. Kohler PF, Muller-Eberhard HJ. Immunochemical quantitation of the third, fourth and fifth components of human complement: concentrations in the serum of healthy adults. J Immunol 1967; 99:1211–1216.

156. Geng L, Iwabuchi K, Sakai S, Ogasawara M, Fujita M, Noguchi M, Good RA, Morikawa K, Onoe K. A study on location of synthetic site which mainly synthesizes and delivers fifth component of complement system in vivo. Microbiol Immunol 1986; 30:1281–1290.

157. Colten HR. Ontogeny of the human complement system: in vitro biosynthesis of individual complement components by fetal tissues. J Clin Invest 1972; 51:725–730.

158. Whaley K. Biosynthesis of the complement components and the regulatory proteins of the alternative complement pathway by the human peripheral blood monocytes. J Exp Med 1980; 151:501–516.

159. Beatty DW, Davis AEI, Cole FS, Einstein LP, Colten HR. Biosynthesis of complement by human monocytes. Clin Immunol Immunopathol 1981; 18:334–343.

160. Cole FS, Schneeberger EE, Lichtenberg NA, Colten HR. Complement biosynthesis in human breast-milk macrophages and blood monocytes. Immunology 1982; 46:429–441.

161. Hetland G, Johnson E, Falk RJ, Eskeland T. Synthesis of complement components C5, C6, C7, C8, and C9 in vitro by human monocytes and assembly of the terminal complement complex. Scand J Immunol 1986; 24:421–428.

162. Cole FS, Matthews WJJ, Rossing TH, Gash DJ, Lichtenberg NA, Pennington JE. Complement biosynthesis by human bronchoalveolar macrophages. Clin Immunol Immunopathol 1983; 27:153–159.

163. Strunk RC, Eidlen DM, Mason RJ: Pulmonary alveolar type II epithelial cells synthesize and secrete proteins of the classical and alternative complement pathways. J Clin Invest 1988; 81:1419–1426.

164. Ooi YM. Histamine suppresses in vitro synthesis of precursor (pro-C5) of the fifth complement component (C5) by mouse peritoneal macrophages. J Immunol 1982; 129:200–205.

165. Rosenfeld SI, Kelly ME, Leddy JP. Hereditary deficiency of the fifth component of complement in man. I. Clinical, immunochemical, and family studies. J Clin Invest 1976; 57:1626–1634.

166. Rosenfeld SI, Baum J, Steigbigel RT, Leddy JP. Hereditary deficiency of the fifth component of complement in man. II. Biological properties of C5-deficient human serum. J Clin Invest 1976; 57:1635–1643.

167. Rosenfeld SI, Weitkamp LR, Ward F. Hereditary C5 deficiency in man: genetic linkage studies. J Immunol 1977; 119:604–608.

168. Snyderman R, Durack DT, McCarty GA, Ward FE, Meadows L. Deficiency of the fifth component of complement in human subjects. Clinical, genetic and immunologic studies in a large kindred. Am J Med 1979; 67:638–645.

169. Peter G, Weigert MB, Bissel AR, Gold R, Kreutzer D, McLean RH. Meningococcal meningitis in familial deficiency of the fifth component of complement. Pediatrics 1981; 67:882–886.

170. McLean RH, Peter G, Gold R, Guerra L, Yunis EJ, Kreutzer DL. Familial deficiency of C5 in humans: intact but deficient alternative complement pathway activity. Clin Immunol Immunopathol 1981; 21:62–76.

171. Cesbron JY, Maillet F, Valance J, Langlet N, Kazatchkine M. [Homozygotic C5 deficiency disclosed by purulent *Neisseria meningitidis* meningitis]. [French]. Presse Med 1985; 14:2287–2289.

172. Haeney MR, Ball AP, Thompson RA. Recurrent bacterial meningitis due to genetic deficiencies of terminal complement components (C5 and C6). Immunobiology 1980; 158:101–106.

173. Gianella-Borradori A, Borradori L, Schneider PM, Gautier E, Spath PJ. Combined complete C5 and partial C4 deficiency in humans: clinical consequences and complement-mediated functions in vitro. Clin Immunol Immunopathol 1990; 55:41–55.

174. Ross SC, Densen P. Complement deficiency states and infection: epidemiology, pathogenesis and consequences of neisserial and other infections in an immune deficiency. Medicine 1984; 63:243–273.

175. Wang X, Fleischer DT, Whitehead WT, Haviland DL, Rosenfeld SI, LeddyJP, Snyderman R, Wetsel RA. Inherited human complement C5 deficiency. Nonsense mutations in exons 1 (Gln1 to Stop) and 36 (Arg1458 to Stop) and compound heterozygosity in three African–American families. J Immunol 1995; 154:5464–5471.

176. Rosenberg LT, Tachibana DK: Activity of mouse complement. J Immunol 1962; 89:861–867.

177. Cinader B, Dubiski S, Wardlaw AC. Distribution, inheritance, and properties of an antigen, MuB1, and its relation to hemolytic complement. J Exp Med 1964; 120:897–924.

178. Hobart MJ, vaz Guedes MA, Lachmann PJ. Polymorphism of human C5. Ann Hum Genet 1981; 45:1–4.

179. Becherer JD, Alsenz J, Servis C, Myones BL, Lambris JD. Cell surface proteins reacting with activated complement components. Comple Inflam 1989; 6:142–165.

180. Fearon DT, Ahearn JM. Complement receptor type 1 (C3/C4b receptor; CD35) and complement receptor type 2 (C3d/Epstein-Barr virus receptor; CD21). Curr Top Microbiol Immunol 1990; 153:83–98.

181. Hugli TE. The anaphylatoxin C3a. Curr Top Microbiol Immunol 1990; 153:181–208.

182. Gerard C, Gerard NP. C5a anaphylatoxin and its seven transmembrane-segment receptor. Annu Rev Immunol 1994; 12775:808–808.

183. Wetsel RA: Structure, function, and cellular expression of complement anaphylatoxin receptors. Curr Opin Immunol 1995; 7:48–53.

184. Gerard NP, Gerard C. The chemotactic receptor for human C5a anaphylatoxin. Nature 1991; 349:614–617.

185. Boulay F, Mery L, Tardif M, Brouchon L, Vignais P. Expression cloning of a receptor for C5a anaphylatoxin on differentiated HL-60 cells. Biochemistry 1991; 30:2993–2999.

186. Roglic A, Prossnitz ER, Cavanagh SL, Pan Z, Zou A, Ye RD. cDNA cloning of a novel G protein-coupled receptor with a large extracellular loop structure. Biochem Biophys Acta 1996; 1305:39–43.

187. Huey R, Hugli TE. C5a receptor. Methods Enzymol 1987; 150:615–627.

188. Haviland DL, Mccoy RL, Whitehead WT, Akama H, Molmenti EP, Brown AH, JC, Parks WC, Perlmutter DH, Wetsel RA. Cellular expression of the C5a anaphylatoxin receptor (C5aR): demonstration of C5aR on nonmyeloid cells of the liver and lung. J Immunol 1995; 154:1861–1869.

189. Lacy M, Jones J, Whittlemore SR, et al: Expression of the receptors for the C5 anaphylatoxin, interleukin-8, and fMLP by human astrocytes and microglia. J Neuroimmunol 1995; 61:71–78.

190. Matsubara S, Yamamoto T, Tsuruta T, Takagi K, Kambara T. Complement C4-derived monocyte-directed chemotaxis-inhibitory factor. A molecular mechanism to cause polymorphonuclear leukocyte-predominant infiltration in rheumatoid arthritis synovial cavities. Am J Pathol 1991; 138:1279–1291.

191. Tsuruta T, Yamamoto T, Matsubara S, Nagasawa S, Tanase S, Tanaka JT, K, Kambara T. Novel function of C4a anaphylatoxin. Release from monocytes of protein which inhibits monocyte chemotaxis. Am J Pathol 1993; 142:1848–1857.

192. Murakami Y, Yamamoto T, Imamichi T, Nagasawa S. Cellular responses of guinea-pig macrophages to C4a; inhibition of C3a-induced O2-generation by C4a. Immunol Lett 1993; 36:301–304.

193. Becherer JD, Lambris JD. Identification of the C3b receptor-binding domain in third component of complement. J Biol Chem 1988; 263:14586–14591.

194. Ross GD, Polley MJ. Specificity of human lymphocyte complement receptors. J Exp Med 1975; 141:1163–1180.

195. Reynes M, Aubert JP, Cohen JHM, Audouin J, Tricottet V, Diebold J, Kazatchkine MD. Human follicular dendritic cells express CR1, CR2, and CR3 complement receptor antigens. J Immunol 1985; 135:2687–2694.

196. Fischer E, Delibrias C, Kazatchkine MD. Expression of CR2 (the C3dg/EBV receptor, CD21) on normal human peripheral blood lymphocytes. J Immunol 1991; 146:865–869.

197. Watry D, Hedrick JA, Siervo S, Rhodes G, Lamberti JJ, Lambris JDT, CD. Infection of human thymocytes by Epstein-Barr virus. J Exp Med 1991; 173:971–980.

198. Ross GD, Newman SL, Lambris JD, Devery-Pocius JE, Cain JA, Lachmann PJ. Generation of three different fragments of bound C3 with purified factor I or serum. II. Location of binding sites in the C3 fragments for factors B and H, complement receptors, and bovine conglutinin. J Exp Med 1983; 158:334–352.

199. Kalli KR, Ahearn JM, Fearon DT. Interaction of iC3b with recombinant isotypic and chimeric forms of CR2. J Immunol 1991; 147:590–594.

200. Lambris JD, Ganu VS, Hirani S, Muller-Eberhard HJ. Mapping of the C3d receptor (CR2)-binding site and a neoantigenic site in the C3d domain of the third component of complement. Proc Natl Acad Sci USA 1985; 82:4235–4239.

201. Nemerow GR, Houghten RA, Moore MD, Cooper NR. Identification of an epitope in the major envelope protein of Epstein-Barr virus that mediates viral binding to the B lymphocyte EBV receptor (CR2). Cell 1989; 56:369–377.

202. Hasty LA, Lambris JD, Lessey BA, Pruksananonda K, Lyttle CR. Hormonal regulation of complement components and receptors throughout the menstrual cycle. Am J Obstet Gynecol 1994; 170:168–175.

203. Diefenbach RJ, Isenman DE. Mutation of residues in the C3dg region of human complement component C3 corresponding to a proposed binding site for complement receptor type 2 (CR2, CD21) does not abolish binding of iC3b or C3dg to CR2. J Immunol 1995; 154:2303–2320.

204. Esparza I, Becherer JD, Alsenz J, Delahera A, Lao Z, Tsoukas CD, Lambris JD. Evidence for multiple sites of interaction in C3 for complement receptor type-2 (C3d/EBV receptor, CD21). Eur J Immunol 1991; 21:2829–2838.

205. Tanner J, Whang Y, Sample J, Sears A, Kieff E. Soluble gp350/220 and deletion mutant glycoprotein block Epstein-Barr virus adsorption to lymphocytes. J Virol 1988; 62:4452–4464.

206. Delcayre AX, Salas F, Mathur S, Kovats K, Lotz M, Lernhardt W. Epstein Barr virus complement C3d receptor is an interferon-alpha receptor. EMBO J 1991; 10:919–926.

207. Melchers F, Erdei A, Schulz T, Dierich MP. Growth control of activated, synchronized murine B cells by the C3d fragment of human complement. Nature 1985; 317:264–267.

208. Bohnsack JF, Cooper NR. CR2 ligands modulate human B cell activation. J Immunol 1988; 141:2569–2576.

209. Carter RH, Fearon DT. Polymeric C3dg primes human B lymphocytes for proliferation induced by anti-IgM. J Immunol 1989; 143:1755–1760.

210. Tsokos GC, Lambris JD, Finkelman FD, Anastassiou ED, June CH. Monovalent ligands of complement receptor 2 inhibit whereas polyvalent ligands enhance anti-Ig-induced human B cell intracytoplasmic free calcium concentration. J Immunol 1990; 144:1640–1645.

211. Changelian PS, Fearon DT. Tissue-specific phosphorylation of complement receptors CR1 and CR2. J Exp Med 1986; 163:101–115.

212. Barel M, Vazquez A, Charriaut C, Aufredou MT, Galanaud P, Frade R. gp 140, the C3d/EBV receptor (CR2), is phosphorylated upon in vitro activation of human peripheral B lymphocytes. FEBS Lett 1986; 197:353–356.

213. Lyamani F, Gauffre A, Barel M, Fiandinotirel A, Hermann J, Frade R. A 16 amino-acid synthetic peptide, derived from human C3d, carries regulatory activity on in vitro phosphorylation of a cellular component of the human B-lymphoma cells, Raji. Biochem Biophys Res Commun 1991; 175:823–830.

214. Matsumoto AK, Kopickyburd J, Carter RH, Tuveson DA, Tedder TF, Fearon DT. Intersection of the complement and immune systems: a signal transduction complex of the lymphocyte-B containing complement receptor type-2 and CD19. J Exp Med 1991; 173:55–64.

215. Pezzuto A, Dorken B, Rabinovitch PS, Ledbetter JA, Moldenhauer G, Clark EA. CD19 monoclonal antibody HD37 inhibits anti-immunoglobulin-induced B cell activation and proliferation. J Immunol 1987; 138:2793–2799.

216. Tuveson DA, Ahearn JM, Matsumoto AK, Fearon DT. Molecular interactions of complement receptors on B lymphocytes: A CR1/CR2 complex distinct from the CR2/CD19 complex. J Exp Med 1991; 173:1083–1089.

217. Hebell T, Ahearn JM, Fearon DT. Suppression of the immune response by a soluble complement receptor of B lymphocytes. Science 1991; 254:102–105.

218. Wiersma EJ, Kinoshita T, Heyman B. Inhibition of immunological memory and T-independent humoral responses by monoclonal antibodies specific for murine complement receptors. Eur J Immunol 1991; 21:2501–2506.

219. Thyphronitis G, Kinoshita T, Inoue K, Schweinle JE, Tsokos GC, Metcalf ES, Finkelman FD, Balow JE. Modulation of mouse complement receptor-1 and receptor-2 suppresses antibody responses in vivo. J Immunol 1991; 147:224–230.

220. Dempsey PW, Allison MED, Akkaraju S, Goodnow CC, Fearon DT. C3d of complement as a molecular adjuvant: bridging innate and acquired immunity. Science 1996; 271:348–350.

221. Hynes RO. Integrins: a family of cell surface receptors. Cell 1987; 48:549–554.

222. Wright SD, Reddy PA, Jong MT, Erickson BW. C3bi receptor (complement receptor type 3) recognizes a region of complement protein C3 containing the sequence Arg-Gly-Asp. Proc Natl Acad Sci USA 1987; 84:1965–1968.

223. Sekizawa A, Fujii T, Tochinai S. Membrane receptors on *Xenopus* macrophages for two classes of immunoglobulins (IgM and IgY) and the third complement component (C3). J Immunol 1984; 133:1431–1435.

224. Grossberger D, Marcuz A, Du Pasquier L, Lambris JD. Conservation of structural and functional domains in complement component C3 of Xenopus and mammals. Proc Natl Acad Sci USA 1989; 86:1323–1327.

225. Becherer JD, Alsenz J, Lambris JD. Molecular aspects of C3 interactions and the structural/functional analysis of C3 from different species. Curr Top Microbiol Immunol 1990; 153:45–72.

226. Taniguchi-Sidle A, Isenman DE. Mutagenesis of the Arg-Gly-Asp triplet in human complement component-C3 does not abolish binding of iC3b to the leukocyte integrin complement receptor type-III (CR3, CD11b/CD18). J Biol Chem 1992; 267:635–643.

227. Taniguchi-Sidle A, Isenman DE. Interactions of human complement component C3 with factor B and with complement receptors type 1 (CR1, CD35) and type 3 (CR3, CD11b/CD18) involve an acidic sequence at the N-terminus of C3 α-chain. J Immunol 1994; 153:5285–5302.

228. Gaither TA, Vargas I, Inada S, Frank MM. The complement fragment C3d facilitates phagocytosis by monocytes. Immunology 1987; 62:405–411.

229. Law SKA, Gagnon J, Hildreth JEK, Wells CE, Willis AC, Wong AJ. The primary structure of the β-subunit of the cell surface adhesion glyproteins LFA-1, CR3 and p150,95 and its relationship to the fibronectin receptor. EMBO J 1987; 6:915–919.

230. Kishimoto TK, O'Connor K, Lee A, Roberts TM, Springer TA. Cloning of the β subunit of the leukocyte adhesion proteins: homology to an extracellular matrix receptor defines a novel supergene family. Cell 1987; 48:681–690.

231. Lublin DM, Atkinson JP. Decay-accelerating factor and membrane cofactor protein. Curr Top Microbiol Immunol 1990; 153:123–145.

232. Medof ME, Walter EI, Rutgers JL, Knowles DM, Nussenzweig V. Identification of the complement decay-accelerating factor (DAF) on epithelium and glandular cells and in body fluids. J Exp Med 1987; 165:848–864.

233. Post TW, Liszewski MK, Adams EM, Tedja I, Miller EA, Atkinson JP. Membrane cofactor protein of the complement system: alternative splicing of serine/threonine/proline rich exons and cytoplasmic tails produces multiple isoforms that correlate with protein phenotype. J Exp Med 1991; 174:93–102.

234. Russell SM, Sparrow RL, Mckenzie IFC, Purcell DFJ. Tissue-specific and allelic expression of the complement regulator CD46 is controlled by alternative splicing. Eur J Immunol 1992; 22:1513–1518.

235. Pryzdial ELG, Isenman DE. Alternative complement pathway activation fragment Ba binds to C3b. J Biol Chem 1987; 262:1519–1525.

236. Ganu VS, Müller-Eberhard HJ. Inhibition of factor B and factor H binding to C3b by synthetic peptide corresponding to residues 749–789 of human C3 (abstr). Complement 1985; 2:27.

237. O'Keefe MC, Caporale LH, Vogel CW. A novel cleavage product of human complement components C3 with structural and functional properties of cobra venom factor. J Biol Chem 1988; 263:12690–12697.

238. Burger R, Deubel U, Hadding U, Bitter-Suermann D. Identification of functionally relevant determinants on the complement component C3 with monoclonal antibodies. J Immunol 1982; 129:2042–2050.

239. Koistinen V, Wessberg S, Leikola J. A common binding region of complement factors B and H on C3b revealed by monoclonal anti-C3d (abstr). Compl Inflamm 1989; 6:270–280.

240. Lambris JD, Avila D, Becherer JD, Muller-Eberhard HJ. A discontinuous factor H binding site in the third component of complement as delineated by synthetic peptides. J Biol Chem 1988; 263:12147–12150.

241. Becherer JD, Alsenz J, Esparza I, Hack CE, Lambris JD. A segment spanning residues 727–768 of the complement C3 sequence contains a neoantigenic site and accommodates the binding of CR1, factor H, and factor B. Biochemistry 1992; 31:1787–1794.

242. Alsenz J, Avila D, Huemer HP, Esparza I, Becherer JD, Kinoshita TW, Y, Oppermann S, Lambris JD. Phylogeny of the third component of complement, C3: Analysis of the conservation of human CR1, CR2, H, and B binding sites, concanavalin A binding sites, and thiolester bond in the C3 from different species. Dev Comp Immunol 1992; 16:63–76.

243. Alsenz J, Becherer JD, Nilsson B, Lambris JD. Structural and functiuonal analysis of C3 using monoclonal antibodies. Curr Top Microbiol Immunol 1989; 153:235–248.

244. Tamerius JD, Pangburn MK, Müller-Eberhard HJ. Selective inhibition of functional sites of cell-bound C3b by hybridoma-derived antibodies. J Immunol 1982; 128:512–514.

245. Wörner I, Burger R, Lambris JD. Localization and functional characterization of epitopes on α and β chains of C3 (abstr). Compl Inflamm 1989; 6:416–417.

246. Klickstein LB, Bartow TJ, Miletic V, Rabson LD, Smith JA, Fearon DT. Identification of distinct C3b and C4b recognition sites in the human C3b/C4b receptor (CR1, CD35) by deletion mutagenesis. J Exp Med 1988; 168:1699–1717.

247. Sanchez-Corral P, Garcia OC, Rodriguez de Cordoba S. Isoforms of human C4b-binding protein I: molecular basis for the C4BP isoform pattern and its variations in human plasma. J Immunol 1995; 155:4030–4036.

248. Garcia OC, Sanchez-Corral P, Rodriguez de Cordoba S. Isoforms of human C4b-binding protein II: differential modulation of the *C4BPA* and *C4BPB* genes by acute phase cytokines. J Immunol 1995; 155:4037–4043.

249. Chung LP, Bentley DR, Reid KBM. Molecular cloning and characterization of the cDNA coding for C4b-binding protein, a regulatory protein of the classical pathway of the human complement system. Biochem J 1985; 230:133–141.

250. Chapitis J, Lepow IH. Multiple sedimenting species of properdin in human and interaction of purified properdin with the third component of complement. J Exp Med 1976; 143:241–257.

251. Lambris JD, Alsenz J, Schulz TF, Dierich MP. Mapping of the properdin-binding site in the third component of complement. Biochem J 1984; 217:323–326.

252. Daoudaki ME, Becherer JD, Lambris JD. A 34-amino acid peptide of the third component of complement mediates properdin binding [published erratum appears in J. Immunol. 1988,141:1788]. J Immunol 1988; 140:1577–1580.

253. Braconier JH, Sjoholm AG, Soderstrom C. Fulminant meningococcal infections in a family with inherited deficiency of properdin. Scand J Infect Dis 1983; 15:339–344.

254. Lachmann PJ, Elias DE, Moffett A. Conglutinin and immunoconglutinins. In: Ingram DG, ed. Biological Activities of Complement. Basel:Karger, 1972:202–226.

255. Loveless RW, Feizi T, Childs RA, Mizuochi T, Stoll MS, Oldroyd RG, Lachmann PJ. Bovine serum conglutinin is a lectin which binds non-reducing terminal N-acetylglucosamine, mannose and fucose residues. Biochem J 1989; 258:109–113.

256. Hirani S, Lambris JD, Muller-Eberhard HJ. Localization of the conglutinin binding site on the third component of human complement. J Immunol 1985; 134:1105–1109.

257. Giclas PC, King TE, Baker SL, Russo J, Henson PM. Complement activity in normal rabbit bronchoalveolar fluid description of an inhibitor of C3 activation. Am Rev Respir Dis 1987; 135:403–411.

258. Oxvig C, Haaning J, Kristensen L, Wagner JM, Rubin I, Stigbrand T, Gleich GJ, Sottrup-Jensen L. Identification of angiotensinogen and complement C3dg as novel proteins binding the proform of eosinophil major basic protein in human pregnancy serum and plasma. J Biol Chem 1995; 270:13645–13651.

259. Dierich MP, Huemer HP, Prodinger WM. C3 binding proteins of foreign origin. Curr Top Microbiol Immunol 1990; 153:163–180.

260. Cooper NR. Complement evasion strategies of microorganisms. Immunol Today 1991; 12:327–331.

261. Friedman HM, Cohen GH, Eisenberg RJ, Seidel CA, Cines DB. Glycoprotein C of herpes simplex virus 1 acts as a receptor for the C3b complement component on infected cells. Nature 1984; 309:633–635.

262. Seidel-Dugan C, Ponce de Leon M, Friedman HM, Fries LF, Frank MM, Cohen GH, Eisenberg RJ. C3b receptor activity on transfected cells expressing glycoprotein C of herpes simplex virus types 1 and 2. J Virol 1988; 62:4027–4036.

263. McNearney TA, Odell C, Holers VM, Spear PG, Atkinson JP. Herpes simplex virus glycoproteins gC-1 and gC-2 bind to the third component of complement and provide protection against complement mediated neutralization of viral infectivity. J Exp Med 1987; 166:1525–1535.

264. Eisenberg RJ, Ponce de Leon P, Friedman HM, Fries LF, Frank MM, Hastings JC, Cohen GH. Complement component C3b binds directly to purified glycoprotein C of herpes simplex virus types 1 and 2. Microbial Pathol 1987; 3:423–435.

265. Hung SL, Peng C, Kostavasili I, Friedman HM, Lambris JD, Eisenberg RJ, Cohen GH. The interaction of glycoprotein C of herpes simplex virus types 1 and 2 with the alternative complement pathway. Virology 1994; 203:299–312.

266. Kostavasili I, Sahu A, Friedman HM, Eisenberg RJ, Cohen GH, Lambris JD. Mechanism of complement inactivation by glycoprotein C of herpes simplex virus. J Immunol 1997; 158:1763–1771.

267. Mold C, Bradt BM, Nemerow GR, Cooper NR. Epstein-Barr virus regulates activation and processing of the third component of complement. J Exp Med 1988; 168:949–969.

268. Kotwal GJ, Moss B. Vaccinia virus encodes a secretory polypeptide structurally related to complement control proteins. Nature 1988; 335:176–178.

269. Mckenzie R, Kotwal GJ, Moss B, Hammer CH, Frank MM. Regulation of complement activity by vaccinia virus complement-control protein. J Infect Dis 1992; 166:1245–1250.

270. Joiner KA, daSilva WD, Rimoldi MT, Hammer CH, Sher A, Kipnis TL. Biochemical characterization of a factor produced by trypomastigotes of *Trypanosoma cruzi* that accelerates the decay of complement C3 convertases. J Biol Chem 1988; 263:11327–11335.

271. Norris KA, Bradt B, Cooper NR, So M. Characterization of a *Trypanosoma-cruzi* C3 binding protein with functional and genetic similarities to the human complement regulatory protein, decay-accelerating factor. J Immunol 1991; 147:2240–2247.

272. Calderone RA, Linehan L, Wadsworth E, Sandberg AL. Identification of C3d receptors on *Candida albicans*. Infect Immun 1988; 56:252–258.

273. Heidenreich F, Dierich MP. *Candida albicans* and *Candida stellatoidea*, in contrast to other candida species, bind iC3b and C3d but not C3b. Infect Immun 1985; 50:598–600.

274. Gustafson KS, Vercellotti GM, Bendel CM, Hostetter MK. Molecular mimicry in *Candida albicans*. Role of an integrin analogue in adhesion of the yeast to human endothelium. J Clin Invest 1991; 87:1896–1902.

275. Minkoff MS, Wong WW, Silberstein DS. Identification of C3 beta-chain as the human serum eosinophil cytotoxicity inhibitor. J Exp Med 1991; 174:1267–1270.

276. Jack RM, Ward PA. The role in vivo of C3 and the C3b receptor in babesial infection in the rat. J Immunol 1980; 124:1574–1578.

277. Hautanen A, Keski-Oja J. Interaction of fibronectin with complement component C3. Scand J Immunol 1983; 17:225–230.

278. Bartok I, Erdei A, Mouzaki A, Osawa H, Szolosi A, Eigentler A, Diamantstein T, Dierich MP, Gergely J. Interaction between C3 and IL-2: Inhibition of C3b binding to CR1 by IL-2. Immunol Lett 1989; 21:131–138.

279. Leivo I, Engvall E. C3d fragment of complement interacts with laminin and binds basement membranes of glomerulus and trophoblast. J Cell Biol 1986; 103:1091–1100.

6

Proteins of the Membrane Attack Complex

MNASON E. PLUMB and JAMES M. SODETZ
University of South Carolina, Columbia, South Carolina

I. INTRODUCTION

Complement-mediated cell lysis is a consequence of terminal pathway activation and interaction among components C5b, C6, C7, C8, and C9. These interactions lead to formation of C5b-9, a cytolytically active, macromolecular complex commonly referred to as the membrane attack complex (MAC) (Fig. 1). MAC assembly begins with proteolytic cleavage of C5 by either the alternative or classical pathway C5 convertase. The cleavage product C5b interacts with C6 through a metastable binding site to form a soluble C5b-6 dimer. Subsequent binding of C7 produces C5b-7, a trimeric complex that expresses a transient, high-affinity lipid-binding site. In the presence of a target cell, C5b-7 physically associates with the membrane where it subsequently binds C8 to form tetrameric C5b-8 on the surface. This complex functions as a receptor by promoting binding and polymerization of C9 to form the porelike structure characteristic of a lytically active MAC. Association of C5b-7 with host cell membranes is inhibited primarily by vitronectin (S protein), a multifunctional plasma protein that blocks the lipid-binding site on C5b-7. Binding of C8 and C9 to SC5b-7 produces SC5b-9, the lytically inactive, soluble counterpart of the MAC.

Other than the initial bond cleavage in C5, all steps in the MAC assembly process are nonenzymatic. Individually, the MAC components have properties of hydrophilic

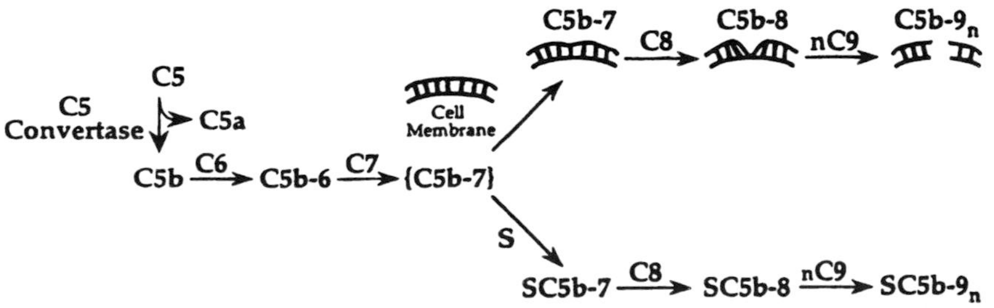

Figure 1 Assembly of the membrane attack complex. Activation by C5 convertase leads to formation of lytically active C5b-9 (MAC) on target cell membranes or the inactive, soluble SC5b-9 complex.

proteins but when combined they form an amphipathic complex capable of disrupting membrane organization. Lipids in the target membrane are not degraded but instead undergo a disruptive rearrangement as a result of MAC insertion. This rearrangement increases local membrane permeability that results in osmotic lysis of simple cells such as erythrocytes and triggers a variety of intracellular signaling events in nucleated cells. In bacteria, MAC disrupts the outer membrane, thereby increasing permeability and inducing lethal changes in the inner membrane.

All five MAC components circulate independently yet they interact in a sequential manner once C5b is formed. As each complex is assembled, binding specificity changes so as to recognize the next component in the pathway. The molecular basis for this specificity is still unknown; however, once associated, the affinity between components is high despite the noncovalent nature of their interaction. Dissociation can only be accomplished by solubilization of the membrane and denaturation of the complexes.

Of the five MAC components, C6, C7, C8, and C9 share structural features not found in C5b. Therefore they are considered together in this chapter, whereas properties of C5 and C5b are described elsewhere in this book.

II. PHYSICAL PROPERTIES AND STRUCTURE

A. General Features of the MAC Components

Table 1 lists some physical properties of the MAC proteins. Human C6 is a single-chain protein with reported molecular weights of 120,000 by sodium dodecyl sulfate polyacrylamide gel electrophoresis (SDS-PAGE) and 104,800 by sedimentation equilibrium; it has a sickle-like shape (1–3). C6 purified from pooled serum exhibits multiple electrophoretic forms ranging from pI 6.15 to 6.55 (4). Mature human C6 contains 64 Cys residues, all of which form intrachain disulfide bonds (2, 3). There are two N-glycosylation sites at Asn[303] and Asn[834] and both contain complex-type oligosaccharide chains totaling ~5% (w/w) (3). There is no evidence of any O-linked sugars.

Human C7 is also a single-chain protein and is similar in size to C6. Reported molecular weights are 105,000 (SDS-PAGE) and 92,400 (sedimentation equilibrium) (1). Its shape as determined by electron microscopy is that of a flexible, elongated molecule (5). Purified C7 consists of four major isoelectric forms ranging from pI 6.05 to 6.40. The amino acid sequence of mature C7 contains 56 Cys residues, all of which are internally linked by disulfide bonds (5). Carbohydrate composition as well as analysis of C7 fragments indicate that Asn[180] and Asn[732] contain complex-type oligosaccharide chains totaling 6% (w/w). As with C6, there is no evidence of O-linked sugars. Amino acid sequences for C6 and C7 from species other than human have not been reported.

Human C8 is an oligomeric protein composed of three nonidentical subunits (α, β, γ) encoded by separate genes. The subunits are arranged as a disulfide-linked α-γ dimer and a noncovalently associated β chain (6). C8 purified from pooled serum contains a 1:1 ratio of α-γ and β for a total molecular weight of 151,000, and it exhibits multiple isoelectric forms ranging from pI 6.2 to 7.5. Its overall shape is predicted to be globular (7). C8α-γ and C8β can be dissociated and purified in the presence of denaturing or high ionic strength buffers (8). Apparent molecular weights are ~86,000 and 64,000 (SDS-PAGE), respectively. The affinity of C8α–γ for C8β is remarkably high. The purified subunits physically recombine when mixed at dilute concentrations (<1 ng/ml) and at

Table 1 Properties of Human MAC Components

| Subunit | Serum Concentration (~µg/ml) | Molecular Weight | | Amino Acids | | Carbohydrate (~%w/w) | Isoelectric Point | Extinction Coefficient[c] (280nm, 1%, 1cm) | Genetic Locus |
		Apparent[a]	Calculated[b]	Leader Sequence	Mature Protein				
C6	45	120,000	102,469	21	913	5	6.15–6.55	9.3	5p13
C7	55	105,000	91,111	22	821	6	6.05–6.40	9.9	5p13
C8	80	151,000[d]	142,981	—	—	3	6.20–7.50	14.9	—
C8α	—	64,000	61,711	30	554	4	—	11.8[e]	1p32
C8β	—	64,000	60,943	54	537	4	—	13.7	1p32
C8γ	—	22,000	20,327	20	182	0	—	—	9q34.3
C9	60	71,000	60,978	21	538	8	4.95	9.9	5p13

[a]SDS-PAGE.
[b]Based on amino acid sequences in Swiss Protein Sequence Data Bank
[c]Experimentally determined
[d]Sedimentation equilibrium
[e]Value for C8α-γ

only slight molar excesses (1:2) relative to each other (9,10). C8 formed by recombination of C8α-γ and C8β has physical and functional characteristics similar to native C8.

Amino acid sequences of the human C8 subunits were determined from cDNA clones (11–14). Mature C8α contains 29 Cys, all of which form intrachain disulfide bonds except one (Cys^{164}), which forms an interchain bond to C8γ (15). Mature C8β contains 28 Cys that are all internally linked. Carbohydrate compositions indicate that C8α and C8β each contain one N-linked, complex-type oligosaccharide chain but no O-linked sugars (11,12). C8α contains two possible sites (Asn^{13,407}) for N-linked carbohydrate. Peptide sequencing suggests that Asn^{13} is utilized (11); however, Asn^{407} is also a candidate because it is the only site conserved in rabbit C8α (16). C8β has three potential sites (Asn^{47,189,499}) but only Asn^{47} is conserved in rabbit C8β. Thus far, rabbit is the only other species for which C8 sequence is available.

Mature human C8γ contains three Cys, two of which form a single intrachain disulfide (Cys^{76,168}) while the third (Cys^{40}) is linked to C8α (14,17). The protein has a pyroglutamyl residue at the N-terminus and contains no carbohydrate. In other species, C8γ may be N-glycosylated. Rabbit C8γ has one possible N-glycosylation site (Asn^{153}) and a higher apparent molecular weight of 25,000 (16).

Human C9 is a single-chain protein similar in size to C8α and C8β. Reported molecular weights are 70–77,000 (sedimentation equilibrium), 71,000 (SDS-PAGE), and 73,000 (small angle neutron scattering) (7). The calculated extinction coefficient is 8.0 (18) and the experimentally determined one is 9.9 (19). The N-terminus is blocked by a pyroglutamyl residue. Amino acid sequence deduced from cDNA clones indicates that C9 contains 24 Cys, all of which form intrachain disulfide bonds (20,21). C9 contains 8% (w/w) carbohydrate consisting of complex-type chains linked to each of two possible N-glycosylation sites (Asn^{256,394}) (22). It remains uncertain whether C9 contains small amounts of O-linked carbohydrate. C9 is cleaved once by α-thrombin at position 244–245 to produce an N-terminal (C9a) and a C-terminal (C9b) fragment with apparent molecular weights of ~34,000 and 37,000, respectively (23). These fragments remain tightly associated after cleavage. C9 is capable of binding 1 mol/mol Ca^{2+} at a site located within C9a (24). Calcium is not required for C9 activity but does enhance its thermal stability. The shape of monomeric C9 was originally considered to be globular but appears to be more elongated (7,18). Amino acid sequences have also been reported for mouse (25), rabbit (26), horse (27), trout (28), and rat (29) C9.

C9 is unique among the MAC components because it is capable of self-polymerization. Monomeric C9 can be induced to polymerize by divalent cations such as Zn^{2+} (30), elevated temperature (31), or partial digestion with trypsin (32). Poly C9 nominally contains 12–18 C9 monomers arranged as a hollow cylindrical structure rimmed with a torus at one end (22, 31, 33, 34). Polymers of this size are SDS resistant, possibly because of disulfide exchange between C9 monomers (35). Poly C9 is estimated to have an inner diameter of ~10 nm, outer diameters of ~21 nm (torus) and ~18 nm (cylinder), and an overall length of ~15 nm (22,34). The ultrastructure of poly C9 resembles that of the porelike structure formed by the MAC. Poly C9 alone is not normally cytolytic but it can lyse reduced and alkylated sheep erythrocytes (36). There are conflicting reports as to whether polymerized C9 can lyse phospholipid vesicles (37,38).

B. Modular Structure of C6, C7, C8α, C8β, and C9

Sequence comparisons indicate that human C6, C7, C8α, C8β, and C9 constitute a family of structurally related proteins. The similar-sized members C6 and C7 exhibit 33.7%

sequence identity and 53.5% similarity. Likewise, C8α and C8β exhibit 34.7% identity and 53.6% similarity to each other. C9 is 31.7% and 28.7% identical and 51.9% and 50.9% similar to C8α and C8β, respectively. Since the amino acid sequences were originally published, several errors and discrepancies have been identified and resolved. These revisions are annotated in the Swiss Protein Sequence Databank.

The structural organization of all five proteins is highly conserved and modular in design (Fig. 2). Each protein contains cysteine-rich modules ~40–80 residues in length that exhibit significant sequence similarity to modules found in a number of functionally unrelated proteins (39). Included is the thrombospondin type I (TSP1) module repeated three times in thrombospondin (40). C6 contains two copies in the N-terminus whereas the other family members have one. With the exception of C9, all have a second TSP1 module located towards the C-terminus. Also conserved is the low-density lipoprotein-receptor class A (LDLRA) module repeated seven times in the LDL receptor (41). Towards the C-terminus of each protein is an epidermal growth factor (EGF) module that exhibits

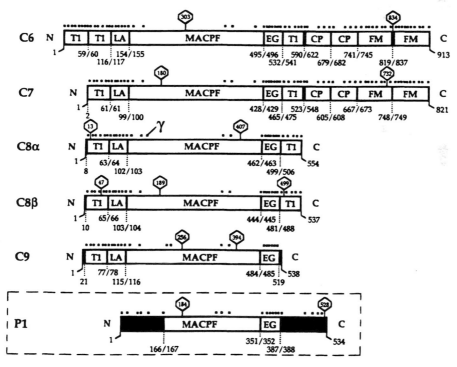

Figure 2 Structural organization of the MAC protein family. Shown are protein maps based on amino acid sequences and module boundaries listed in the Swiss Protein Sequence Data Bank. Module abbreviations correspond to TSP1 (T1), LDLRA (LA), EGF (EG), CCP (CP), and FIM (FM) modules (39). The membrane attack complex/perforin segment (MACPF) is an extended region of sequence similarity found within all family members and perforin (P1). A map of perforin is included to emphasize conservation of the MACPF region and the EGF module. Residue numbers under each map correspond to module boundaries in the mature proteins. In C7, the N-terminal TSP1 and the LDLRA module overlap by one residue (position 61). Hexagonal symbols identify Asn residues that are possible N-glycosylation sites. Approximate location of Cys residues is designated by (■) above each protein. C8γ is shown as linked to Cys[164] in C8α.

sequence similarity to epidermal growth factor (42). Both C6 and C7 contain additional tandemly repeated modules in their C-terminal regions. The complement control protein (CCP) module (also known as the short consensus repeat [SCR], or Sushi module) is repeated multiple times in several of the complement control proteins while the factor I module (FIM) module occurs once in factor I (43). Although not strictly a module, the internal region of each protein is designated MACPF to emphasize sequence similarity between members of the MAC protein family and perforin (44). Perforin is a 70 kDa protein released from the secretory granules of cytotoxic T lymphocytes. During lympho-cyte-mediated cytolysis, perforin self-polymerizes in the presence of Ca^{2+} to form trans-membrane lesions on target cells. Polyperforin and poly C9 have similar physical and functional characteristics.

The disulfide-bond pattern in C9 has recently been determined, and those Cys residues located within the modules were found to be internally cross-linked (Fig. 3) (45). Also significant is the location of disulfide bonds within the MACPF region of C9. These involve Cys residues located in close proximity to each other. This feature and the small number of disulfide bonds suggest minimal conformational constraints within the relatively large MACPF segment.

C. C8γ: A Member of the Lipocalin Family

Although human C8γ is an integral part of C8 and therefore of the MAC, it is not considered a member of the MAC protein family. It is not structurally related to any complement protein but instead exhibits sequence similarity to the α-2μ-globulin or "lipocalin" family of proteins (46). More than 25 members of this family have been identified, primarily on the basis of sequence comparisons (47,48). Members are widely distributed in both vertebrates and invertebrates. They have similar molecular weights of ~20,000, generally weak pairwise sequence identities averaging ~20%, and a common ability to bind small hydrophobic ligands (49). Unlike C8γ, most are independently secreted proteins. Examples are serum retinol-binding protein, milk β-lactoglobulin, and LCN1 from tears, all of which bind retinol; α-2μ-globulin and mouse urinary protein, both of which bind pheromones; the odorant-binding protein of the nasal mucosa that binds odorants; and insecticyanin and bilin-binding protein from insect hemolymph that bind biliverdin for coloration and camouflage. As described in Section III.B, the genomic structure of C8γ is consistent with its relationship to the lipocalin family; however, it is unclear whether it has the related function of binding small, hydrophobic ligands.

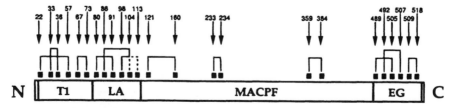

Figure 3 Disulfide bonds within human C9. Shown is the experimentally determined disulfide-bond pattern in human C9. Cys[86] and Cys[98] are unassigned and linked to either Cys[104] or Cys[113].

III. GENOMIC ORGANIZATION

A. MAC Protein Family

Genes for C6 (50), C7 (51), C8α (52), C8β (53), and C9 (54) have been isolated and characterized. Although introns were not fully characterized, minimum lengths of the genes are estimated to be ~80 kb, 80 kb, 70 kb, 40 kb, and 90 kb, respectively. Close correspondence between restriction maps of genomic clones and human genomic DNA suggests that all are single-copy genes.

Features of the genes are consistent with the ancestral relationship predicted from sequence similarities and structural homologies of the proteins. C6 and C7 contain 18 exons whereas C8β has 12 and C8α and C9 have 11 (Fig. 4). The total number of exons in each gene is still tentative because transcription initiation sites have not been identified. The first exon in C6 and C7 is designated exon "0" for historical reasons and to emphasize the close alignment of exons 1–11 with the other family members (51). For the most part, corresponding exons in each protein are similar in length. Exceptions include exons 1 and 2 in all the genes, exon 5 in C8α, exon 6 in C9, and exon 16 in C6. Also, exon 10 in C8β is interrupted by an intron, the result being two exons (exons 10 and 11) that span what corresponds to exon 10 in the other proteins. Exon phases are highly conserved except for the boundaries between exons 0–1 in C6 and C7. When module boundaries are superimposed on the genes, there is a general lack of correspondence with exon boundaries. Most modules extend over two exons, the exceptions being the EGF module in all but C8β and the second CCP module in C6 and C7. Lack of boundary correspondence along with highly conserved phases suggests that this family arose by gene duplication rather than exon shuffling.

Polymorphisms at both the protein and DNA level have been identified for members of the MAC protein family. Segregation of polymorphic markers in informative families established that C6, C7, and C9 are closely linked on chromosome 5p13 (56–58). Analysis of human genomic DNA by pulsed-field gel electrophoresis and characterization of YAC clones later revealed that C6 and C7 are within 160 kb and oriented 3'-3' relative to transcription (51,59,60). A physical map of this region has been developed from characterization of the YAC clones. Although genetically linked, C9 is not physically linked to C6 or C7 and is estimated to be more than 2.5 Mb away. For C8, genetic studies of protein polymorphisms (61,62), analysis of somatic cell hybrids (63) and in situ hybridizations (64) established that C8α and C8β are closely linked on chromosome 1p32. Based on analysis of genomic DNA digests using large cDNA probes, the genes were originally reported to be physically linked (<2.5 kb) and in a 5'α–β3' orientation (63). However, when probes specific for the 5' and 3' ends of the genes were used, these results were found to be artifactual (52). Analysis of isolated YAC clones later confirmed that C8α and C8β are indeed physically linked (<23 kb), but in a 3'-3' orientation with respect to transcription (65).

Conservation of genomic organization further suggests that C6, C7, C8α, C8β, and C9 are derived from a common ancestral gene. Based on the relative sizes of the proteins, it has been hypothesized that deletions from the ends of a more complex ancestral gene at least as large as C6 may have occurred (50). The 3'-3' arrangement of C6 and C7 as well as C8α and C8β makes details of subsequent evolutionary events difficult to reconstruct. One possibility is that a single, ancestral gene was duplicated in such a way as to assume a tail-to-tail arrangement. This gene pair then evolved into the contemporary C6 and C7 genes on chromosome 5 and subsequently was transposed as a unit to produce

```
EXON
          C6   1  MARRSVLYFI LLNALINKGQ ACFCDHYAWT QWTSCSKTCN SGTQSRHAr       2
          C7   0  .......... .......... .....(MK)V ISLFILVGFI GEFQSFSSe        2
     1    C8α     .......... .......... ..MFAVVFFI LSLMTCQPGV TAQEKVNGl       2
          C8β     .......... .......MXN SRTWAWRAPV ELFLLCAALG CLSLPGSAr       2
          C9      .......... .......... .MSACRSFAV .AICILEISI LTAQYTTSe       2

                               T1
          C6   gQI VVDKYYQENF CEQICSKQET RECMWQRCPI NCLLGDFGPW SDCDPCIEKQ      0
          C7   .......... .......... ...rASSPV NCQWDFYAPW SECNGCTKTQ           0
     2    C8α  nR VRRAATPAAVI TCQLSNWSEW TDCFPCQDKK                           0
          C8β  gGE RPHSFGSNAV NKSFAKSRQM RSVDVTLMPI DCELSSWSSW TTCDPCQKKR      0
          C9   rYDPEL TESSGSASHI DCRMSPWSEW SQCDPCLRQM                        0
                                                    T1

          C6   SKVRSVLRPS QFGGQPCTEP LVAFQPCIPS KLCKIEBADC KNKFRC.DSG         1
          C7   TRRRSVAVYG QYGGQPCVGN AFETQSCEPT RGCPTEB.GC GERFRC.FSG         1
     3    C8α  YRHRSLLQPN KFGGTICSGD IWDQASCSSS TTCVRQ.AQC GQDFQCKETG         1
          C8β  YRYAYLLQPS QFHGEPCNFS DKEVEDCVTN RPCGSQ.VRC                    1
          C9   FRSRSIEVFG QFNGKRCTDA VGDRRQCVPT EPCEDAEDDC GNDFQC.STG         1
                    T1                                          LA

          C6   lyRCIARKLECN GENDCGD.NS .DERDCGRT. .KAV.CT.RK YNPIPSVQLM GNGl   2
          C7   lyQCISKSLVCN GDSDC.DEDS ADEDRCEDSE RRPS.CDIDK ..PPPNIELT GNGl   2
     4    C8α  lyRCLKRHLVCN GDQDCLD.GS .DEDDCEVR AIDEDCS.Q. YEPIPGSQKA ALGl    2
          C8β  lyRCVNRRLLCN GDNDCGD.QS .DEANCRHIY KK...CQ.HE MDQYWGIGSL ASGl   2
          C9   lyRCIKMRLRCN GDNDCGD.FS .DEDDCESEP RPP..CRDRV VEESELARTA GYGl   2
                         LA

          C6   y FHFLAGEPRG EVLDNSFTGG ICKTVKSSRT SNP....... .......... YRVPANLENV GFE   0
          C7   y YNELTGQFRN RVINTKSFGG QCRKVFSGDG KDF....... .......... YRLSGNVLSY TFQ   0
     5    C8α  y YNILTQEDAQ SVYDASYYGG QCETVYNGEW RELRYDSTCE RLYYGDDEKY FRKPYNFLKY HFE   0
          C8β  y INLFTNSFEG PVLDHRYYAG GCSPHYILNT R......... .......... FRKPYNVESY TPQ   0
          C9   y INILGMDPLS TPFDNEFYNG LCNRDRDGNT .......... .......LTY YRRPWNVASL IYE   0

          C6   VQTAEDD LKTDFYKDLT SLGHNENQQG SFSSQGGSSF SVP.IFYS.. .......... ......SKRS ENINHNSAFK QAIQASHKK   0
          C7   VKI.NND FNYEFYNSTW SYVKHTSTEH TSSSRKRSFF RSS.S..S.. .......... ......SSRS YTSHTNEIHK G.......K   0
     6    C8α  AL.ADTG ISSEFYDNAN DLLSKVKKDK SDSFGVTIGI GPAGSPLL.. .......... ......VGVG VSHSQDTSFL NELNKYNEK   0
          C8β  TQ.GKYE FILKEYESYS DFERNVTEKM ASKSGFSFGF KIPG1.FE.. .......... ......LGIS SQSDRGKHYI RRTKRFSHT   0
          C9   TK.GEKN FRTEHYEEQI EAFKSIIQEK TSNFNAAISL KFTPTETNKA EQCCEETASS ISLHGKGSFR FSYSKNETYQ LFLSYSSKK   0

          C6   D SSFIRIHKVM KVLNFTTKAK D.LHLSDVFL KALNHLPLEY NSALYSRIFD DFGTHYFTSG SLGGVYDLLY QFSSEELKNS G   1
          C7   S YQLLVVENTV EVAQFINNNP EFLQLAEPFW KELSNLPSLY DYSAYRRLID QYGTHYLQSG SLGGEYRVLF YVDSEKLKQN A   1
     7    C8α  K FIFTRIFTKV QTAHFKMRKD DIM.LDEGML QSLMELPDQY NYGMYAKFIN DYGTHYITGS SMGGIYEYIL VIDKAKMESL G   1
          C8β  K SVFLHARSDL EVAHYKLKPR SLM.LHYEFL QRVKRLPLEY SYGEYRDLFR DFGTHYITEA VLGGIYEYTL VMNKEAMERG A   1
          C9   E KMFLHVKGEI HLGRFVMRNR DVV.LTTTFV DDIKALPTTY EKGEYFAFLE TYGTHYSSSG SLGGLYELIY VLDKASMKRK G   1

          C6   lyLTEEEAKHC VRIETKKRV. ...LFAKKTK VEHRCTINKL SEKHE.G   1
          C7   spFNSVEEKKC KSSGWHFVV. ...KFSSHG. ....CKELEN ALKAASG   1
     8    C8α  lyITSRDITTC FGGSLGIQYE .DKINVGGGL SGDHCKKFGG G.KT..G   1
          C8β  spYTLNNVHAC AKNDFKIGGA IEEVYVSLGV SVGKCRGILN EIK...A   1
          C9   lyVELKDIKRC LGYHLDVSLA FSEISVGAEF NKDDCVKRGE G.RA..V   1

          C6   lySFI.Q.GAEKSISLIR GGRSEYGAAL AW.EKGSSGL EEKTFSEWLE SVKENPAVID FE   0
          C7   lyT...QNNVLRGEPFIR GGGAGFISGL SYLELDNPAG NKRRYSAWAE SVTNLPQVIK QK   0
     9    C8α  luRARKAMAVEDIISRVR GGSSGWSGGL A.QNRSTITY .R...S.WGR SLKYNPVVID FE   0
          C8β  spRNKRDTMVEDLVVLVR GGASEHITTL AYQELPTADL MQ....EWGD AVQYNPAIIK VK   0
          C9   aJNITSENLIDDVVSLIR GGTRKYAFEL KEKLLRGTVI DVTDFVNWAS SINDAPVLIS QK   0
```

Figure 4 Exon organization of the MAC protein family. Amino acid sequences from the Swiss Protein Sequence Data Bank were aligned using the Genetics Computer Group (GCG) Wisconsin Sequence Analysis Package, Version 8. Minor adjustments were made by introducing gaps to align Cys residues. Exon boundaries were determined from the published gene structures and are depicted in an arrangement similar to that described elsewhere (51). Included are the recently revised boundaries for C9 exons 4–5, 5–6 and 10–11 (55). Sequences begin with the predicted initiation Met. The N-terminus of each mature protein is underlined. Where exon boundaries occur within a codon, amino acids are designated by the three letter code in italics. Exon boundary phases are in the right column. Not shown is "exon 0" of C6, which contains only 5′ untranslated sequence (50). Exon 0 of C7 contains two residues (MK) of translated sequence; for clarity these residues are

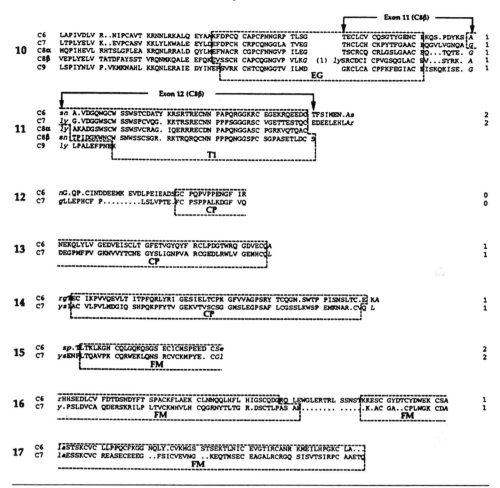

included within exon 1. Phases for exon 0 in C6 and C7 are indicated to the left of their respective exon 1 sequences. Within C8β, exon 10 is interrupted by an intron that produces an additional exon. The phase for the exon 10–11 boundary of C8β is shown in parentheses. Dotted lines show the module boundaries as defined in Figure 2.

the contemporary C8α and C8β genes on chromosome 1. Although plausible, such an explanation makes it difficult to understand the duplication event that produced C9. One alternative possibility is that C6 or C7 and C8α or C8β are products of independent tandem duplications that resulted in a tail-to-tail orientation because of some intrinsic feature of these genes. Without additional structural information from flanking sequence, one cannot predict the exact mechanism.

B. C8γ

The human C8γ gene has been completely sequenced and the transcription initiation site identified (46). The gene contains seven exons spanning ~1.8 kb. Comparison of the C8γ genomic structure to other members of the lipocalin family reveals a striking similarity in exon numbers, lengths, boundaries, and phases. Furthermore, the human C8γ locus is located near a cluster of other lipocalin genes. Analysis of somatic cell hybrids initially localized C8γ to chromosome 9q (63) while PCR of sorted translocation chromosomes further localized it to 9q22.3–q32 (66). However, recent identification of DNA polymorphisms and genotyping of informative families have revised the location to 9q34.3 (67). It is interesting that the region 9q34.2–q34.3 contains genes for the lipocalins LCN1 (tear lipocalin), LCN2 (lipocalin 2 or neutrophil gelatinase associated lipocalin, the human counterpart of mouse 24p3 oncogene), placental protein 14 (the human homologue of β-lactoglobulin), and the brain form of prostaglandin D2 synthase (67). Nearby at 9q32–q33 are genes encoding the lipocalins α-1-acid glycoprotein and α-1-microglobulin (protein HC). Location of C8γ within this cluster provides compelling evidence that it arose by duplication of a lipocalin gene.

IV. ASSEMBLY OF MAC

A. Formation and Properties

Assembly of the MAC is initiated by a single enzymatic event in which C5 is cleaved by C5 convertase to form C5a and C5b. The latter contains a cleaved α chain (α') of ~150 kDa and a disulfide-linked β chain of ~75 kDa. Newly formed C5b interacts with C6 to form C5b-6, a stable dimer that can be purified from complement-activated serum (68, 69). The complex is stable in high ionic strength buffer but is irreversibly dissociated by chaotropic agents. Cross-linking studies indicate that within C5b-6, C6 is in close proximity to the α' chain of C5b (70).

Interaction of fluid-phase C5b-6 with C7 generates the C5b-7 trimer. Crosslinking of C5b-7 indicates C7 is in close proximity to the C5bα' chain; therefore, this chain may mediate binding of both C6 and C7 (70). This step in MAC formation involves a hydrophilic to amphiphilic transition of the constituent proteins that produces a complex with a high affinity for lipid (e.g., phospholipid and detergent micelles, synthetic lipid vesicles, lipoproteins, and membranes) (71). In the absence of lipid or inhibitory proteins, C5b-7 self-aggregates through its hydrophobic membrane binding site to form inactive protein micelles. Although relatively nonspecific towards lipid, C5b-7 deposition on simple cells such as erythrocytes may be localized to specific structures on the surface. Recent evidence indicates C5b-6 binds through ionic interactions to sialic acid on surface molecules such as gangliosides or glycophorin (72). Subsequent binding of C7 disrupts this transient interaction, resulting in the exposure of hydrophobic domains and direct association of C5b-7 with the membrane bilayer. Consistent with this interpretation is the binding preference of C5b-6 for synthetic vesicles containing acidic phospholipids and the ability of fluid-phase gangliosides and glycophorin to compete for C5b-6 and limit its uptake by target membranes (73,74). Specificity of C5b-6 and C5b-7 for substructures on target cell membranes remains a poorly understood aspect of the MAC assembly process.

A model for ultrastructural changes that occur during C5b-7 formation has been proposed based on electron microscopy data (5). This model depicts membrane-bound C5b-7 as an extended hooklike structure. C5b is exposed to the aqueous phase while C6 and C7 form a stalklike structure that penetrates into the bilayer; however, penetration is not sufficient for membrane lysis. Data from electron paramagnetic resonance studies of planar lipid bilayers containing spin-labeled probes determined that C5b-7 associates with the outer lipid surface and only minimally penetrates into the hydrocarbon phase (75). In contrast, binding of C8 and C9 to C5b-7 induces structural changes suggestive of deeper bilayer penetration, which is required for MAC lytic activity.

In the next step of MAC assembly, C8 binds to a site on C5b-7 to form the tetrameric C5b-8 complex. Evidence indicates that C8 binding is mediated strictly by the C8β chain and appears to involve a recognition site on C5b (10). Studies performed in solution demonstrated that C8 binds to C5 or C5b-6 but not C6 or C7 (76). Similar binding was observed using purified C8β instead of C8. Cross-linking of membrane-bound C5b-8 corroborated these findings and indicated that C8β is physically associated with C5b in this complex. Immunochemical analysis of purified MAC suggests that C5b and C8β are also closely associated within C5b-9 (77).

C5b-8 can cause leakage from synthetic lipid vesicles (78), promote slow osmotic lysis of erythrocytes (79), and induce responses in nucleated cells (80). Labeling of C5b-8 by aqueous phase and membrane-restricted probes identified C8 as a major contributor to membrane perturbation. When synthetic phospholipid vesicles were used as targets, C8α-γ was found to be the predominant component in contact with the hydrocarbon phase (81). C6 and C7 were labeled by both probes but to a lesser extent, whereas C5b and C8β were found to be primarily exposed to the aqueous phase. Distribution of label between the aqueous and hydrocarbon phases changed significantly as C5b-7 was converted to C5b-8, indicating rearrangement of C5b, C6, and C7 during the process. Results obtained with synthetic vesicles were extended using erythrocyte membranes as targets for C5b-8 (82). Again C8α-γ was the predominant component labeled by a membrane-restricted probe, and further analysis determined that the label was exclusively in C8α. Other constituents were labeled to a lesser extent, while C8γ was not labeled under any conditions.

The primary function of membrane-bound C5b-8 is to serve as a receptor for C9 in the final step of MAC formation (83). Binding to C5b-8 is a two-stage process. First, C9 interacts with a binding site on the C8α chain. This is a reversible interaction at 0°C but becomes irreversible at 37°C when C9 unfolds and inserts into the membrane (84). Binding of the first C9 mediates incorporation of additional C9 molecules, presumably through C9–C9 interactions. Evidence that C9 undergoes conformational changes in the process comes largely from studies of poly C9 and includes changes in ultrastructure (22), loss or gain of epitopes for anti-C9 antibodies (85,86), and accessibility to proteases (33) or labeling reagents (36). The number of C9 molecules required to form a lytically active MAC and the mechanism by which the MAC disrupts membrane organization have been the subject of debate for years. The substance of this debate is addressed in several reviews (87–90).

One area of agreement concerns the fact that heterogeneity exists in the composition and ultrastructure of the MAC. These properties vary with the number of C9 molecules incorporated, which is determined by the characteristics of the target (membranes, vesicles, liposomes, etc.) and the amount of C9 available to C5b-8. When C9 input is high, MAC formed on erythrocytes or synthetic vesicles may contain as many as 12 C9 molecules (91,92). Here, the ultrastructure resembles that of Zn^{2+}-induced poly C9 (91–93). Indeed, this form of MAC consists of a tubular-shaped, pore-like structure composed primarily of polymerized C9 with C5b-8 attached as a club-like appendage (91). Photolabeling by membrane-restricted probes confirmed that C9 is in close association with the lipid bilayer in MAC as well as in poly C9 (94). The pore diameter of this MAC is ~10 nm, which agrees with that for poly C9. Based on these results, it is apparent that C5b-8 functions much like Zn^{2+} by promoting C9 unfolding and formation of poly C9.

One controversial aspect is whether formation of a tubular-shaped polymer of C9 is necessary for MAC lytic activity. Several lines of evidence indicate that poly C9 contributes to MAC-mediated lysis but is not absolutely required. MAC formed on erythrocytes at typical serum concentrations of C9 contains an average of three to six C9 molecules (19,95,96). Under these conditions, some complexes contain more or less than the average number of C9 molecules and accordingly may or may not appear as ringlike tubular structures. In either case, photolabeling of MAC indicates a direct interaction between C9 and the membrane (94). This is consistent with evidence that MAC has lytic potential independent of poly C9 formation. Thrombin-cleaved C9 under certain conditions does not form tubular structures but is able to lyse membrane vesicles (97). Other studies have shown that MAC containing as few as one C9 per C5b-8 is hemolytically active at 37°C (84). Lesions with ultrastructural characteristics of poly C9 were completely absent on these erythrocyte targets. Pore diameters of these complexes were only ~1–3 nm but sufficient to promote osmotic lysis. Thus, the pore "size" of the MAC is variable and depends on the number of C9 molecules incorporated.

Another controversial aspect of MAC is how the "pore" itself is formed. The concept of a transmembrane channel lined with amphipathic helices contributed by poly C9 is compatible with most available experimental data. More difficult to understand is how MAC containing nontubular or only one C9 can alter local membrane permeability and promote lysis. Evidence from freeze-etch electron microscopy indicates that tubular C5b-9 binds and thereby restructures lipid organization within its immediate environment (98). This has also been proposed to occur with nontubular forms of MAC, which may form smaller transmembrane channels or pores that are restricted in size because of the amount of C9 available (94). Also of importance may be the role of C8α. This subunit along with C9 are the two MAC components predominantly labeled by membrane-restricted probes and therefore both are likely to perturb lipid organization. Thus, in complexes containing only one or a few C9 molecules, C8α may contribute directly to lysis whereas in complexes that contain poly C9, its contribution may be less significant. Regardless of the mechanism by which the MAC components collectively perturb membrane organization, it is clear that one or more of them acquires the ability to bind lipid upon incorporation into the complex.

B. Inhibitors

MAC activity towards autologous cells is regulated by serum proteins vitronectin (S protein) and clusterin (SP40-40), and the membrane-associated protein CD59 that is expressed on a variety of cell types. Vitronectin is a 75 kDa protein that mediates cell attachment and cell–cell adhesion through interaction with integrin receptors (99). It also contains a high-affinity heparin-binding site that mediates nonreceptor attachment of vitronectin–protein complexes. It has a regulatory function in both the coagulation and fibrinolytic systems because of its heparin-binding capability and its ability to modulate thrombin activity and plasminogen activation. Several of vitronectin's functions have been assigned to specific structural domains (100).

Vitronectin exerts its complement inhibitory activity primarily by binding to C5b-7 and blocking its interaction with the target membrane (101,102). The result is formation of soluble SC5b-7 containing an estimated three or four molecules of vitronectin (103). SC5b-7 binds one C8 and three C9 molecules to form SC5b-8 and SC5b-9, respectively. Based on experiments using synthetic peptides, the inhibitory activity of vitronectin was initially attributed to interaction between a short segment of highly basic residues in its heparin-binding domain and a segment of acidic residues within the LDLRA modules of MAC proteins (104). However, more recent data suggest the C5b-7 binding site is not contained within the heparin-binding domain (105). An internal 43 kDa fragment of vitronectin that lacks the heparin-binding site was shown to compete with C5b-7 for binding to immobilized vitronectin. This fragment also blocks C5b-7 attachment to erythrocytes, and inhibits C5b-8 mediated polymerization of C9. In addition, SC5b-9 has been shown to bind immobilized heparin (106). This suggests the heparin-binding site is accessible in this complex and is not likely to be in direct contact with the MAC proteins.

Clusterin is a multifunctional protein composed of disulfide-linked α and β subunits each with a molecular weight of $\sim$35,000–40,000 (107,108). It is a hydrophobic protein that circulates in a complex with lipid and apolipoprotein A-1. Clusterin is typically found along with vitronectin in soluble MAC complexes. It inhibits MAC formation by binding to C5b-7, C5b-8, and C5b-9, and it also inhibits Zn^{2+}-induced C9 polymerization. Ligand blotting assays indicate that it binds to C7, C8β, and the C9b domain of C9 and thus may interact specifically with these proteins in SC5b-9. Four amphipathic helices predicted from the amino acid sequence of clusterin may mediate its interaction with the hydrophobic membrane-binding site on the nascent MAC. It has been suggested that these interact with two amphipathic helices that are conserved in all the MAC components and that form the presumptive membrane-binding site in C9 (108).

Human CD59 is an $\sim$20 kDa protein that functions to protect blood and vascular cells from lysis by human MAC. It inhibits MAC activity by interacting with C8 and C9 during assembly of the nascent complex on target cells (109). This interaction limits the number of C9 molecules bound by C5b-8 and restricts formation of a functional MAC complex. The inhibitory activity of human CD59 is species-selective and is most effective towards primate C8 and C9. This selectivity has been useful in identifying CD59-binding sites in human C8 and C9.

V. STRUCTURE-FUNCTION RELATIONSHIPS

A. C6 and C7

Hydropathic analyses of C6 and C7 do not reveal any extended segments of hydrophobic residues that might function as membrane-binding domains (3,5). Multiple, short hydrophobic segments are distributed throughout, and occur most frequently in the C-terminal half of each protein. Regions of C6 and C7 in contact with membrane lipid have not been experimentally identified but it is likely that multiple sites of contact are involved.

The C5b-binding site in C6 and C7 is believed to reside in the C-terminal region containing the tandemly arranged CCP and FIM modules (Fig. 2). This would be consistent with the role of these modules in mediating interactions between complement regulatory proteins and C3b and C4b, the homologues of C5b (43). Evidence of a role for these modules in binding C5b was initially obtained using a 34 kDa C-terminal proteolytic fragment of C6 that contains the intact CCP and FIM modules (2). When immobilized on a solid support, this fragment bound C5b from activated serum. These results were corroborated when the corresponding fragment of C7 was independently shown to bind to immobilized C5 (70). These studies also attempted to localize further the C5b binding site in C6. A fragment containing residues 1–610 and fragments containing both CCP modules (residues 611–747) or the tandem FIM modules (residues 748–913) were each tested for binding to immobilized C5. Only intact C6 and the fragment containing the FIM modules bound specifically. Thus, it was concluded that C6 and C7 interaction with C5b is mediated by the FIM modules.

More recent evidence suggests the binding site is not located in the FIM modules. Humans with subtotal C6 deficiency synthesize a truncated form of C6 lacking two-thirds of the first FIM and the entire second FIM module (110). An important finding is that this truncated C6 is functional despite the absence of these modules. Also, a monoclonal antibody that inhibits C5b-6 formation has been mapped to a site in the third TSPI module of C6 (111). Because of the close proximity of this site to the CCP modules and the functionality of a truncate lacking the FIM modules, it has now been suggested that binding of C6 to C5b is mediated by the CCP modules.

B. C8

The ability to isolate C8α-γ and C8β in stable form has facilitated efforts to assign functional roles to the C8 subunits (112). Selective cleavage of the interchain disulfide bond in C8α-γ has also enabled the individual roles of C8α and C8γ to be studied. From these efforts, a model has emerged that recognizes the existence of distinct functional sites on C8 (Fig. 5A).

C8β fulfills several roles and is envisioned as having several different functional sites. Deciphering the location of these sites should now be possible since recombinant forms of human C8β have been expressed in both mammalian and nonmammalian systems (113). One site is recognized by C5b-7 and is the site that mediates incorporation of C8 into the nascent MAC. Studies using purified subunits showed that C8β alone binds to C5b-7 on erythrocyte membranes (114). Binding is specific and inhibited by intact C8.

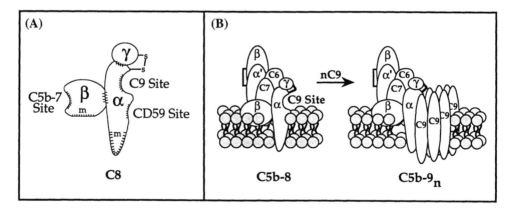

Figure 5 Functional sites in human C8. (*A*) Schematic representation of the functional sites identified for each subunit of C8. These are depicted as distinct, nonoverlapping sites (identified as I I ſ I I I) because they function simultaneously within the MAC. Their location within the primary structure of each subunit is unknown, the exception being the CD59 site. Membrane-binding sites are designated "m". (*B*) Relative locations of the C8 subunits within membrane-bound C5b-8 and C5b-9. Spatial arrangement of the subunits in relation to the other MAC proteins is based on cumulative data described in the text. The α′ and β chains of C5b are shown as a disulfide-linked dimer. C9 is shown as a polymer composed of an arbitrary number of monomeric units.

Whether a conformationally defined domain or a specific sequence on C8β is recognized remains to be determined. As noted earlier, within C5b-7 it is likely that C5b provides the binding site for C8β. Although C8α-γ has no affinity for C5b-7, it is required for MAC formation because complexes of C5b-7 and C8β do not bind C9.

A second functional site on C8β mediates its interaction with the C8α chain. This was determined in experiments using purified C8α and C8γ obtained after cleavage of the interchain disulfide bond in C8α-γ (115). C8α alone associates with C8β and produces a stable C8α·C8β dimer referred to as C8'. This analogue is functionally similar to C8 with respect to binding C5b-7, mediating C9 incorporation, and promoting cell lysis. Thus, C8γ is not directly involved in interactions with C8β nor is it required for C8 activity.

A third functional site on C8β consists of one or more segments that interact directly with the target membrane bilayer. Evidence for this comes from photolabeling experiments using membrane-restricted probes to identify C5b-8 and C5b-9 components inserted in the membrane bilayer (81,82,94). C8β was only moderately labeled in these experiments; therefore, it is in contact with the membrane but only to a limited extent.

Several functional sites have also been identified in C8α. One mediates C8α-γ association with C8β. As described above, C8α forms a stable dimer with C8β in the absence of C8γ. A second site appears to interact with lipid bilayers. As noted earlier, C8α is one of the predominant components of C5b-8 and C5b-9 inserted in target membranes. A third site directs binding and incorporation of C9 into the MAC. Evidence for this comes from the observation that C8, C8α-γ, or C8α can associate with C9 in solutions of low ionic strength (116). The same study demonstrated that a C5·C8·C9 trimeric complex can also form in solution. More recently, small-angle neutron scattering experiments determined that C8 and C9 form a dimer at physiological ionic strength (7). Together, these data support a mechanism for MAC formation in which C8 binds to C5b-7 by association of C8β with C5b while C8α interacts with and directs incorporation of C9 into C5b-8.

A fourth site in C8α is involved in interactions with C8γ. C8α and C8γ retain a high affinity for each other after cleavage of the interchain disulfide bond (117). This suggests that C8α expresses a stable binding site for C8γ and C8γ likewise has a binding site for C8α. The significance of these sites may relate to the fact that unlike disulfide-linked subunits that are synthesized as single-chain precursors, C8α and C8γ are synthesized independently and, therefore, must associate co- or posttranslationally for disulfide bond formation to occur. Interestingly, the Cys to which C8γ is attached resides in exon 5 of C8α. This exon is significantly longer than exon 5 of the other MAC proteins because of an insertion of 18 residues that includes Cys[164] (Fig. 4). Thus, it is likely this insertion uniquely confers binding specificity toward C8γ and in fact may encode the binding site itself. There is no dependence of C8α on C8γ for synthesis and secretion. Recombinant forms of each can be produced independently in mammalian and nonmammalian cells (118). Recombinant C8α is hemolytically active when combined with purified C8β, thus confirming that C8γ is not essential for C8 activity.

A fifth site on C8α functions as a CD59-binding site. It was initially observed that human CD59 binds specifically to surface-adsorbed human C8α-γ and C8α but not the corresponding subunits from rabbit, a species that exhibits unrestricted lytic activity towards human erythrocytes (119). Functional evidence in support of the binding data was obtained using human erythrocytes as target cells and comparing lytic activities of human and rabbit C8 to a hybrid composed of human β and rabbit α-γ (16). Activity of the hybrid C8 was comparable to rabbit C8, indicating that restriction of lysis depends primarily on the species of C8α-γ. Together, these results established that the site recognized by CD59 is located in C8α.

A likely location for the CD59-binding site was revealed by comparing sequences of human and rabbit C8α, which identified a single segment of significant sequence dissimilarity (human 349–385 vs. rabbit 349–386) (16). Recombinant peptides spanning these sequences were expressed, purified, and tested for CD59 binding (120). CD59 specifically bound to the human peptide and required an intact disulfide-bond between Cys^{345}–Cys^{369}. Binding to the corresponding peptide from rabbit C8α was not observed. Functional evidence that this region is selectively recognized by CD59 was provided in this same study by preparing chimeric C8α cDNA in which segments containing these sequences were exchanged between human and rabbit. The chimeric C8α cDNA was used along with cDNAs for human or rabbit C8β and C8γ to cotransfect COS cells. Hemolytic activity of expressed chimeric C8 was measured using heterologous target cells reconstituted with CD59. Results confirmed that CD59 recognizes a conformationally sensitive site internal to residues 320–415 of human C8α. These data also suggested that interaction of CD59 is influenced by sequence immediately N-terminal to this segment in C8α and by human C8β but is unaffected by C8γ.

The CD59-binding site in C8α is inaccessible in intact C8 and is only expressed when the protein is surface-adsorbed or denatured (119). During MAC assembly, this site presumably becomes exposed as a consequence of conformational changes associated with C8 binding to C5b-7. It has been suggested that C5b-8 may contain two sites of contact with C9 (121). One is on C8α and mediates initial binding while the second promotes proper unfolding of C9 for insertion into the membrane. At this second site CD59 could exert its inhibitory function by sterically hindering the unfolding of the first C9, thereby restricting binding of additional C9 molecules. If so, this second site would likely be at or near the CD59-binding site.

The function of C8γ remains unknown. It is not required for MAC assembly, function, or interaction with inhibitors. Because it is a lipocalin, it likely has a tertiary structure similar to other members of this family and may bind an as yet unidentified small ligand. Three-dimensional structures have been determined for several lipocalins including human retinol-binding protein, bovine β-lactoglobulin, mouse urinary protein, and insecticyanin (122). Despite low sequence identity, these proteins have highly conserved folding patterns consisting of a core of eight antiparallel β-strands arranged into two orthogonal sheets to form a β-barrel structure with a cup-shaped ligand-binding site. This site is lined with apolar residues that confer specificity toward hydrophobic ligands. Members of the fatty acid-binding protein family, which also bind small hydrophobic ligands, have a similar β-barrel structure. Thus, it has been suggested that both families form part of a larger "structural superfamily" that might appropriately be named the calycins to reflect the cup-shaped structure of its members (123). Molecular modeling of C8γ against bovine β-lactoglobulin indicates it is capable of forming a β-barrel structure with a distinct binding site (15). Consistent with this is the close correlation between exons in C8γ and those exons containing conserved structural elements that define the β-barrel in other lipocalins (46).

Several possible functions for C8γ have been suggested. Initially it was proposed to be the target of C8-binding protein, an as yet uncharacterized membrane-associated protein thought to interact with C8 and inhibit C5b-9 mediated lysis of homologous cells (124). However, later experiments established that the presence or absence of C8γ had no effect on homologous restriction of C5b-9 (125). C8α-γ was also shown to bind retinol/

retinoic acid and, consequently, C8γ was proposed to be a retinol-binding protein (15). The validity of this proposal is tempered by the fact that binding was only observed with intact C8α-γ and in the presence of 2M NaCl. In a recent study using recombinant C8γ, retinol binding was not observed under a variety of conditions including physiological ionic strength (118). If C8γ does indeed have a binding site for small ligands it may recognize a specific structure on C8α, possibly one that serves as a "docking" site prior to intracellular disulfide-bond formation. As an alternative, it may function to shield C8α from premature membrane interaction during biosynthetic processing or secretion. An argument against the latter is the fact that recombinant C8α can be synthesized and secreted from transfected mammalian cells independently of C8γ.

The various C8 functional sites depicted in Figure 5A are placed within the context of C5b-8 and C5b-9 in Figure 5B. This topographical model emphasizes the location of these sites in relation to the other MAC proteins and the membrane. C8β is shown in close proximity to C5bα', C6, and C7 based on cross-linking data and the fact that it alone binds to C5b-7. C8α is depicted as inserted in the bilayer in both C5b-8 and C5b-9. Binding of the first C9 to C8α promotes unfolding, insertion, and polymerization of C9. Not shown is the CD59 binding site, which is likely located near the membrane and/ or C9 binding site(s). Within both complexes, the site of contact between C8α and C8γ is on the periphery. Evidence for this includes the ability of C8γ to bind C5b-8' and C5b-(8')9, two analogues of the MAC that contain C8' instead of C8 (117). This could only occur if the C8γ-binding site is accessible in C5b-8' and remains so after incorporation of C9. Furthermore, photolabeling experiments failed to detect interaction of C8γ with membrane bilayers (82). This result and the observation that C8γ is not essential for lytic function are consistent with a peripheral location.

C. C9

Because thrombin cleavage of C9 is restricted to a single site, early efforts to define structure–function relationships focused on the C9a and C9b fragments. Thrombin-cleaved C9 retains hemolytic (97) and bactericidal (126) activity and the ability to self-polymerize (36). C9b is significantly more hydrophobic than C9a and can independently express some of the functions of C9. Purified C9b releases markers from lipid vesicles, alters the conductance of synthetic lipid bilayers, and depolarizes inner membrane vesicles from gram-negative bacteria (127,128). Recently C9b was shown to lyse sheep erythrocytes in the absence of C5b-8 and to inhibit growth of sensitive bacterial spheroblasts (129). The activity of C9b and the fact that C9 alone is toxic when osmotically introduced into the periplasm of serum-sensitive *E. coli* has led to the suggestion that the "lethal" component in complement killing of some gram-negative bacteria may be a C9-derived product that acts on the inner membrane (90,130).

A distinguishing feature of C9 is the absence of a C-terminal TSP1 module (Fig. 2). Lack of such a module was originally thought to confer on C9 the unique ability to self-polymerize. This notion was supported by the fact that C9 from species other than human also lack this module. One exception is trout, whose C9 sequence deduced from a cDNA clone was found to contain a C-terminal TSP1 module (28). Formation of classical ringlike lesions on erythrocytes exposed to trout serum was interpreted as evidence that trout C9 can polymerize despite the presence of this module. A concern with respect to this conclusion remains, however, and that is whether the deduced amino acid sequence is that of trout C9 or a subunit of trout C8 (28).

It has been proposed that human C9 contains five distinct structural domains arranged in a cluster resembling a globular ellipsoid (131). TSP1 and LDLRA modules make up domains 1 and 2, respectively, while MACPF residues 117–226 form domain 3 (Fig. 6). These are followed by the "hinge" region that extends from residues 227 to 266 and includes the thrombin cleavage site. Domain 4 extends from 267 to 364 and contains a putative membrane-binding region. Domain 5 extends from residue 365 in MACPF to the C-terminus. Folding of C9 is presumed to involve interaction between N-terminal domains 1–3 and the C-terminal domains 4–5. Upon incorporation into the MAC, C9 undergoes conformational changes that reorient these domains so as to form an elongated structure with the membrane-interacting segment (domain 4) located at one end for penetration into the bilayer. By functioning as a structural linker, the hinge facilitates unfolding and reorientation of these domains. Interestingly, the hinge is located in exon 6 and corresponds to inserted sequence not found in the other MAC proteins (Fig. 4). Thus, the function of the hinge may be unique to C9.

Experimental evidence supports a rearrangement of domains 4 and 5 during membrane insertion. C9 contains two discontinuous segments of sequence (residues 293–296 in domain 4 and 528–532 in domain 5) that are identical to a single continuous sequence in mellitin (residues 8–11 and 12–16), the hemolytic peptide from bee venom (132). Antibodies against mellitin inhibit C9 hemolytic activity, whereas antibodies against the individual C9 sequences do not. In contrast, antibodies against a composite peptide containing both sequences (simulating mellitin residues 8–16) compete for the same epitope as antimellitin and inhibit C9 hemolytic activity. Thus, these segments of domains 4 and 5 together must form a discontinuous epitope that, when bridged by an antibody, prevents C9 unfolding.

In the folded state, interaction between the N- and C-terminal regions of C9 may involve a cluster of acidic residues located within the LDLRA module (residues 100–115) and a cluster of basic residues in domain 5 (residues 415–425). The former exhibit sequence similarity to the ligand-binding domains within the LDL receptor, while the latter are similar to the putative receptor-binding domain within the apoB-100/apoE ligands

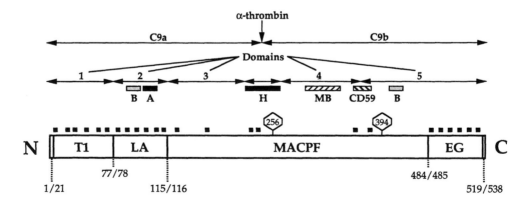

Figure 6 Functional sites in human C9. The five domains and hinge region (H) of C9 are shown in relation to the protein map described in Figure 2. Functional sites described in the text include the α-thrombin cleavage site, membrane-binding site (MB), CD59 recognition site (CD59), a cluster of acidic residues within the LDLRA module (A), and two clusters of basic residues with sequence similarity to apoB-100/apoE (B).

(131). Thus, folding of C9 may mimic a receptor–ligand-type interaction between these regions. Also potentially significant is a second cluster of basic residues resembling the apoB-100/apoE receptor-binding domain located immediately N-terminal (residues 90–97) to the acidic residues in LDLRA. While these clusters of acidic and basic residues may be important for C9 folding, they may also mediate lateral protein–protein interactions during MAC assembly and/or C9 polymerization. Experimental evidence does, in fact, suggest that electrostatic interactions are important. It has been shown that negatively charged molecules such as heparin, chondroitin-sulfate A, and suramin and positively charged molecules such as protamine and poly-L-lysine that inhibit LDL receptor–ligand interaction also inhibit poly C9 formation and MAC assembly (133).

The acidic cluster within LDLRA also contains sequence similar to the consensus sequence found in EF-hand motifs in a number of calcium-binding proteins (134). When this region was targeted for mutagenesis by substituting Ala for four adjacent acidic residues (DEDD) at positions 109–112, the mutant C9 was expressed by insect cells and exhibited hemolytic activity comparable to wild-type C9. Because calcium is not required for C9 hemolytic activity and because direct binding of calcium to recombinant C9 was not measured, these results are inconclusive with respect to whether this sequence encodes a calcium-binding site. However, the targeted residues are in the same acidic cluster believed to be involved in C9 folding and intermolecular interactions during MAC assembly. Substituting them with uncharged residues does not abolish C9 activity. Therefore, one can at least conclude that a negative charge at these four positions is not essential for function.

The membrane-interaction site in C9 was initially localized to C9b using membrane-restricted photosensitive probes (135). Subsequent studies suggested that the site is centered on residues 287–345 (136). Within this segment, two amphipathic α-helices (residues 292–308 and 313–333) separated by a turn (residues 309–312) were proposed to align in an antiparallel manner to form the membrane-spanning domain of C9 (136). Conservation of these sequences across the MAC protein family suggested that they fulfill a common function by forming the walls of a transmembrane channel. However, it has been noted that because the helices are amphipathic rather than hydrophobic and the turn itself is hydrophilic, insertion into a membrane bilayer from the aqueous milieu is unlikely (90). The alternative mechanism proposes that amphipathic helices or β-structures lie parallel to the membrane surface with their hydrophobic faces embedded in the membrane. How this arrangement would produce the porelike structure characteristic of the fully assembled MAC is unclear. These helices are nevertheless important for proper C9 folding. Characterization of recombinant mutants in which the amphipathic nature of these helices was altered by successive substitutions on their hydrophobic surfaces revealed that some conservative substitutions were tolerated, and a hemolytically active C9 was produced (137). However, nonconservative substitutions produced an improperly folded C9 that failed to be secreted.

Human C9 contains a cryptic CD59-binding site that is only exposed upon denaturation or incorporation into the MAC. This site was initially localized to C9b by ligand-blotting assays (119). Binding of CD59 to proteolytic fragments and C9-derived peptides spanning the entire C9b domain further narrowed the site to within residues 359–411 (138). This site lies within one of two extended regions of sequence dissimilarity between human and rabbit C9. Because the latter species exhibits unrestricted lysis towards human erythrocytes, recombinant C9 chimeras were prepared in which these segments were exchanged between human and rabbit (26). Assays revealed that CD59 inhibits hemolytic activity of chimeras containing human C9 sequence between residues 334 and 415, irrespective of whether the remainder of the protein contains human or rabbit sequence. By contrast, when this segment of human C9 contains rabbit sequence, lytic activity is unaffected by CD59. Further analysis of chimeras with substitutions internal to this segment determined that the CD59 recognition site is centered on those residues within the disulfide loop formed by Cys^{359}–Cys^{384}, with an additional contribution by residues C-terminal to this segment (139). Mutant human C9 in which Ala is substituted for $Cys^{359,384}$ is fully inhibited by CD59, indicating that a disulfide bond between these residues is not required for interaction with CD59. This segment recognized by CD59 is adjacent to the membrane-binding site in C9. By binding near this site, CD59 may prevent its exposure during MAC formation and thereby interfere with C9 insertion into the membrane.

When the sequences of human C8α and C9 are aligned, there is an overlap between those segments that encode the respective CD59-binding sites (120). However, the sequences at these sites are suprisingly dissimilar. This suggests either that both proteins fold so as to align their conserved residues into a common structural motif recognized by CD59 or that binding sites expressed by each consist of distinct motifs that are recognized equally well by this inhibitor. With respect to the latter, it is of interest that whereas CD59 binding to C9 does not require a disulfide bond between $Cys^{359,384}$, binding to C8α depends on the integrity of the disulfide bond between the corresponding residues $Cys^{345,369}$.

A second segment of sequence divergence among species is located in the hinge domain. It was reported that a synthetic peptide corresponding to residues 247–261 within this region binds to CD59, enhances MAC-mediated lysis of human erythrocytes by inhibiting CD59, and therefore encodes a CD59 binding site (140). Others subsequently determined that binding of this peptide to CD59 is nonspecific (138). In assays performed in the presence and absence of CD59 on target cells, this peptide as well as several unrelated peptides enhanced MAC-mediated lysis irrespective of whether CD59 was present. Presumably this was the result of sublytic perturbation of the target membrane, which makes it more susceptible to lysis. The role of the hinge as a CD59-binding site was also examined in a functional context by preparing and characterizing recombinant chimeras of C9 (26). Introducing the hinge sequence from rabbit into human C9 failed to overcome inhibition by CD59. Although still considered controversial (141), these data suggest that the hinge does not contain a functional CD59 recognition site.

D. The Modules

Modules found in the MAC components are known to mediate protein–protein interactions in a variety of other proteins (39, 42). Thus, it is reasonable to assume they have a similar function in the MAC assembly process. A comparison of corresponding modules from each of the MAC proteins indicates that they have a high degree of sequence similarity to each other and to consensus sequences derived from the same modules in other proteins (Fig. 7). With the exception of the first C6 TSP1 and the C9 EGF modules, all Cys residues within the MAC modules are conserved. When the disulfide bond pattern in each of the C9 modules is aligned in relation to Cys residues in the other proteins, it is apparent that all corresponding modules are likely to have the same pattern.

One can also predict the EGF module in C9 folds to form a structural motif similar to the EGF protein. As with some EGF modules and EGF itself (142,143), C9 has a six-Cys backbone and a 1–3, 2–4, and 5–6 disulfide bond pattern. EGF modules with this cross-

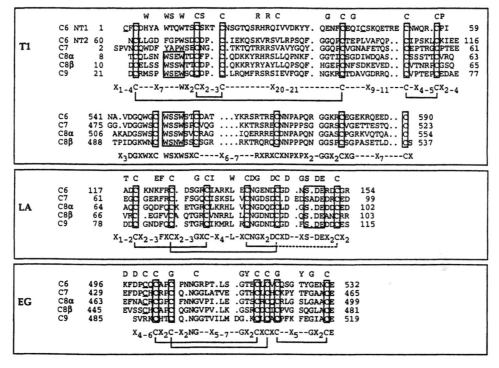

Figure 7 Alignment of modules in the MAC proteins. Module sequences were aligned using the Genetics Computer Group (GCG) Wisconsin Sequence Analysis Programs Version 8 with some minor spacing modifications. Residue numbers correspond to module boundaries in Figure 2. Consensus Cys residues are boxed and those not found in all five proteins are underlined. The WSxW and SDE sequences described in the text are shaded. Above the modules are consensus sequences typically found in other proteins. Below each is the consensus sequence found in the MAC protein family, along with the disulfide bond pattern for C9.

linking pattern are predicted to have similar secondary and tertiary structures (144–146). In contrast, EGF modules in the other MAC proteins contain an additional Cys not found in C9. Furthermore, they contain five Cys in their C-terminal TSP1 module rather than the six typically found in other proteins (147). This suggests that the additional Cys in the EGF module is linked to one in the C-terminal TSP1 module. Also noteworthy are two nonconserved Cys in the first TSP1 of C6, which are likely to be linked to each other.

LDLRA modules in all the MAC proteins contain a cluster of acidic residues located near the C-terminal end. As noted previously (Section V.C.), this region is proposed to be involved in C9 folding and possibly in protein-protein interactions during MAC assembly. These residues along with an invariant SDE sequence are also conserved in all seven LDLRA modules of the LDL receptor (41). Structural analyses and the disulfide bond pattern predict the SDE triplet and flanking acidic residues to be located within a single loop that interacts with a highly basic region of the apoprotein ligands (148–150). Interestingly, the SDE sequence is also conserved in the MAC LDLRA modules. Furthermore, the disulfide bond pattern for modules in the LDL receptor agrees with one of two possible patterns for the C9 LDLRA module (e.g., Cys^{80}-Cys^{91}, Cys^{86}-Cys^{104} and Cys^{98}-Cys^{113} in Fig. 3) (149). This suggests the LDLRA modules of all the MAC proteins may be folded similar to those in the LDL receptor, with the acidic cluster mediating a receptor-ligand type interaction between the components.

Another significant feature is the cluster of basic residues located in the center of the TSP1 modules. Nearby is a WSxW sequence that is conserved in all the MAC TSP1 modules except those at the N-terminus of C6 and C7. The WSxW sequence is also found in TSP1 modules in thrombospondin. This sequence in conjunction with flanking basic residues mediates thrombospondin binding to transforming growth factor β (151), fibronectin (152), and heparin (153). With the exception of C7, all the MAC components bind heparin (154). Thus, it is possible this interaction involves the region near the WSxW sequence. If so, this region may normally function by binding negatively charged segments of adjacent proteins during MAC assembly.

VI. PERSPECTIVE

In view of the conserved structures and common genetic origin of the MAC proteins, several specific questions can be asked with respect to the mechanism of MAC assembly and function. Perhaps most intriguing is why seven different gene products are required to produce a complex whose primary function is to disrupt lipid organization, particularly when the complex is relatively nonspecific in its action. With respect to this, the bactericidal action of MAC appears to involve a more complex mechanism than simple disruption of the outer membrane, while induction of responses in nucleated cells may likewise require more than local perturbation of the lipid bilayer. As details of these mechanisms are deciphered, a rationale for the evolution of a multiprotein complex such as the MAC may become apparent. Also of interest is the function of C8γ and the related questions of why this protein evolved from a lipocalin gene to become an integral part of C8, why it is located on the periphery of the MAC, and why it has no apparent role in the *in vitro* expression of MAC lytic activity. The discovery of additional biological functions of MAC may provide answers to these and other questions.

With regard to molecular aspects of MAC assembly, a relevant question concerns the basis for the unusual ability of these hydrophilic proteins to bind lipid when incorporated into the MAC. This suggests that each contains one or more cryptic lipid-binding sites that are expressed as a result of conformational changes during the assembly process. Equally interesting is the basis for the specificity of interactions between the components. All components share common structural features (e.g., the modules), therefore one can compare formation of MAC to the assembly of a heteropolymer with monomeric units joined together by common structural elements, which logically must be the modules. However, there is an order to the assembly process and the specificity of interaction is most likely dictated by differences in surface features or sequences within the fine-structure of the modules. With the ability to express recombinant forms of the MAC proteins, progress towards identifying lipid binding sites as well as deciphering the role of the modules should advance rapidly.

REFERENCES

1. DiScipio RG, Gagnon J. Characterization of human complement components C6 and C7. Mol Immunol 1982; 19:1425–1431.

2. Haefliger JA, Tschopp J, Vial N, Jenne DE. Complete primary structure and functional characterization of the sixth component of the human complement system: identification of the C5b-binding domain in complement C6. J Biol Chem 1989; 264:18041–18051.

3. DiScipio RG, Hugli TE. The molecular architecture of human complement component C6. J Biol Chem 1989; 264:16197–16206.

4. Podack ER, Kolb WP, Esser AF, Müller-Eberhard HJ. Structural similarities between C6 and C7 of human complement. J Immunol 1979; 123:1071–1077.

5. DiScipio RG, Chakravarti DN, Müller-Eberhard HJ, Fey GH. The structure of human complement component C7 and the C5b-7 complex. J Biol Chem 1988; 263:549–560.

6. Steckel EW, York RG, Monahan JB, Sodetz JM. The eighth component of human complement: purification and physiochemical characterization of its unusual subunit structure. J Biol Chem 1980; 255:11997–12005.

7. Esser AF, Thielens NM, Zaccai G. Small angle neutron scattering studies of C8 and C9 and their interactions in solution. Biophys J 1993; 64:743–748.

8. Rao AG, Sodetz JM. Purification of functional subunits of the eighth component of human complement (C8) under nondenaturing conditions. Complement 1984; 1:182–186.

9. Monahan JB, Stewart JL, Sodetz JM. Studies of the association of the eighth and ninth components of human complement within the membrane-bound cytolytic complex. J Biol Chem 1983; 258:5056–5062.

10. Monahan JB, Sodetz JM. Binding of the eighth component of human complement to the soluble cytolytic complex is mediated by its β-subunit. J Biol Chem 1980; 255:10579–10582.

11. Rao AG, Howard OMZ, Ng SC, Whitehead AS, Colten HR, Sodetz JM. Complementary DNA and derived amino acid sequence of the α subunit of human complement protein C8: evidence for the existence of a separate α subunit mRNA. Biochemistry: 1987; 26:3556–3564.

12. Howard OMZ, Rao AG, Sodetz JM. Complementary DNA and derived amino acid sequence of the β subunit of human complement protein C8: identification of a close structural and ancestral relationship to the α subunit and C9. Biochemistry 1987; 26:3565–3570.

13. Haefliger J-A, Tschopp J, Nardelli D, Wahli W, Kocher HP, Tosi M, Stanley KK. Complementary DNA cloning of complement C8 beta and its sequence homology to C9. Biochemistry 1987; 26:3551–3556.

14. Ng SC, Rao AG, Howard OMZ, Sodetz JM. The eighth component of human complement (C8): evidence that it is an oligomeric serum protein assembled from products of three different genes. Biochemistry 1987; 26:5229–5233.

15. Haefliger J-A, Peitsch MC, Jenne DE, Tschopp J. Structural and functional characterization of complement C8γ, a member of the lipocalin protein family. Mol Immunol 1991; 28:123–131.

16. White RV, Kaufman KM, Letson CS, Platteborze PL, Sodetz JM. Characterization of rabbit complement component C8: functional evidence for the species-selective recognition of C8α by homologous restriction factor (CD59). J Immunol 1994; 152:2501–2508.

17. Haefliger J-A, Jenne D, Stanley KK, Tschopp J. Structural homology of human complement component C8γ, and plasma protein HC: identity of the cysteine bond pattern. Biochem Biophys Res Comm 1987; 149:750–754.

18. DiScipio RG. The size, shape and stability of complement component C9. Mol Immunol 1993; 30:1097–1106.

19. Stewart JL, Monahan JB, Brickner A, Sodetz JM. Measurement of the ratio of the eighth and ninth components of human complement on complement-lysed membranes. Biochemistry 1984; 23:4016–4022.

20. DiScipio RG, Gehring MR, Podack ER, Kan CC, Hugli TE, Fey GH. Nucleotide sequence of cDNA and derived amino acid sequence of human complement component C9. Proc Natl Acad Sci USA 1984; 81:7298–7302.

21. Stanley KK, Kocher P-H, Luzio JP, Jackson P, Tschopp J. The sequence and topology of human complement component C9. EMBO J 1985; 4:375–382.

22. DiScipio RG, Hugli TE. The architecture of complement component C9 and poly(C9). J Biol Chem 1985; 260:14802–14809.

23. Biesecker G, Gerard C, Hugli TE. An amphiphilic structure of the ninth component of human complement: evidence from analysis of fragments produced by α-thrombin. J Biol Chem 1982; 257:2584–2590.

24. Thielens NM, Lohner K, Esser AF. Human complement protein C9 is a calcium binding protein: structural and functional implications. J Biol Chem 1988; 263:6665–6670.

25. Stanley KK, Herz J. Topological mapping of complement component C9 by recombinant DNA techniques suggests a novel mechanism for its insertion into target membranes. EMBO J 1987; 6:1951–1957.

26. Hüsler T, Lockert DH, Kaufman KM, Sodetz JM, Sims PJ. Chimeras of human complement C9 reveal the site recognized by complement regulatory protein CD59. J Biol Chem 1995; 270:3483–3486.

27. Esser AF, Tarnuzzer RW, Tomlinson S, Tatar LD, Stanley KK. Horse complement protein C9: primary structure and cytotoxic activity. Mol Immunol 1996; 33:725–733.

28. Tomlinson S, Stanley KK, Esser AF. Domain structure, functional activity, and polymerization of trout complement protein C9. Dev Comp Immunol 1993; 17:67–76.

29. O'Hara LC, Lassitar HA, Feldhoff RC. Complement component C9: nucleotide sequence of rat C9 cDNA; interspecies comparisons of amino acid sequences. Mol Immunol 1996; 33(Suppl. 1):26.

30. Tschopp J. Circular polymerization of the membranolytic ninth component of complement: dependence on metal ions. J Biol Chem 1984; 259:10569–10573.

31. Podack ER, Tschopp J. Polymerization of the ninth component of complement (C9): formation of poly (C9) with a tubular ultrastructure resembling the membrane attack complex of complement. Proc Natl Acad Sci USA 1982; 79:574–578.

32. Tschopp J, Amiguet P, Schäfer S. Increased hemolytic activity of the trypsin-cleaved ninth component of complement. Mol Immunol 1986; 23:57–62.

33. Podack ER, Tschopp J. Circular polymerization of the ninth component of complement: ring closure of the tubular complex confers resistance to detergent dissociation and to proteolytic degradation. J Biol Chem: 1982; 257:15204–15212.

34. Tschopp J, Engel A, Podack ER. Molecular weight of poly(C9): 12 to 18 C9 molecules form the transmembrane channel of complement. J Biol Chem 1984; 259:1922–1928.

35. Yamamoto K-I, Migita S. Mechanisms for the spontaneous formation of covalently linked polymers of the terminal membranolytic complement protein (C9). J Biol Chem 1983; 258:7887–7889.

36. DiScipio RG. The relationship between polymerization of complement component C9 and membrane channel formation. J Immunol 1991; 147:4239–4247.

37. Tschopp J, Müller-Eberhard HJ, Podack ER. Formation of transmembrane tubules by spontaneous polymerization of the hydrophilic complement protein C9. Nature 1982; 298:534–538.

38. Dankert JR, Shiver JW, Esser AF. Ninth component of complement: self-aggregation and interaction with lipids. Biochemistry 1985; 24:2754–2762.

39. Doolittle RF. The multiplicity of domains in proteins. Annu Rev Biochem 1995; 64:287–314.

40. Lawler J, Hynes RO. The structure of human thrombospondin, an adhesive glycoprotein with multiple calcium-binding sites and homologies with several different proteins. J Cell Biol 1986; 103:1635–1648.

41. Hobbs HH, Russell DW, Brown MS, Goldstein JL. The LDL receptor locus in familial hypercholesterolemia: mutational analysis of a membrane protein. Annu Rev Genet 1990; 24:133–170.

42. Campbell ID, Bork P. Epidermal growth factor-like modules. Curr Opin Struct Biol 1993; 3:385–392.

43. Liszewski MK, Farries TC, Lublin DM, Rooney IA, Atkinson JP. Control of the complement system. Adv Immunol 1996; 61:201–283.

44. Lichtenheld MG, Olsen KJ, Lu P, Lowrey DM, Hameed A, Hengartner H, Podack ER. Structure and function of human perforin. Nature 1988; 335:448–451.

45. Lengweiler S, Schaller J, Rickli EE. Identification of disulfide bonds in the ninth component (C9) of human complement. FEBS Lett 1996; 380:8–12.

46. Kaufman KM, Sodetz JM. Genomic structure of the human complement protein C8γ: homology to the lipocalin gene family. Biochemistry 1994; 33:5162–5166.

47. Pervaiz S, Brew K. Homology and structure-function correlations between α_1-acid glycoprotein and serum retinol-binding protein and its relatives. FASEB J 1987; 1:209–214.

48. Igarashi M, Nagata A, Toh H, Urade Y, Hayaishi O. Structural organization of the gene for prostaglandin D synthase in the rat brain. Proc Natl Acad Sci USA 1992; 89:5376–5380.

49. North ACT. Structural homology in ligand-specific transport proteins. Biochem Soc Symp 1990; 57:35–48.

50. Hobart MJ, Fernie B, DiScipio RG. Structure of the human C6 gene. Biochemistry 1993; 32:6198–6205.

51. Hobart MJ, Fernie BA, DiScipio RG. Structure of the human C7 gene and comparison with the C6, C8A, C8B, and C9 genes. J Immunol 1995; 154:5188–5194.

52. Michelotti GA, Snider JV, Sodetz JM. Genomic organization of human complement protein C8α and further examination of its linkage to C8β. Hum Genet 1995; 95:513–518.

53. Kaufmann T, Rittner C, Schneider PM. The human complement component C8B gene: structure and phylogenetic relationship. Hum Genet 1993; 92:69–75.

54. Marizziti D, Eggertsen G, Fey GH, Stanley KK. Relationships between the gene and protein structure in human complement component C9. Biochemistry 1988; 27:6529–6534.

55. Witzel-Schlömp K, Späth P, Hobart M, Fernie B, Rittner C, Kaufmann T, Schneider PM. The human complement C9 gene: identification of two mutations causing deficiency and revision of the gene structure. J Immunol 1997; 158:5043–5049.

56. Hobart MJ, Joysey V, Lachmann PJ. Inherited structural variation and linkage relationships of C7. J Immunogenet 1978; 5:157–163.

57. Coto E, Martínez-Naves E, Domínguez O, DiScipio RG, Urra JM, López-Larrea C. DNA polymorphism and linkage relationship of the human complement component C6, C7 and C9 genes. Immunogenetics 1991; 33:184–187.

58. Rogde S, Myklebost O, Olving JH, Kyrkjebo HT, Jonassen R, Olaisen B, Gedde-Dahl T. The human genes for complement components 6 (C6) and 9 (C9) are closely linked on chromosome 5. J Med Genet 1991; 28:587–590.

59. Setién F, Alvarez V, Coto E, DiScipio RG, López-Larrea C. A physical map of the human complement component C6, C7, and C9 genes. Immunogenetics 1993; 38:341–344.

60. Hobart MJ, Fernie BA, DiScipio RG, Lachmann PJ. A large-scale molecular map of the C6 and C7 complement component gene region on chromosome 5p13. Hum Mol Genet 1993; 2:1035–1036.

61. Rittner CW, Hargesheimer W, Stradmann B, Bertrams J, Baur MP, Petersen BH. Human C81(α-γ) polymorphism: detection of the α-γ subunit on SDS-PAGE, formal genetics and linkage relationship. Am J Hum Genet 1986; 38:482–491.

62. Rogde S, Olaisen B, Gedde-Dahl T, Teisberg P. The C8A and C8B loci are closely linked on chromosome 1. Ann Hum Genet 1986; 50:139–144.

63. Kaufman KM, Snider JV, Spurr NK, Schwartz CE, Sodetz JM. Chromosomal assignment of genes encoding the α, β, and γ subunits of human complement component C8: identification of a close physical linkage between the α and β loci. Genomics 1989; 5:475–480.

64. Theriault A, Boyd E, Whaley K, Sodetz JM, Connor JM. Regional chromosomal assignment of genes encoding the α and β subunits of human complement protein C8 to 1p32. Hum Genet 1992; 88:703–704.

65. Platteborze PL, Hobart MJ, Sodetz JM. Physical linkage and orientation of the human complement C8α and C8β genes on chromosome 1p32. Hum Genet 1996; 98:443–446.

66. Yuille MAR, Goudie DG, Zhou CY, Carter NP, Affara NA, Ferguson-Smith MA. Physical mapping of cDNAs assigned to chromosome 9. Ann Hum Genet 1992; 56:214.

67. Dewald G, Cichon S, Bryant SP, Hemmer S, Nöthen MM, Spurr NK. The human complement C8G gene, a member of the lipocalin gene family: polymorphisms and mapping to chromosome 9q34.3. Ann Hum Genet 1996; 60:281–291.

68. Podack ER, Kolb WP, Müller-Eberhard HJ. The C5b-6 complex: formation, isolation, and inhibition of its activity by lipoprotein and the S-protein of human serum. J Immunol 1978; 120:1841–1848.

69. Podack ER, Biesecker G, Kolb WP, Müller-Eberhard HJ. The C5b-6 complex: reaction with C7, C8, C9. J Immunol 1978; 121:484–490.

70. DiScipio RG. Formation and structure of the C5b-7 complex of the lytic pathway of complement. J Biol Chem 1992; 267:17087–17094.

71. Podack ER, Biesecker G, Müller-Eberhard HJ. Membrane attack complex of complement: generation of high-affinity phospholipid binding sites by fusion of five hydrophilic plasma proteins. Proc Natl Acad Sci USA 1979; 76:897–901.

72. Marshall P, Hasegawa A, Davidson EA, Nussenzweig V, Whitlow M. Interaction between complement proteins C5b-7 and erythrocyte membrane sialic acid. J Exp Med 1996; 184:1225–1232.

73. Silversmith RE, Nelsestuen GL. Interaction of complement proteins C5b-6 and C5b-7 with phospholipid vesicles: effects of phospholipid structural features. Biochemistry 1986; 25:7717–7725.

74. Tomita A, Radike E, Parker CJ. Isolation of erythrocyte membrane inhibitor of reactive lysis type II: identification as glycophorin A. J Immunol 1993; 151:3308–3323.

75. Esser AF, Kolb WP, Podack ER, Müller-Eberhard HJ. Molecular reorganization of lipid bilayers by complement: a possible mechanism for membranolysis. Proc Natl Acad Sci USA 1979; 76:1410–1414.

76. Stewart JL, Kolb WP, Sodetz JM. Evidence that C5b recognizes and mediates C8 incorporation into the cytolytic complex of complement. J Immunol 1987; 139:1960–1964.

77. Podack ER. Molecular composition of the tubular structure of the membrane attack complex of complement. J Biol Chem 1984; 259:8641–8647.

78. Zalman LS, Müller-Eberhard HJ. Comparison of channels formed by poly C9, C5b-8 and the membrane attack complex of complement. Mol Immunol 1990; 27:533–537.

79. Ramm LE, Whitlow MB, Mayer MM. Size of the transmembrane channels produced by complement proteins C5b-8. J Immunol 1982; 129:1143–1146.

80. Seeger W, Suttorp N, Hellwig A, Bhakdi S. Noncytolytic terminal complement complexes may serve as calcium gates to elicit leukotriene B4 generation in human polymorphonuclear leukocytes. J Immunol 1986; 137:1286–1293.

81. Podack ER, Stoffel W, Esser AF, Müller-Eberhard HJ. Membrane attack complex of complement: distribution of subunits between the hydrocarbon phase of target membranes and water. Proc Natl Acad Sci USA 1981; 78:4544–4548.

82. Steckel EW, Welbaum BE, Sodetz JM. Evidence of direct insertion of terminal complement proteins into cell membrane bilayers during cytolysis: labeling by a photosensitive membrane probe reveals a major role for the eighth and ninth components. J Biol Chem 1983; 258:4318–4324.

83. Podack ER, Tschopp J, Müller-Eberhard HJ. Molecular organization of C9 within the membrane attack complex of complement: induction of circular C9 polymerization. J Exp Med 1982; 156:268–282.

84. Bhakdi S, Tranum-Jensen J. C5b-9 assembly: average binding of one C9 molecule to C5b-8 without poly-C9 formation generates a stable transmembrane pore. J Immunol 1986; 136:2999–3005.

85. Laine RO, Esser AF. Detection of refolding conformers of complement protein C9 during insertion into membranes. Nature 1989; 341:63–65.

86. Kontermann R, Deppisch R, Rauterberg EW. Several epitopes on native human complement C9 are involved in interaction with the C5b-8 complex and other C9 molecules. Eur J Immunol 1990; 20:623–628.

87. Bhakdi S, Tranum-Jensen J. Damage to mammalian cells by proteins that form transmembrane pores. Rev Physiol Biochem Pharmacol 1987; 107:147–223.

88. Esser AF. Big MAC attack: complement proteins cause leaky patches. Immunol Today 1991; 12:316–318.

89. Bhakdi S, Tranum-Jensen J. Complement lysis: a hole is a hole. Immunol Today 1991; 12:318–320.

90. Esser AF. The membrane attack complex of complement: assembly, structure and cytotoxic activity. Toxicology 1994; 87:229–247.

91. Tschopp J. Ultrastructure of the membrane attack complex of complement: heterogeneity of the complex caused by different degree of C9 polymerization. J Biol Chem 1984; 259:7857–7863.

92. Tschopp J, Podack ER, Müller-Eberhard HJ. The membrane attack complex of complement: C5b-8 complex as accelerator of C9 polymerization. J Immunol 1985; 134:495–499.

93. Tranum-Jensen J, Bhakdi S, Freeze-fracture analysis of the membrane lesion of human complement. J Cell Biol 1983; 97:618–626.

94. Amiguet P, Brunner J, Tschopp J. The membrane attack complex of complement: lipid insertion of tubular and nontubular polymerized C9. Biochemistry 1985; 24:7328–7334.

95. Bhakdi S, Tranum-Jensen J. Molecular weight of the membrane C5b-9 complex of human complement: characterization of the terminal complex as a C5b-9 monomer. Proc Natl Acad Sci USA 1981; 78:1818–1822.

96. Bhakdi S, Tranum-Jensen J. On the cause and nature of C9-related heterogeneity of terminal complement complexes generated on target erythrocytes through the action of whole serum. J Immunol 1984; 133:1453–1463.

97. Dankert JR, Esser AF. Proteolytic modification of human complement protein C9: loss of poly(C9) and circular lesion formation without impairment of function. Proc Natl Acad Sci USA 1985; 82:2128–2132.

98. McCloskey MA, Dankert JR, Esser AF. Assembly of complement components C5b-8 and C5b-9 on lipid bilayer membranes: visualization by freeze-etch electron microscopy. Biochemistry 1989; 28:534–540.

99. Preissner KT. Structure and biological role of vitronectin. Annu Rev Cell Biol 1991; 7:275–310.

100. Suzuki S, Pierschbacher MD, Hayman EG, Nguyen K, Öhgren Y, Ruoslahti E. Domain structure of vitronectin: alignment of active sites. J Biol Chem 1984; 259:15307–15314.

101. Podack ER, Kolb WP, Müller-Eberhard HJ. The SC5b-7 complex: formation, isolation, properties and subunit composition. J Immunol 1977; 119:2024–2029.

102. Podack ER, Müller-Eberhard HJ. Binding of desoxycholate, phosphatidylcholine vesicles, lipoprotein and of the S-protein to complexes of terminal complement components. J Immunol 1978; 121:1025–1030.

103. Bhakdi S, Tranum-Jensen J. Terminal membrane C5b-9 complex of human complement: transition from an amphiphilic to a hydrophilic state through binding of the S protein from serum. J Cell Biol 1982; 94:755–759.

104. Tschopp J, Masson D, Schäfer S, Peitsch M, Preissner KT. The heparin binding domain of S-protein/vitronectin binds to complement components C7, C8, and C9 and perforin from cytolytic T-cells and inhibits their lytic activities. Biochemistry 1988; 27:4103–4109.

105. Sheehan M, Morris CA, Pussell BA, Charlesworth JA. Complement inhibition by human vitronectin involves non-heparin binding domains. Clin Exp Immunol 1995; 101:136–141.

106. Høgåsen K, Mollnes TE, Harboe M. Heparin-binding properties of vitronectin are linked to complex formation as illustrated by in vitro polymerization and binding to the terminal complement complex. J Biol Chem 1992; 267:23076–23082.

107. Jenne DE, Tschopp J. Clusterin: the intriguing guises of a widely expressed glycoprotein. Trends Biochem Sci 1992; 17:154–159.
108. Tschopp J, Chonn A, Hertig S, French LE. Clusterin, the human apolipoprotein and complement inhibitor, binds to complement C7, C8β, and the b domain of C9. J Immunol 1993; 151:2159–2165.
109. Rollins SA, Zhao J, Ninomiya H, Sims PJ. Inhibition of homologous complement by CD59 is mediated by a species-selective recognition conferred through binding to C8 within C5b-8 or C9 within C5b-9. J Immunol 1991; 146:2345–2351.
110. Würzner R, Hobart MJ, Fernie BA, Mewar D, Potter PC, Orren A, Lachmann PJ. Molecular basis of subtotal complement C6 deficiency: a carboxy-terminally truncated but functionally active C6. J Clin Invest 1995; 95:1877–1883.
111. Würzner R, Mewar D, Fernie BA, Hobart MJ, Lachmann PJ. Importance of the third thrombospondin repeat of C6 for terminal complement complex assembly. Immunology 1995; 85:214–219.
112. Sodetz JM. Structure and function of C8 in the membrane attack sequence of complement. Curr Top Microbiol Immunol 1989; 140:19–31.
113. Letson CS, Kaufman KM, Sodetz JM. In vitro expression of the beta subunit of human complement component C8. Mol Immunol 1996; 33:1295–1300.
114. Monahan JB, Sodetz JM. Role of the β-subunit in the interaction of the eighth component of human complement with the membrane-bound cytolytic complex. J Biol Chem 1981; 256:3258–3262.
115. Brickner A, Sodetz JM. Function of subunits within the eighth component of human complement: selective removal of the γ chain reveals it has no direct role in cytolysis. Biochemistry 1984; 23:832–837.
116. Stewart JL, Sodetz JM. Analysis of the specific association of the eighth and ninth components of human complement: identification of a direct role for the α subunit of C8. Biochemistry 1985; 24:4598–4602.
117. Brickner A, Sodetz JM. Functional domains of the α-subunit of the eighth component of human complement: identification and characterization of a distinct binding site for the γ chain. Biochemistry 1985; 24:4603–4607.
118. Kaufman KM, Letson CS, Platteborze PL, Schreck SF, Plumb ME, Sodetz JM. Characterization of recombinant forms of human C8α and C8γ. Mol Immunol 1996; 33(Suppl.1):10.
119. Ninomiya H, Sims PJ. The human complement regulatory protein CD59 binds to the α-chain of C8 and to the "b" domain of C9. J Biol Chem 1992; 267:13675–13680.
120. Lockert DH, Kaufman KM, Chang C-P, Hüsler T, Sodetz JM, Sims PJ. Identity of the segment of human complement C8 recognized by complement regulatory protein CD59. J Biol Chem 1995; 270:19723–19728.
121. Meri S, Morgan BP, Davies A, Daniels RH, Olavesen MG, Waldmann H, Lachmann PJ. Human protectin (CD59), an 18,000–20,000 MW complement lysis restricting factor, inhibits C5b-8 catalysed insertion of C9 into lipid bilayers. Immunology 1990; 71:1–9.
122. Newcomer ME. Retinoid-binding proteins: structural determinants important for function. FASEB J 1995; 9:229–239.
123. Flower DR, North ACT, Attwood TK. Structure and sequence relationships in the lipocalins and related proteins. Protein Sci 1993; 2:753–761.
124. Hänsch GM. The homologous species restriction of the complement attack: structure and function of the C8 binding protein. Curr Top Microbiol Immunol 1989; 140:109–118.
125. Davé SJ, Sodetz JM. Regulation of the membrane attack complex of complement: evidence that C8γ is not the target of homologous restriction factors. J Immunol 1990; 144:3087–3090.
126. Esser AF. C9-mediated cytotoxicity and the function of poly(C9). In Membrane-Mediated Cytotoxicity, Vol. 45. Bonavida B, Collier RJ, eds. UCLA Symposia on Molecular and Cellular Biology, New Series. New York: Alan R. Liss, 1987:411–422.

127. Shiver JW, Dankert JR, Donovan JJ, Esser AF. The ninth component of human complement (C9): functional activity of the b fragment. J Biol Chem 1986; 261:9629–9636.

128. Dankert JR, Esser AF. Complement-mediated killing of *Escherichia coli*: dissipation of membrane potential by a C9-derived peptide. Biochemistry 1986; 25:1094–1100.

129. Gu X, Dankert JR. Isolation of the C9b fragment of human complement component C9 using urea in the absence of detergents. J Immunol Methods 1996; 189:37–45.

130. Dankert JR, Esser AF. Bacterial killing by complement: C9-mediated killing in the absence of C5b-8. Biochem J 1987; 244:393–399.

131. Stanley KK. The molecular mechanism of complement C9 insertion and polymerisation in biological membranes. Curr Top Microbiol Immunol 1989; 140:49–65.

132. Laine RO, Esser AF. Identification of the discontinous epitope in human complement protein C9 recognized by anti-melittin antibodies. J Immunol 1989; 143:553–557.

133. Tschopp J, Masson D. Inhibition of the lytic activity of perforin (cytolysin) and of late complement components by proteoglycans. Mol Immunol 1987; 24:907–913.

134. Taylor KM, Morgan BP, Campbell AK. Altered glycosylation and selected mutation in recombinant human complement component C9: effects on haemolytic activity. Immunology 1994; 83:501–506.

135. Ishida B, Wisnieski BJ, Lavine CH, Esser AF. Photolabeling of a hydrophobic domain of the ninth component of human complement. J Biol Chem 1982; 257:10551–10553.

136. Peitsch MC, Amiguet P, Guy R, Brunner J, Maizel Jr JV, Tschopp J. Localization and molecular modeling of the membrane-inserted domain of the ninth component of human complement and perforin. Mol Immunol 1990; 7:589–602.

137. Dupuis M, Peitsch MC, Hamann U, Stanley KK, Tschopp J. Mutations in the putative lipid-interaction domain of complement C9 result in defective secretion of the functional protein. Mol Immunol 1993; 30:95–100.

138. Chang C-P, Hüsler T, Zhao J, Wiedmer T, Sims PJ. Identity of a peptide domain of human C9 that is bound by the cell-surface complement inhibitor, CD59. J Biol Chem 1994; 269:26424–26430.

139. Hüsler T, Lockert DH, Sims PJ. Role of a disulfide-bonded peptide loop within human complement C9 in the species-selectivity of complement inhibitor CD59. Biochemistry 1996; 35:3263–3269.

140. Tomlinson S, Whitlow MB, Nussenzweig V. A synthetic peptide from complement protein C9 binds to CD59 and enhances lysis of human erythrocytes by C5b-9. J Immunol 1994; 152:1927–1934.

141. Tomlinson S, Wang Y, Ueda E, Esser AF. Chimeric horse/human recombinant C9 proteins identify the amino acid sequence in horse C9 responsible for restriction of hemolysis. J Immunol 1995; 155:436–444.

142. Højrup P, Magnusson S. Disulphide bridges of bovine factor X. Biochem J 1987; 245:887–892.

143. Savage Jr RC, Hash JH, Cohen S. Epidermal growth factor: location of disulfide bonds. J Biol Chem 1973; 248:7669–7672.

144. Cooke RM, Wilkinson AJ, Baron M, Pastore A, Tappin MJ, Campbell ID, Gregory H, Sheard B. The solution structure of human epidermal growth factor. Nature 1987; 327:339–341.

145. Baron M, Norman DG, Harvey TS, Handford PA, Mayhew M, Tse AGD, Brownlee GG, Campbell ID. The three-dimensional structure of the first EGF-like module of human factor IX: comparison with EGF and TGF-α. Protein Sci 1992; 1:81–90.

146. Rao Z, Handford P, Mayhew M, Knott V, Brownlee GG, Stuart D. The structure of a Ca^{2+}-binding epidermal growth factor-like domain: its role in protein-protein interactions. Cell 1995; 82:131–141.

147. Smith KF, Nolan KF, Reid KBM, Perkins SJ. Neutron and X-ray scattering studies on the human complement protein properdin provide an analysis of the thrombospondin repeat. Biochemistry 1991; 30:8000–8008.

148. Daly NL, Scanlon MJ, Djordjevic JT, Kroon PA, Smith R. Three-dimensional structure of a cysteine-rich repeat from the low-density lipoprotein receptor. Proc Natl Acad Sci USA 1995; 92:6334–6338.

149. Bieri S, Djordjevic JT, Daly NL, Smith R, Kroon PA. Disulfide bridges of a cysteine-rich repeat of the LDL receptor ligand-binding domain. Biochemistry 1995; 34:13059–13065.

150. Dyer DA, Cistola DP, Parry GC, Curtiss LK. Structural features of synthetic peptides of apolipoprotein E that bind the LDL receptor. J Lipid Res 1995; 36:80–88.

151. Schultz-Cherry S, Chen H, Mosher DF, Misenheimer TM, Krutzsch HC, Roberts DD, Murphy-Ullrich JE. Regulation of transforming growth factor-β activation by discrete sequences of thrombospondin 1. J Biol Chem 1995; 270:7304–7310.

152. Sipes JM, Guo N-H, Nègre E, Vogel T, Krutzsch HC, Roberts DD. Inhibition of fibronectin binding and fibronectin-mediated cell adhesion to collagen by a peptide from the second type I repeat of thrombospondin. J Cell Biol 1993; 121:469–477.

153. Guo N-H, Krutzsch HC, Nègre E, Zabrenetzky VS, Roberts DD. Heparin-binding peptides from the type I repeats of thrombospondin: structural requirements for heparin binding and promotion of melanoma cell adhesion and chemotaxis. J Biol Chem 1992; 267:19349–19355.

154. Sahu A, Pangburn MK. Identification of multiple sites of interaction between heparin and the complement system. Mol Immunol 1993; 30:679–684.

7

Regulatory Proteins of Complement

M. KATHRYN LISZEWSKI and JOHN P. ATKINSON
Washington University School of Medicine, St. Louis, Missouri

I. OVERVIEW OF REGULATION

The ability of the complement system to destroy and facilitate removal of infecting microbes must be tightly regulated in order to avoid injury to self. This is most clearly evidenced by deficiencies of its control proteins that cause excessive complement consumption leading to pathologic states. That nearly half of complement proteins serve in regulation further attests to the potency of this system and the importance of appropriate control. In effect, the regulatory proteins provide complement with the ability to recognize "self" from "nonself." That is, foreign materials lacking control proteins are attacked while host tissues bearing these proteins are protected (1).

The general design of this control system is to prevent complement damage on host cells/tissues (i.e., inappropriate targets) and activation in fluid phase (i.e., no target) (see Table 1). As a result, overlapping activities are found between the plasma and membrane inhibitors. Regulatory proteins accomplish their task by inhibiting or destabilizing activation complexes and by mediating specific proteolytic cleavages that degrade "activated" components.

The complement system is regulated at the key steps of initiation, amplification (convertase formation), and membrane attack.

II. CONTROL OF COMPLEMENT INITIATION

A. Control of Classical Pathway Initiation

Control of the initiation step of the classical pathway is accomplished by C1 inhibitor (C1-Inh). This protein will be discussed in detail in Chapter 21 and will be only briefly noted here.

The classical pathway is initiated when antibody binds to antigen, triggering the attachment of C1 to the Fc portion of antibody. Thus, antibody selects the target in this pathway. C1-Inh forms equimolar (probably covalent) complexes and dissociates C1r and C1s from the antibody–C1 complex. C1-Inh does not inhibit appropriate activation but blocks fluid phase activation and excessive activation on a target.

Table 1   Regulatory Proteins of Complement

	Molecular mass (kDa)	Serum concentration (μg/ml)	Function
Initiation Step			
C1 inhibitor (C1-INH)	105	120–200	Inactivates C1r and C1s; a "serpin"
Amplification Step			
Factor I	88	35	Cleaves C3b/C4b in the presence of a cofactor protein
Membrane cofactor protein (MCP)	51–68	Membrane	Cofactor for factor I-mediated cleavage of C4b and C3b
Decay accelerating factor (DAF)	70	Membrane	Accelerates decay of C3/C5 convertases
C4b-binding protein (C4BP)	560	250	Cofactor for factor I cleavage of C4b; destabilizes CP C3/C5 convertases
Factor H	150	500	Cofactor for factor I cleavage of C3b; destabilizes AP C3/C5 convertases and CP C5 convertase
Complement receptor type one (CR1)	190–280	Membrane	Receptor for C3b/C4b; inhibitory profile similar to MCP and DAF
Properdin, P	112–224	25	Stabilizes AP convertases
Membrane Attack Step			
CD59	18	Membrane	Blocks MAC on host cells
Clusterin	80	35–105	Blocks fluid phase MAC
S protein	75–80	250–450	Blocks fluid phase MAC
Other			
Anaphylatoxin inactivator	305	35	Inactivates C3a, C4a, C5a

CP, classical pathway; AP, alternative pathway; MAC, membrane attack complex.

B.   Control of Activation of the Alternative Pathway

Contrary to the classical pathway, the alternative pathway has no initiating factor equivalent to antibody. Rather, the firing of the alternative pathway is intimately associated with the autoactivation of C3 via cleavage of its thioester bond. The thioester moiety of C3 is subject to continuous, spontaneous, low-level hydrolysis. This "tickover" activates C3 such that it can bind to hydroxyl or amino groups (in essence, almost any biological surface). C3 bound to nonspecific acceptor molecules in plasma (such as water) or to cell surfaces may then form convertases and create a feedback loop. Thus, control of the alternative pathway is aimed at preventing inappropriate convertase assembly (the amplification step), either in the fluid phase or on self-tissue.

III. CONTROL OF THE AMPLIFICATION PHASE: CONVERTASE REGULATION

A. Overview

The classical and alternative pathway convertases can rapidly (<5 min) deposit large amounts of clustered C3b on the target, thereby marking the material for destruction. The activities of convertases are dependent on the association of multiple components: C4b with C2a (classical pathway C3 convertase) and C3b with Bb and properdin (alternative pathway C3 convertase). Binding of C3b to each of the above convertases also transforms them into C5 convertases, which are the gateway to formation of the terminal, lytic membrane attack complex (MAC).

Regulatory proteins tightly control the convertase step. Eight proteins are involved in regulating C3/C5 convertases: plasma proteins, C4b-binding protein (C4BP), factors H and I, and cellular proteins membrane cofactor protein (MCP; CD46), decay accelerating factor (DAF; CD55), complement receptors type (CR1; CD35) and 2 (CR2; CD21). The plasma protein, properdin, serves as a positive regulator (i.e., it stabilizes the two alternative pathway convertases).

Six of these proteins belong to a family of genetically, structurally, and functionally related proteins called the regulators of complement activation (RCA) group (2) (see Fig. 1). The genes are tightly clustered on the long arm of chromosome one (1q3.2). At the protein level each is composed largely or entirely of contiguous repeats called complement control protein modules (CCP) (also called short consensus repeats; SCR) (Fig. 1). These are the domains for C3b and C4b interaction. Each CCP is composed of approximately 60 amino acids, with 4 invariant cysteines and 10–18 other highly conserved residues. The pairing of the cysteines within each module forms the characteristic "double-loop" structure of the CCP. These repeats mediate ligand binding and decay accelerating and cofactor activities.

The RCA proteins employ two physiological mechanisms for regulation: decay-accelerating activity and/or cofactor activity. Decay-accelerating activity refers to the dissociation of convertase components, while cofactor activity refers to the process of proteolytic degradation of C3b and C4b as directed by factor I and the cofactor protein. Cofactor activity may be mediated by the same protein that serves as a decay accelerator or by a different one (Table 2).

The sites in C3 that are recognized by members of the RCA are related, although the exact binding sites appear to be different. During cleavage of iC3 by factor I and CR1 or H, CR1 and H bind to at least two sites on C3 that are partially or entirely contained within residues 727–768 of the alpha chain. While the MCP-binding site(s) on C3b have not been elucidated, they are different from those for CR1 (3).

B. Convertase Control on Host Cells

1. Membrane Cofactor Protein

Almost every cell, except erythrocytes, expresses membrane cofactor protein (MCP; CD46; measles virus receptor). As its name implies, it serves as a cofactor to the serine protease factor I for the proteolytic cleavage of C3b and C4b deposited on host cells (4,5).

MCP has an unusual electrophoretic characteristic. On sodium dodecyl sulfate polyacrylamide gel electrophoresis (SDS-PAGE) it appears as two broad heterogeneous protein species of 51–58 kDa ("lower" band) and 59–68 kDa ("upper" band). Most individuals

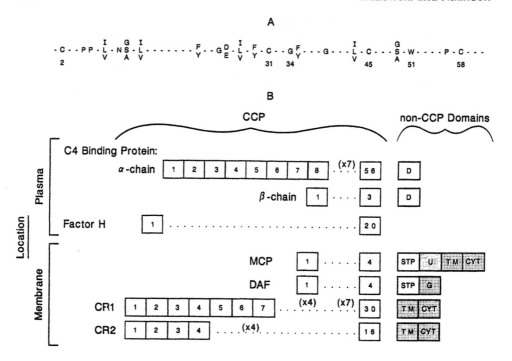

Figure 1 (A) The conserved amino acids in the repeating motif called a complement control protein module (CCP) are illustrated. Each CCP consists of ~60 amino acids. (B) A schematic representation of the six members of the regulators of complement activation (RCA) family. The number of blocks indicates the CCP modules that compose the protein. In the case of CR1 and CR2, larger homologous groupings of CCP are found. TM, transmembrane domain; CYT, cytoplasmic domain; STP, serine-threonine-proline-enriched area; G, glycolipid anchor; U, domain of unknown functional significance; D, disulfide bridge-containing domain. (Adapted from ref. 77.)

express variable quantities of both bands. However, there is a predominance of "upper" band in 65% of the population, equivalence of both bands in 29% and "lower" band predominance in 6% of the population (6).

    MCP is usually expressed as four isoforms that differ in two regions secondary to alternative splicing (Fig. 2) (7,8). Each isoform is composed of four CCP modules with

Table 2 Comparison of Fluid Phase and Membrane Convertase Regulators

	DAA	CA	Substrate[a]
C4BP	+	+	C4b
Factor H	+	+	C3b
DAF	+	−	C3b/C4b
MCP	−	+	C3b/C4b
CR1	+	+	C3b/C4b

DAA, decay-accelerating activity (i.e., the ability to dissociate convertases).
CA, cofactor activity (the participation of the regulator with factor I to cleave and thereby inactivate C3b/C4b).
C4BP and factor H are plasma proteins, while DAF, MCP and CR1 are membrane-anchored.
[a]C4b and C3b are part of a convertase for DAA.

Ser/Thr/Pro-Enriched (STP) Domain

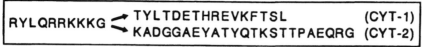

B: - VSTSSTTKSPASSAS -
C: - GPRPTYKPPVSNYP -

Cytoplasmic Domain

| RYLQRRKKKG | TYLTDETHREVKFTSL | (CYT-1) |
| | KADGGAEYATYQTKSTTPAEQRG | (CYT-2) |

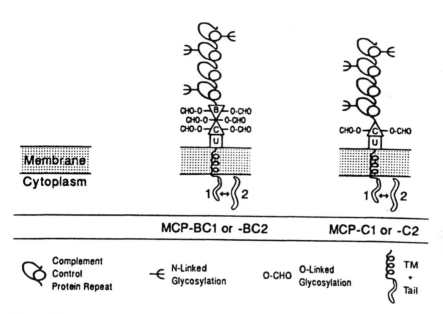

CHO-O—B—O-CHO
CHO-O—╳—O-CHO
CHO-O—C—O-CHO
U

Membrane
Cytoplasm

1 ↔ 2

MCP-BC1 or -BC2

CHO-O—C—O-CHO
U

1 ↔ 2

MCP-C1 or -C2

Complement Control Protein Repeat

N-Linked Glycosylation

O-CHO O-Linked Glycosylation

TM + Tail

Figure 2 Schematic representation of the structure and alternatively spliced amino acids of the four common isoforms of MCP. MCP consists of four CCP modules; three of which bear sites for N-glycosylation. Following this is the variably spliced STP segment that is a site for extensive O-glycosylation. This is flanked by a small segment of undefined function, a transmembrane domain (TM) and one of two alternatively spliced cytoplasmic tails of 16 or 23 amino acids. (From ref. 20.)

three sites for N-linked glycosylation. The alternatively spliced O-glycosylation area (called the STP domain because it is enriched in serines, threonines, and prolines) consists of 14 or 29 amino acids depending upon whether or not exon 8, which encodes 15 amino acids (segment B), is present in the mRNA. The upper molecular weight forms result from splicing in of the "B" segment, which increases the molecular mass by 10–15 kDa. Following the STP domain lies a small segment of 15 amino acids of unknown functional significance. Next is a transmembrane segment, intracytoplasmic anchor, and then a cytoplasmic tail of 16 or 23 amino acids. Alternative splicing of the regions that code for the STP domain and cytoplasmic tails produces the four common isoforms bearing the B + C or C only regions with either of the two cytoplasmic tails. Thus designations for the four common isoforms are MCP-BC1, MCP-BC2, MCP-C1, and MCP-C2. Other forms have been noted (7,9).

The single-copy gene for MCP, consisting of 14 exons and 13 introns, is found in the RCA cluster (1q3.2) (7,10,11). The phenotypic pattern of MCP is under autosomal dominant control and is associated with a Hind III RFLP (6,10,12,13). The promoter for MCP lies within a GC-rich region in the first several hundred nucleotides upstream from the transcriptional start site (14). The gene lacks typical TATA or CAAT sequences. An MCP-like element was found that is a partial duplication consisting of sequences homologous to the 5' end of MCP (i.e., the signal peptide and CCP 1–3) (14). It is unknown if this species produces a protein.

MCP is a cofactor for the factor I-mediated cleavage of C3b (to iC3b) and C4b (to C4c and C4d) deposited on host cells. MCP performs this role intrinsically (i.e., it protects only the cell on which it is attached, not neighboring cells) (15). The second, third, and fourth CCP modules of MCP are necessary for cofactor activity for C3b and C4b. Interesting is that while the second, third, and fourth CCP mediate C4b binding, only CCP 3 and 4 are necessary for C3b binding. Thus, binding and cofactor activity are not always synonymous (16).

The distribution of MCP may be important for its function of inhibiting complement activation and serving as measles virus receptor. MCP is transported to the basolateral surface of epithelial cells. This activity is mediated by the cytoplasmic tails (17).

Structural variations among MCP isoforms may provide for functional variations. Isoform precursors with cytoplasmic tail 1 (CYT-1) are processed into their mature forms approximately fourfold faster than those with CYT-2 (18,19). MCP isoforms with a larger O-glycosylation domain (BC) also protect better against the classical pathway as compared to C isoforms probably in part related to preferential binding to C4b (20). Two additional findings suggest that MCP structure affects function. First, tissue-specific expression differences of isoforms have been found in brain (C2), kidney (BC), salivary gland (BC) (9), and fetal heart (C) (21). Second, there is a surprising variability within a tissue as to the pattern of MCP expression. Kidney, skin, reproductive, synovial, eye, thyroid, and liver tissues have been examined in some detail (22).

2. Decay-Accelerating Factor

Decay-accelerating factor (DAF; CD55) and MCP are sister proteins with complementary regulatory activities. Like MCP, DAF has a very wide tissue distribution. It functions as a regulator of the alternative and classical pathway C3/C5 convertases. DAF also possesses four CCP modules followed by an STP domain. However, it is attached to cells by a glycosylphosphatidyl inositol (GPI) anchor and serves to accelerate the dissociation of convertases rather than regulate by proteolytic cleavage.

Pro-DAF contains a 34 amino acid signal peptide. The mature protein consists of 347 amino acids (23). There is one site for N-linked glycosylation on CCP 1. Following the four CCP modules there is a 67 amino acid STP domain that is the site for extensive O-glycosylation (adding ~26,000 kDa to the mol wt). The carboxyl terminus concludes with 24 amino acids of markedly hydrophobic character, which are excised in the endoplasmic reticulum concomitant with the addition of a preassembled GPI anchor. This type of anchoring (shared also by the MAC regulator CD59) may increase mobility in the membrane, allow for phospholipase-mediated shedding, facilitate apical targeting, and promote transmembrane signaling (24).

The 40 kb DAF gene consists of 11 exons and lies within a 900 kb fragment within the RCA locus on chromosome 1 at position q3.2 (22). Three RFLPs of the DAF gene have been reported (25,26). DAF promoter activity is contained within the first several hundred nucleotides upstream from the transcriptional start site in a GC-rich island. DAF lacks typical TATA and CAAT promoter sequences; however, there are several potential *cis*-acting elements corresponding to Sp1, Ap-1, AT-2, and cAMP-responsive elements (27,28).

The functional role of DAF is to dissociate C3 and C5 convertases. It does not prevent the initial binding of C2 to C4b or B to C3b, but rather disengages C2a or Bb from the convertases (29). The remaining C4b or C3b retains the ability to reform convertases. Similar to MCP, DAF performs its protective role intrinsically (30).

CCP 2, 3, and 4 of DAF are responsible for its regulatory activities (31). Specifically, the classical pathway C3 convertase regulatory activity resides within CCP 2–3, while alternative pathway C3 convertase regulatory activity lies within CCP 2–4 (32). The STP domain also influences functional activity, acting in part as a nonspecific "spacer" (31). The exact binding site of DAF on the convertase is unclear, although there is a weak association with C4b and C3b, not requiring C2 or factor B (33). Fluid phase inhibition studies, however, suggest that the binding affinity is much greater for the convertase than for C3b or C4b alone (34).

3. Complement Receptors Type 1 and 2

Complement receptors are more fully discussed in chapter 8. The role of CR1 as a complement regulator relates more to immune complex binding, processing, and removal than to protection of host tissues from complement attack. CR1 interacts with clustered derivatives of C3 (C3b, iC3b) and C4 (C4b) in immune complexes. Although CR1 possesses both decay accelerating and cofactor activities, its very limited distribution (primarily on peripheral blood cells) suggests a primary role in immune complex handling rather than in host cell protection.

CR2 binds several C3-derived ligands including C3dg and, to a lesser extent, iC3b and C3b. CR2 probably plays only a minor role, if any, in complement regulation due to its limited regulatory profile and restricted tissue distribution (primarily on B lymphocytes).

C. Convertase Control in Plasma

1. Factor H

Factor H is an abundant (0.3–0.5 mg/ml) plasma glycoprotein synthesized primarily in the liver. Because of its decay-accelerating activities for the alternative pathway convertase and cofactor activity converting C3b to iC3b, factor H prevents fluid-phase activation of the alternative pathway. This is clearly illustrated by the rare syndrome of factor H deficiency. Inherited deficiency of factor H leads to uncontrolled complement activation with a secondary deficiency (consumption) of plasma C3, often resulting in membranoproliferative glomerulonephritis (see chapter 26).

Factor H (150 kDa) consists of a polypeptide of 1213 amino acids formed entirely into 20 contiguous CCP (Fig. 1). The factor H gene also found in the RCA gene cluster (1q3.2) is tightly linked to the b subunit of coagulation factor XIII and has yet to be physically linked to the RCA cluster.

The binding site for C3b probably lies in the amino portion of factor H. Electron micrographs indicate that C3b binds near one end of factor H, and an amino terminal 38 kDa tryptic fragment consisting of CCP 1–5 was found to possess cofactor activity for

C3b. A highly homologous, truncated version of factor H (CCP 1–7) possesses both C3b-binding and cofactor activities (35,36). Lastly, transfection of a series of deletion mutants lacking each of the first five CCP demonstrated CCP 1–4 are required for full activity, although CCP 1–3 were sufficient for cofactor activity (36,37).

2. C4b-Binding Protein

C4b-binding protein (C4BP) is a plasma protein (0.2 mg/ml) whose synthesis in the liver is upregulated by interleukin-6 and tumor necrosis factor (38). It possesses both decay-accelerating and cofactor activities for C4b. Just as occurs with C3, the thioester moiety of C4 may "tickover" and cause activation of C4. In addition, C4 is cleaved during classical pathway activation to form C4b that deposits on immune complexes and nearby surfaces. Unlike C3b, however, there is no feedback loop for activated C4. Rather, the activation of the classical pathway is dependent on the fixation of C1 when antibody binds to antigen, triggering subsequent activation of C4 and C2. Contrary to the alternative pathway, the classical pathway has an earlier control protein, C1 inhibitor, to prevent fluid phase activation of C1 that would result in unchecked cleavage of C4 and C2 as is observed in hereditary angioedema.

C4BP consists of seven identical 75 kDa α chains and one 45 kDa β chain held together by disulfide bonds near their carboxyl termini and forming a spiderlike arrangement of chains (see Fig. 3) (38). In addition to this common plasma form of C4BP, there are other minor species differing in the number of α chains or in the lack of a β chain.

Each α chain consists of 549 amino acids divided into eight CCP followed by a 58 residue segment at the carboxyl end. A study of proteolytic fragments indicated that CCP

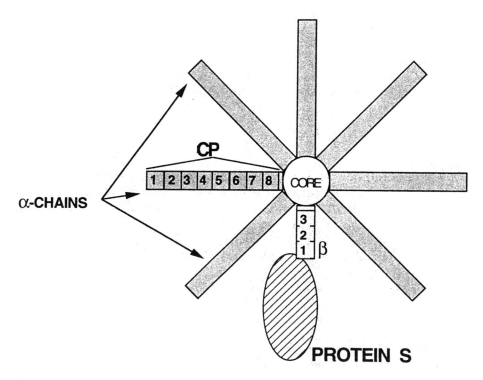

Figure 3   Schematic representation of the structure of C4BP. (From ref. 22.)

6 was involved in ligand binding. Electron micrographs also demonstrate that the outer ends of the arms bind C4b (39). The β chain consists of 3 CCP with the first module including at least part of the binding site for S protein.

The C4BP α and β chain genes are closely linked in a head-to-tail arrangement in the RCA cluster. The α chain gene (C4BPA) consists of 12 exons including a separate one for each of the eight CCP except for CCP 2, which is a split exon (similar to other RCA members). For the β chain, the first two CCP are encoded by individual exons, while CCP 3 is encoded by a split exon. Two α chain-related pseudogenes, C4BPAL1 (40) and C4BPAL2 (41), lie proximal to C4BP. In hepatic cells, the C4BPA promoter is found within the first 369 base pairs upstream from the transcription start site. The hepatic transcription factor HNF1 interacts at −38 base pairs and is critical for promoter activity (42).

C4BP regulates fluid phase C4b2a, the C3 convertase. It performs this role in three basic ways:

1. Binding to C4b. Because C4BP has several interactive chains, one C4BP molecule may simultaneously bind four to six C4b fragments.
2. Displacement of C2a from the convertase. Displacement of C2a occurs analogously to the activity of factor H against C3bBb. Once C2a is dissociated, it cannot rebind.
3. Cofactor activity for factor I cleavage of C4b. C4BP in conjunction with factor I degrades C4b into C4c and C4d fragments.

Finally, more than 50% of plasma protein S, a vitamin K-dependent regulator of the coagulation system, is complexed with C4BP via the β chain. The function of this interaction is unknown.

3. Properdin

In contrast to the negative regulators discussed above, properdin is a positive regulator that stabilizes the alternative pathway convertase (see (22) for a detailed review with more complete references). Such an activity is highly desirable on a foreign surface (e.g., on a microbe), but deleterious in the fluid phase or on a host cell. The unusual polymeric structure of properdin ensures that its activities are highly selective for C3b molecules clustered on a target. Properdin, unlike other plasma complement proteins, which are primarily of hepatocyte origin, is largely synthesized by blood mononuclear cells.

Properdin consists of identical, noncovalently linked 56 kDa chains that form dimers (30%), trimers (45%), tetramers (10%), or larger species (16%). Each subunit carries a single N-linked glycosylation site that is not necessary for function. The precursor contains 469 amino acids with a 27 residue signal peptide. Residues 77-437 form six modules (known as thrombospondin type 1 [TSP1]) enriched in cysteines, glycines, prolines and serines (see Fig. 4). Mutagenesis studies indicate that TSP1-4 may be important for the stabilization of the C3 convertase (C3bBb) (43). In addition, a TSP1-6 deletion mutant was unable to form oligomers and one lacking TSP1-5 could not bind C3b. Properdin is assembled into functional oligomers prior to secretion by a process that is poorly understood.

The properdin gene lies on the X chromosome within band Xp11.23–Xp21.1 (44). It contains 10 exons including (1 each for TSP1-1-5 and two exons for TSP1-6 (45). As would be anticipated, properdin deficiency is inherited as a sex-linked trait.

Properdin stabilizes the alternative pathway convertase by its binding to and then protection of C3b in the convertase. A weak interaction with factor B alone has been

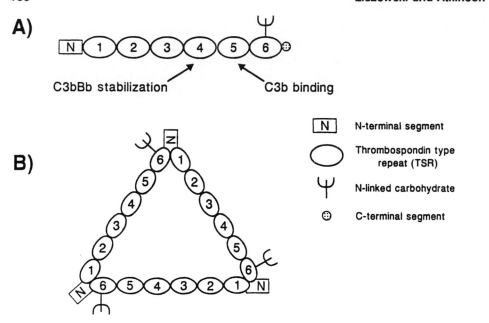

Figure 4 (A) Model of human properdin monomer. (B) Trimeric model of properdin showing head-to-tail orientation at junctions. (Adapted from ref. 43.)

detected, indicating some association with both C3b and B. It is interesting that properdin inhibits binding of C5 to C3b. In order of affinity, properdin binds C3bBb > C3bB > C3b (46). Binding to C3b also enhances the affinity for factor B. After properdin attaches, the rates of spontaneous and factor H-dependent dissociation of the convertase are dramatically slowed.

IV. CONTROL OF THE MEMBRANE ATTACK COMPLEX

A. Regulators of Deposited MAC

1. CD59

This 18–20 kDa GPI-linked membrane protein is widely expressed on host cells and is an inhibitor of MAC formation on the same cell on which it is tethered (i.e., intrinsic activity). Because it was simultaneously identified by several groups, it bears a number of names: MAC inhibitory factor (MACIF), membrane inhibitor of reactive lysis (MIRL), protectin, homologous restriction factor 20 (HRF20), and p18 (22).

The precursor to CD59 consists of 128 amino acids containing a 25 residue signal peptide. A hydrophobic sequence of 26 amino acids at the carboxyl terminus provides the signal for the GPI substitution which occurs at Asn77 (47). There is a single N-linked glycosylation site at Asn18 as well as extensive intrachain disulfide bonding by the 10 cysteine residues. Nuclear magnetic resonance spectroscopy has determined that CD59 is folded into a disc-shaped domain with the disulfide bonds clustered in the hydrophobic center with four looped extensions protruding from the disc (48,49).

The CD59 gene is located on chromosome 11 at position 11p13 (50,51). The gene encompasses >20 kb and contains four exons. Expression of CD59 may be upregulated by cytokines, phorbol myristate acetate, and calcium ionophore(52–55). There is experimental evidence that CD59 is upregulated at the level of transcription (55) and that some cells may possess intracellular pools that can be rapidly mobilized (54).

CD59 binds C8 and C9, inhibiting formation of the MAC on host cells (Fig. 5). Thus, CD59 inhibits MAC assembly after the stage of C5b-7 insertion into cell membranes (56). CD59 possesses binding sites for both the β chain of C8 and the b domain of C9 (57). Precise regions of contact are being elucidated. One study used a series of CD59 peptides and found that residues 27–38 possessed the site binding to C8 and C9 (58). CD59 was found specifically to bind residues 334–385 of the alpha chain of C8 and to require the disulfide bond between Cys345 and Cys369 (59). Using synthetic peptides from C9, residues 247–261 (the "hinge" region of C9 that unfolds during insertion) had CD59-binding activity (60). However, another report (57) found that peptides 359–411 of C9 and not the hinge region were able to bind CD59. In confirmation of the latter study, residues 334–415 of C9 also were found to contain a site recognized by CD59 (61).

B. Regulation of Fluid-Phase MAC

1. S Protein/Vitronectin

S protein (site-specific protein) is a 75–80 kDa glycoprotein synonymous with vitronectin (serum spreading factor). The plasma concentration is 0.25–0.45 mg/ml with the liver being the primary site for synthesis.

S protein is a single-chain polypeptide consisting of 478 residues (62,63). The precursor has a signal peptide of 19 residues. The amino terminus of the mature protein begins with a somatomedin B domain (containing eight interlinked cysteines with a characteristic folding pattern). Next lies a linear region, the connecting segment, bearing an RGD sequence (for binding to integrins), a highly acidic domain (residues 53–64), a

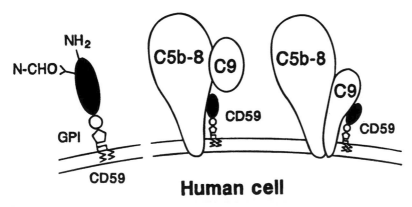

Figure 5 Schematic representation of CD59 structure and function. CD59 is a GPI-anchored protein that binds C8 and C9 to inhibit the further assembly of the membrane attack complex on host cells.

putative cross-linking site, and a collagen binding site. The carboxyl terminus bears a heparin-binding domain represented by a 40 amino acid segment enriched in basic residues.

S protein is processed differentially in individuals due to an allelic variation. Some individuals express plasma S protein as a single chain whereas others express a two-chain form or a mixture of both (heterozygotes) as a result of differential proteolytic cleavage at position 381 (64). At this site some individuals have a methionine to threonine substitution that results in a different susceptibility to proteolysis (65).

The S protein gene has been mapped to the centromeric region of chromosome 17 (66). It consists of eight exons with a single mRNA transcript of 1.7 kb (62).

S protein functions as a regulator by binding to a metastable binding site on the C5b-7 complex, thereby preventing its insertion into cell membranes (67). Although the resulting SC5b-7 complex can still incorporate C8 and C9, these complexes are lytically inactive. It appears that S protein acts via the heparin-binding site to inhibit C9 polymerization but has an even greater, though unspecified, effect on preventing insertion of C5b-7 into cell membranes (68).

2. Clusterin

This MAC-inhibitory protein also possesses several names: SP-40,40, cytolysis inhibitor (CLI), sulfated glycoprotein 2 (SGP2), and apolipoprotein J. It is an 80 kDa heterodimeric glycoprotein with multiple functions. It is present in plasma at a concentration of 0.035–0.105 mg/ml and it associates with lipoproteins to form ApoA1–clusterin–lipoprotein complexes (69,70). Clusterin has been identified in a wide variety of cells and tissues.

Two nonidentical α and β subunits of approximately equal size (35–40 kDa) make up clusterin. The single chain precursor consists of 445 amino acids with the first 21 residues incorporated into a signal peptide (71). Proteolytic cleavage between Arg205 and Ser206 generates the two subunit structure. Each chain possesses three N-linked glycosylation sites and five cysteines. The amino terminus forms an α-helix followed by a segment (amino acids 77–98) bearing homology to the cysteine-rich thrombospondin type 1 modules (TSP1) found in terminal complement proteins (71).

The single-copy clusterin gene is found on chromosome 8 at 8p21, proximal to the lipoprotein lipase (LPL) gene (72–75).

Similar to S protein, clusterin also inhibits MAC assembly after the C5b-7 step. It prevents insertion of C5b-7 into cell membranes and produces hemolytically inactive, soluble complexes. The relative importance of S protein versus clusterin remains to be determined. The mechanism of its interaction is dependent on the thrombospondin-like unit of the amino terminus. This segment promotes interactions with hydrophobic regions of MAC proteins. Thus, clusterin binds avidly to C7, and β chain of C8 and the b domain of C9.

Also, C8 itself has been shown to inhibit C5b-7 activity and thus serves a dual function in complement-mediated cytolysis. That is, at the cell surface C8 is required for the lytic action of the C5b-9 complex, while in the fluid phase binding of C8 to soluble C5b-7 prevents attachment to a target membrane (76).

V. CONTROL OF ANAPHYLATOXINS

When complement proteins C3, C4, and C5 are activated, small peptides of 74–77 amino acids are released from the splitting of single Arg-X bonds at the amino terminus of the α chain. The resulting anaphylatoxins (C3a, C4a, and C5a) possess reactive potencies that significantly differ. The anaphylatoxins are inactivated rapidly by a plasma enzyme called carboxypeptidase N that removes a carboxyl-terminal arginyl residue. This subject is discussed more fully in Chapter 11.

REFERENCES

1. Farries TC, Atkinson JP. Separation of self from non-self in the complement system. Immunol Today 1987; 8:212–215.
2. Hourcade D, Holers VM, Atkinson JP. The regulators of complement activation (RCA) gene cluster. Adv Immunol 1989; 45:381–416.
3. Lambris JD, Lao Z, Oglesby TJ, Atkinson JP, Hack CE, Becherer JD. Dissection of CR1, Factor H, membrane cofactor protein, and factor B binding and functional sites in the third complement component. J Immunol 1996; 156:4821–4832.
4. Seya T, Atkinson JP. Functional properties of membrane cofactor protein of complement. Biochemistry 1989; 264:581–588.
5. Seya T, Turner JR, Atkinson JP. Purification and characterization of a membrane protein (gp45–70) that is a cofactor for cleavage of C3b and C4b. J Exp Med 1986; 163:837–855.
6. Ballard L, Seya T, Teckman J, Lublin DM, Atkinson JP. A polymorphism of the complement regulatory protein MCP (membrane cofactor protein or gp 45–70). J Immunol 1987; 138:3850–3855.
7. Post TW, Liszewski MK, Adams EM, Tedja I, Miller EA, Atkinson JP. Membrane cofactor protein of the complement system: alternative splicing of serine/threonine/proline-rich exons and cytoplasmic tails produces multiple isoforms which correlate with protein phenotype. J Exp Med 1991; 174:93–102.
8. Russell SM, Sparrow RL, McKenzie IFC, Purcell DFJ. Tissue-specific and allelic expression of the complement regulator CD46 is controlled by alternative splicing. Eur J Immunol 1992; 22:1513–1518.
9. Johnstone RW, Russell SM, Loveland BE, McKenzie IFC. Polymorphic expression of CD46 protein isoforms due to tissue-specific RNA splicing. Mol Immunol 1993; 30:1231–1241.
10. Bora NS, Post TW, Atkinson JP. Membrane cofactor protein of the complement system: a Hind III restriction fragment length polymorphism that correlates with the expression polymorphism. J Immunol 1991; 146:2821–2825.
11. Bora NS, Lublin DM, Kumar BV, Hockett RD, Holers VM, Atkinson JP. Structural gene for MCP maps to within 100 kb of the 3' end of the C3b/C4b receptor (CR1) gene. J Exp Med 1989; 169:597–602.
12. Wilton AN, Johnstone RW, McKenzie IFC, Purcell DFJ. Strong associations between RFLP and protein polymorphisms for CD46. Immunogenetics 1992; 36:79–85.
13. Risk JM, Flanagan BF, Johnson PM. Polymorphism of the human CD46 gene in normal individuals and in recurrent spontaneous abortion. Hum Immunol 1991; 30:162–167.
14. Cui W, Hourcade D, Post TW, Greenlund AC, Atkinson JP, Kumar V. Characterization of the promoter region of the membrane cofactor protein (CD46) gene of the human complement system and comparison to a membrane cofactor protein-like genetic element. J Immunol 1993; 151:4137–4146.
15. Oglesby TJ, Allen CJ, Liszewski MK, White DJG, Atkinson JP. Membrane cofactor protein (MCP, CD46) protects cells from complement-mediated attack by an intrinsic mechanism. J Exp Med 1992; 175:1547–1551.
16. Adams EM, Brown MC, Nunge M, Krych M, Atkinson JP. Contribution of the repeating domains of membrane cofactor protein (CD46) of the complement system to ligand binding and cofactor activity. J Immunol 1991; 147:3005–3011.

17. Maisner A, Liszewski MK, Atkinson JP, Schwartz-Albiez R, Herrler G. Two different cytoplasmic tails direct isoforms of the membrane cofactor protein (MCP; CD46) to the basolateral surface of Madin-Daby canine kidney (MDCK) cells. J Biol Chem 1996; 271:18853–18858.

18. Liszewski MK, Tedja I, Atkinson JP. Membrane cofactor protein (CD46) of complement: processing differences related to alternatively spliced cytoplasmic domains. J Biol Chem 1994; 269:10776–10779.

19. Ballard LL, Bora NS, Yu GH, Atkinson JP. Biochemical characterization of membrane cofactor protein of the complement system. J Immunol 1988; 141:3923–3929.

20. Liszewski MK, Atkinson JP. Membrane cofactor protein (MCP; CD46): Isoforms differ in protection against the classical pathway of complement. J. Immunol 1996; 156:4415–4421.

21. Gorelick A, Oglesby TJ, Rashbaum W, Atkinson JP, Buyon JP. Ontogeny of membrane cofactor protein: phenotypic divergence in the fetal heart. Lupus 1995; 4:293–296.

22. Liszewski M, Farries T, Lublin D, Rooney I, Atkinson J. Control of the complement system. Adv Immunol 1996; 61:201–283.

23. Lublin DM, Atkinson JP. Decay-accelerating factor: biochemistry, molecular biology, and function. Annu Rev Immunol 1989; 7:35–58.

24. Englund PT. The structure and biosynthesis of glycosyl-phosphatidylinositol protein anchors. Annu Rev Biochem 1992; 62:121–138.

25. Rey-Campos J, Rubinstein P, DeCordoba SR. Decay-accelerating factor. Genetic polymorphism and linkage to the RCA (regulator of complement activation) gene cluster in humans. J Exp Med 1987; 166:246–252.

26. Stafford HA, Tykocinski ML, Lublin DM, et al. Normal polymorphic variations and transcription of the decay accelerating factor gene in paroxysmal nocturnal hemoglobinuria cells. Proc Natl Acad Sci USA 1988; 85:880–884.

27. Ewulona UK, Ravi L, Medof ME. Characterization of the decay-accelerating factor gene promoter region. Proc Natl Acad Sci USA 1991; 88:4675–4679.

28. Thomas DJ, Lublin DM. Identification of 5′ flanking regions affecting the expression of the human decay accelerating factor gene and their role in tissue-specific expression. J Immunol 1993; 150:151–160.

29. Fujita T, Inoue T, Ogawa K, Iida K, Tamura N. The mechanism of action of decay-accelerating factor (DAF). DAF inhibits the assembly of C3 convertases by dissociating C2a and Bb. J Exp Med 1987; 166:1221–1228

30. Medof ME, Kinoshita T, Nussenzweig V. Inhibition of complement activation on the surface of cells after incorporation of decay-accelerating factor (DAF) into their membranes. J Exp Med 1984; 160:1558–1578.

31. Coyne KE, Hall SE, Thompson ES, et al. Mapping of epitopes, glycosylation sites, and complement regulatory domains in human decay accelerating factor. J Immunol 1992; 149:2906–2913.

32. Brodbeck WG, Liu D, Sperry J, Mold C, Medof ME. Localization of classical and alternative pathway regulatory activity within the decay-accelerating factor. J Immunol 1996; 156:2528–2533.

33. Kinoshita T, Medof ME, Nussenzweig V. Endogenous association of decay-accelerating factor (DAF) with C4b and C3b on cell membranes. J Immunol 1986; 136:3390–3395.

34. Pangburn MK. Differences between the binding sites of the complement regulatory proteins DAF, CR1 and factor H on C3 convertases. J Immunol 1986; 136:2216–2221.

35. Misasi R, Huemer HP, Schwaeble W, Solder E, Larcher C, Dierich MP. Human complement factor H: an additional gene product of 43 kDa isolated from human plasma shows cofactor activity for the cleavage of the third component of complement. Eur J Immunol 1989; 19:1765–1768.

36. Kuhn S, Skerka C, Zipfel PF. Mapping of the complement regulatory domains in the human Factor H-like protein 1 and in Factor H. J Immunol 1995; 155:5663–5670.

37. Gordon DL, Kaufman RM, Blackmore TK, Kwong J, Lublin DM. Identification of complement regulatory domains in human Factor H. J Immunol 1995; 155:348–356.

38. Barnum SR, Dahlback B. C4b-binding protein, a regulatory component of the classical pathway of complement, is an acute-phase protein and is elevated in systemic lupus erythematosus. Compl Inflamm 1990; 7:71–77.

39. Dahlback B, Smith CA, Muller-Eberhard HJ. Visualization of human C4b-binding protein and its complexes with vitamin K-dependent protein S and complement protein C4b. Proc Natl Acad Sci USA 1983; 80:3461–3465.

40. Sanchez-Corral P, Pardo-Manuel-de-Villena F, Rey-Compos J, Rodriguez-de-Cordoba S. C4BPAL1, a member of the human regulator of complement activation (RCA) gene cluster that resulted from the duplication of the gene coding for the alpha-chain of C4b-binding protein. Genomics 1993; 17:185–193.

41. Devillena FPM, Rodriguez-de-Cordoba S. C4BPAL2: a second duplication of the C4BPA gene in the human RCA gene cluster. Immunogenetics 1995; 41:139–143.

42. Arenzana N, Rodriguez de Cordoba S, Rey-Campos J. Expression of the human gene coding for the alpha-chain of C4b-binding protein, C4BPA, is controlled by an HNF1-dependent hepatic-specific promoter. Biochem J 1995; 308:613–621.

43. Higgins JM, Wiedemann H, Timpl R, Reid KB. Characterization of mutant forms of recombinant human properdin lacking single thrombospondin type I repeats. Identification of modules important for function. J Immunol 1995; 155:5777–5785.

44. Goundis D, Holt SM, Boyd Y, Reid KBM. Localization of properdin structural locus to Xp11.23–Xp21.1. Genomics 1989; 5:56–60.

45. Nolan KF, Kaluz S, Higgins JM, Goundis D, Reid KBM. Characterization of the human properdin gene. Biochem J 1992; 287:291–297.

46. Farries TC, Lachmann PJ, Harrison RA. Analysis of the interaction between properdin and factor B components of the alternative-pathway C3 convertase of complement. Biochem J 1988; 252:667–675.

47. Sugita Y, Nakano Y, Oda E, et al. Determination of carboxyterminal residue and disulfide bonds of MACIF (CD59) a glycosylphosphatidylinositol anchored membrane protein. J Biochem 1993; 114:473–477.

48. Fletcher CM, Harrison RA, Lachmann PJ, Neuhaus D. Structure of a soluble, glycosylated form of the complement regulatory protein CD59. Structure 1994; 2:185–199.

49. Kieffer B, Driscoll PC, Campbell ID, Willis AC, van der Merwe PA, Davis SJ. Three dimensional solution structure of the extracellular region of the complement regulatory protein CD59, a new cell-surface protein domain related to snake venom neurotoxins. Biochemistry 1994; 33:4471–4482.

50. Hekhl-Ostreicher B, Ragg S, Drechsler M, Scherthan H, Royer-Pokora B. Localization of the human CD59 gene by fluorescence in situ hybridization and pulsed-field gel electrophoresis. Cytogenet Cell Genet 1993; 63:144–146.

51. Tone M, Walsh LA, Waldmann H. Gene structure of human CD59 and demonstration that discrete mRNAs are generated by alternative polyadenylation. J Mol Biol 1992; 227:971–976.

52. Moutabarrik A, Nakanishi I, Namiki M, et al. Cytokine-medicated regulation of the surface expression of complement regulatory proteins CD46 (MCP), CD55 (DAF) and CD59 on human vascular endothelial cells. Lymphokine Cytokine Res 1993; 12:167–172.

53. Meri S, Nattila P, Renkonken R. Regulation of CD59 expression on the human endothelial cell line EAhy 926. Eur J Immunol 1993; 23:2511–2516.

54. Gordon DL, Papazaharoudakis H, Sadlon TA, Arellano A, Okada N. Upregulation of human neutrophil CD59, a regulator of the membrane attack complex of complement, following cell activation. Immunol Cell Biol 1994; 72:222–229.

55. Holguin MH, Martin CB, Weis JH, Parker CJ. Enhanced expression of the complement regulatory protein membrane inhibitor of reactive lysis (CD59) is regulated at the level of transcription. Blood 1993; 82:968–977.

56. Avies A, Simmons DL, Hale G, et al. CD59, an LY6-like protein expressed in human lymphoid cells, regulates the action of the complement membrane attack complex on homologous cells. J Exp Med 1989; 170:637–654.

57. Chang CP, Hulser T, Zhao J, Wiedmer T, Sims PJ. Identity of a peptide domain of C9 that is bound by cell-surface complement inhibitor CD59. J Biol Chem 1994; 269:26424–26430.

58. Nakano Y, Tozaki T, Kikuta N, et al. Determination of the active site of CD59 with synthetic peptides. Mol Immunol 1995; 32:241–247.

59. Lockert DH, Kaufman KM, Chang CP, Husler T, Sodetz JM, Sims PJ. Identity of the segment of human complement C8 recognized by complement regulatory protein CD59. J Biol Chem 1995; 270:19723–19728.

60. Tomlinson S, Whitlow B, Nussenzweig V. A synthetic peptide from complement component C9 binds to CD59 and enhances lysis of human erythrocytes by C5b-9. J Immunol 1994; 152:1927–1934.

61. Husler T, Lockert DH, Kaufman KM, Sodetz JM, Sims PJ. Chimeras of human complement C9 reveal the site recognized by complement regulatory protein CD59. J Biol Chem 1995; 270:3483–3486.

62. Jenne D, Stanley KK. Nucleotide sequence and organization of the human S-protein gene: Repeating peptide motifs in the "pexin" family and a model for their evolution. Biochemistry 1987; 26:6735–6742.

63. Barnes DW, Reing J. Human spreading factor: synthesis and response by Hep G2 cells in culture. J Cell Physiol 1985; 125:207–214.

64. Dahlback B, Podack ER. Characterization of human S-protein, an inhibitor of the membrane attack complex of complement. Demonstration of a free reactive thiol group. Biochemistry 1985; 24:2368–2374.

65. Kubota K, Hayashi M, Oishi N, Sakaki Y. Polymorphism of the human vitronectin gene causes vitronectin blood type. Biochem Biophys Res Commun 1990; 167:1355–1360.

66. Fink TM, Jenne DE, Lichter P. The human vitronectin (complement S-protein) gene maps to the centromeric region of 17q. Human Genet 1992; 88:569–572.

67. Podack ER, Kolb WP, Muller-Eberhard HJ. The SC5b-7 complex: formation, isolation, properties and subunit composition. J Immunol 1977; 119:2024–2029.

68. Milis L, Morris CA, Sheehan MC, Charlesworth JH, Pussel BA. Vitronectin-mediated inhibition of complement: evidence for different binding sites for C5b-7 and C9. Clin Exp Immunol 1993; 92:114–119.

69. deSilva HV, Stuart WD, Duvic CR, et al. A 70 kDa lipoprotein designated ApoJ is a marker for subclasses of human plasma high density lipoproteins. J Biol Chem 1990; 265:13240–13247.

70. Jenne DE, Lowin B, Peitsch MC, Bottcher A, Schmidt G, Tschopp J. Clusterin (complement lysis inhibitor) forms a high density lipoprotein complex with apolipoprotein A-1 in human plasma. J Biol Chem 1991; 226:11030–11036.

71. Jenne DE, Tschopp J. Molecular structure and functional characterization of a human complement cytolysis inhibitor found in blood and seminal plasma: identity to sulfated glycoprotein 2, a constituent of rat testis fluid. Proc Natl Acad Sci USA 1989; 86:7123–7127.

72. Slawin K, Sawszuk IS, Olsson CA, Buttyan R. Chromosomal assignment of the human homologue encoding SGP2. Biochem Biophys Res Commun 1990; 172:160–164.

73. Purello M, Bettuzzi S, DiPietro C, et al. The gene for SP-40,40 human homolog of rat sulfated glycoprotein 2, rat clusterin and rat testosterone repressed message 2 maps to chromosome 8. Genomics 1991; 10:151–161.

74. Tobe T, Minoshima S, Yamase S, Choi NH, Tomita M, Shimizu N. Assignment of a human serum glycoprotein SP-40,40 gene (CLI) to chromosome 8. Cytogenet Cell Genet 1991; 57:193.

75. Fink TM, Zimmer M, Tschopp J, Etienne J, Jenne DE, Lichter P. Human clusterin (CLI) maps to 8p21 in proximity to the lipoprotein lipase (LPL) gene. Genomics 1993; 16:526–528.
76. Nemerow GR, Yamamoto K-I, Lint TF. Restriction of complement-mediated membrane damage by the eighth component of complement: a dual role for C8 in the complement attack sequence. J Immunol 1979; 123:1245–1252.
77. Liszewski MK, Post TW, Atkinson JP. Membrane cofactor protein (MCP or CD46): newest member of the regulators of complement activation gene cluster. Annu Rev Immunol 1991; 9:431–455.

8

Complement Receptors

JOSEPH M. AHEARN
University of Pittsburgh School of Medicine, Pittsburgh, Pennsylvania

ARIELLA M. ROSENGARD
Johns Hopkins University School of Medicine, Baltimore, Maryland

I. COMPLEMENT RECEPTOR TYPE 1

Complement receptor type 1 (CR1, CD35) is a type I transmembrane glycoprotein expressed on erythrocytes, mononuclear phagocytes, eosinophils, B lymphocytes, T lymphocytes, glomerular podocytes, and follicular dendritic cells (1–5). Four CR1 allotypes have been identified, making it the most polymorphic among known complement receptors (6–10). All four allotypes share the same 25 residue transmembrane domain and 43 amino acid cytoplasmic tail, and all of the allotypes have extracytoplasmic domains composed entirely of short consensus repeats (SCR) arranged in tandem. The allotypes differ from one another structurally by multiples of seven SCR, referred to as long homologous repeats (LHR) (11), and have been designated A (F), B(S), C(F′) and D. Thus, allotypes A (F), B(S), C(F′), and D, have extracytoplasmic domains that consist of four, five, three, and (presumably) six LHR, respectively, as well as two additional SCRs that separate the last LHR from the transmembrane domain in each allotype. The extracellular domains of allotypes A, B, C, and D, are therefore composed entirely of 30, 37, 23, and (presumably) 44 SCR, respectively.

The primary, functional role of CR1 is phagocytosis and clearance of immune complexes, which is mediated by its capacity to bind complement ligands C3b, iC3b, and C4b, and its capacity to inactivate C3 and C5 convertases of the alternative and classical complement pathways through decay accelerating and factor I cofactor functions (12–14). CR1 has also recently been shown to serve as a receptor for the variant surface protein of *Plasmodium falciparum,* PfEMP1 (15).

A. Gene Organization

A single copy gene encoding CR1 maps to band q32 of chromosome 1, within the regulators of complement activation (RCA) gene cluster that spans 750 kb (16). This RCA cluster contains genes encoding complement receptor type 2 (CR2,CD21), decay accelerating factor (DAF,CD55), membrane cofactor protein (MCP,CD46), factor H, and C4-binding protein (16–21). These six RCA proteins are functionally related by their shared capacity to bind ligands derived from complement proteins C3 and/or C4, and they are structurally related by the shared presence of tandem domains of ~60 amino acids each, known as short consensus repeats (SCR) or complement control protein (CCP) modules.

The CR1 gene encoding the S allele spans 158 kb and contains 47 exons (22,23). A single exon encodes the signal sequence and part of the 5′ UT region. The seven SCRs within each of the five LHR (A,B/A,B,C,D) are encoded by eight exons; within each LHR, SCR-1, -5, and -7 are each encoded by a single exon; SCR-2 and -6 are each encoded by a pair of exons; and a single exon encodes SCR-3 and -4 (22). Of the eight different SCR each encoded by two exons, the intron that splits each exon pair occurs at the same position within each SCR: between the second and third nucleotide of the glycine codon that occurs three residues after the second conserved cysteine (22). This pattern is consistent among other RCA family members, including human CR2 (24), murine factor H (25), human interleukin-2 (26), murine C4b-binding protein (27,28), the α chain of human C4b-binding protein (29), the β chain of human C4b-binding protein (30), human decay accelerating factor (31), and murine Crry (32). The carboxyl-terminal two SCRs that are not part of an LHR are encoded by two exons. One exon encodes residues 1969–1976 that link the last SCR to the transmembrane region. Two exons encode the transmembrane domain. Single exons encode the cytoplasmic domain and the 3′ UT region, respectively (22). A crossover event between LHR-A and LHR-B that produced the LHR unique to allotype S (LHR-A/B; LHR-S) is thought to have occurred between nucleotide 68 of the fifth exons in the respective LHRs, and 383 bp downstream at the site of a 17 bp insertion in LHR-B (22). The crossover event between LHR-A and LHR-C that presumably gave rise to LHR-B is likewise thought to have occurred within the fourth exons of these LHR, based upon inspection of intronic sequences within the three LHR (22).

Approximately 2 kb of the 5′ end of the CR1 gene has been sequenced and characterized (22). The transcription start site of the CR1 gene is 111 bp upstream of the translation initiation codon ATG, and a second possible start site has been identified 29 bp further upstream. No TATA box is present. However, a sequence at position −87 matches the octamer sequence ATGCAAAT, which has been determined to bind OTF-1 and OTF-2 (33). At position +22, a seven of eight nucleotide match for the Y box of class II MHC genes is present (34). The functional relevance of these elements has not been determined. Four potential polyadenylation signals have been identified, and it has been determined that the second of these is actually used (22).

The CR1 allotypes are not the products of alternative splicing. The F allele spans 133 kb, and it is composed of 39 exons (22). It does not contain the genomic region of the S allele that encodes LHR-B/A. The gene encoding the S allotype can be differentiated from the F allele by a 14.5 kb BamHI RFLP present only in the former (35). The F′ allele differs from the F allele in that it lacks LHR-B (36). All of the introns in the F allele are type 1 or type 2, and the pattern of intron type is consistent among all four LHR (22). The frequencies of the A(F), B(S), C(F′), and D allotypes are 0.82, 0.18, <0.01, and <0.01, respectively, being named alphabetically in order of decreasing gene frequency (9).

Erythrocytes from different normal individuals vary by as much as 10-fold in the number of CR1 molecules expressed on the membrane (37), and this variability has been shown to be due to a *cis*-acting tissue-specific regulatory element within the CR1 gene (38). Polymorphic HindIII restriction fragments of 7.4 and 6.9 kb, which are closely associated with high (H) or low (L) expression, respectively, of CR1 on erythrocytes (38), are caused by a single transversion in an intron between exons encoding SCR-2 in LHR-D (AAGCAT [H] vs. AAGCTT [L]); the allelic HindIII fragments extend from the 3' region of LHR-C to LHR-D (23).

Additional genomic polymorphisms have been identified (39) and mapped to a region that appears to be a partially duplicated CR1 allele near the CR1 locus (23). This region spans 40 kb and contains at least 10 potential exons, with 95% homology to CR1 at the nucleotide level and 91% homology at the amino acid level (40). The potential coding sequences correspond to the CR1 signal peptide and SCRs 1–6, and SCR-9. No sequences similar to SCR-7 and -8 appear to be present in this duplicated region, and a protein product of this region has not been detected. This CR1-like region and the CR1 gene are thought to have been generated by a gene duplication event (40).

B. Protein Structure and Function

The four CR1 allotypes have Mr under reducing/nonreducing conditions of ~250,000/190,000 (A,F), 290,000/220,000 (B,S), 210,000/160,000 (C,F'), and >290,000/250,000 (D) (41). These differences reflect variations in the numbers of LHRs within the proteins, with each LHR encoding a polypeptide of 46,000–52,000 Da.

The F allotype is composed of 2,039 residues, including a 41 amino acid signal peptide, and a 1930 amino acid extracellular domain composed entirely of 30 SCRs (42,43). The amino-terminal 28 SCRs are arranged in four LHRs (-A, -B, -C, -D) of seven SCRs each, and two additional SCRs link LHR-D with a 25 residue transmembrane region and a 43 amino acid cytoplasmic domain (42).

The sequences of LHR-A and LHR-B are 61% identical within SCR-1 and SCR-2, and >99% identical in the remaining five SCRs (42). The tandem alignment of 30 SCRs in the F allotype of CR1 creates a flexible, filamentous structure 80–90 nm in length, as determined by electron microscopic analysis (44).

Whereas amino acid homology between adjacent SCRs ranges from 30–40%, homologies between SCRs that occupy the same relative positions in two different LHRs range from 56 to 100% (11,42). For example, alignment of residues within SCR-3 through SCR-7 of LHR-A and residues within SCR-10 through SCR-14 of LHR-B reveals only one difference among the 327 positions. SCR-8 through SCR-11 of LHR-B and SCR-15 through SCR-18 of LHR-C likewise differ at 3 of 253 positions. It has also been demonstrated that the 28 SCRs within LHR-A,-B,-C, and -D of the F allotype are of four different types based upon amino acid sequence homology (45). According to this nomenclature, the composition of the four LHRs is LHR-A (a-a-a-a-a-a-a), LHR-B (b-b-a-a-a-a-a), LHR-C (b-b-a-a-c-c-c), and LHR-D (d-d-d-d-c-c-c).

Three additional homology regions have been identified in CR1 allotype A. Homology region I is composed of SCR-1 and SCR-2. Homology region II, extending from SCR-3 to SCR-18, exhibits greater than 99% sequence conservation among 7-SCR repeating units within the 16 SCRs. Homology region III, extending from SCR-19 to SCR-28, exhibits 91% fidelity of sequence repetition.

There are 25 potential N-linked glycosylation sites in the amino acid sequence of the F allotype (42), of which 6–8 appear to be modified by tri- and tetraantennary complex type oligosaccharides (46,47). Differences in glycosylation account for differences in

CR1 size observed between erythrocytes and polymorphonuclear leukocytes in the same individual (46). Nonglycosylated CR1 binds iC3 with 41% efficiency as compared with receptor-bearing carbohydrate (47). CR1 does not bear O-linked carbohydrates (47).

A naturally occurring, soluble form of CR1 has been demonstrated in plasma of normal individuals (48,49), and in culture supernatants of monocytes, lymphocytes, and neutrophils (49). The mean serum concentration in 31 normal individuals ranged from 17.8 to 55.7 ng/ml, with a mean of 31.4 ng/ml, and serum levels, which are identical to plasma levels, have been demonstrated to fluctuate widely in a variety of pathological states (49). It has not been determined whether this soluble form of the receptor is secreted or shed from plasma membranes; and it is not known if levels correlate with in vivo complement activation. These studies also demonstrated that, in contrast to the repeated epitopes recognized by mAb Yz-1 (50), anti-CR1 mAb 3D9 recognizes a single CR1 epitope and is therefore a direct quantitation of E CR1 (49). The biological $t_{1/2}$ of endogenous CR1 was estimated to be 2–3 days.

The ligand-binding domains of CR1 have been mapped through deletion mutagenesis (42), substitution mutagenesis (51,52), and creation and characterization of chimeric receptors (53). Early studies had suggested that the CR1 allotypic variants do not differ functionally in their cofactor activities or in their capacities to inhibit fluid phase classical and alternative pathway C3 convertases (54). These findings were based upon studies of purified forms of the endogenous F, S, and F′ proteins. Subsequent studies involved creation and characterization of a panel of six deletion mutants in which one, two, or three LHRs, respectively, were deleted from the F allotype (ABCD) (42). This panel included recombinant receptors ABCD, AD, BD, CD, and D, in which the nomenclature reflects the LHRs remaining in the deletion mutant. Recombinant full length receptor (ABCD) formed rosettes with erythrocytes bearing methylamine-treated C3 (EC3[ma]) or C4 (EC4[ma]). However, only mutants BD and CD were capable of binding (EC3[ma]), demonstrating independent C3-binding sites in LHR-B and LHR-C but not in LHR-A or LHR-D. Deletion mutant AD was likewise most capable of binding (EC4[ma]) suggesting that the primary C4-binding site is located within LHR-A.

Characterization of additional mutants demonstrated that the C4b-binding site of CR1 resides primarily in SCR-1 and SCR-2 of LHR-A (42). Inspection of amino acid sequence homologies led to the mapping of the two C3-binding sites to the amino-terminal pair of SCRs within LHR-B (SCR-8 and SCR-9) and LHR-C (SCR-15 and SCR-16), respectively. A deletion mutant containing LHR-D alone bound neither C3b nor C4b, demonstrating that the carboxyl-terminal 9 SCRs common to all CR1 allotypes lack an intact ligand-binding domain. Although the amino-terminal pair of SCRs within LHR-A, LHR-B, and LHR-C was shown to be a primary binding site for C4, C3, and C3, respectively, each of the three domains also appeared to be a secondary binding site for C3, C4, and C4, respectively.

Thus, these studies identified three distinct and independent ligand-binding domains within the F allotype of CR1, each of which is capable of binding both C3 and C4 fragments (42). SCR-1 and SCR-2 of LHR-A is a primary C4-binding site and a secondary C3-binding site, and the amino-terminal pair of SCRs within both LHR-B and LHR-C are primary C3-binding sites and secondary C4-binding sites. Later studies were unable to detect binding of C3b dimers to receptors containing SCR1-4 of LHR-A, suggesting that this secondary affinity may be considerably lower than that of the primary recognition sites (55). These studies also determined that the epitope recognized by the anti-CR1 mAb Yz-1 (50) is repeated within LHR-A,-B and-C (42).

Potential functional differences among the CR1 allotypes were also explored through studies of soluble, recombinant forms of the F, S, and F′ allotypes, which contained LHR-ABCD, -ABBCD, and -ACD respectively (36). All three soluble forms of the receptor were shown to be equally capable of binding monomeric C3b and serving as cofactors for factor-I mediated conversion of C3b to iC3b and C3dg (36). In contrast to these studies using monomeric C3b, the three variant forms of CR1, which contain zero, one, and two LHR-B domains, respectively, differed considerably in their capacities to bind dimeric C3b. The concentrations of soluble LHR-ACD, -ABCD, and -ABBCD required to achieve 50% inhibition of the interaction between C3b dimer and erythrocyte CR1 were 100 nM, 10 nM, and 1 nM, respectively (36). Consistent with these observations was the finding that these three variants also differed in their capacities to inhibit the alternative pathway C3 and C5 convertases, with the -ABBCD and the -ABCD forms being 30-fold more effective than the -ACD form of soluble CR1 (36). In contrast, the three variants had similar capacities to inhibit the classical pathway C3 and C5 convertases, suggesting that they have similar affinities for C4b (36). These findings together supported a model in which tandem ligand-binding domains contained within adjacent LHRs of a single CR1 molecule promote multivalent receptor–ligand interactions (23,36).

Although the amino-terminal pair of SCRs within LHR-A,-B, and-C were initially shown to determine ligand specificity, it was subsequently shown that the first four SCRs of an LHR are required to bind C3b with an affinity indistinguishable from that of the wild type receptor. This was demonstrated by studies of recombinant membrane-bound CR1-CR2 chimeric receptors, in which the ligand-binding domain of human CR2 (SCR-1 and SCR-2) was replaced with different LHRs and SCRs of CR1 (53). Polymeric and dimeric forms of C3b were used as ligands. In these investigations, the dissociation constants for polymeric C3b (tetrameric and greater) of wild type CR1 and recombinant chimeric receptors bearing LHR-BD and -CD were 1.0–2.7 nM. Chimeric receptors that contained SCRs 1–4, 1–3, or 2–4 of LHR-B or LHR-C had Kd of 1.8–2.4, 6–9, and 22–36 nM, respectively. The factor I cofactor activity of CR1 maps coordinately with C3b binding (53,54).

Further investigations demonstrated that the C4b ligand-binding domain of CR1 also consists of four SCR. These studies demonstrated that SCR 1–4 of LHR-A bind C4b dimers with an affinity ($K_d \sim 4 \times 10^{-7}$ M) similar to wild type receptor, whereas SCR 1–2 alone bind C4b dimers with lower affinity ($K_d = 1.4 \times 10^{-6}$ M) (56). The first four SCR of LHR-C (SCR 15–18) were shown to be less effective in binding C4b dimers ($K_d = 1.2 \times 10^{-6}$ M) than the first four SCR of LHR-A (SCR 1–4). (In comparison, the affinity of CR1 for C3b dimers is $K_d = 1-2 \times 10^{-8}$ M [55].)

Efforts to begin to identify amino acids within these domains that determine ligand specificity involved studies in which residues from C3-binding sites were substituted for those in C4-binding sites and vice versa (51). The rationale in these studies was that SCR-1 and SCR-8 are 55% homologous and SCR-2 and SCR-9 are 70% homologous, yet SCR-1 and SCR-2 determine C4b-binding specificity and SCR-8 and SCR-9 determine C3b-binding specificity. Recombinant CR1 mutants were therefore created in which residues that differed between SCR-1 and SCR-8 and between SCR-2 and SCR-9 were substituted and characterized for changes in ligand-binding specificity (51). Several of the substitutions resulted in no functional change. Other substitutions resulted in loss of ligand binding that could reflect loss of receptor–ligand contact sites or disruption of a receptor conformation required for ligand binding. The most interesting and informative results of these studies were derived from characterization of a mutant in which five amino acids at the carboxyl-terminus of SCR-2 (*DNETPICD*) were replaced by the five corresponding residues of SCR-9 (*STKPPICQ*). These substitutions resulted in the acquisition of iC3 binding without alteration of C4b binding, suggesting that these residues are critical in determining the C3 binding specificity of LHR-B and LHR-C in which they naturally occur, and these amino acid positions may be critical in ligand discrimination. This is one of only two model systems in which the sequences of individual SCRs have been manipulated to result in a gain of function.

Further dissection of the structural requirements for ligand binding to CR1 was accomplished through studies of soluble, recombinant forms of CR1 consisting of 8-1/2 SCRs (52). These investigations first compared a deletion mutant consisting of SCR NH$_2$-1-2-3-4-5-6-7-8-(9$_{1/2}$)-COOH, with a mutant in which SCR-8 and SCR-9 were substituted for SCR-1 and SCR-2, creating a protein composed of SCR NH$_2$-8-9-3-4-5-6-7-8-(9$_{1/2}$)-COOH. The construct containing CR1-4, bound mainly to C4b, consistent with previous studies, whereas the substitution of SCR-8,9 for SCR-1,2 resulted in a receptor, CR1–4(8,9) that bound iC3 as well as C4b. In addition, C4b bound more avidly to CR1–4(8,9) than to CR1–4. This latter result was in contrast to previous studies (42), which had indicated that the SCR-8,9 domain is not a primary C4b-binding site. The two studies differed, however, in that the former report (42) was based upon characterization of a chimeric construct in which the amino-terminal half of SCR-8 was replaced by the corresponding portion of SCR-1. This subsequent report (52) suggests that the amino-terminal portion of SCR-8 does influence C4b binding specificity. Studies of similar receptors composed of only the amino-terminal 7 SCRs produced indistinguishable results. Although not tested directly, substitution of SCR-15 and SCR-16 for SCR-1 and SCR-2 was predicted to generate identical results because the sequence of this SCR pair differs from that of SCR-8 and SCR-9 by only a single residue. Thus, these findings further demonstrated that the amino-terminal pair of SCRs within LHR-A (SCR-1,2), LHR-B (SCR-8,9), and LHR-C (SCR-15,16) determine ligand specificity, although they suggest that each domain does not necessarily bind primarily C3 or C4.

These studies were extended to investigate the effects of exchanging residues that differed between SCR-1,2 (site 1) and SCR-8,9 (site 2) yet occupied homologous positions in the sequences (52). Similar to previous work, 11 of the substitutions resulted in no detectable effect on C3/C4 binding or cofactor activity. Characterization of the other mutants led to several interesting observations. First, regions were identified in corresponding locations within SCR-1 and SCR-8 that, when exchanged, led to reduced binding of iC3 and C4b to site 2 and enhanced binding of both ligands to site 1. Second, residues were identified in corresponding locations within SCR-2 and SCR-9 that, when exchanged, led to reduced binding of iC3 and C4b to site 2 and enhanced binding of ligands to site 1. Third, site 2 was shown to be a more potent cofactor for factor I-mediated ligand cleavage than is site 1, and the cofactor activity of site 2 is higher for C3b than it is for C4b. Fourth, changes in cofactor activity observed following substitutions were generally accompanied by parallel changes in ligand-binding capacity. However, certain substitutions did alter cofactor activity more than ligand binding. Fifth, and of most interest, transfer of four amino acids—Gly[35] from SCR-1 and Arg,[64] Asn,[65] Tyr,[94] from SCR-2, to corresponding locations in SCR-8 and SCR-9—created a ligand-binding domain with greater iC3 and C4b-binding activity than any wild-type site, and enhanced cofactor activity for both ligands. It was subsequently demonstrated that replacement of Ser[37] of SCR-1 with Tyr from the homologous position of SCR-9, and replacement of Gly[79] of SCR-2 with

Asp from the corresponding position of SCR-16 resulted in acquisition of C3b binding by the C4b binding site of CR1 (57). Neither substitution alone had this effect.

Efforts to identify the region of C3 involved in binding to CR1 have identified a sequence near the N-terminus of the a'-chain of C3, which includes the charged residues ^{730}DE and ^{736}EE (58).

These findings, and similar mutagenesis studies of other RCA proteins such as CR2 (59) that have demonstrated gain of function, represent the foundation for elucidating the structure–function relationships of these proteins. Further mutagenesis studies, together with complementary three-dimensional structural determinations, will undoubtedly lead to determination of how the hypervariable regions of the SCR mediate the multifunctional capacities of complement regulatory proteins. In addition, the demonstration that function can be enhanced beyond the capacity of wild-type receptors (52), holds great promise for rational design and development of novel therapeutic agents based on an understanding of RCA protein structure–function relationships.

II. COMPLEMENT RECEPTOR TYPE 2

Complement receptor type 2 (CR2, CD21) is a 140 kDa type I transmembrane glycoprotein expressed on late pre- and mature B lymphocytes (60–66), B cell lines (60), some T cell lines (67–70), thymocytes (71), and follicular dendritic cells (5,72). Approximately 40% of peripheral blood T cells express CR2; however, the level of expression is 10-fold lower than that found on human peripheral blood B lymphocytes (73).

Short (CD21S) and long (CD21L) forms of CR2 have been identified composed of a 954 amino acid extracellular domain or a 1013 amino acid extracellular domain, respectively (72,74–76). Both forms have the same 24 residue transmembrane region, and 34 amino acid cytoplasmic tail. The extracellular domain is composed entirely of either 15 (CD21S) or 16 (CD21L) tandem short consensus repeats (SCR) or complement control protein (CCP) modules. CR2 is a receptor for the C3b, iC3b, and C3dg cleavage fragments of C3 (60,61,66,77–80), an interaction involved in B-cell activation and proliferation. CR2 has been reported to serve as a cofactor for factor I-mediated cleavage of particle-bound iC3b (81), but not for soluble iC3b (82). CR2 expressed on human B lymphocytes can activate the alternative pathway of complement and serve as a primary acceptor site for C3 during this process (83,84). CR2 is also the B lymphocyte receptor for Epstein-Barr virus (77,85–87). CD23 (88–90) and interferon α (91) are also reported to be ligands for CR2.

A. Gene Organization

A single copy gene encoding CR2 spans 35 kb (92) and maps to band q32 of chromosome 1, within the regulators of complement activation (RCA) gene cluster. Inspection of the exon–intron organization of the *CR2* gene reveals a general pattern in which 16 SCRs are encoded by four groups of exons (24). Group 1 encodes SCR 1–4, group 2 encodes SCR 5–8, group 3 encodes SCR 9–12, and group 4 encodes SCR 13–16. In each group, the first pair of SCRs is encoded by a single exon, the third SCR is encoded by a single exon, and the fourth SCR is encoded by two exons. The only exception to this pattern is that SCR-16 is encoded by a single exon. This repeated pattern in genomic organization is paralleled by coding sequence homology revealed by inspection of the cDNA (75) (see below). The transmembrane domain is encoded by two exons, and the cytoplasmic domain is encoded by a single exon (24). It has been proposed that the current *CR2* gene evolved from a primordial locus in which each of four exons encoded a single SCR (24).

Whereas human CR1 and human CR2 are structurally distinct and encoded by different genes, murine CR1 and murine CR2 are the products of alternative splicing of transcripts generated by the *Cr2* locus (93,94). Murine CR2, like the human CR2 homolog, consists of a 15 SCR extracellular domain. However, murine CR1, unlike human CR1, is identical to murine CR2 except for an additional six SCRs added to the amino terminus of murine CR2. A search for human sequences homologous to those that encode SCR 1–6 of murine CR1 has identified such genomic sequence located between nucleotides encoding the human CR2 signal peptide and the exon encoding SCR-1 of human CR2 (95). However, these sequences were not detected in mature transcripts derived from the locus, suggesting that they are pseudoexons: remnants of a more primitive gene product that may have been a homolog of murine CR1.

Restriction fragment length polymorphisms of the *CR2* gene have been identified for TaqI and HaeIII (24). Two Taq I allelic fragments are located near the SCR-1 and SCR-2 encoding exon, with frequencies of 0.7 and 0.3 in normal whites (24). Three HaeIII allelic fragments are generated by polymorphic sites located near the SCR-15 exon, with frequencies of 0.93, 0.05, and 0.02 in normal whites (24).

The CR2 promoter has been identified and partially characterized (92,96). The exon encoding the CR2 signal peptide and 5' untranslated sequence is more than 10 kb upstream of the exon encoding SCR-1 and SCR-2. Two transcription initiation sites have been located at a CA dinucleotide, 92 bp upstream from the initiator methionine codon. Inspection of the promoter region has identified potential regulatory elements including an SP1 site (−142), an AP-2 site (−80), TATTTAA (−29), and two AP-1 sites (−87)(−987). Preliminary studies have suggested that this promoter region does not mediate tissue-specific expression of CR2 (92).

B. Protein Structure and Function

CR2 was initially cloned from a human tonsillar cDNA library using a human CR1 cDNA probe at low stringency hybridization (74,75), and from a Raji B lymphoblastoid cell cDNA library using a synthetic oligonucleotide probe based upon amino acid sequence of tryptic peptides generated from CR2 purified from Raji cells (76). Amino acid sequence derived from cDNA cloned from the tonsil library revealed a 20 amino acid signal peptide, a 954 residue extracellular domain organized into 15 SCR of 57–74 amino acids each, a 24 residue transmembrane region, and a 34 amino acid cytoplasmic tail (75). One of five cDNA clones generated from the tonsil library encoded a 16th SCR referred to as 10a because of its location between SCR-10 and SCR-11 of the 15 SCR form of CR2 (75). The single cDNA cloned from the Raji cell library also encoded 16 SCRs (76), and SCR-11 in this clone is identical to SCR-10a from the 15 SCR clone. It has been demonstrated that every fourth SCR in CR2 belongs to a homology group such that the 16 SCRs can be aligned into four homology groups of four SCR each (1,5,9,13; 2,6,10,14; 3,7,11,15; 4,8,12,16) (75,76). The degree of amino acid identity between SCRs in homologous groups ranges from 35% to 51% (76). This is consistent with the exon–intron organization of the gene described above, and further support for the hypothesis that CR2 evolved from a primordial four-SCR unit.

The 15 SCR (CD21S) and 16 SCR (CD21L) forms of CR2 represent alternatively spliced transcripts (97). In one study, both transcripts were detected in all of seven B lymphoblastoid cell lines examined, as well as in human tonsillar tissue, although the ratio of the two transcripts varied considerably (97). The 15 SCR transcript was more abundant in most of the cell lines; however, they were present in approximately equal amounts in each of two tonsils (97). Ligand-binding studies of the 15 SCR and 16 SCR forms of CR2 have demonstrated identical affinities of the two proteins for iC3b and for gp350/220 (98). Therefore, SCR-10a plays no role in these interactions.

The cytoplasmic domain contains four tyrosine, four serine, and two threonine residues (75,76), and it has been determined that CR2 is phosphorylated in tonsillar B cells and in Raji cells following exposure to PMA (99). There are 11 potential N-linked glycosylation sites in the 15 SCR form of CR2 and two additional sites in SCR-10a (75,76). It has been demonstrated that 8–11 of these sites are modified on mature CR2 polypeptides in SB B lymphoblastoid cells (100). It has also been determined that glycosylation is required for stability of CR2, but glycosylation is not required for CR2 to bind C3-Sepharose (100).

Three alleles of CR2 that differ in primary structure have been identified, and referred to as forms I, II, and III (97). Form I is the 15 SCR form described above and forms II and III each contain the 16th SCR 10a. Form I also differs from forms II and III by the presence of alanine at position 3237 within the cytoplasmic domain, in contrast to the glutamic acid found in forms II and III. Several other amino acid substitutions within SCR-7, SCR-10, SCR-10a, and SCR-12 differentiate the three forms from one another (97). Functional differences have not been correlated with the three forms of CR2. However, it has recently been demonstrated that follicular dendritic cells selectively express the 16 SCR or "long" form of CR2 (CD21L), while B cells selectively express the 15 SCR or "short" form of CR2 (CD21S) (72). CR2 thus becomes the first human FDC-specific molecule to be characterized. Three anti-human FDC mAbs 7D6, DRC-1 and KiM4, which are specific for FDC networks on tonsillar and splenic tissue, were shown to recognize CD21L (72). Low levels of the 7D6 antigen were also detected on Raji cells, consistent with the successful cloning of the 16 SCR form of CR2 from the Raji cDNA library as described above (76). Two amino acid differences were detected in this report as compared with the sequence originally reported from Raji cells: Ser to Asn at position 1979, and Arg to His at position 2075. It has not been determined whether the epitope(s) recognized by the CD21L-specific mAbs are encoded by SCR-10a or whether they represent conformational changes in epitopes encoded elsewhere that are induced by incorporation of 10a into the protein (72). The functional significance of this interesting and unexpected observation, and the transcriptional machinery responsible for FDC-specific and B cell-specific forms of CR2, have not been determined.

CR2 expressed by the Jurkat T cell line has a larger apparent molecular weight of 155 kDa, compared with 145 kDa CR2 found in B cells and the HPB-ALL T cell line, although the mRNAs are all 4.7 kb (70). The slower electrophoretic mobility of Jurkat CR2 appears to be due to differential glycosylation (70).

Release of soluble forms of CR2 from lymphocytes has been reported (101,102). A 72 kD C3d-binding protein was first identified in Raji B lymphoblastoid cell culture media, and suspected to represent the product of CR2 proteolysis because of the presence of the CR2-specific epitope recognized by mAb OKB7 (101). More recently, a 135 kDa soluble form of CR2 representing the extracytoplasmic portion of the molecule has been identified in culture supernatants from both the Raji B lymphoblastoid cell line and the

HPB-ALL acute T cell leukemia line, and in normal human serum (102). This 135 kD protein was demonstrated to bind iC3b as well as a soluble, recombinant form of CD23 (102)

Hydrodynamic and electron microscopic studies of soluble, recombinant CR2 have demonstrated that the molecule is highly extended (f/f_o=2.1) and highly flexible. The soluble form of the 16 SCR receptor has a contour length of 386 $\pm$ 35 Å, and each of the 16 SCRs appears as a discrete domain with a calculated length of 24.1 $\pm$ 2 Å (103).

Four specific functions have been mapped to different structural domains of CR2. First, SCR-1 and SCR-2 are both necessary (104) and together sufficient (104,105) for binding ligands C3b, iC3b, and C3dg. The affinities of the intact receptor for polymeric C3dg (pC3dg) and gp350 are the same as the affinities of SCR-1 and SCR-2 alone for the two ligands: 0.7 nM for the polymeric natural ligand and an approximately 10-fold weaker affinity for the monomeric viral ligand. Studies on the interaction between soluble recombinant CR2 and monomeric C3dg have demonstrated that the affinity of the receptor for monomeric C3dg (K_d = 27.5 μm) is 10^4-fold less under physiological conditions than the affinity of the receptor for monomeric gp350 (K_d = 3.2 nM) (103). The affinity for monomeric C3dg is enhanced at reduced ionic strength (103).

Second, SCR-1 and SCR-2 are both necessary (104) and together sufficient (104,105) for binding Epstein-Barr virus (EBV) and EBV ligand gp350/220. It has been determined that CR2 binds directly to the external domain of gp350/220, an interaction that does not involve other viral or cellular proteins (106). Homologous peptides have been identified in C3 (EDPGKQLYNVEA; residues 1199–1210 of mature C3)) and gp350/220 (EDPGFF-NVE) (106,107,65), and these regions of the natural and viral ligands have been shown, through peptide studies, to participate in the binding of the respective ligands to CD21 (108–110). It should be noted, however, that rigorous mutagenesis studies have failed to corroborate a role for this region of C3 in binding to CR2. (111). The basis for these contradictory and surprising observations is not clear.

Soluble, recombinant forms of the ligand-binding domain of CD21 have been created in which SCR-1 and SCR-2 are fused to *Staphylococcus aureus* protein A (112), to murine complement factor H (112), or to IgG1 (113). Each of these soluble fusion proteins blocked binding of gp350/220 to the receptor and infection of B cells by EBV, as has been reported for soluble recombinant full-length CR2 (114). The viral ligand gp350/220, like its receptor, is a highly extended protein (f/f_o = 2.4/2.2), whereas the natural ligand C3dg is more compact (f/fo = 1.5) (103).

Third, CD23 (FcεR2), a low-affinity receptor for IgE, is reported to bind to CD21 (88), an interaction that may influence the survival of B cells in germinal centers (90). This interaction was initially shown to be partially inhibited by mAb HB-5, and completely inhibited by anti-CR2 mAb BU-33 (88). Other anti-CR2 mABs were also reported to block the CD21-CD23 interaction, including BU-32, BU-34, and BU-42 (88). Anti-CR2 mAb B-2 did not block the interaction. Additional studies have suggested that SCR-5-8 of CR2 may be involved in this interaction with CD23, and N-linked oligosaccharides within this domain may participate (89).

Fourth, CD21 and CD19 participate in a multimolecular B-cell membrane complex (115) in which CD21 interacts with CD19 on the B-cell membrane via its transmembrane and extracellular domains (116). CR2 also interacts in a bimolecular complex with CD35 (117) via the extracellular domains of the two receptors (116). The domains of CR2 responsible for the formation of multimolecular complexes observed in T cells (68,118) have not been determined.

In addition to these functional domains, the epitopes recognized by several monoclonal antibodies have been mapped to sites throughout the extracellular domain of the receptor. SCR-1 and SCR-2 are both necessary (104) and together sufficient (104,105) for binding mAb OKB7 (119), which blocks binding of CR2 to C3d and to EBV (120). The mAb HB-5, which does not block binding of either ligand to the receptor, binds to an epitope within SCR-3 and SCR-4, and mAb B2 has been mapped to an epitope contained within SCR 11–14 by one study (104) and within SCR 9–11 by a second study (105), suggesting that the epitope may reside within SCR-11. Anti-CR2 monoclonal antibodies 1C8, 1F8, 2G7, and 6F7 (121) have been shown to recognize epitopes located within SCR 12–15 (105).

Together, these studies indicated that SCR-1 and SCR-2 of CR2 are both necessary and together sufficient for binding natural ligands derived from C3, the viral ligand gp350, and mAb OKB7 that blocks binding of both ligands to the receptor. One early indication that the sites for binding natural and viral ligands are overlapping but distinct was the successful generation of anti-CR2 monoclonal antibodies capable of specifically blocking binding of either the natural ligand or the viral ligand to the receptor (122). Subsequent studies that utilized human–murine CR2 chimeras demonstrated that the requirements for binding C3dg versus gp350 were actually distinct. These studies took advantage of the differential capacities of murine CD21 and human CD21 to bind EBV. Murine CR2, like human CR2, is composed of 15 SCRs, and the ligand-binding domains of the two receptors (SCR-1 and SCR-2) share 61% amino acid identity (123). Although both receptors have been shown to have the same affinity for polymeric human C3dg (124), only the human receptor is capable of binding EBV. Anti-human CD21 mAb OKB7 (119) and anti-murine CD21 mAb 7G6 (125), specifically block binding of ligand to their respective receptors.

These observations facilitated the design of an experimental system to dissect the structural requirements for binding of natural and viral ligands to human CD21 (59), to determine the structural basis for differential binding of EBV to the human receptor versus the mouse receptor (59), to map the binding sites for mAbs OKB7 and 7G6 (59), and to determine the requirements of the non-ligand-binding domains of human CD21 during cellular infection by EBV (126).

Creation and characterization of a panel of 24 human-murine CD21 chimeric receptors demonstrated that preferential binding of EBV to human CR2 is not due to unique amino acids capable of binding the virus, because it is possible to substitute murine for human sequence throughout SCR-1 and SCR-2 and still retain the capacity to bind EBV (59). Specificity of EBV for the human receptor instead reflects a distinct conformation of the human receptor that can be achieved in murine CR2 with single amino acid substitutions in two discontinuous regions of the primary structure: replacement of proline at position 15 with the corresponding serine from human CR2, and elimination of a potential N-linked glycosylation site between SCR-1 and SCR-2. In addition, species-specific binding of mAb 7G6, mAb OKB7, and EBV, can all be manipulated by interspecies sequence substitutions within the sequence PILNGRIS, residues 8–15 of the human receptor. These studies have also demonstrated that the OKB7 and 7G6 epitopes are mutually exclusive, the C3d- and gp350-binding epitopes are distinct, and the epitopes recognized by OKB7 and by EBV are distinct. Thus, species-specific epitopes within murine CD21 and human CD21 are influenced by critical linear as well as nonlinear determinants, all of which appear to involve the same amino-terminal octapeptide.

The three-dimensional structure of CR2 has not yet been determined. However, additional insight into CR2 structure–function relationships can be gained from consideration of related studies of other RCA family members. The tertiary structures of single SCRs (127,128) and SCR pairs (129–130) have been solved through studies of factor H (127–129) and vaccinia virus complement control protein (VCP) (130) (Fig. 1). The dimensions of an individual SCR are approximately 40Å × 16Å × 12Å (127), and SCR pairs interface at the extremes of the long axes of the modules (129,130). The framework of an SCR consists of a β sandwich in which the NH2 and the COOH termini are at opposite ends of the module, and β strands lie parallel with the long axis of the module. This structure is stabilized by a pair of disulfide bonds between C1-C3 and C2-C4. The

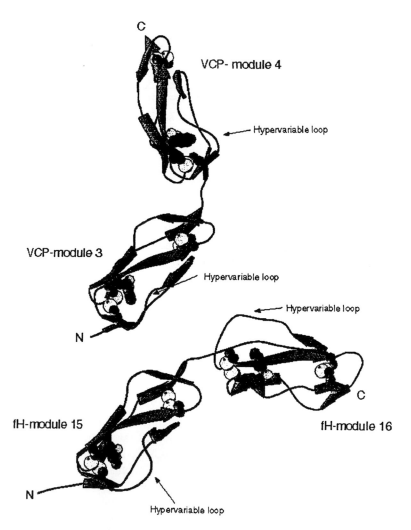

Figure 1 Two examples of short consensus repeat (SCR) pairs, also referred to as complement control protein (CCP) module pairs. The SCR-3 and SCR-4 pair from vaccinia complement control protein (VCP) (130) is shown above, and the SCR-15 and SCR-16 pair from human factor H (129) is shown below. A MOLSCRIPT representation is used to show the backbones. (Figure courtesy of Dr. Paul Barlow, The University of Edinburgh.)

two faces contribute side chains, which are highly conserved among SCRs, to form a globular, compact, hydrophobic core. Sequences that are less conserved among SCRs are inserted as loops and turns within this framework. One such loop protrudes 15 Å laterally to the long axis and is called the hypervariable loop (127–130). Studies of the SCR-15, SCR-16 pair of modules from factor H have demonstrated that these two modules are aligned end-to-end and do not make extensive contacts with one another (129). Structural potential for intermodular flexibility was also apparent from these studies. In contrast, studies of the SCR-3 and SCR-4 pair from VCP demonstrate a more extensive interface between the two modules, and a more rigid structure (130). Curious is that the hypervariable loops of VCP SCR-3 and SCR-4 are situated on the same side of the molecule, representing a potential ligand-binding surface (130).

Thus, although the hypervariable loops of the modules are undoubtedly involved in determining the multifunctional nature of this family of proteins, additional structural studies of individual SCRs and SCR arrays will be required before confident predictions of function can be made from inspection and modeling of structure. These studies are already, however, supportive of conclusions regarding CR2 structure–function generated from the mutagenesis experiments described above. The orientation of SCR-1 and SCR-2 of CR2 to one another may be critical for generating a receptor conformation that will bind EBV. Perhaps limited substitution of human sequence with mouse residues maintains this conformation. However, more extensive incorporation of murine sequence disrupts the alignment of SCR-1 and SCR-2 such that the domain will no longer bind the virus, even though the residues that mediate receptor–ligand contact are still present.

It has been demonstrated that the specific role of CR2 during EBV infection of B lymphoblastoid cells is to capture virions at the cell surface, after which cofactors not associated with CR2 mediate postbinding events (126). In these studies, the ligand-binding domain of ICAM-1 (CD54), the rhinovirus receptor, was replaced with SCR-1 and SCR-2, the EBV-binding domain of CR2. This CD21-CD54 chimera was capable of mediating infection of three B lymphoblastoid cell lines, demonstrating that the extracytoplasmic, transmembrane, and cytoplasmic non-ligand-binding domains of CR2 are not required for EBV infection of these cells. It is presumed that other B-cell-specific factors in addition to CR2 are responsible for the narrow tropism of EBV. This conclusion is also supported by observations that expression of high levels of recombinant human CR2 on cell types other than human B cells is not accompanied by efficient infection of these by EBV (131).

III. COMPLEMENT RECEPTOR TYPE 3

Complement receptor type 3 (CR3, CD11b/CD18, Mac-1, Mo1, OKM-1, α_M/β_2) is an α/β heterodimeric adhesion molecule that was the first member of the leukocyte-restricted integrin family to be discovered (132). A common 95-kD β subunit is shared with CD11a/CD18 (LFA-1, α_L/β_2) and CD11c/CD18 (CR4, p150,95, α_x/β_2), whereas the α subunits are related but individually distinct, and differentiate the three heterodimers from one another. Expression of CR3 is restricted to leukocytes (133–135). CR3 is expressed primarily on mononuclear phagocytes and natural killer (NK) cells, and expression of CR3 on activated granulocytes is considerably higher than either of the other two leukocyte-restricted heterodimers (6–8×10^5 molecules/cell) (133). In resting monocytes, expression of CR3 is greater than expression of CR4, whereas in tissue macrophages the opposite is true (134,135).

iC3b is the only complement ligand for CR3 (136–138), which is also a receptor for coagulation factor X (139), fibrinogen (140–142), lipopolysaccharide (143), zymosan (144), soluble Fcγ receptor type III (FcγRIII; CD16) (145), the counterreceptor ICAM-1 (CD54) (146,147), filamentous hemagglutinin of *Bordetella pertussis* (148), and *Leishmania promastigote* surface glycoprotein gp63 (149). CR3 has also recently been reported to serve as a receptor for the acute phase protein, haptoglobin (150). The diverse ligand-binding capabilities of CR3 make it the most functionally versatile complement receptor. CD11b/CD18 participates in mediating adhesion of mononuclear phagocytes to endothelial cells (146,151–153), cellular extravasation and chemotaxis to sites of inflammation (146), phagocytosis of CR3-ligand opsonized particles (154), and enhancement of NK cell activity for C3-coated targets (155).

A. Gene Organization

The CD11b gene is clustered with the other CD11 α subunits on chromosome 16, band p11–p11.2 (156,157). The single copy CD11b gene spans 55 kb, encodes a single 4.8 kb mRNA, and contains 30 exons separated by introns ranging in size from 84 bp to 9.1 kb (158). The exons are arranged in seven clusters in a pattern similar to that demonstrated for CD11c (159). In particular, the intron/exon junctions in CD11b and CD11c are nearly identical, suggesting that the two genes are the products of a recent duplication event (158,159). Exon 1 encodes 83 bp of the 5′ untranslated sequence, and the first nine residues of the signal peptide. Exon 2 encodes the remaining 7 amino acids of the signal sequence and the first 29 residues of the mature protein (158). An I domain, also referred to as an L domain or a von Willebrand factor type A (VWFA) module, is encoded by exons 6, 7, 8, and 9. This I domain, which is absent in most other integrins besides the leukocyte integrins, is thought to have arisen by insertion of exons 6 through 9 into a primordial integrin gene (158).

Three tandem repeats of a putative divalent cation-binding "EF-hand loop" domain are encoded by exons 13, 14, and 15, respectively, which are thought to have arisen through gene duplication events (158). Exon 29 encodes the first 22 residues of the putative transmembrane domain, and exon 30 encodes the remaining 4 amino acids of the transmembrane region, the 19 amino acid cytoplasmic tail, and the entire 1158-bp of the 3′ untranslated region.

The predominant transcriptional start site is located 83 bp upstream from the initiator methionine codon, and a weaker start site is located at position +4 (158). Characterization of the CD11b promoter by deletion mutagenesis demonstrated that the sequence extending from −412 to bp +83 is three times more active in U937 cells than the sequence extending from −1704 to +83 (160). However, further deletions 3′ of −412 resulted in diminished transcriptional activity, indicating the presence of positive regulatory elements in this region. These studies also demonstrated that 92 bp of promoter sequence upstream of the transcriptional start site can direct myeloid-specific gene expression, although it is 100-fold less active that the −412 to +83 sequence (160). The CD11b promoter contains two Sp1 consensus binding sites at −64 and −103, respectively, and a purine-rich potential PU.1 site at −134 (160). The promoter lacks TATAA and CCATT boxes.

The CD18 gene maps to chromosome 21, band q22.3 (156,161) and encodes a single 3.0 kb mRNA (162).

B. Protein Structure and Function

CR3 is a heterodimer with α and β subunits of 165,000 and 95,000 M_r, respectively, and a 1:1 stoichiometry. The α subunit, CD11b, is a 165 kD type I transmembrane glycoprotein that associates noncovalently with the 95-kDa CD18 β chain to form CR3. The primary structure of the mature CD11b polypeptide contains 1136 (163) or 1137 (164,165) amino acids. The one residue difference is a Gln^{484}, located between two conserved cysteines at 478 and 489, which is encoded by two independently reported human cDNA clones (164,165) that contain an extra codon, CAG, between bp 1580 and 1581 of the third independently derived clone (163). No functional difference has been ascribed to this polymorphism, or alternative form of the receptor. CD11b consists of a 16 residue signal peptide, a 1092 (or 1091) residue extracellular domain, a 26 residue transmembrane region, and a 19 amino acid cytoplasmic tail (164). The cytoplasmic domain contains one serine constitutively phosphorylated in resting human leukocytes (166,167).

The extracellular domain of CD11b contains seven homologous tandem repeats, each of which contains approximately 60 amino acids. Repeats V through VII show the highest degree of similarity to one another, and contain the consensus sequence DXDXDGXXDXXE, characteristic of EF-loop metal-binding proteins. The putative divalent cation-binding sites of CD11b are 87% identical to those of CD11c, and 38% identical to integrin α subunits in general (164), making this region the most conserved between CD11b and other integrin α subunits (164). Repeats I–IV lack the metal-binding consensus sequences, but contain the sequences YFGAS/AL and LVTVGAP that are conserved in other integrins (164). An I domain, consisting of 187 amino acids (residues 150–338), is inserted between the second and third homologous repeats of CD11b. This I domain is homologous to the VWFA mondules A domains of von Willebrand factor, factor B, and C2. The I domain of CD11b shares 64% amino acid identity with the corresponding domain in CD11c, yet these two proteins share only 36% amino acid identity with the I domain of CD11a.

There are 19 potential N-linked glycosylation sites in the CD11b sequence, which have been partially characterized. Treatment of the αM precursor of M_r ~160,000 with either Endo H or N-glycanase results in a product of M_r~137,000, and the mature αM subunit of ~167,000 is partially sensitive to Endo H (M_r~153,000) and completely susceptible to N-glycanase (Mr~137,000)(168).

CD11b also shares approximately 25% amino acid identity (164) with the α subunits of platelet glycoprotein IIb/IIIa (169), vitronectin receptor (170), and fibronectin receptor (171), which are 40% identical to one another. Each of the latter three integrins contains a cleavage site involved in proteolytic processing of the α subunits into a light chain that is membrane anchored and a heavy chain that is entirely extracellular and linked by disulfide bond to the α chain. The structure of CD11b is differentiated from those of these three receptors, and similar to that of CD11c (the α chain of CR4) in lacking this cleavage site. The transmembrane domains of CD11b and CD11c are 88% identical (164,172), suggesting that these sequences serve an important function shared by the two molecules, in addition to simply providing a hydrophobic membrane-spanning segment.

A polymorphic determinant in CD11b has been identified by mAb RM.184 (173). This epitope appears to be in the α chain of the receptor, is dependent upon association with CD18, and was present in 14% of the Australian population studied.

Cloning and characterization of the CD18 cDNA have determined that the primary structure of CD18 is that of a type I transmembrane protein consisting of 747 amino acids

(162,174). This includes a 22 residue signal peptide, an extracellular domain of 678 amino acids, a 23 residue transmembrane domain, and a 46 amino acid cytoplasmic tail. The cytoplasmic domain contains one tyrosine, three threonine, and four serine residues. Although CD18 is not constitutively phosphorylated, induction with either PMA or FMLP generates primarily phosphoserine, with small amounts of phosphothreonine and phospho-tyrosine (166,167). There are six potential N-linked glycosylation sites.

CD18 has an unusually high cysteine content (7.4%), and all 56 cysteines of the mature polypeptide are located in the extracellular domain. A region of the extracellular domain extending from amino acids 445 to 631 contains four tandem repeats of an 8-cysteine motif. This cysteine-rich (20%) region is thought to be involved in extensive intrachain, rather than interchain, disulfide bond formation because the α and β chains of the receptor are noncovalently associated (162). It has been determined that the CD18 subunit of CR3 is glycosylated in a different site-specific pattern compared with the identical CD18 subunit that is associated with CD11a, the α_L chain of LFA-1 (175). These studies, which were performed with a cell line that expresses both heterodimers simultaneously, indicate that the quaternary structure of the leukocyte integrins influences site-specific glycosylation of CD18 (175). There is no homology between CD11b and CD18.

Mapping of the binding sites for the numerous CR3 ligands has proven challenging. Initial studies utilized experimental systems based upon ligand-coated particles, ligand-derived peptides, monoclonal antibodies, and CR3 expressed on live phagocytes. These studies can be summarized as follows.

Intercellular adhesion molecule 1 (ICAM-1, CD54) a counterreceptor for both LFA-1 (CD11a/CD18) (176) and CR3 (CD11b/CD18) (147), has an extracellular region that consists of five tandem immunoglobulin-like domains (177,178). Whereas LFA-1 binds to the amino-terminal immunoglobulin-like domain of ICAM-1 (179), CR3 binds to the third immunoglobulin-like domain (180), which does not contain an RGD sequence (177,178). Elimination of potential N-linked glycosylation sites in the third immunoglobu-lin-like domain of ICAM-1 or inhibition of the biosynthesis of N-linked oligosaccharides on ICAM-1, enhances binding of ICAM-1 to purified CR3, but not to LFA-1 (180). This observation suggests that glycosylation of ICAM-1 may regulate differential adhesion to LFA-1 versus CR3 in vivo (180).

Anti-CR3 mAb OKM10 (181), directed against the I domain of the α chain, a decapeptide derived from the carboxyl terminus of the γ chain of fibrinogen (LGGAK-QAGDV), and proteolytic fragments of fibrinogen, all block binding of both fibrinogen and iC3b to CR3 (140). Attachment of Leishmania gp63 to CR3 is also inhibited by mAb OKM10, and gp63 competes with iC3b for binding to CR3 (140). Together, these observations suggested that the binding sites for fibrinogen, iC3b, and gp63 on CR3 are overlapping, if not identical (140).

Factor X and iC3b likewise compete for binding to CR3, suggesting a common binding site (139). Homologous sequences in human C3 (**LEICTRYRGD**) (1386–1395), fibrinogen (**LGGAKQAGD**) (402–410), leishmania gp63 (**PGGLQQGRGD**) (367–376), and filamentous hemagglutinin of *Bordetella pertussis* (TV**GRGD**PHQ) (1094–1102) were initially thought to mediate these interactions based upon the capacity of peptides based upon these sequences to inhibit binding of the respective ligands to CR3 (140,148,149,182).

Subsequent studies utilized CR3 purified to homogeneity from PMN derived from human peripheral blood (183). These investigations confirmed the specific interaction of CR3 with fibrinogen, gp63 of *Leishmania mexicana,* LPS from *Escherichia coli,* lipophosphoglycan, and filamentous hemagglutinin of *Bordetella pertussis*. Soluble forms of these ligands at μg/ml concentrations effectively inhibited binding of EC3bi to purified CR3. However, these studies were not able to confirm interaction of CR3 with zymosan or its major component β-glucan, at ligand concentrations as high as 1 mg/ml. More surprising was that these studies demonstrated that RGD-containing peptides, at concentrations as high as 10 mg/ml, are unable to block the interaction of C3bi with CR3. Instead, RGD peptides appeared to affect CR3 function indirectly by binding to leukocyte-response integrin (LRI), a β3 integrin known to enhance the phagocytic capacity of PMN (184,185). This conclusion is supported not only by the failure of RGD peptides to block binding of EC3bi to CR3 but also by the demonstration that ligation of LRI with anti-β3 mAb enhances binding of EC3bi to CR3, and blockade of LRI with Fab of polyclonal anti-β3 inhibits binding of EC3bi to CR3 in a manner quantitatively similar to the inhibitory effects of RGD peptides (183).

Additional studies supported an indirect effect of the RGD ligand sequence in mediating binding to CR3. First, site-directed mutagenesis of the RGD region of C3bi to AAA did not affect its interaction with CR3 (186). Second, proteolytic fragments of fibrinogen that lack the carboxyl-terminal RGD-containing dodecapeptide of the γ chain, as well as the RGD sequences of the A chain, were capable of binding to CR3 (187). Third, RGD affinity chromatography successfully isolated integrins from monocytes. However, CR3 was not one of the proteins isolated (184).

Additional investigations to map the ligand-binding domains of CR3 utilized CR3/CR4 chimeric receptors (188). These studies demonstrated that the I domain is a major recognition site for iC3b, ICAM-1, and fibrinogen. These studies also successfully mapped the epitopes recognized by a panel of 34 anti-CR3 mAbs. Of these, 19 recognized the I domain, 11 bound to the carboxyl-terminal region, and 1 bound to the divalent cation repeat domain (188). Two of the mAb recognized a discontinuous epitope formed by the amino-terminal region and the divalent cation domain, and one of these, CBRM1/32, blocked binding of the receptor to iC3b, ICAM-1, and fibrinogen (188). This was the only mAb that bound outside of the I domain that blocked binding of these ligands to CR3.

Further investigations have indicated that CR3 is expressed in an inactive state on resting leukocytes, and high avidity ligand-binding by CR3 occurs only following stimulation of cells via heterologous receptors such as LRI (189–192). A novel mAb (CBRM1/5) binds to an activation-specific neoepitope of CR3 on a subset (10–30%) of stimulated neutrophils (192). This unique probe, which blocks CR3-dependent adhesion to fibrinogen and ICAM-1, recognizes an epitope in the I domain on neutrophils and monocytes following stimulation with chemoattractants or phorbol esters, but not on resting myeloid cells. Another molecular reporter of the activated conformation of CR3, mAb 7E3, recognizes CD11b/CD18 only following stimulation of monocytes with adenosine diphosphate (ADP) or with agonists that induce transients in cytosolic Ca^{2+} such as FMLP (190). ADP is known to induce rapidly a high-avidity state of CR3 for factor X (139) and for fibrinogen (141).

In contrast to the binding domain for these ligands, soluble Fc$_\gamma$ receptor type III (F$_\gamma$RIII; sCD16) is thought to bind outside the I domain, near the lectin-like region of CR3, based upon mAb inhibition studies (145). The binding site for lipopolysaccharide (143) is also distinct from the C3bi/fibrinogen/gp63 binding domain as shown by the capacity of mAb OKM10 to block specifically binding of C3bi but not lipid IVa, and the capacity of mAb 904 to block specifically the binding of lipid IVa but not C3bi (193). These two mAbs both recognize the α chain of CR3, and appear to recognize differentially epitopes of two distinct ligand-binding domains. In addition, a dodecapeptide corresponding to the CR3-binding site of C3 (residues 1390–1401), was shown to compete effectively with C3bi but not with lipid IVa for binding to CR3 (193). Presence of this peptide actually enhanced significantly binding of lipid IVa to the receptor. Studies using a decapeptide based upon the CR3-binding site of the γ chain of fibrinogen (residues 402–411) produced similar results, demonstrating inhibition of C3bi binding and enhancement of lipid IVa binding (193).

Although the β-glucan binding capacity of CR3 is controversial (183), a β-glucan-binding site of CR3 has been mapped through studies based upon CR3/CR4 chimeric receptors, and ligands that included a soluble, low-molecular-mass (10 kDa) mannose-rich polysaccharide isolated from zymosan (SZP), and β-glucan preparations from mushroom, seaweed, barley, and yeast (194). These studies demonstrated that CR3 is probably the only leukocyte β-glucan receptor, CR3 has only one type of lectin site, this ligand-binding domain has broad sugar specificity, and the CR3 lectin-site is cation independent. Although the efforts to map this lectin-binding domain were inconclusive, the data suggested that one or two such sites are located C-terminal to the I domain.

CR3, like the other leukocyte integrins, requires Ca^{2+} or Mg^{2+} for ligand binding. Whereas the classical EF-loop metal-binding domains contain a glutamic acid in the $-Z$ position that is coordinated with metal, this residue is absent in CD11b, and other integrins. It is thought that the aspartic acid of the Arg-Gly-Asp (RGD) sequence in some CR3 ligands, or a similar residue in other ligands, may coordinate with metal bound to the receptor (195). Surprising was that a novel divalent cation-binding site has been identified in the A (I) domain of CR3 that is essential for binding iC3b (196). A recombinant peptide encoding the A domain, expressed in *E. coli,* binds Mn^{2+} with high affinity, and Mg^{2+}, Zn^{2+}, Ni^{2+}, Co^{2+}, and Cd^{2+}, but not Ca^{2+} or Ba^{2+} compete effectively with Mn^{2+} for binding. Targeted mutagenesis of aspartic acid residues at positions 140 and 242 eliminated metal binding and abolished the capacity of the mutant receptors to bind iC3b, without affecting heterodimer formation, expression of the receptor, or recognition of the receptor by a panel of mAbs (196). These findings suggest that the capacity of CD11b to bind iC3b, and perhaps other ligands, is dependent upon divalent cation binding to the A domain.

Determination of the secondary structure and the crystal structure of the A domain has confirmed and extended these observations (197,198). The A domain consists of one antiparallel and five parallel β strands that form a central sheet surrounded by seven α helices, a classical "Rossmann" fold. A single metal-binding site, containing a Mg^{2+} ion in these studies, sits at the top of the β sheet, on the surface of the A domain. The metal ion has coordination sites for six ligands. However, the two aspartate, at positions 140 and 242 identified in the above studies do not coordinate the metal directly but indirectly through hydrogen bonds to a coordinated water molecule. One of the coordination sites is occupied by a carboxylate oxygen atom from a glutamate residue provided by a neighboring A domain. This metal-binding site, with a free coordination site, has been termed the metal ion-dependent adhesion site (MIDAS) motif (198). The MIDAS consensus sequence is DXSXS (residues 140–144 in CD11b), and T^{209} and D^{242} from discontinuous regions of the polypeptide. Inspection of A domain sequences in numerous other proteins has identified MIDAS motifs (198). Furthermore, although the α subunit A domain and integrin β domains are not homologous, comparison of hydropathy profiles suggests that integrin β subunits do contain MIDAS motifs with a three-dimensional fold similar to the A domain of CD11b (198).

Recent data suggest that CR3 may associate noncovalently with a 16 kD intracellular protein. However, the subunit and residues involved in this interaction have not been determined (199). There is evidence to suggest, however, that a C-terminal domain of CR3, recognized by mAb VIM12, might be involved in complex formation between CR3 and glycophosphatidylinositol (GPI)-anchored FcγRIIIB (CD16) on human granulocytes (189). A lectin-like interaction between these two molecules has been proposed (200), and this C-terminal domain contains 15 of the 19 potential N-linked glycosylation sites in CD11b.

IV. COMPLEMENT RECEPTOR TYPE 4

Complement receptor type 4 (CR4; CD11c/CD18; p150,95; α_x/β_2) is an α/β heterodimeric adhesion molecule that was the third member of the leukocyte-restricted integrin family to be discovered (201–203). A common 95 kD β subunit is shared with CD11a/CD18 (LFA-1; α_L/β_2) and CD11b/CD18 (Mac-1α_M/β_2), whereas the α subunits are related but individually distinct, and differentiate the three heterodimers from one another. CR4 is expressed primarily on myeloid cells (134), dendritic cells (204), NK cells (205), activated B lymphocytes (206), some cytotoxic T cells (134,207), and platelets (208). Myeloid cell activation leads to a rapid increase in membrane expression of CR4, apparently due to translocation of intracellular pools since protein synthesis is not required (205). It has also been determined that myeloid cell differentiation is accompanied by coordinate expression of CR3 and CR4 (134). CR4 is a marker for hairy cell leukemias, as determined by reactivity with monoclonal antibody αS-HCL 3 (αLeu-M5) (209), and for certain B-cell lymphoproliferative disorders (210,211).

iC3b is the primary complement ligand for CR4, which is also reported to be a receptor for fibrinogen (212), lipopolysaccharide (143), soluble Fcγ receptor type III (FcγRIII; CD16) (145), and CD23 (213).

A. Gene Organization

The gene encoding CD11c is located on the short arm of chromosome 16, together with the genes encoding CD11a and CD11b, between 16p11 and 16p13.1 (156,161). Each of the three genes is present as a single copy (156), and the CD11c gene generates a single 4.7 kb mRNA (172). The gene encoding the common β subunit, CD18, is located on chromosome 21, band q22.3 (156,161). The α chain locus has been identified as a breakpoint in acute myelomonocytic leukemia (214), and the β chain locus has been identified as a breakpoint in translocations associated with the blast phase of chronic myelogenous leukemia (215).

The CD11c polypeptide, consisting of 1144 amino acids, is encoded by 31 exons that are grouped in five clusters and extend over 25 kilobases (159). Exon 2 encodes 52 bp of 5′ untranslated sequence and the amino-terminal 12 residues of the signal peptide, and exon 3 encodes the carboxyl-terminal 7 residues of the signal sequence and the first 28 residues of the mature protein (159). Exons 7–10 (43, 48, 50, and 51 residues) encode residues 125–318, which form an I domain. Examination of the intronic sequence within and flanking the exons encoding the I domain have led to interesting speculation regarding its evolution. Splice sites flanking exons 7–10 are conserved as phase class I, yet splice sites within the I domain are not conserved. It has been proposed that "the I domain was inserted as a primordial exon into ancestral genes for a number of different protein families. Subsequent evolution occurred by duplication and diversification of the entire gene to yield gene families (integrin α subunits, complement factor B and C2), duplication of the I domain within the gene (the repeats of von Willebrand factor and chicken cartilage matrix protein), and intron insertion and deletion within the I domain (159). This process may have contributed to the structural basis for functional diversity that has been reported for I domains.

Each of three divalent cation-binding repeats is encoded by exons 14, 15, and 16, respectively (159). Exon 30 encodes the last 15 amino acids of the extracellular domain and the first 22 amino acids of the transmembrane region. Exon 31 encodes the last 4 residues of the transmembrane domain, the 30 residue cytoplasmic tail, and 434 bp of 3'-untranslated sequence (159).

Expression of CD18 on all leukocytes suggests that transcriptional regulatory elements are responsible for the more restricted distribution of CD11c/CD18 among leukocyte subsets, as well as for the coordinated expression of CR4 that accompanies myeloid cell differentiation along monocytic and granulocytic pathways. The 5' region of the gene has been characterized for the presence of tissue-specific transcriptional regulatory elements (216,217). Several interesting observations have been made. There are multiple transcription initiation sites, including two major start sites at 66 bp (+2) and 67 bp (+1) upstream from the initiator methionine codon. There are no TATA or CAAT boxes in the promoter; however, an "initiator sequence" (Inr) 5'-TTCCTCA-3', which has been described in several other genes (218), immediately precedes the +1 cap site. The promoter has been localized to a 1 kb fragment extending from −960 to +40, and this region has been shown to confer tissue-specific expression in myeloid cells that parallels endogenous CD11c differential expression (217). Multiple putative binding sequences have been identified for both ubiquitous and leukocyte-specific transcription factors, including consensus sequences for Sp1, c-myc, AP-1, AP2, NF-kB, OCT, HEPT, and PU.1, a B-cell- and macrophage-specific factor. Regions −42 to −34 and −13 to −5 contain consensus sequences for Ets factors (219). Six potential retinoic acid responsive elements (220) are also present.

One of the AP-1 binding sites (AP1-60) in the proximal promoter region of the CD11c gene has been further characterized. Differential binding of Fos family members to this element appears to be involved in transcriptional regulation of basal as well as developmental expression of CD11c/CD18 among myeloid cells (216). Additional studies have demonstrated that Sp1-binding sites at −70 and at −120 contribute to regulation of CD11c expression (221,222). In particular, the regions −72 to −63 and −132 to −104 of the CD11c promoter bind to Sp1, these sites are essential for Sp1-dependent expression of CD11c, and elements in these regions participate in regulation of phorbol-ester induced differentiation of HL60 myeloid cells (222). Further studies have demonstrated that myeloid-specific expression of CD11c involves myeloid-restricted binding of Sp1 to the CD11c promoter and a cooperative interaction between the Sp1 and AP-1-binding sites (222). First, Sp1 contacts the promoter within regions −69 to −63 and −116 to −105 in differentiated but not in undifferentiated HL60 cells (222). Second, both Sp1 sites are capable of cooperating with AP1, and Sp1 acts synergistically with AP1 to activate CD11c (222). Third, Sp1 binding facilitates binding of c-jun (222). Fourth, the −62 to −44 region contains two consensus sequences for AP1 that bind purified c-jun (219). Fifth, the Ets site described above from −42 to −34 (Ets C) cooperates with the two AP1 sites located immediately adjacent (219). The proteins that bind to the Ets sites have not been determined.

B. Protein Structure and Function

The α subunits of the leukocyte-restricted integrins, CD11a, CD11b, and CD11c, are structurally related, and presumably evolved from common gene and polypeptide origins. CD11c, a type I transmembrane glycoprotein, consists of a 1081 amino acid extracellular domain, a 26 residue transmembrane region, and a 30 amino acid cytoplasmic tail (172). The extracellular domain contains three tandem repeated sequences of 58, 70 and 68 amino acids, respectively, which are located between residues 424 and 619. Centered in each of the repeats is a putative divalent cation-binding motif that resembles sequences found in metal-binding proteins such as calmodulin, parvalbumin, and troponin C (223), which are thought to have a common evolutionary origin (224). This motif has been determined to form a helix–loop–helix conformation referred to as an "EF hand," a term that arose from studies of carp muscle calcium-binding protein (parvalbumin) (225). In this configuration, the calcium-binding domain resembles a right hand with the thumb (helix f) and the forefinger (helix E) extended, and fingers three through five clenched. The middle finger represents the calcium-binding loop. It has been determined from three-dimensional studies of other proteins in this family that functional differences are made possible, in part, by changes in the orientation of the helices to one another as well as in differences in the linker regions (223).

Residues 125–318 form an I domain, the structure and function of which has been described above for CR3. There are 10 N-X-S/T sites (172), of which 5 or 6 appear to be glycosylated (168). CD11c contains no O-linked oligosaccharides (168).

CD11c shares 35% and 67% amino acid identity with CD11a and CD11b, respectively (172). CD11c also shares approximately 25% amino acid identity with the α subunits of platelet glycoprotein IIb/IIIa (169), vitronectin receptor (170), and fibronectin receptor (171). The structure of CD11c is differentiated from the structures of these three RGD receptors by the absence of the cleavage sites involved in the proteolytic processing of each of the other three integrin α subunits into a light chain that is membrane anchored and a heavy chain that is entirely extracellular and linked by disulfide bond to the α chain.

Although the function of CR4 has not been completely elucidated, it is known to share with CD11a/CD18 and CD11b/CD18 the capacity to mediate adhesion of leukocytes to endothelium (151,226). It has been demonstrated that CR4 has a counterreceptor on human umbilical vein endothelial cells, and inhibition of the interaction by monoclonal antibodies to different regions of CR4 suggest that more than one ligand mediate the interaction (226). Adhesion of TNF-α-stimulated neutrophils to fibrinogen has been shown to occur via binding of CR4 to the sequence Gly-Pro-Arg, which represent residues 17–19 in the amino-terminal domain of the A chain of fibrinogen (212). Monoclonal antibodies to the CD11c α subunit of the receptor block this interaction (212).

Shortly after its discovery, several studies suggested that CR4, like CR3, had the capacity to bind complement ligand iC3b (138,151,227,228). However, these studies were not conclusive. In particular, although CD11c/CD18 was identified via iC3b-Sepharose chromatography (138), neither COS nor CHO cells expressing recombinant CD11c/CD18 were found to be capable of binding iC3b (183). Further investigations led to the surprising discovery that although COS cells expressing human CD11c/CD18 did not bind erythrocytes bearing iC3b, COS cells bearing a human CD11c/chicken CD18 hybrid were capable of binding the iC3b-coated particles (229). In this same study, purified CD11c/CD18 coated onto plastic was shown to bind iC3b-opsonized erythrocytes. Together, these studies suggested that the α subunit, CD11c, must adopt a particular conformation to acquire the capacity to bind iC3b (229). Presumably the chicken β subunit facilitates this in transfected cells whereas the human CD18 subunit does not. Purified, soluble heterodimer must also more readily adopt the ligand-binding conformation than endogenous membrane-bound receptor (229).

The epitopes recognized by several anti-CR4 monoclonal antibodies have been determined in studies employing a panel of transfectants expressing recombinant CR4 or CR3/CR4 chimeras (229). Monoclonal antibodies CBRp150/2C1 and CBRp150/4G1 have been mapped to the C-terminal region of CD11c, mAb SHCL3 recognizes a discontinuous epitope composed of both the amino-terminal domain and the divalent cation-binding regions, and mAbs 3.9 and BL-4H4 have been localized to the I domain of CD11c (229). The capacity of mAbs 3.9 and BL-4H4 also to block binding of iC3b to CR4 suggests that the I domain of the α subunit of CR4 contains the iC3b recognition site.

More recently, soluble Fcγ receptor type III (FcγRIII, CD16) has been identified as a ligand for CR4 (145). The location of the binding site for CD16 has not been mapped on CR4; however, attempts to block binding with monoclonal antibodies suggest that it does not bind to the I domain of CR4 (145). CR4 is also reported to serve as a monocyte receptor for CD23 (213). The physiological consequences of these interactions have not been determined, although it has been shown that ligation of CR4 with CD11c monoclonal antibodies activates neutrophil spreading and neutrophil respiratory burst (230).

V. COMPLEMENT RECEPTOR C1qR$_p$

C1q, the first component of the classical complement pathway, serves to recognize antigen-antibody complexes and other non-immunoglobulin activators of the classical pathway of complement activation through binding of its globular (head) domains. The collagen-like (tail) domains of C1q then stimulate a variety of responses through interaction with numerous cell types including mononuclear phagocytes, lymphocytes, fibroblasts, and endothelial cells. C1q is a member of the structurally and functionally related collectin family of proteins, which includes mannose-binding protein (MBP) and pulmonary surfactant protein A (SP-A). They are composed of an amino-terminal collagen-like domain and a carboxyl-terminal non-collagenous lectin domain. These collectins have been shown to enhance monocyte phagocytosis mediated by FcR as well as by CR1 (231–234), and the capacity of MBP to inhibit partially the binding of C1q to monocytes and neutrophils suggests that they may share a receptor involved in collectin-mediated mononuclear phagocytosis (234).

The first phagocytic cell surface protein conclusively shown to modulate C1q-triggered responses was C1qR$_p$ (235). C1qR$_p$ was initially identified by affinity chromatography using 176 kDa C1q collagen-like domain fragments coupled to Sepharose to isolate C1q-tail-binding proteins from mononuclear phagocytes (236). Monoclonal antibody R139, generated by immunization with the C1q-binding fractions and specific for one of the C1q-binding proteins, was shown to recognize a protein of apparent molecular mass (Mr) of 126,000 under reducing conditions, and to inhibit C1q-mediated, and MBP-mediated, enhancement of mononuclear cell phagocytosis (234,237). Subsequent investigations have recently led to the identification and characterization of the C1qR$_p$ protein and cloning of the cDNA (235). The location and structure of the C1qR$_p$ gene have not been reported, although it has been determined that it is present as a single copy and encodes a single mRNA species of 6.7 kb (235).

A. Protein Structure and Function

The primary structure of C1qRp has been deduced through partial amino acid sequence analysis of protein purified from detergent extracts of U937 cells and complete nucleotide sequence analysis of cDNA generated from U937 mRNA (235). The C1qR$_p$ cDNA encodes a 652 amino acid precursor that contains the 631 residue mature protein with a predicted molecular mass of 66,495 Da and a pI of 5.24. The putative primary structure of the mature receptor consists of a 559 amino acid extracellular domain, a 25 amino acid transmembrane region, and a 47 residue cytoplasmic tail that contains the sequence RAMENQY (638–644) that represents a tyrosine kinase recognition motif. The amino terminus of the extracellular region contains a 156 amino acid sequence with some similarity to a C-type (calcium-dependent) carbohydrate recognition domain (CRD). Of the 18 "nearly invariant" residues found within the 130 amino acid CRD domain consensus, 7 are conserved in C1qR$_p$, including the four cysteines that form intrachain disulfide bonds (235,238,239). Contained within this CRD is the sequence FWIGLQREK that is similar to sequences found in other membrane receptors believed to modulate endocytosis, including the human mannose macrophage receptor (235,240).

Carboxyl-terminal of the C-type CRD are five epidermal growth factor (EGF)-like modules (241), each of which consists of 40–43 amino acids including 6 cysteines that have been shown in other proteins to form intrachain disulfide bonds in the pattern: C1-C3, C2-C4, C5-C6. EGF-like modules 3–5 each contain an asparagine hydroxylation motif D/N-X-D/N-Q/E-C-X$_{4-7}$-C-X$_3$-C-X-D*/N*-X$_4$-Y/F, in which the asterisks represent hydroxylated residues. Such calcium-binding EGF-like domains are present in a variety of extracellular proteins such as the vitamin K-dependent plasma proteins factors IX and X, protein C, and protein S, the connective tissue component fibrillin-1, and complement proteins C1r and C1s (242). A high-resolution x-ray crystallographic structure of the first calcium-binding EGF-like domain from factor IX has been determined (243). These studies suggest that calcium bound to EGF-like modules functions both to stabilize the structure of the module and to mediate directly protein–protein interactions either between EGF-like modules or between EGF modules and other domain types, which may be diverse among this structurally related but functionally diverse group of proteins (243). These structural data also suggest that in proteins such as C1qRp with multiple tandem EGF-like domains, the domains are unlikely to function independent of one another (243).

One potential N-linked glycosylation site is present at position 325 (235). Preliminary evidence suggests that modification at this site as well as extensive O-linked glycosylation are responsible for the discrepancy between the predicted molecular mass (66,495 Da) of C1qR$_p$ and the apparent molecular weight of the receptor as determined by sodium dodecyl sulfate–polyderylamide gel electrophoresis (SDS-PAGE) (126,000) (235).

Monoclonal antibodies R3, R139, and U40.3 recognize distinct epitopes of the receptor (236,237). Of these, only R3 blocks C1q binding, whereas R139 and R3 both inhibit C1q-mediated enhancement of phagocytosis (237). The structural domains recognized by the antibodies and responsible for these functions have not yet been identified.

In summary, C1qR$_p$ is a novel type I membrane glycoprotein with a putative primary structure that includes a C-type CRD domain, five EGF-like modules of which three are likely to bind calcium, and a cytoplasmic tyrosine phosphorylation motif. These features are consistent with the demonstrated capacity of this C1q receptor to transduce cellular activation signals, including enhancement of phagocytosis, following capture of C1q-containing complexes. Further studies of this recently cloned receptor will undoubtedly generate additional important and unanticipated insights into multiple biological processes.

REFERENCES

1. Fearon DT. Identification of the membrane glycoprotein that is the C3b receptor of human erythrocyte, polymorphonuclear leukocyte, B lymphocyte, and monocyte. J Exp Med 1980; 152:20–30.
2. Wilson JG, Tedder TF, Fearon DT. Characterization of human T lymphocytes that express the C3b receptor. J Immunol 1983; 131:684–689.
3. Gelfand MC, Frank MM, Green I. A receptor for the third component of complement in the human renal glomerulus. J Exp Med 1975; 142:1029–1034.
4. Kazatchkine MD, Fearon DT, Appay MD, Mandet C, Bariety J. Immunohistochemical study of the human glomerular C3b receptor in normal kidney and in seventy-five cases of renal diseases. J Clin Invest 1982; 69:900–912.
5. Reynes M, Aubert JP, Cohen JHM, Audoin J, Tricottet V, Diebold J, Kazatchkine MD. Human follicular dendritic cells express CR1, CR2, and CR3 complement receptor antigens. J Immunol 1985; 135:2687–2694.
6. Dykman TR, Cole JL, Iida K, Atkinson JP. Polymorphism of human erythrocyte C3b/C4b receptor. Proc Natl Acad Sci USA 1983; 80:1698–1702.
7. Dykman TR, Cole JL, Iida K, Atkinson JP. Structural heterogeneity of the C3b/C4b receptor (CR1) on human peripheral blood cells. J Exp Med 1983; 157:2160–2165.
8. Wong WW, Wilson JG, Fearon DT. Genetic regulation of a structural polymorphism of human C3b receptor. J Clin Invest 1983; 72:685–693.
9. Dykman TR, Hatch JA, Atkinson JP. Polymorphism of the human C3b/C4d receptor. Identification of a third allele and analysis of receptor phenotypes in families and patients with systemic lupus erythematosus. J Exp Med 1984; 159:691–703.
10. Dykman TR, Hatch JA, Aqua MS, Atkinson JP. Polymorphism of the C3b/C4b receptor (CR1): characterization of a fourth allele. J Immunol 1985; 134:1787–1789.
11. Klickstein LB, Wong WW, Smith JA, Weis JH, Wilson JG, Fearon DT. Human C3b/C4b receptor (CR1). Demonstration of long homologous repeating domains that are composed of short consensus repeats characteristic of C3/C4 binding proteins. J Exp Med 1987; 165:1095–1112.
12. Fearon DT. Regulation of the amplification C3 convertase of human complement by an inhibitory protein isolated from the human erythrocyte membrane. Proc Natl Acad Sci USA 1979; 76:5867–5871.
13. Iida K, Nussenzweig V. Complement receptor is an inhibitor of the complement cascade. J Exp Med 1981; 153:1138–1150.
14. Medof ME, Iida K, Mold C, Nussenzweig V. Unique role of the complement receptor CR_1 in the degradation of C3b associated with immune complexes. J Exp Med 1982; 156:1739–1754.
15. Rowe JA, Moulds JM, Newbold CI, Miller LH. Plasmodium falciparum rosetting is mediated by PfEMP1 and requires complement receptor 1. Nature (In press), 1997.
16. Weis JH, Morton CC, Bruns GAP, Weis JJ, Klickstein LB, Wong WW, and Fearon DT. A complement receptor locus: genes encoding C3b/C4b receptor and C3d/Epstein-Barr virus receptor maps to 1q32. J Immunol 1987; 138:312–315.
17. Rodriguez De Cordoba S, Lublin DM, Rubinstein P, Atkinson JP. Human genes for the three complement components that regulate the activation of C3 are tightly linked. J Exp Med 1985; 161:1189–1195.
18. Lublin DM, Liszewski MK, Post TW, Arce MA, LeBeau MM, Rebentisch MB, Lemons RS, Seya T, Atkinson JP. Molecular cloning and chromosomal localization of human membrane cofactor protein (MCP). J Exp Med 1988; 168:181–194.

19. Bora NS, Lublin DM, Kumar BV, Hockett RD, Holers VM, Atkinson JP. Structural gene for human membrane cofactor protein (MCP) of complement maps to within 100 kb of the 3' end of the C3b/C4b receptor gene. J Exp Med 1989; 169:597–602.

20. Carroll MC, Alicot EM, Katzman PJ, Klickstein LB, Smith JA, Fearon DT. Organization of the genes encoding complement receptors type 1 and 2, decay-accelerating factor, and C4-binding protein in the RCA locus on human chromosome 1. J Exp Med 1988; 167:1271–1280.

21. Rey-Campos J, Rubinstein P, Rodriguez de Cordoba. A physical map of the human regulator of complement activation gene cluster linking the complement genes *CR1, CR2, DAF,* and *C4BP.* J Exp Med 1988; 167:664–669.

22. Vik DP, Wong WW. Structure of the gene for the F allele of complement receptor type 1 and sequence of the coding region unique to the S allele. J Immunol 1993; 151:6214–6224.

23. Wong WW, Cahill JM, Rosen MD, Kennedy CA, Bonaccio ET, Morris MJ, Wilson JG, Klickstein LB, Fearon DT. Structure of the human CR1 gene. Molecular basis of the structural and quantitative polymorphisms and identification of a new CR1-like allele. J Exp Med 1989; 169:847–863.

24. Fujisaku A, Harley JB, Frank MB, Gruner BA, Frazier B, Holers VM. Genomic organization and polymorphisms of the human C3d/Epstein-Barr virus receptors. J Biol Chem 1989; 264:2118–2125.

25. Vik DP, Keeney JB, Munoz Canoves P, Chaplin DD, Tack BF. Structure of the murine complement factor H gene. J Biol Chem 1988; 263:16720–16724.

26. Leonard WJ, Depper JM. Kanehisa M, Kronke M, Peffer NJ, Stevlik PB, Sullivan M, Greene WC. Structure of the human interleukin-2 receptor gene. Science 1985; 230:633–639.

27. Barnum SR, Kristensen T, Chaplin DD, Seldin MF, Tack BF. Molecular analysis of the murine C4b-bp protein gene: chromosome assignment and partial gene organization. Biochemistry 1989; 28:8312–8317.

28. Moffat GJ, Vik DP, Noack D, Tack BF. Complete structure of the murine C4b-binding protein gene and regulation of its expression by dexamethasome. J Biol Chem 1992; 267:20400–20406.

29. Rodriguez de Cordoba S, Sanchez-Corral P, Rey-Campos J. Structure of the gene coding for the α polypeptide chain of the human complement component C4b-binding protein. J Exp Med 1991; 173:1073–1082.

30. Hillarp A, Pardo-Manuel F, Ruiz RR, Rodriguez de Cordoba S, Dahlback B. The human C4b-binding protein β-chain gene. J Biol Chem 1993; 268:15017–15023.

31. Post TW, Arce MA, Liszewski MK, Thompson ES, Atkinson JP, Lublin DM. Structure of the gene for human complement protein decay accelerating factor. J Immunol 1990; 144:740–744.

32. Paul MS, Aegerter M, Cepek K, Miller MD, Weis JH. The murine complement receptor gene family. III. The genomic and transcriptional complexity of the Crry and Crry-ps genes. J Immunol 1990; 144:1988–1996.

33. Kemler I, Schaffner W. Octamer transcription factors and the cell-type specificity of immunoglobulin gene expression. FASEB J 1990; 4:1444–1449.

34. Finn PW, Kara CJ, Van TT, Douhan J, Boothby MR, Glimcher LH. The presence of a DNA binding complex correlates with Eβ class II MHC gene expression. EMBO J 1990; 9:1543–1549.

35. Wong WW, Klickstein LB, Smith JA, Weis JH, Fearon DT. Identification of a partial cDNA clone for the human receptor for complement fragment C3b/C4b. Proc Natl Acad Sci USA 1985; 82:7711–7715.

36. Wong WW, Farrell SA. Proposed structure of the F' allotype of human CR1. Loss of a C3b binding site may be associated with altered function. J Immunol 1991; 146:656–662.

37. Wilson JG, Wong WW, Schur PH, Fearon DT. Mode of inheritance of decreased C3b receptors on erythrocytes of patients with systemic lupus erythematosus. N Engl J Med 1982; 307:981–986.

38. Wilson JG, Murphy EE, Wong WW, Klickstein LB, Weis JH, Fearon DT. Identification of a restriction fragment length polymorphism by a CR1 cDNA that correlates with the number of CR1 on erythrocytes. J Exp Med 1986; 164:50–59.

39. Wong WW, Kennedy CA, Bonaccio ET, Wilson JG, Klickstein LB, Weis JH, Fearon DT. Anaylsis of multiple restriction fragment length polymorphisms of the gene for the human complement receptor type 1: duplication of genomic sequences occurs in association with a high molecular weight receptor allotype. J Exp Med 1986; 164:1531–1546.

40. Hourcade D, Miesner DR, Bee C, Zeldes W, Atkinson JP. Duplication and divergence of the amino-terminal coding region of the complement receptor 1 (CR1) gene. An example of concerted (horizontal) evolution within a gene. J Biol Chem 1990; 265:974–980.

41. Wong WW, Fearon DT. Human receptor for C3b/C4b: complement receptor type I. Meth Enzymol 1987; 150:579–585.

42. Klickstein LB, Bartow TJ, Miletic V, Rabson LD, Smith JA, Fearon DT. Identification of distinct C3b and C4b recognition sites in the human C3b/C4b receptor (CR1; CD35) by deletion mutagenesis. J Exp Med 1988; 168:1699–1717.

43. Hourcade D, Miesner DR, Atkinson JP, Holers VM. Identification of an alternative polyadenylation site in the human C3b/C4b receptor (complement receptor type 1) transcriptional unit and prediction of a secreted form of complement receptor type 1. J Exp Med 1988; 168:1255–1270.

44. Weisman HF, Bartow T, Leppo MK, Marsh HC, Carson GR, Concino MF, Boyle MP, Roux KH, Weisfeldt ML, Fearon DT. Soluble human complement receptor type 1: an in vivo inhibitor of complement suppressing post-ischemic myocardial inflammation and necrosis. Science 1990; 249:146–151.

45. Ahearn JM, Fearon DT. Structure and function of the complement receptors CR1 (CD35) and CR2 (CD21). Adv Immunol 1989; 46:183–219.

46. Sim RB. Large scale isolation of complement receptor type 1 (CR1) from human erythrocytes. Proteolytic fragmentation studies. Biochem J 1985; 232:883–889.

47. Lublin DM, Griffith RC, Atkinson JP. Influence of glycosylation on allelic and cell-specific Mr variation, receptor processing and ligand binding of the human complement C3b/C4b receptor. J Biol Chem 1986; 261:5736–5744.

48. Yoon SH, Fearon DT. Characterization of a soluble form of the C3b/C4b receptor (CR1) in human plasma. J Immunol 1985; 134:3332–3338.

49. Pascual M, Duchosal MA, Steiger G, Giostra E, Pechere A, Paccaud J-P. Danielsson C, Schifferli JA. Circulating soluble CR1 (CD35): serum levels in diseases and evidence for its release by human leukocytes. J Immunol 1993; 151:1702–1711.

50. Changelian PS, Jack RM, Collins LA, Fearon DT. PMA induces the ligand-independent internalization of CR1 on human neutrophils. J Immunol 1985; 134:1851–1858.

51. Krych M, Hourcade D, Atkinson JP. Sites within the complement C3b/C4b receptor important for the specificity of ligand binding. Proc Natl Acad Sci USA 1991; 88:4353–4357.

52. Krych M, Clemenza L, Howdeshell D, Hauhart R, Hourcade D, Atkinson JP. Analysis of the functional domains of complement receptor type 1 (C3b/C4b receptor; CD35) by substitution mutagenesis. J Biol Chem 1994; 269:13273–13278.

53. Kalli KR, Hsu P, Bartow TJ, Ahearn JM, Matsumoto AK, Klickstein LB, Fearon DT. Mapping of the C3b-binding site of CR1 and construction of a $(CR1)_2$-F(ab')$_2$ chimeric complement inhibitor. J Exp Med 1991; 174:1451–1460.

54. Seya T, Holers VM, Atkinson JP. Purification and functional analysis of the polymorphic variants of the C3b/C4b receptor (CR1) and comparison with H, C4-binding protein (C4bp), and decay accelerating factor (DAF). J Immunol 1985; 135:2661–2667.

55. Makrides SC, Scesney SM, Ford PJ, Evans KS, Carson GR, Marsh HC. Cell surface expression of the C3b/C4b receptor (CR1) protects Chinese hamster ovary cells from lysis by human complement. J Biol Chem 1992; 267:24754–24761.

56. Reilly BD, Makrides SC, Ford PJ, Marsh HC, Mold C. Quantitative analysis of C4b dimer binding to distinct sites on the C3b/C4b receptor (CR1). J Biol Chem 1994; 269:7696–7701.

57. Subramanian VB, Clemenza L, Krych M, Atkinson JP. Substitution of two amino acids confers C3b binding to the C4b binding site of CR1 (CD35): analysis based on ligand binding by chimpanzee erythrocyte complement receptor. J Immunol 1996; 157:1242–1247.

58. Taniguchi-Sidle A, Isenman DE. Interactions of human complement component C3 with Factor B and with complement receptors type 1 (CR1,CD35) and type 3 (CR3,CD11b/CD18) involve an acidic sequence at the N-terminus of C3 α'-chain. J Immunol 1994; 153:5285–5302.

59. Martin DR, Yuryev A, Kalli KR, Fearon DT, Ahearn JM. Determination of the structural basis for selective binding of Epstein-Barr virus to human complement receptor type 2. J Exp Med 1991; 174:1299–1311.

60. Ross GD, Polley MJ, Rabellino EM, Grey HM. Two different complement receptors on human lymphocytes. One specific for C3b and one specific for C3b inactivator-cleaved C3b. J Exp Med 1973; 138:798–811.

61. Eden A, Miller GW, Nussenzweig V. Human lymphocytes bear membrane receptors for C3b and C3d. J Clin Invest 1973; 52:3239–3242.

62. Bhan AK, Nadler LM, Stashenko P, McCluskey RT, Schlossman SF. Stages of B cell differentiation in human lymphoid tissue. J Exp Med 1981; 154:737–749.

63. Nadler LM, Stashenko P, Hardy R, van Agthoven A, Terhorst C, Schlossman SF. Characterization of a human B cell-specific antigen (B2) distinct from B1. J Immunol 1981; 126:1941–1947.

64. Iida K, Nadler L, Nussenzweig V. Identification of the membrane receptor for the complement fragment C3d by means of a monoclonal antibody. J Exp Med 1983; 158:1021–1033.

65. Tedder TF, Clement LT, Cooper MD. Expression of C3d receptors during human B cell differentiation: immunofluorescence analysis with the HB-5 monoclonal antibody. J Immunol 1984; 133:678–683.

66. Weis JJ, Tedder TF, Fearon DT. Identification of a 145,000 Mr membrane protein as the C3d receptor (CR2) of human B lymphocytes. Proc Natl Acad Sci USA 1984; 81:881–885.

67. Fingeroth JD, Clabby ML, Strominger JD. Characterization of a T-lymphocyte Epstein-Barr virus/C3d receptor (CD21). J Virol 1988; 62:1442–1447.

68. Delibrias C-C, Fischer E, Bismuth G, and Kaga-Tilikine MD. Expression, molecular association, and functions of C3 complement receptors CR1 (CD35) and CR2 (CD21) on the human T cell line NHPB-ALL. J Immunol 1992; 149:768–774.

69. Tsoukas CD, Lambris JD. Expression of EBV/C3d receptors on T cells: biological significance. Immunol Today 1993; 14:56–59.

70. Sinha SK, Todd SC, Hedrick JA, Speiser CL, Lambris JD, Tsoukas. Characterization of the EBV/C3d receptor on the human Jurkat T cell line: evidence for a novel transcript. J Immunol 1993; 150:5311–5320.

71. Tsoukas CD, Lambris JD. Expression of CR2/EBV receptors on human thymocytes detected by monoclonal antibodies. Eur J Immunol 1988; 18:1299–1302.

72. Liu Y-J, Xu J, de Bouteiller O, Parham CL, Grouard G, Djossou O, de Saint-Vis B, Lebecque S, Banchereau J, Moore KW. Follicular dendritic cells specifically express the long CR2/CD21 isoform. J Exp Med 1997; 185:165–170.

73. Fischer E, Delibrias C, and Kazatchkine MD. Expression of CR2 (the C3dg/EBV receptor, CD21) on normal human peripheral blood T lymphocytes. J Immunol 1991; 146:865–869.

74. Weis JJ, Fearon DT, Klickstein LD, Wong WW, Richards SA, de Bruyn Kops A, Smith JA, Weis JH. Identification of a partial cDNA clone for the C3d/Epstein-Barr virus receptor of human B lymphocytes: homology with the receptor for fragments C3b and C4b of the third and fourth components of complement. Proc Natl Acad Sci 1986; 83:5639–5643.

75. Weis JJ, Toothaker LE, Smith JA, Weis JH, Fearon DT. Structure of the human B lymphocyte receptor for C3d and the Epstein-Barr virus and relatedness to other members of the family of C3/C4 binding proteins. J Exp Med 1988; 167:1047–1066.

76. Moore MD, Cooper NR, Tack BF, Nemerow GR. Molecular cloning of the cDNA encoding the Epstein-Barr virus/C3d receptor (complement receptor type 2) of human B lymphocytes. Proc Natl Acad Sci USA 1987; 84:9194–9198.

77. Mold C, Cooper NR, Nemerow GR. Incorporation of the purified Epstein Barr virus/C3d receptor (CR2) into liposomes and demonstration of its dual ligand binding functions. J Immunol 1986; 136:4140–4145.

78. Ross GD, Polley MJ. Specificity of human lymphocyte complement receptors. J Exp Med 1975; 141:1163–1180.

79. Lambris JD, Dobson NJ, Ross GD. Isolation of lymphocyte membrane complement receptor type two (the C3d receptor) and preparation of receptor-specific antibody. Proc Natl Acad Sci USA 1981; 78:1828–1832.

80. Frade R, Myones BL, Barel M, Krikorian L, Charriaut C, Ross GD. Gp140, a C3b-binding membrane component of lymphocytes, is the B cell C3dg/C3d receptor (CR2) and is distinct from the neutrophil C3dg receptor (CR4). Eur J Immunol 1985; 15:1192–1197.

81. Mitomo K, Fujita T, Iida K. Functional and antigenic properties of complement receptor type 2, CR2. J Exp Med 1987; 165:1424–1429.

82. Weis JJ, Richards SA, Smith JA, Fearon DT. Purification of the B lymphocyte receptor for the C3d fragment of complement and the Epstein-Barr virus by monoclonal antibody affinity chromatography, and assessment of its functional capacities. J Immunol Methods 1986; 92:79–87.

83. Mold C, Nemerow GR, Bradt BM, Cooper NR. CR2 is a complement activator and the covalent binding site for C3 during alternative pathway activation by Raji cells. J Immunol 1988; 140:1923–1929.

84. Marquart HV, Svehag S-E, Leslie RGQ. CR2 is the primary acceptor site for C3 during alternative pathway activation of complement on human peripheral B lymphocytes. J Immunol 1994; 153:307–315.

85. Jondal M, Klein G. Surface markers on human B and T lymphocytes. II. Presence of Epstein-Barr virus receptors on B lymphocytes. J Exp Med 1973; 138:1365–1378.

86. Frade R, Barel M, Ehlin-Henriksson B, Klein G. gp140, the C3d receptor of human B lymphocytes, is also the Epstein-Barr virus receptor. Proc Natl Acad Sci USA 1985; 82:1490–1493.

87. Fingeroth JD, Weiss JJ, Tedder TF, Strominger JL, Biro PA, Fearon DT. Epstein-Barr virus receptor of human B lymphocytes is the C3d receptor CR2. Proc Natl Acad Sci USA 1984; 81:4510–4514.

88. Aubry J-P, Pochon S, Graber P, Jansen KU, Bonnefoy J-Y. CD21 is a ligand for CD23 and regulates IgE production. Nature 1992; 358:505–507.

89. Aubry J-P, Pochon S, Gauchat J-F, Nueda-Marin A, Holers VM, Graber P, Siegfried C, Bonnefoy J-Y. CD23 interacts with a new functional extracytoplasmic domain involving N-linked oligosaccharides on CD21. J Immunol 1994; 152:5806–5813.

90. Bonnefoy J-Y, Henchoz S, Hardie D, Holder MJ, Gordon J. A subset of anti-CD21 antibodies promote the rescue of germinal center B cells from apoptosis. Eur J Immunol 1993; 23:969–972.

91. Delcayre AX, Salas F, Mathur S, Kovats K, Lotz M, Lernhardt W. Epstein Barr virus/complement C3d receptor is an interferon α receptor. EMBO J 1991; 10:919–926.

92. Yang L, Behrens M, Weis JJ. Identification of 5′-regions affecting the expression of the human CR2 gene. J Immunol 1991; 147:2404–2410.

93. Molina H, Kinoshita T, Inoue K, Carel J-C, Holers VM. A molecular and immunochemical characterization of mouse CR2. Evidence for a single gene model of mouse complement receptors 1 and 2. J Immunol 1990; 145:2974–2983.

94. Kurtz CB, O'Toole E, Christensen SM, Weis JH. The murine complement receptor gene family. IV. Alternative splicing of Cr2 gene transcripts predicts two distinct gene products that share homologous domains with both human CR2 and CR1. J Immunol 1990; 144:3581–3591.

95. Holguin MH, Kurtz CB, Parker CJ, Weis JJ, Weis JH. Loss of human CR1- and murine crry-like exons in human CR2 transcripts due to CR2 gene mutations. J Immunol 1990; 145:1776–1781.

96. Rayhel EJ, Dehoff MH, Holers VM. Characterization of the human complement receptor 2 (CR2, CD21) promoter reveals sequences shared with regulatory regions of other developmentally restricted B cell proteins. J Immunol 1991; 146:2021–2026.

97. Toothaker LE, Henjes AJ, Weis JJ. Variability of CR2 gene products is due to alternative exon usage and different CR2 alleles. J Immunol 1989; 142:3668–3675.

98. Kalli KR, Ahearn JM, Fearon DT. Interaction of iC3b with recombinant isotypic and chimeric forms of CR2. J Immunol 1991; 147:590–594.

99. Changelian PS, Feaon DT. Tissue-specific phosphorylation of complement receptors CR1 and CR2. J Exp Med 1986; 163:101–115.

100. Weis JJ, Fearon DT. The identification of N-linked oligosaccharides on the human CR2/Epstein-Barr virus receptor and their function in receptor metabolism, plasma membrane expression, and ligand binding. J Biol Chem 1985; 260:13824–13830.

101. Myones BL, Pross GD. Identification of a spontaneously shed fragment of B cell complement receptor type two (CR₂) containing the C3d-binding site. Complement 1987; 4:87–98.

102. Fremeaux-Bacchi V, Bernard I, Maillet F, Mani J-C, Fontaine M, Bonnefoy J-Y, Kazatchkine MD, Fischer E. Human lymphocytes shed a soluble form of CD21 (the C3dg/Epstein-Barr virus receptor, CR2) that binds iC3b and CD23. Eur J Immunol 1996; 26:1497–1503.

103. Moore MD, DiScipio RG, Cooper NR, Nemerow GR. Hydrodynamic, electon microscopic, and ligand-binding analysis of the Epstein-Barr virus/C3dg receptor (CR2). J Biol Chem 1989; 264:20576–20582.

104. Lowell CA, Klickstein LB, Carter RH, Mitchell JA, Fearon DT, Ahearn JM. Mapping of the Epstein-Barr virus and C3dg binding sites to a common damain on complement receptor type 2. J Exp Med 1989; 170:1931–1946.

105. Carel J-C, Myones BL, Frazier B, Holers VM. Structural requirements for C3d,g/Epstein-Barr virus receptor (CR2/CD21) ligand binding, internalization, and viral infection. J Biol Chem 1990; 265:12293–12299.

106. Tanner J, Weis J, Fearon D, Whang Y, Kieff E. Epstein-Barr virus gp350/220 binding to the B lymphocyte C3d receptor mediates adsorption, capping, and endocytosis. Cell 1987; 50:203–213.

107. Nemerow GR, Mold C, Schwend VK, Tollefson V, Cooper NR. Identification of gp350 as the viral glycoprotein mediating attachment of Epstein-Barr virus (EBV) to the EBV/C3d receptor of B cells: Sequence homology of gp350 and C3 complement fragment C3d. J Virol 1987; 61:1416–1420.

108. Lambris JD, Ganu VS, Hirani S, Muller-Eberhard HJ. Mapping of the C3d receptor (CR2) binding site and a neoantigenic site in the C3d domain of the third component of complement. Proc Natl Acad Sci USA 1985; 82:4235–4239.

109. Nemerow GR, Houghten RA, Moore MD, Cooper NR. Identification of an epitope in the major envelope protein of Epstein-Barr virus that mediates viral binding to the B lymphocyte EBV receptor (CR2). Cell 1989; 56:369–377.

110. Esparza I, Becherer JD, Alsenz J, De la Hera A, Lao Z, Tsoukas CD, Lambris JD. Evidence for multiple sites of interaction in C3 for complement receptor type 2 (C3d/EBV receptor, CD21). Eur J Immunol 1991; 21:2829–2838.

111. Diefenbach RJ, Isenman. Mutation of residues in the C3dg region of human complement component C3 corresponding to a proposed binding site for complement receptor type 2 (CR2, CD21) does not abolish binding of iC3b or C3dg to CR2. J Immunol 1995; 154:2303–2320.

112. Moore MD, Cannon MJ, Sewall A, Finlayson M, Okimoto M, Nemerow GR. Inhibition of Epstein-Barr virus infection in vitro and in vivo by soluble CR2 (CD21) containing two short consensus repeats. J Virol 1991; 65:3559–3565.

113. Hebell T, Ahearn JM, Fearon DT. Suppression of the immune response by a soluble complement receptor of B lymphocytes. Science 1991; 254:102–105.

114. Nemerow GR, Mullen JJ, Dickson PW, Cooper NR. Soluble recombinant CR2 (CD21) inhibits Epstein-Barr virus infection. J Virol 1990; 64:1348–1352.

115. Matsumoto AK, Kopicky-Burd J, Carter RH, Tuveson DA, Tedder TF, Fearon DT. Intersection of the complement and immune systems: a signal transduction complex of the B lymphocyte-containing complement receptor type 2 and CD19. J Exp Med 1991; 173:55–64.

116. Matsumoto AK, Martin DR, Carter RH, Klickstein LB, Ahearn JM, Fearon DT. Functional dissection of the CD21/CD19/TAPA-1/Leu-13 complex of B lymphocytes. J Exp Med 1993; 178:1407–1417.

117. Tuveson DA, Ahearn JM, Matsumoto AK, Fearon DT. Molecular interactions of complement receptors on B lymphocytes: A CR1/CR2 complex distinct from the CR2/CD19 complex. J Exp Med 1991; 173:1083–1089.

118. Prodinger WM, Larcher C, Schwendinger M, Dierich MP. Ligation of the functional domain of complement receptor type 2 (CR2, CD21) is relevant for complex formation in T cell lines. J Immunol 1996; 156:2580–2584.

119. Rao PE, Wright SD, Westberg EF, Goldstein G. OKB7, a monoclonal antibody that reacts at or near the C3d binding site of human CR2. Cell Immunol 1985; 93:549–555.

120. Nemerow GR, Wolfert R, McNaughton ME, Cooper NR. Identification and characterization of the EBV receptor on human B lymphocytes and its relationship to the C3d receptor (CR2). J Virol 1985; 55:347–351.

121. Petzer AL, Schulz TF, Stauder R, Eigentler A, Myones B, Dierich. Structural and functional analysis of CR2/EBV receptor by means of monoclonal antibodies and limited tryptic digestion. Immunology 1988; 63:47–53.

122. Barel M, Fiandino A, Delcayre AX, Lyamani F, Frade R. Monoclonal and anti-idiotypic anti-EBV/C3d receptor antibodies detect two binding sites, one for EBV and one for C3d on glycoprotein 140, the EBV/C3dR, expressed on human B lymphocytes. J Immunol 1988; 141:1590–1595.

123. Molina H, Kinoshita T, Inoue K, Carel, J-C, Holers VM. A molecular and immunochemical characterization of mouse CR2. J Immunol 1990; 145:2974–2983.

124. Molina H, Brenner C, Jacobi S, Gorka J, Carel J-C, Kinoshita T Holers VM. Analysis of Epstein-Barr virus-binding sites on complement receptor 2 (CR2/CD21) using human-mouse chimeras and peptides. J Biol Chem 1991; 266:12173–12179.

125. Kinoshita T, Thyphronitis G, Tsokos GC, Finkelman FD, Hoag K, Sakai H, Inoue K. Characterization of murine complement receptor type 2 and its immunological cross-reactivity with type 1 receptor. Int Immunol 1990; 2:651–659.

126. Martin DR, Marlowe RL, Ahearn JM. Determination of the role for CD21 during Epstein-Barr virus infection of B-lymphoblastoid cells. J Virol 1994; 68:4716–4726.

127. Norman DG, Barlow PN, Baron M, Day AJ, Sim RB, Campbell ID. Three-dimensional structure of a complement control protein module in solution. J. Mol. Biol. 1991; 219:717–725.

128. Barlow PJ, Norman DG, Steinkasserer A, Horne TJ, Pearce J, Driscoll PC, Sim RB, Campbell ID. Solution structure of the fifth repeat of factor H: a second example of the complement control protein module. Biochemistry 1992; 31:3626–3634.

129. Barlow PN, Steinkasserer A, Norman DG, Kieffer B, Wiles AP, Sim RB, Campbell ID. Solution structure of a pair of complement modules by nuclear magnetic resonance. J Mol Biol 1993; 232:268–284.

130. Wiles A, Shaw G, Bright J, Perczel A, Campbell ID, Barlow PN. NMR studies of a viral protein that mimics the regulators of complement activation. J Mol Biol (In press).

131. Ahearn JM, Hayward SD, Hickey JC, Fearon DT. Epstein-Barr virus (EBV) infection of murine L cells expressing receombinant human EBV/C3d receptor. Proc Natl Acad Sci USA 1988; 85:9307–9311.

132. Springer T, Galfre G, Secher DS, Milstein C. Mac-1: a macrophage differentiation antigen identified by monoclonal antibody. Eur J Immunol 1979; 9:301–306.

133. Arnaout MA, Spits H, Terhorst C, Pitt J, Todd RF III. Deficiency of a leukocyte surface glycoprotein (LFA-1) in two patients with Mo1 deficiency. Effects of cell activation on Mo1/LFA-1 surface expression in normal and deficient leukocytes. J Clin Invest 1984; 74:1291–1300.

134. Miller LJ, Schwarting R, Springer TA. Regulated expression of the Mac-1, LFA-1, p150,95 glycoprotein family during leukocyte differentiation. J Immunol 1986; 137:2891–2900.

135. Freyer DR, Morganroth ML, Rogers CE, Arnaout MA, Todd RF III. Regulation of surface glycoproteins CD11/CD18 (Mo1, LFA-1, p150,95) by human mononuclear phagocytes. Clin Immunol Immunopathol 1988; 46:272–283.

136. Beller DI, Springer TA, Schreiber RD. Anti-Mac-1 selectively inhibits the mouse and human type three complement receptor. J Exp Med 1982; 156:1000–1009.

137. Arnaout MA, Todd RF, Dana N, Melamed J, Schlossman SF, Colten HR. Inhibition of phagocytosis of complement C3- or immunoglobulin G-coated particles and of C3bi binding by monoclonal antibodies to a monocyte-granulocyte membrane glycoprotein (Mo1). J Clin Invest 1983; 72:171–179.

138. Micklem KJ, Sim RB. Isolation of complement-fragment-iC3b-binding proteins by affinity chromatography. Biochem J 1985; 231:233–236.

139. Altieri DC, Edgington TS. The saturable high affinity association of factor X to ADP-stimulated monocytes defines a novel function of the Mac-1 receptor. J Biol Chem 1988; 263:7007–7015.

140. Wright SD, Weitz JI, Huang AJ, Levin SM, Silverstein SC, Loike JD. Complement receptor type three (CD11b/CD18) of human polymorphonuclear leukocytes recognizes fibrinogen. Proc Natl Acad Sci USA 1988; 85:7734–7738.

141. Altieri DC, Bader R, Mannucci PM, Edgington TS. Oligospecificity of the cellular adhesion receptor MAC-1 encompasses an inducible recognition specificity for fibrinogen. J Cell Biol 1988; 107:1893–1900.

142. Trezzini C, Jungi TW, Kuhnert P, Peterhans E. Fibrinogen association with human monocytes: evidence for constitutive expression of fibrinogen receptors and for involvement of Mac-1 (CD18, CR3) in the binding. Biochem Biophys Res Commun 1988; 156:477–484.

143. Wright SD, Jong MTC. Adhesion-promoting receptors on human macrophages recognize *Escherichia coli* by binding to lipopolysaccharide. J Exp Med 1986; 164:1876–1888.

144. Ross GD, Cain JA, Lachmann PJ. Membrane complement receptor type three (CR$_3$) has lectin-like properties analogous to bovine conglutinin and functions as a receptor for zymosan and rabbit erythrocytes as well as a receptor for iC3b. J Immunol 1985; 134:3307–3315.

145. Galon J, Gauchat J-F, Mazieres N, Spagnoli R, Storkus W, Lotze M, Bonnefoy J-Y, Fridman W-H, Sautes C. Soluble Fcγ receptor type III (FcγRIII,CD16) triggers cell activation through interaction with complement receptors. J Immunol 1996; 157:1184–1192.

146. Smith CW, Marlin SD, Rothlein R, Toman C, Anderson DC. Cooperative interactions of LFA-1 and Mac-1 with intercellular adhesion molecule-1 in facilitating adherence and transendothelial migration of human neutrophils in vitro. J Clin Invest 1989; 83:2008–2017.

147. Diamond MS, Staunton DE, de Fougerolles AR, Stacker SA, Garcia-Aguilar J, Hibbs ML, Springer TA. ICAM-1 (CD54): A counter-receptor for Mac-1 (CD11b/CD18). J Cell Biol 1990; 111:3129–3139.

148. Relman D, Tuomanen E, Falkow S, Golenbock DT, Saukkonen K, Wright SD. Recognition of a bacterial adhesin by an integrin: macrophage CR3 ($\alpha_M\beta_2$, CD11b/CD18) binds filamentous hemagglutinin of Bordetella pertussis. Cell 1990; 61:1375–1382.

149. Russell DG, Wright SD. Complement receptor type 3 (CR3) binds to an Arg-Gly-Asp-containing region of the major surface glycoprotein, gp63, of *Leishmania promastigotes*. J Exp Med 168:279–292.

150. El Ghmati SM, Van Hoeyveld EM, Van Strijp JAG, Ceuppens JL, Stevens EAM. Identification of haptoglobin as an alternative ligand for CD11b/CD18. J Immunol 1996; 156:2542–2552.
151. Anderson DC, Miller LJ, Schmalstieg FC, Rothlein R, Springer TA. Contributions of the Mac-1 glycoprotein family to adherence-dependent granulocyte functions: structure-function assessments employing subunit-specific monoclonal antibodies. J Immunol 1986; 137:15–27.
152. Arnaout MA, Lanier LL, Faller DV. Relative contribution of the leukocyte molecules Mo1, LFA-1, and p150,95 (LeuM5) in adhesion of granulocytes and monocytes to vascular endothelium is tissue- and stimulus-specific. J Cell Physiol 1988; 137:305–309.
153. Lo SK, Van Seventer GA, Levin SM, Wright SD. Two leukocyte receptors (CD11a/CD18 and CD11b/CD18) mediate transient adhesion to endothelium by binding to different ligands. J Immunol 1989; 143:3325–3329.
154. Ezekowitz RAB, Sim RB, Hill M, Gordon S. Local opsonization by secreted macrophage complement components. J Exp Med 1983; 159:244–260.
155. Ramos OF, Kai C, Yefenof E, Klein E. The elevated natural killer sensitivity of targets carrying surface-attached C3 fragments require the availability of the iC3b receptor (CR3) on the effectors. J Immunol 1988; 140:1239–1243.
156. Corbi AL, Larson RS, Kishimoto TK, Springer TA, Morton CC. Chromosomal location of the genes encoding the leukocyte adhesion receptors LFA-1, Mac-1, and p150,95. Identification of a gene cluster involved in cell adhesion. J Exp Med 1988; 167:1597–1607.
157. Arnaout MA, Remold-O'Donnell E, Pierce MW, Harris P, Tenen DG. Molecular cloning of the α subunit of human and guinea pig leukocyte adhesion glycoprotein Mo1: chromosomal localization and homology to the α subunits of integrins. Proc Natl Acad Sci USA 1988; 85:2776–2780.
158. Fleming JC, Pahl HL, Gonzalez DA, Smith TF, Tenen. Structural analysis of the *CD11b* gene and phylogenetic analysis of the α-integrin gene family demonstrate remarkable conservation of genomic organization and suggest early diversification during evolution. J Immunol 1993; 150:480–490.
159. Corbi AL, Garcia-Aguilar J, Springer TA. Genomic structure of an integrin α subunit, the leukocyte p150,95 molecule. J Biol Chem 1990; 265:2782–2788.
160. Pahl HL, Rosmarin AR, Tenen DG. Characterization of the myeloid-specific CD11b promoter. Blood 1992; 79:865–870.
161. Marlin SD, Morton CC, Anderson DC, Springer TA. LFA-1 Immunodeficiency disease: definition of the genetic defect and chromosomal mapping of alpha and beta subunits of the lymphocyte function-associated antigen 1 (LFA-1) by complementation in hybrid cells. J Exp Med 1986; 164:855–867.
162. Kishimoto TK, O'Connor K, Lee A, Roberts TM, Springer TA. Cloning of the β subunit of the leukocyte adhesion proteins: homology to an extracellular matrix receptor defines a novel supergene family. Cell 1987; 48:681–690.
163. Arnaout MA, Gupta SK, Pierce MW, Tenen DG. Amino acid sequence of the alpha subunit of human leukocyte adhesion receptor Mo1 (complement receptor type 3). J Cell Biol 1988; 106:2153–2158.
164. Corbi AL, Kishimoto TK, Miller LJ, Springer TA. The human leukocyte adhesion glycoprotein Mac-1 (complement receptor type 3, CD11b) α subunit. Cloning, primary structure, and relation to the integrins, von Willebrand factor and factor B. J Biol Chem 1988; 263:12403–12411.
165. Hickstein DD, Hickey MJ, Ozols J, Baker DNM, Back AL, Roth GJ. cDNA sequence for the αM subunit of the human neutrophil adherence receptor indicates homology to integrin α subunits. Proc Natl Acad Sci USA 1989; 86:257–261.
166. Chatila TA, Geha RS, Arnaout MA. Constitutive and stimulus-induced phosphorylation of CD11/CD18 leukocyte adhesion molecules. J Cell Biol 1989; 109:3435–3444.
167. Buyon JP, Slade SG, Reibman J, Abramson SB, Philips MR, Weissmann G, Winchester R. Constitutive and induced phosphorylation of the α-and β-chains of the CD11/CD18 leukocyte integrin family. Relationship to adhesion-dependent functions. J Immunol 1990; 144:191–197.

168. Miller LJ, Springer TA. Biosynthesis and glycosylation of p150,95 and related leukocyte adhesion proteins. J Immunol 1987; 139:842–847.

169. Poncz M, Eisman R, Heidenreich R, Silver SM, Vilaire G, Surrey S, Schwartz E, Bennett. Structure of the platelet membrane glycoprotein IIb. J Biol Chem 1987; 262:8476–8482.

170. Suzuki S, Argraves WS, Arai H, Languino LR, Pierschbacher MD, Ruoslahti E. Amino acid sequence of the vitronectin receptor α subunit and comparative expression of adhesion receptor mRNAs. J Biol Chem 1987; 262:14080–14085.

171. Argraves WS, Suzuki, S, Arai H, Thompson K, Pierschbacher MD, Ruoslahti E. Amino acid sequence of the human fibronectin receptor. J Cell Biol 1987; 105:1183–1190.

172. Corbi AL, Miller LJ, O'Connor K, Larson RS, Springer TA. cDNA cloning and complete primary structure of the α subunit of a leukocyte adhesion glycoprotein, p150,95. EMBO J 1987; 6:4023–4028.

173. Russ GR, Haddad AP, Tait BD, d'Apice JF. Polymorphism of the complement receptor for C3bi. J Clin Invest 1985; 76:1965–1970.

174. Law SKA, Gagnon J, Hildreth JEK, Wells CE, Willis AC, Wong AJ. The primary structure of the β-subunit of the cell surface adhesion glycoproteins LFA-1, CR3 and p150,95 and its relationship to the fibronectin receptor. EMBO J 1987; 6:915–919.

175. Dahms NM, Hart GW. Influence of quaternary structure on glycosylation. J Biol Chem 1986; 261:13186–13196.

176. Marlin SD, Springer TA. Purified intercellular adhesion molecule-1 (ICAM-1) is a ligand for lymphocyte function-associated antigen 1 (LFA-1). Cell 1987; 51:813–819.

177. Simmons D, Makgoba MW, Seed B. ICAM1, an adhesion ligand of LFA-1, is homologous to the neural cell adhesion molecule NCAM. Nature 1988; 331:624–627.

178. Staunton DE, Marlin SD, Stratowa C, Dustin ML, Springer TA. Primary structure of intercellular adhesion molecule 1 (ICAM-1) demonstrates interaction between members of the immunoglobulin and integrin supergene families. Cell 1988; 52:925–933.

179. Staunton DE, Dustin ML, Erickson HP, Springer TA. The arrangement of the immunoglobulin-like domains of ICAM-1 and the binding site for LFA-1 and rhinovirus. Cell 1990; 61:243–254.

180. Diamond MS, Staunton DE, Marlin SD, Springer TA. Binding of the integrin Mac-1 (CD11b/CD18) to the third immunoglobulin-like domain of ICAM-1 (CD54) and its regulation by glycosylation. Cell 1991; 65:961–971.

181. Wright SD, Rao PE, Van Voorhis WC, Craigmyle LS, Iida K, Talle MA, Westberg EF, Goldstein G, Silverstein SC. Identification of the C3bi receptor of human monocytes and macrophages by using monoclonal antibodies. Proc Natl Acad Sci USA 1983; 80:5699–5703.

182. Wright SD, Reddy PA, Jong MTC, Erickson BW. C3bi receptor (complement receptor type 3) recognizes a region of complement protein C3 containing the sequence Arg-Gly-Asp. Proc Natl Acad Sci USA 1987; 84:1965–1968.

183. Van Strijp JAG, Russell DG, Tuomanen E, Brown EJ, Wright SD. Ligand specificity of purified complement receptor type three (CD11b/CD18, $\alpha_M\beta_2$,Mac-1). Indirect effects of an ARG-GLY-ASP (RGD) sequence. J Immunol 1993; 151:3324–3336.

184. Brown EJ, Goodwin JL. Fibronectin receptors of phagocytes. Characterization of the Arg-Gly-Asp binding proteins of human monocytes and polymorphonuclear leukocytes. J Exp Med 1988; 167:777–793.

185. Gresham HD, Goodwin JL, Allen PM, Anderson DC, Brown EJ. A novel member of the integrin receptor family mediates Arg-Gly-Asp-stimulated neutrophil phagocytosis. J Cell Biol 1989; 108:1935–1943.

186. Taniguchi-Sidle A, Isenman DE. Mutagenesis of the Arg-Gly-Asp triplet in human complement component C3 does not abolish binding of iC3b to the leukocyte integrin complement receptor type III (CR3, CD11b/CD18). J Biol Chem 1992; 267:635–643.

187. Altieri DC, Agbanyo FR, Plescia J, Ginsberg MH, Edgington TS, Plow EF. A unique recognition site mediates the interaction of fibrinogen with the leukocyte integrin Mac-1 (CD11b/CD18). J Biol Chem 1990; 265:12119–12122.

188. Diamond MA, Garcia-Aguilar J, Bickford JK, Corbi AL, Springer TA. The I domain is a major recognition site on the leukocyte integrin Mac-1 (CD11b/CD18) for four distinct adhesion ligands. J Cell Biol 1993; 120:1031–1043.

189. Stockl J, Majdic O, Pickl WF, Rosenkranz A, Prager E, Gschwantler E, Knapp W. Granulocyte activation via a binding site near the C-terminal region of complement receptor type 3 α-chain (CD11b) potentially involved in intramembrane complex formation with glycosylphosphatidylinositol-anchored FcγRIIIB (CD16) molecules. J Immunol 1995; 154:5452–5463.

190. Altieri DC, Edgington. A monoclonal antibody reacting with distinct adhesion molecules defines a transition in the functional state of the receptor CD11b/CD18 (Mac-1). J Immunol 1988; 141:2656–2660.

191. Buyon JP, Abramson SB, Philips MR, Slade SG, Ross GD, Weissman G, Winchester RJ. Dissociation between increased surface expression of Gp165/95 and homotypic neutrophil aggregation. J Immunol 1988; 140:3156–3160.

192. Diamond MS, Springer TA. A subpopulation of Mac-1 (CD11b/CD18) molecules mediates neutrophil adhesion to ICAM-1 and fibrinogen. J Cell Biol 1993; 120:545–556.

193. Wright SD, Levin SM, Jong MTC, Chad Z, Kabbash LG. CR3 (CD11b/CD18) expresses one binding site for Arg-Gly-Asp-containing peptides and a second site for bacterial lipopolysaccharide. J Exp Med 1989; 169:175–183.

194. Thornton BP, Vetvicka V, Pitman M, Goldman RC, Ross GD. Analysis of the sugar specificity and molecular location of the β-glucan-binding lectin site of complement receptor type 3 (CD11b/CD18). J Immunol 1996; 156:1235–1246.

195. Larson RS, Springer TA. Structure and function of leukocyte integrins. Immunol Rev 1990; 114:181–217.

196. Michishita M, Videm V, Arnaout MA. A novel divalent cation-binding site in the A domain of the β2 integrin CR3 (CD11b/CD18) is essential for ligand binding. Cell 1993; 72:857–867.

197. Perkins SJ, Smith KF, Williams SC, Haris PI, Chapman D, Sim RB. The secondary structure of the von Willebrand factor type A domain in factor B of human complement by Fourier transform infrared spectroscopy. Its occurrence in collagen types VI, VII, XII, and XIV, the integrins and other proteins by averaged structure predictions. J Mol Biol 1994; 238:104–119.

198. Lee J-O, Rieu P, Arnaout MA, Liddington R. Crystal structure of the A domain from the α subunit of integrin CR3 (CD11b/CD18). Cell 1995; 80:631–638.

199. Messika EJ, Avni O, Gallily R, Yefenof E, Baniyash M. Identification and characterization of a novel protein associated with macrophage complement receptor 3. J Immunol 1995; 154:6563–6570.

200. Zhou M-j, Todd RF, van de Winkel JGJ, Petty HR. Cocapping of the leukoadhesion molecules complement receptor type 3 and lymphocyte function-associated antigen-1 with Fcγ receptor III on human neutrophils. Possible role of lectin-like interactions. J Immunol 1993; 150:3030–3041.

201. Sanchez-Madrid, F, Nagy JA, Robbins E, Simon P, and Springer TA. A human leukocyte differentiation antigen family with distinct α-subunits and a common β-subunit: the lymphocyte-function associated antigen (LFA-1), the C3bi complement receptor (OKM1/Mac-1), and the p150,95 molecule. J Exp Med 1983; 158:1785–1803.

202. Lanier LL, Arnaout MA, Schwarting R, Warner NL, Ross GD. P150/95, third member of the LFA-1/CR₃ polypeptide family identified by anti-Leu M5 monoclonal antibody. Eur J Immunol 1985; 15:713–718.

203. Springer TA, Miller LJ, Anderson DC. P150,95, the third member of the MAC-1, LFA-1 human leukocyte adhesion glycoprotein family. J Immunol 1986; 136:240–245.

204. Freudenthal PS, Steinman RM. The distinct surface of human blood dendritic cells, as observed after an improved isolation method. Proc Natl Acad Sci USA 1990; 87:7698–7702.

205. Werfel T, Witter W, Gotze O. CD11b and CD11c antigens are rapidly increased on human natural killer cells upon activation. J Immunol 1991; 147:2423–2427.

206. Postigo AA, Corbi AL, Sanchez-Madrid F, de Landazuri MO. Regulated expression and function of CD11c/CD18 integrin on human B lymphocytes. Relation between attachment to fibrinogen and triggering of proliferation through CD11c/CD18. J Exp Med 1991; 174:1313–1322.

207. Keizer GD, Borst J, Visser W, Schwarting R, de Vries JE, Figdor CG. Membrane glycoprotein p150,95 of human cytotoxic T cell clones is involved in conjugate formation with target cells. J Immunol 1987; 138:3130–3136.

208. Vik DP, Fearon DT. Cellular distribution of complement receptor type 4 (CR4): expression on human platelets. J Immunol 1987; 138:254–258.

209. Schwarting R, Stein HH, Wang CY. The monoclonal antibodies αS-HCL 1 (αLeu-14) and αS-HCL 3 (αLeu-M5) allow the diagnosis of hairy cell leukemia. Blood 1985; 65:974–983.

210. De la Hera A, Alvarez-Mon M, Sanchez-Madrid F, Martinez-A C, Durantez A. Co-expression of Mac-1 and p150,95 on CD5+ B cells. Structural and functional characterization in human chronic lymphocytic leukemia. Eur J Immunol 1988; 18:1131–1134.

211. Hanson CA, Gribbin TE, Schnitzer B, Schlegelmilch JA, Mitchell BS, Stoolman LM. CD11c (LEU-M5) expression characterizes a B-cell chronic lymphoproliferative disorder with features of both chronic lymphocytic leukemia and hairy cell leukemia. Blood 1990; 76:2360–2367.

212. Loike JD, Sodeik B, Cao L, Leucona S, Weitz JI, Detmers PA, Wright SD, Silverstein SC. CD11c/CD18 on neutrophils recognizes a domain at the N terminus of the Aα chain of fibrinogen. Proc Natl Acad Sci USA 1991; 88:1044–1048.

213. Lecoanet-Henchoz S, Gauchat JF, Aubry JP, Graber P, Life P, Paul-Eugene N, Ferrua B, Corbi AL, Dugas B, Plater-Zyberk C, et al. CD23 regulates monocyte activation through a novel interaction with the adhesion molecules CD11b-CD18 and CD11c-CD18. Immunity 1995; 3:119–125.

214. Le Beau MM, Diaz MO, Karin M, Rowley JD. Metallothionein gene cluster is split by chromosome 16 rearrangements in myelomonocytic leukaemia. Nature (Lond) 1985; 313:709–711.

215. Rubin CM, Larson RA, Bitter MA, Carrino JJ, Le Beau MM, Diaz MO, Rowley JD. Association of a chromosomal 3;21 translocation with the blast phase of chronic myelogenous leukemia. Blood 1987; 70:1338–1342.

216. Lopez-Rodriguez C, Kluin-Nelemans HC, Corbi AL. AP-1 regulates the basal and developmentally induced transcription of the CD11c leukocyte integrin gene. J Immunol 1996; 156:3780–3787.

217. Lopez-Cabrera M, Nueda A, Vara A, Garcia-Aguilar J, Tugores A, Corbi AL. Characterization of the p150,95 leukocyte integrin α subunit (CD11c) gene promoter. J Biol Chem 1993; 268:1187–1193.

218. Smale ST, Baltimore D. The "initiator" as a transcription control element. Cell 1989; 57:103–113.

219. Noti JD, Reinemann BC, Petrus MN. Regulation of the leukocyte integrin gene CD11c is mediated by AP1 and Ets transcription factors. Mol Immunol 1996; 33:115–127.

220. Glass CK, Lipkin SM, Devary OV, Rosenfeld MG. Positive and negative regulation of gene transcription by a retinoic acid-thyroid hormone receptor heterodimer. Cell 1989; 59:697–708.

221. Lopez-Rodriguez C, Chen H-M, Tenen DG, Corbi AL. Identification of Sp-1 binding sites in the CD11c (p150,95α) and CD11a (LFA-1α) integrin subunit promoters and their involvement in the tissue-specific expression of CD11c. Eur J Immunol 1995; 25:3496–3503.

222. Noti JD, Reinemann BC, Petrus MN. Sp1 binds two sites in the CD11c promoter in vivo specifically in myeloid cells and cooperates with AP1 to activate transcription. Mol Cell Biol 1996; 16:2940–2950.

223. Szebenyi DME, Obendorf SK, Moffat K. Structure of vitamin D-dependent calcium-binding protein from bovine intestine. Nature 1981; 294:327–332.

224. Tufty RM, Kretsinger RH. Troponin and parvalbumin calcium binding regions predicted in myosin light chain and T4 lysozyme. Science 1975; 187:167–169.

225. Kretsinger RH, Nockolds CE. Carp muscle calcium-binding protein. II. Structure determination and general description. J Biol Chem 1973; 248:3313–3326.

226. Stacker ASA, Springer TA. Leukocyte integrin p150,95 (CD11c/CD18) functions as an adhesion molecule binding to a counter-receptor on stimulated endothelium. J Immunol 1991; 146:648–655.

227. Malhotra V, Hogg N, Sim RB. Ligand binding by the p150,95 antigen of U937 cells: properties in common with complement receptor type 3 (CR3). Eur J Immunol 1986; 16:1117–1123.

228. Myones BL, Dalzell JG, Hogg N, Ross GD. Neutrophil and monocyte cell surface p150,95 has iC3b-receptor (CR$_4$) activity resembling CR3. J Clin Invest 1988; 82:640–651.

229. Bilsland CAG, Diamond MS, Springer TA. The leukocyte integrin p150,95 (CD11c/CD18) as a receptor for iC3b. Activation by a heterologous β subunit and localization of a ligand recognition site to the I domain. J Immunol 1994 152:4582–4589.

230. Berton G, Laudanna C, Sorio C, Rossi F. Generation of signals activating neutrophil functions by leukocyte integrins: LFA-1 and gp150/95, but not CR3, are able to stimulate the respiratory burst of human neutrophils. J Cell Biol 1989; 109:1341–1349.

231. Bobak DA, Gaither TG, Frank MM, Tenner AJ. Modulation of FcR function by complement: subcomponent C1q enhances the phagocytosis of IgG-opsonized targets by human monocytes and culture-derived macrophages. J Immunol 1987; 138:1150–1156.

232. Bobak DA, Frank MM, Tenner AJ. C1q acts synergistically with phorbol dibutyrate to activate CR1-mediated phagocytosis by human mononuclear phagocytes. Eur J Immunol 1988; 18:2001–2007.

233. Tenner AJ, Robinson, SL, Borchelt J, Wright JR. Human pulmonary surfactant protein (SP-A), a protein structurally homologous to C1q, can enhance FcR- and CR1-mediated phagocytosis. J Biol Chem 1989; 264:13923–13928.

234. Tenner AJ, Robinson, SL, Ezekowitz RAB. Mannose binding protein (MBP) enhances mononuclear phagocyte function via a receptor that contains the 126,000 Mr component of the C1q receptor. Immunity 1995; 3:485–493.

235. Nepomuceno RR, Henschen-Edman AH, Burgess WNH, Tenner AJ. cDNA cloning and primary structure analysis of C1qR$_p$, the human C1q/MBL/SPA receptor that mediates enhanced phagocytosis in vitro. Immunity 1997; 6:119–129.

236. Guan E, Burgess WH, Robinson S, Goodman EB, McTigue KJ, Tenner AJ. Phagocytic cell molecules that bind the collagen-like region of C1q. J Biol Chem 1991; 266:20345–20355.

237. Guan E., Robinson SL, Goodman EB, Tenner AJ. Cell-surface protein identified on phagocytic cells modulates the C1q-mediated enhancement of phagocytosis. J Immunol 1994; 152:4005–4016.

238. Drickamer K. Two distinct classes of carbohydrate-recognition domains in animal lectins. J Biol Chem 1988: 263:9557–9560.

239. Drickamer K. Membrane receptors that mediate glycoprotein endocytosis: Structure and biosynthesis. Kidney Int 1987: 32:S167.

240. Ezekowitz RAB, Sastry K, Bailly P, Warner A. Molecular characterization of the human macrophage mannose receptor: demonstration of multiple carbohydrate recognition-like domains and phagocytosis of yeasts in cos-1 cells. J Exp Med 1990; 172:1785–1794.

241. Cooke RM, Wilkinson, AJ, Baron M, Pastore A, Tappin MJ, Campbell ID, Gregory H, Sheard B. The solution structure of human epidermal growth factor. Nature 1987; 327:339–341.

242. Rees DJG, Jones IM, Handford, PA, Walter, SJ, Esnouf MP, Smith, KJ, Brownlee GG. The role of β-hydroxyaspartate and adjacent carboxylate residues in the first EGF domain of human factor IX. EMBO J 1988: 7:2053–2061.

243. Rao Z, Handford P, Mayhew M, Knott V, Brownlee GG, Stuart D. The structure of a Ca^{2+}-binding epidermal growth factor-like domain: its role in protein–protein interactions. Cell 1995; 82:131–141.

9

Phylogeny of the Complement System

MASARU NONAKA

Nagoya City University Medical School, Nagoya, Japan

I. INTRODUCTION

Gene duplication and exon-shuffling appear to have been important in establishing the complement system in its present form in the mammalian species (1,2). Bf/C2, C1r/C1s are typical examples of gene duplication, which followed the development of the mosaic modular structure that resulted from exon shuffling. On the other hand, C6, C7, C8α, C8β, and C9 appear to have arisen from sequential addition/deletion of three different kinds of domains, indicating that alternate gene duplication and exon shuffling occurred frequently. Therefore, it appears that complement started as a simple system comprising a small number of components with restricted functions, and later developed further with the acquisition of new components through gene duplication and of new functions by modification of the gene duplication products by exon shuffling. Phylogenetic studies of the complement system have been carried out to address the following questions. At what point during evolution was the complement system established? What was the compositional makeup and function of the original complement system? Finally, how did the original complement system develop into the modern sophisticated system observed in mammalian species? Another interesting aspect of the mammalian complement system is the close linkage of the C4, Bf, and C2 genes within the class III region of the major histocompatibility complex (MHC) (3,4). Although the possible physiological significance of the linkage among these complement genes and their linkage to the MHC, is still not understood, one possible implication of the former linkage, especially that between the C4 and C2 genes, may be that it contributed to the evolution of the complement system and the establishment of the classical pathway. Phylogenetic studies of the origin of the classical pathway as well as the origin of linkage of these genes will contribute to verifying this hypothesis. Although definitive answers to the above questions are still forthcoming, recent contributions to our knowledge brought about by using molecular approaches to investigating complement phylogeny have made it possible to outline broadly the evolutionary history of the complement system. In this chapter, the molecular evolution of the complement system with emphasis on the central component C3 is discussed.

II. FUNCTIONAL ASPECTS

Complement-dependent hemolytic activity has been demonstrated in all jawed vertebrate classes (mammals, birds, reptiles, amphibians, bony fish, and cartilaginous fish), whereas its presence in jawless fish (cyclostomes; lamprey and hagfish) or invertebrates has not been demonstrated unambiguously in spite of many reports describing complement-like lytic activity in invertebrates (1). Intrinsic problems encountered in phylogenetic interpretation of hemolytic assays have been discussed (1). In contrast, complement-dependent opsonic activity, which is simpler to assess than hemolytic activity, has been identified not only in jawed vertebrates but also in the jawless fish, lamprey and hagfish (5,6). As described below, it is only recently that definitive evidence was reported demonstrating the presence of the C3 gene in invertebrates (7). The presence of a complement-dependent opsonic system, and a hemolytic system if any, in invertebrates remains to be demonstrated. Since strong evidence for complement-dependent hemolytic activity has only been reported for jawed vertebrates, it is highly probable that opsonic activity predated hemolytic activity.

The presence or absence of two activation pathways, the classical and alternative pathways, has been studied in many vertebrate species mainly using methods involving antibody dependence and Ca^{2+} activation as criteria for the classical pathway. All jawed vertebrate groups analyzed showed evidence of the presence of both pathways (1). However, no evidence for a classical pathway was obtained for jawless fish, indicating again the primitive nature of its complement system (5). The complement system in these fish seems to be very similar to the mammalian alternative pathway functioning as an opsonic system, although its details remain to be clarified. It is noteworthy that definitive molecular evidence demonstrating the presence of both activation pathways in lower vertebrates (e.g., the simultaneous presence of Bf and C2, or C1s and factor D), is still lacking. The apparent presence of both pathway activities in lower vertebrates would not necessarily imply the presence of all the components involved in the mammalian system. Recent progress in analysis of the mammalian complement system has suggested the presence of a third activation pathway called the lectin pathway (8,9). This pathway is initiated by the binding of MBL (mannan-binding lectin) to a bacterial surface, which then activates MASP (MBL associated serine protease), leading to proteolytic activation of C4 and C2. MBL and MASP are structurally related to C1q and C1r/C1s, respectively, suggesting a close genetic relationship between the classical and lectin pathways. It is possible that the lectin pathway is older than the classical pathway, since initiation of this pathway is dependent on a lectin and lectins without doubt are quite ancient in origin. Furthermore, this pathway does not require the involvement of antibodies, which are believed to be restricted to the jawed vertebrates. The bactericidal activity considered to be dependent on the lectin pathway has been demonstrated for all jawed vertebrates examined (10). However, the possible presence of the lectin pathway including the presence of MBL or MASP in cyclostomes or invertebrates remains to be determined.

III. MOLECULAR ASPECTS

This section focuses on the molecular information concerning the primary structure in nonmammalian species of each complement component except for C3/C4/C5, which will be dealt with separately in the next section.

With respect to C1, no cDNA cloning has been reported for C1q, C1r, and C1s from nonmammalian species, although the C1 complex and/or C1q proteins have been isolated from nurse shark (cartilaginous fish) (11), carp (bony fish) (12), bullfrog (amphibian) (13), and chicken (bird) (14), indicating that the basic architecture of C1 has been conserved during vertebrate evolution.

cDNA clones for Bf or C2 have been isolated from lamprey (cyclostome) (15), Medaka fish (15a), zebra fish (bony fish) (Mayer WE, Seeger A, Klein J. Genbank accession number U34662), and *Xenopus* (amphibians) (16,17). Among these only the *Xenopus* sequence was clearly identified as Bf, while all other sequences showed almost the same similarity to both mammalian Bf and C2. These results imply that Bf/C2 gene duplication did not occur before the divergence of bony fish and are in sharp contrast with funtional studies which indicate the presence of both the classical and alternative activation pathways in all jawed vertebrates (1). Even in *Xenopus* with duplicated Bf genes, only suggestive evidence for the presence of the C2 gene was reported (16), and a clear demonstration of the C2 gene remains to be presented. Thus, the point at which Bf/C2 gene duplication occurred during the vertebrate evolution is still not clear. An intriguing possibility is that in lower vertebrates a single Bf/C2 molecule may function in both the classical and alternative pathways. The chicken Bf-like protein has also been suggested to be involved in the classical pathway, and one possible explanation is that Bf/C2 gene duplication occurred along the lineage leading to mammals (18). However, the existing sequence diversity between mammalian Bf and C2 with less than 40% amino acid identity (19), seems to be too large to be explained by diversification after recent gene duplication. Further molecular searching for C2 is required in lower vertebrates.

Concerning late-acting components, C5–C9, the only available nonmammalian cDNA sequence is that of rainbow trout C9 (20), the amino acid sequence of which shows a high degree of identity (36%) with that of human C9. C5 protein and MAC (membrane attack complex) have also been isolated from rainbow trout (21,22). Rainbow trout C5 essentially has the same subunit chain structure as that of mammalian C5, while rainbow trout MAC showed a very similar composition to that of mammalian MAC, although the relative ratio of C9 to other components seemed higher in trout MAC than in mammalian MAC. Regarding receptors and regulatory proteins; since C3-dependent opsonic activity was identified in jawless fish (5,6), bony fish (23), and amphibians (24), the presence of C3 receptors was predicted for all vertebrate groups. Two major mammalian C3 receptors involved in C3-mediated phagocytosis are complement receptor type 1 (CR1) and CR3. CR1 belongs to the RCA (regulators of complement activation) family, whose members are composed mainly of repeats of a 60 amino acid-long module termed complement control protein (CCP), whereas CR3 is a member of the integrin family. The RCA genes, CR1, CR2, C4BPA, C4BPB, H, DAF, and MCP, seem to be extremely unstable, and gross structural differences of these proteins have been reported, even among mammalian species. Thus, human CR1 is a huge molecule composed of 30 CCP modules (25), whereas its mouse and rat genetic homologue, Crry, has only five and six or seven CCP, respectively (26–28). Human C4BPα has likewise eight CCP modules (29), whereas mouse C4BPα is composed of six CCP (30).

These instabilities of CCP-containing complement regulatory genes suggest a relatively recent origin for these genes, rendering CR3 a more probable candidate than CR1 as an opsonic receptor in lower vertebrates or invertebrates. The only report on molecular cloning of nonmammalian CCP-containing complement regulatory proteins describes the isolation of a cDNA clone for the sand bass (bony fish) H-like protein containing 17 CCP modules (31). In addition, *Xenopus* factor I was isolated and characterized (32). Functional studies have indicated a wide distribution of factor I-like C3/C4 cleaving activity in serum of many vertebrate species down to bony fish (33).

IV. EVOLUTION OF C3/C4/C5

Most of the mammalian complement components consist of protein modules, either relatively simple repeats of a single kind, as CCP-containing receptors and regulatory proteins, or mosaic structures of multiple domains as found in C6, which consists of seven different types of modules. All of these complement component modules are also present in noncomplement proteins, and it is conceivable that the complement system utilized already available structures to derive proteins with new functions. In contrast, no obvious domain or repeating structure has been found for C3/C4/C5 in spite of their large molecular sizes consisting of up to 1600–1700 amino acid residues. These proteins show a significant amino acid sequence identity to each other throughout their entire length. Moreover, there is weaker but significant sequence similarity between C3/C4/C5 and α-2-macroglobulin (α2M), a serum protease inhibitor, with the exception of the C-terminal region of C3/C4/C5 (C345C), suggesting that the main structures of C3/C4/C5 and α2M originated from a common ancestor through gene duplication (34). C3/C4/C5 are synthesized as single chain precursors, and are then proteolytically processed to generate disulfide-bonded two subunit chain structures, C3 and C5, or a three subunit chain structure in C4. C3, C4, and α2M have a unique among blood proteins internal thioester bond, formed between a Cys and a Gln residue in the sequence Cys-Gly/Ala-Glu-Gln. C5 lacks this intrachain bond since the Cys and Gln residues are substituted by Ser and Ala, respectively. The exon–intron organization of the mammalian C3, C4, C5, and α2M genes show a close similarity to each other (35–38), supporting the common ancestry of C3/C4/C5 and α2M. Thus, C3, C4, and C5 genes have 41 exons, and the location and phase of the 40 intron insertion positions are perfectly conserved among these genes. Out of the 35 intron insertion positions of the α2M gene, 29 have a common position and phase as those of the C3, C4, and C5 genes.

Since the role played by C3 is so pivotal, it is difficult to imagine the complement system without it. Therefore, a search for the origin of the complement system may yield findings similar to those obtained by searching for the origin of C3. As described above, it is highly probable that the common ancestor of C3, C4, and C5 was generated by gene duplication from α2M, which has been identified in arthropod species (39,40). However, the immediate result of simple gene duplication of the α2M gene would be the formation of two α2M genes. One of the duplicated α2M genes could then have been modified to become the C3/C4/C5 common ancestor. As to what was the most critical change, the answer may be obtained by a structural comparison of mammalian C3, C4, C5, and α2M, as shown schematically at the top of Figure 1. The most important difference may be in the reactivity of the thioester bond itself. The reactivity of the thioester was analyzed in detail using human C4A and C4B as models (41). C4A and C4B have different amino acid residues at only a few positions, although they show quite different binding properties. C4A binds predominantly to amino groups, while C4B binds to both amino and hydroxyl groups (42,43). The residue responsible for this difference in binding properties was identified as His(C4B) or Asp(C4A) located about 100 residues C-terminal to the thioester (44). The presence of a nucleophilic His at this position makes the thioester highly reactive with an activated state half-life of significantly less than 1 s. On the other hand, when

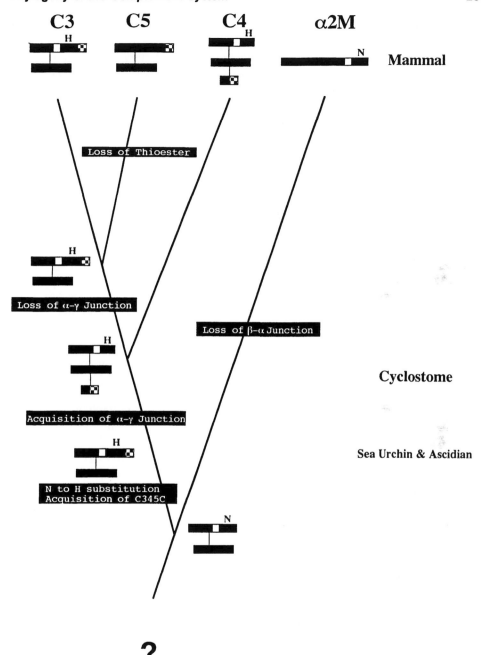

Figure 1 A hypothetical C3, C4, C5, and α2M phylogenetic tree. The evolutionary relationship among C3, C4, C5, and α2M is presented schematically. Structures of mammalian components as well as putative ancestor molecules at branching points are shown. Horizontal black bars indicate polypeptide chains while the thin vertical lines represent disulfide bonds between subunit chains. White areas and checkered areas represent the thioester bond and C345C, respectively. Amino acid residues critical for the reactivity of the thioester bond are shown.

the position is occupied by a nonnucleophilic residue such as Asp in C4A, the reaction is slower with a half-life in the order of 10 s. A quick reaction may be essential for opsonic activity, which requires efficient tagging of biological targets, such as invading microorganisms, and rapid inactivation to avoid binding to bystander host cells. This critical His residue is present in all C3 and C4 sequences so far determined except for C4A molecules found in certain mammalian species (45,46). Covalent binding of α2M to proteases, on the other hand, is believed to be a secondary mechanism for ensuring the trapping effect brought about by a conformational change (47). A slow reactive thioester may be adequate for this purpose. α2M proteins from most species harbor a nonnucleophilic Asn at this position and are believed to show the C4A-type reactivity. Thus, the Asn to His substitution at this position, which could be accomplished by a single A to C nucleotide substitution at the first position of the codon, in one of the duplicated α2M genes may have been the most critical event in the history of the complement system. The second prominent feature of C3, C4, and C5 compared to α2M is the C-terminal extension of C3/C4/C5 (C345C), which is absent from α2M (48). This is a region of about 150 amino acids encoded by the last five exons of the C3, C4, and C5 genes (34–36). To date, no other protein is known to have sequence similarity to this region, and therefore the evolutionary origin of this region is still unknown. The third significant difference between C3/C4/C5 and α2M is their subunit chain structure. In mammalian species, α2M is a single-chain structure, whereas C3 and C5 are both two-subunit chain structures and C4 is a three-subunit chain structure. However, as will be discussed below, these subunit structures are not stable during vertebrate evolution, and the physiological significance of the multiple chain structures of C3/C4/C5 is not known. The fourth difference, although not obvious from Figure 1, is the activating protease. Although α2M harbors a bait region susceptible to many kinds of proteolytic attack, C3/C4/C5 have respective highly specific activating enzymes. It is tempting to hypothesize that this change in cleaving protease was accompanied by a change in the target for covalent binding. Whereas α2M binds directly to the attacking proteases, C3 and C4 mainly bind to the surface of foreign particles that initiate complement activation. This change in binding specificity seems to be a prerequisite for C3 and C4 to function as an opsonin.

Several studies have analyzed C3 cDNA, which has been isolated from at least one species of five major classes of nonmammalian vertebrates, birds (49), reptiles (50), amphibians (51), bony fish (46), and cyclostomes (52,53). The only major vertebrate class on which there is no information on the C3 primary structure is cartilaginous fish. These structural analyses revealed conservation of the basic structure of C3 throughout vertebrate evolution. However, the isolated lamprey C3 protein showed a three-subunit chain structure, and α–γ as well as β–α processing signals were confirmed in a cDNA study (5). On the other hand, some discrepancy was noted in the subunit chain structure of hagfish C3, since purified hagfish C3 protein is reported to have only two subunit chains (54), although the hagfish C3 sequence also harbors possible processing signals at the region corresponding to the α-γ junction of mammalian C4. Only a single C3/C4-like cDNA has been identified in both lamprey and hagfish, and their primary structures showed almost the same similarity to those of mammalian C3 and C4. Therefore, the proteins encoded by these cDNAs are considered to reflect a state before C3/C4 gene duplication, suggesting that the common ancestor of C3 and C4 had a three-subunit chain structure. Recently, C3 of the sea urchin, *Strongylocentrotus purpuratus,* has been cloned, demonstrating the presence of the complement system in invertebrates (7). Although the published sequence represents only about one-third of the C-terminal side of the molecule, it contains the C3/C4/C5 specific C-terminal structure described above, showing its identity to C3/C4/C5 rather than α2M. We have recently identified C3 cDNA from a tunicate, *Halocynthia roretzi,* confirming the presence of the complement system in invertebrates (Nonaka M, unpublished result). The evolutionary origin of C3 remains to be determined.

After establishment of a common ancestor of the C3, C4, and C5 genes, branching among these genes likely followed. Figure 1 represents a hypothetical phylogenetic tree of C3/C4/C5 and α2M whose construction is mainly based on information on the subunit chain structures of these proteins in mammals as well as in lower animals, while also considering functional, thus indirect, evidence for their presence. The main assumption in constructing this tree was that the generation of the β-α and α-γ processing signals most probably occurred only once during the evolution of thioester-containing proteins, since the possibility of generating these signals twice at the same position by chance would be extremely small. In contrast, the loss of these signals could have occurred several times. Since the C3 gene has been identified in a sea urchin (echinoderm) and an ascidian (protochordata), gene duplication between C3/C4/C5 and α2M should have occurred before the emergence of vertebrates. α2M with a two-subunit chain structure has been identified in some lower vertebrates, a bony fish plaice (55), and lamprey (Nonaka M, unpublished finding), although arthropod and higher vertebrate α2M are single subunit chain molecules (39,40). Duplication between α2M and complement C3/C4/C5 most probably occurred in a species whose α2M harbored a two-subunit chain structure, implying the presence of a two-subunit chain α2M in certain invertebrates. There is no α-γ processing signal in the published sea urchin C3 sequence at the position corresponding to the α-γ junction of mammalian C4 (7), suggesting an α-β chain structure. It is conceivable, therefore, that the α-γ processing signal was acquired later, converting the common ancestor of C3/C4/C5 to a three-chain molecule by the time of emergence of cyclostomes. By the time of divergence of cartilaginous fish, C4 should have been generated from the three-chain C3/C4/C5 by gene duplication, since C3 and C4 proteins have been isolated from the nurse shark (Dodds A, Smith SL, personal communication). Here, C3/C4/C5 seems to have lost the α-γ processing signal, once again becoming a two-subunit chain molecule. Final gene duplication between C3 and C5 might have also occurred just after C3/C4 gene duplication, although strong evidence for the presence of C5 is available only for the bony fish (22) and higher vertebrates, and there is still no definitive evidence demonstrating the presence of C5 in cartilaginous fish. C5, accordingly, lost the thioester bond. There is, however, another proposed scenario for the C3/C4/C5 sequential branching pattern based solely on sequence comparisons (56). According to this scheme, C5 was the first component to diverge among the three. Sequence alignment, however, suggests that two sequential branching events are required to generate three genes from a single common ancestor gene, and it seems very difficult to obtain a reliable phylogenetic tree just from sequence comparison. The critical questions that still remain to be answered are, first, when did the first gene duplication between α2M and C3/C4/C5 occur? and, second, from where was the C3/C4/C5-specific C-terminal sequence recruited?

As described above, the C4 genes of certain mammalian species are duplicated. Thus, there are two C4 genes termed C4A and C4B in humans, and C4 and Slp (sex-limited protein) in mouse (57). Both human C4A and C4B proteins are hemolytically active, although the physiological significance of C4A is still not clear (58). In contrast, mouse Slp is resistant to C1s activation due to amino acid sequence diversity in the region near the C1s cleavage site of C4 including a three amino acid deletion (59), and is therefore hemolytically inactive. In addition to primates and rodents, some ungulates such as sheep and cattle have multiple C4 genes of both the C4A and C4B types (46). On the other hand, cat, dog, guinea pig, Syrian hamster, and whale seem to have single C4 genes. These findings can be explained either by multiple independent gene duplications occurring in primates, rodents, and ungulates, or by a single gene duplication event in a common mammal ancestor, followed by multiple gene deletion events occurring in many mammalian groups. The latter explanation appears to be more probable, since there is no obvious reason for such frequent C4 gene duplication in mammalian species. On the other hand, once duplicated, genes could be very unstable and subject to further duplication or deletion by homologous recombination. The only nonmammalian species analyzed so far for the copy number of the C4 gene is *Xenopus* (60). The *Xenopus* C4 gene seems to be single copy, although the *Xenopus* Bf gene is duplicated (17). Recently, multiple C3 genes have been identified in at least three teleost species, trout (61), carp (Nakao M, personal communication), and sea bream (Lambris JD, personal communication). Although trout and carp are qausitetraploid fish, sea bream is a diploid fish. The multiple copy number of the C3 gene, therefore, does not seem to have resulted from tetraploidization. Duplication of various complement genes therefore seems to have occurred several times during vertebrate evolution. However, there is still no clear evidence showing that the extra copy of gene duplication products acquired a new function beneficial to the host.

V. EVOLUTION OF THE CLASSIC PATHWAY AND THE MHC

As has been discussed above, the initial complement system seems to have emerged in invertebrates although its molecular architecture has yet to be defined. The cyclostome complement system seems to be very similar to the mammalian alternative pathway, functioning as an opsonin, while lacking the classic and lytic pathways. There is clear evidence for the presence of the classic and lytic pathways in cartilaginous fish, indicating

	Complement System			Immuno-globulin	T Cell Receptor	MHC Class I, II	RAG	LMP2/7
	Alternative Pathway	Classical Pathway	Lytic Pathway					
Bony Fish	+	+	+	+	+	+	+	+
Cartilaginous Fish	+	+	+	+	+	+	+	+
Jawless Fish	+							

Figure 2 Complement and noncomplement host defense systems in lower vertebrates. + indicates the presence of strong molecular evidence, whereas blanks indicate the absence of molecular evidence in spite of attempts to determine the presence of these systems.

that these pathways arose over a relatively short period of time after the emergence of cyclostomes and before the emergence of cartilaginous fish, which is considered to have occurred about 400 million years ago. Figure 2 summarizes the molecular evidence for the other immunologically important molecules in lower vertebrates and invertebrates. Immunoglobulin (62), T-cell antigen receptor (63), recombination activating gene (RAG) (64), MHC class IA (65), class IIA (66), class IIB (67), and low molecular mass proteinase (LMP) 7 (68) are present in cartilaginous fish, however, all attempts to identify their counterparts in cyclostomes have not as yet succeeded. Therefore, these genes critical in the mammalian immune system, as well as genes involved in the classical and lytic pathways of the complement system seem to have evolved simultaneously at a very early stage of vertebrate evolution. Prior to this, the C3-dependent opsonic system might have been a major host defense mechanism for a long time period, although details of the activation mechanism in the primitive complement system of some invertebrates remain to be clarified. An intriguing point concerning relatively recent immunological genes considered to have been established around the time of the emergence of the cartilaginous fish is the linkage of some of these genes to each other. Thus, the MHC class IA, class IIA, class IIB, LMP2, LMP7, complement C4 and C2 genes reside in the mammalian MHC, suggesting the possibility that close linkage among these genes played some role in establishment of the immune system in more highly evolved life forms. LMP2 and LMP7 are believed to be involved in generation of peptides from endogenous antigens (69,70), which are transported into the ER lumen by the heterodimeric TAP transporter encoded by the TAP1 and TAP2 genes whose counterparts in nonmammalian species have not yet been studied. These genes show a close linkage to each other in the class II region of mammalian MHC, in order from the centromere LMP2, TAP1, LMP7, and TAP2 (71). Thus, class IA, LMP2, LMP7, TAP1, and TAP2 genes provide us with an intriguing example of the linkage of genes that are closely functionally related but structurally totally unrelated. Linkage between the C4 and C2 genes may be another example of this phenomenon. To elucidate the possible roles of these linkages in establishing the class I-dependent antigen presentation system and the classical complement pathway, phylogenetic studies of MHC were performed. Thus, amphibian *Xenopus laevis* MHC was shown to harbor one class IA (72,73), three class IIB (74), one LMP7 (75), one C4 (60), and duplicated Bf genes (16,17). Moreover, two intra-MHC recombinants found during these mapping studies suggested the possibility that the order of these genes is also conserved between humans and *Xenopus* (60,75). Although the *Xenopus* C2 gene remains to be elucidated, these results indicate that the basic structure of the MHC was established before mammals and amphibians last shared a common ancestor about 350 million years ago. Molecular analysis of the possible presence of the MHC structure in bony and cartilaginous fish should provide us with more information concerning the origin and evolution of the classical pathway.

REFERENCES

1. Dodds AW, Day AJ. The phylogeny and evolution of the complement system. In: Whaley K, Loos M, Weiler JM, eds. Complement in Health and Disease. London: Kluwer Academic Publishers, 1993:39–88.
2. Gilbert W. Genes-in-pieces revisited. Science 1985; 228:823–824.

3. Caroll MC, Campbell RD, Bentley DR, and Porter RR. A molecular map of the human major histocompatibility complex class III region linking complement genes C4, C2 and factor B. Nature 1984; 307:237–241.

4. Chaplin DD, Woods DE, Whitehead AS, Goldberger G, Colten HR, Seidman JG. Molecular map of the murine S region. Proc Natl Acad Sci USA 1983; 80:6947–6951.

5. Nonaka M, Fujii T, Kaidoh T, Natsuume-Sakai S, Nonaka M, Yamaguchi N, Takahashi M. Purification of a lamprey complement protein homologous to the third component of the mammalian complement system. J Immunol 1984; 133:3242–3249.

6. Hanley PJ, Hook JW, Raftos DA, Gooley AA, Trent R, Raison RL. Hagfish humoral defense protein exhibits structural and functional homology with mammalian complement components. Proc Natl Acad Sci USA 1992; 89:7910–7914.

7. Smith LC, Chang L, Britten RJ, Davidson EH. Sea urchin genes expressed in activated coelomocytes are identified by expressed sequence tags. J Immunol 1996; 156:593–602.

8. Sato T, Endo Y, Matshushita M, Fujita T. Molecular characterization of a novel serine protease involved in activation of the complement system by mannose-binding protein. Int Immunol 1994; 6:665–669.

9. Takayama Y, Takada F, Takahashi A, Kawakami M. A 100-kDa protein in the C4-activating component of Ra-reactive factor is a new serine protease having module organization similar to C1r and C1s. J Immunol 1994; 152:2308–2316.

10. Kawakami M, Ihara I, Ihara S, Suzuki A, Fukui K. A group of bactericidal factors conserved by vertebrates for more than 300 million years. J Immunol 1984; 132:2578–2581.

11. Ross GD, Jensen JA. The first component (C1n) of the complement system of the nurse shark. I. Hemolytic characteristics of partially purified C1n. J Immunol 1973; 11:175–182.

12. Yano T, Matsuyama H, Nakao M. Isolation of the first component of complement (C1) from carp serum. Nippon Suisan Gakkaishi 1988; 54:851–859.

13. Alexander RG, Steiner LA. The first component of complement from the bullfrog, *Rana catesbeina:* functional properties of C1 and isolation of subcomponent C1q. J Immunol 1980; 124:1418–1425.

14. Yonemasu K, Sasaki T. Purification, identification and characterization of chicken C1q, a subcomponent of the first component of complement. J Immunol Methods 1986; 88:245–253.

15. Nonaka M, Takahashi M, Sasaki M. Molecular cloning of a lamprey homologue of the mammalian MHC class III gene, complement factor B. J Immunol 1994; 152:2263–2269.

15a. Kuroda N, Wada H, Naruse K, Shimado A, Shima A, Sasaki M, Nonaka M. Molecular cloning and linkage analysis of the Japanses medaka fish complement Bf/C2 gene. Immunogenetics 1996; 44:459–467.

16. Kato Y, Salter-Cid L, Flajnik MF, Kasahara M, Namikawa C, Sasaki M, Nonaka M. Isolation of the *Xenopus* complement factor B complementary DNA and linkage of the gene to the frog MHC. J Immunol 1994; 153:4546–4554.

17. Kato Y, Salter-Cid L, Flajnik MF, Namikawa C, Sasaki M, Nonaka M. Duplication of the MHC-linked *Xenopus* complement factor B gene. Immunogenetics 1995; 42:196–203.

18. Kjalke M, Welinder KG, Koch C. Structural analysis of chicken factor B-like protease and comparison with mammalian complement proteins factor B and C2. J Immunol 1993; 151:4147–4152.

19. Ishikawa N, Nonaka M, Wetsel RA, Colten HR. Murine complement C2 and factor B genomic and cDNA cloning reveals different mechanisms for multiple transcripts of C2 and B. J Biol Chem 1990; 265:19040–19046.

20. Stanley KK, Herz J. Topological mapping of complement component C9 by recombinant DNA techniques suggests a novel mechanism for its insertion into target membranes. EMBO J 1987; 6:1951–1957.

21. Nonaka M, Yamaguchi N, Natsuume-Sakai S, Takahashi M. The complement system of rainbow trout (*Salmo gairdneri*) I. Identification of the serum lytic system homologous to mammalian complement. J Immunol 1981; 126:1489–1494.

22. Nonaka M, Natsuume-Sakai S, Takahashi M. The complement system of rainbow trout (*Salmo gairdneri*) II. Purification and characterization of the fifth component (C5). J Immunol 1981; 126:1495–1498.

23. Jonson H, Smith P. Attachment and phagocytosis by salmon macrophages of agarose beads coated with human C3b and iC3b. Dev Comp Immunol 1984; 8:623–630.

24. Sekizawa A, Fujii T, Tochinai S. Membrane receptors on *Xenopus* macrophages for two classes of immunoglobulins (IgM and IgY) and the third complement component (C3). J Immunol 1984; 133:1431–1435.

25. Klickstein LB, Wong WW, Smith JA, Weis JH, Wilson JG, Fearon DT. Human C3b/C4b receptor (CR1). Demonstration of long homologous repeating domains that are composed of the short consensus repeats characteristic of C3/C4 binding proteins. J Exp Med 1987; 165:1095–1112.

26. Paul MS, Aegerter M, O'Brien SE, Kurtz CB, Weis JH. The murine complement receptor gene family. Analysis of mCRY gene products and their homology to human CR1. J Immunol 1989; 142:582–589.

27. Sakurada C, Seno H, Dohi N, Takizawa H, Nonaka M, Okada N, Okada H. Molecular cloning of the rat complement regulatory protein, 5I2 antigen. Biochem Biophys Res Commun 1994; 198:819–826.

28. Quigg RJ, Lo CF, Alexander JJ, Sneed AE, Moxley G. Molecular characterization of rat Crry: widespread distribution of two alternative forms of Crry mRNA. Immunogenetics 1995; 42:362–367.

29. Chung LP, Bentley DR, Reid KB. Molecular cloning and characterization of the cDNA coding for C4b-binding protein, a regulatory protein of the classical pathway of the human complement system. Biochem J 1985; 230:133–141.

30. Kristensen T, Ogata RT, Chung LP, Reid KB, Tack BF. cDNA structure of murine C4b-binding protein, a regulatory component of the serum complement system. Biochemistry 1987; 26:4668–4674.

31. Dahmen A, Kaidoh T, Zipfel PF, Gigli I. Cloning and characterization of a cDNA representing a putative complement-regulatory plasma protein from barred sand bass (*Parablax neblifer*). Biochem J 1994; 301:391–397.

32. Kunnath-Muglia LM, Chang GH, Sim RB, Day AJ, Ezekowitz RA. Characterization of *Xenopus laevis* complement factor I structure: conservation of modular structure except for an unusual insert not present in human factor I. Mol Immunol 1993; 30:1249–1256.

33. Kaidoh T, Gigli I. Phylogeny of C4b-C3b cleaving activity: Similar fragmentation patterns of human C4b and C3b produced by lower animals. J Immunol 1987; 139:194–201.

34. Sottrup-Jensen L, Stepanik TM, Kristensen T, Lonblad PB, Jones CM, Wierzbick DM, Magnusson S, Domdey H, Wetsel RA, Lundwall A, Tack BF, Fey GH. Common evolutionary origin of α2-macroglobulin and complement C3 and C4. Proc Natl Acad Sci USA 1985; 82:9–13.

35. Hattori M, Kusakabe S, Ohgusu H, Tsuchiya Y, Ito T, Sakaki Y. Structure of the rat α2-macroglobulin-coding gene. Gene 1989; 77:333–340.

36. Vik DP, Amguet P, Moffat GJ, Fey M, Amguet-Barras F, Wetsel RA, Tack BF. Structural features of the human C3 gene: Intron/exon organization, transcriptional start site, and promoter region sequence. Biochemistry 1991; 30:1080–1085.

37. Ogata RT, Rosa PA, Zepf NE. Sequence of the gene for murine complement component C4. J Biol Chem 1989; 264:16565–16572.

38. Carney DF, Haviland DL, Noack D, Wetsel RA, Vik DP, Tack BF. Structural aspects of the human C5 gene. Intron/exon organization, 5'-flanking region features, and characterization of two truncated cDNA clones. J Biol Chem 1991; 266:18786–18791.

39. Quigley JP, Armstrong PB. A homologue of α2 macroglobulin purified from the haemolymph of the horseshoe crab *Limulus polyphemus*. J Biol Chem 1985; 260:12715–12719.

40. Spycher SE, Arya S, Isenman DE, Painter RH. A functional thioester containing α2 macroglobulin homologue isolated from the haemolymph of the American lobster *Homarus americanus*. J Biol Chem 1987; 262:14606–14611.

41. Dodds AW, Ren X-D, Willis AC, Law SKA. The reaction mechanism of the internal thioester in the human complement component C4. Nature 1996; 379:177–179.

42. Isenman DE, Young JR. The molecular basis for the difference in immune hemolysis activity of the Chido and Rodgers isotypes of human complement component C4. J Immunol 1984; 132:3019–3027.

43. Law SKA, Dodds AW, Porter RR. A comparison of the properties of two classes, C4A and C4B, of the human complement component C4. EMBO J 1984; 3:1819–1823.

44. Carroll MC, Fathallah DM, Bergamaschini L, Alicot EM, Isenman DE. Substitution of a single amino acid (aspartic acid for histidine) converts the functional activity of human complement C4B to C4A. Proc Natl Acad Sci USA 1990; 87:6868–6872.

45. Lambris JD, Lao Z, Pang J, Alsenz J. Third component of trout complement. cDNA cloning and conservation of functional sites. J Immunol 1993; 151:6123–6134.

46. Ren X-D, Dodds AW, Law SKR. The thioester and isotypic sites of complement component C4 in sheep and cattle. Immunogenetics 1993; 37:120–128.

47. Chu CT, Pizzo SV. Alpha 2-macroglobulin, complement, and biologic defence: Antigens, growth factors, microbial proteases, and receptor ligation. Lab Invest 1994; 71:792–812.

48. Bork P, Bairoch A. Extracellular protein modules: A proposed nomenclature. Suppl TIBS 1995; 20 (3).

49. Mavroidis M, Sunyer JO, Lambris JD. Isolation, primary structure, and evolution of the third component of chicken complement and evidence for a new member of the α2-macroglobulin family. J Immunol 1995; 154:2164–2174.

50. Fritzinger DC, Petrella EC, Connelly MB, Bredehorst R, Vogel CW. Primary structure of cobra complement component C3. J Immunol 1992; 149:3554–3562.

51. Lambris JD, Pappas J, Mavroidis M, Wang Y, Manzone H, Swager J, Du Pasquier L, Silibovsky R. The third component of *Xenopus* complement: cDNA cloning, structural and functional analysis, and evidence for an alternate C3 transcript. Eur J Immunol 1995; 25:572–578.

52. Nonaka M, Takahashi M. Complete complementary DNA sequence of the third component of complement of lamprey. Implication for the evolution of thioester containing proteins. J Immunol 1992; 148:3290–3295.

53. Ishiguro H, Kobayashi K, Suzuki M, Titani K, Tomonaga S, Kurosawa Y. Isolation of a hagfish gene that encodes a complement component. EMBO J 1992; 11:829–837.

54. Fujii T, Nakamura T, Sekizawa A, Tomonaga S. Isolation and characterization of a protein from hagfish serum that is homologous to the third component of the mammalian complement system. J Immunol 1992; 148:117–123.

55. Starkey PM, Barrett AJ. Evolution of α2macroglobulin: the structure of a protein homologous with human α2macroglobulin from plaice (*Pleuronectes platessa*) plasma. Biochem J 1982; 205:105–115.

56. Hughes AL. Phylogeny of the C3/C4/C5 complement-component gene family indicates that C5 diverged first. Mol Biol Evol 1994; 11:417–425.

57. Campbell RD, Law SKA, Reid KBM, Sim RB. Structure, organization, and regulation of the complement genes. Annu Rev Immunol 1988; 6:161–195.

58. Law SKA, Dodds AW. Catalysed hydrolysis—the complement quickstep. Immunol Today 1996; 17:105.

59. Ogata RT, Cooper NR, Bradt BM, Mathias P, Picchi MA. Murine complement component C4 and sex-limited protein: identification of amino acid residues essential for C4 function. Proc Natl Acad Sci USA 1989; 86:5575–5579.

60. Mo R, Kato Y, Nonaka M, Nakayama K, Takahashi M. Fourth component of *Xenopus laevis* complement: cDNA cloning and linkage analysis of the frog MHC. Immunogenetics 1996; 43:360–369.

61. Sunyer JO, Zarkadis IK, Sahu A, Lambris JD. Multiple forms of complement C3 in trout that differ in binding to complement activators. Proc Natl Acad Sci USA 1996; 93:8546–8551.

62. Hinds KR, Litman GW. Major reorganization of immunoglobulin V_H segmental elements during vertebrate evolution. Nature 1986; 320:546–549.

63. Rast JP, Litman GW. T-cell receptor gene homologs are present in the most primitive jawed vertebrates. Proc Natl Acad Sci USA 91; 1994:9248–9252.

64. Thompson CB. New insights into V(D)J recombination and its role in the evolution of the immune system. Immunity 1995; 3:531–539.

65. Hashimoto K, Nakanishi T, Kurosawa Y. Identification of a shark sequence resembling the major histocompatibility complex class I α3 domain. Proc Natl Acad Sci USA 1992; 89:2209–2212.

66. Kasahara M, Vazquez M, Sato K, McKinney EC, Flajnik MF. Evolution of the major histocompatibility complex: Isolation of class II A cDNA clones from the cartilaginous fish. Proc Natl Acad Sci USA 1992; 89:6688–6692.

67. Bartl S, Weissman IL. Isolation and characterization of major histocompatibility complex class IIB genes from the nurse shark. Proc Natl Acad Sci USA 1994; 91:262–266.

68. Kandil E, Namikawa C, Nonaka M, Greenberg AS, Flajnik MF, Ishibashi T, Kasahara M. Isolation of low molecular mass polypeptide cDNA clones from primitive vertebrates: Implications for the origin of MHC class I-restricted antigen presentation. J Immunol 1996; 156:4245–4253.

69. Van Kaer L, Ashton-Rickardt PG, Eichelberger M, Gaczynska M, Nagashima K, Rock KL, Goldberg AL, Doherty PC, Tonegawa S. Altered peptidase and viral-specific T cell response in LMP2 mutant mice. Immunity 1994; 1:533–541.

70. Fehling HJ, Swat W, Laplace C, Kuhn R, Rajewsky K, Muller U, von Boehmer H. MHC class I expression in mice lacking the proteasome subunit LMP-7. Science 1994; 265:1234–1237.

71. Beck S, Kelly A, Radley E, Khurshid F, Alderton RP, Trowsdale J. DNA sequence analysis of 66 kb of the human MHC class II region encoding a cluster of genes for antigen processing. J Mol Biol 1992; 228:433–441.

72. Flajnik MF, Canel C, Kramer J, Kasahara M. Evolution of the major histocompatibility complex: molecular cloning of major histocompatibility complex class I from the amphibian *Xenopus*. Proc Natl Acad Sci USA 1991; 88:537–541.

73. Shum BP, Avila D, Pasquier LD, Kasahara M, Flajnik, MF. Isolation of a classical MHC class I cDNA from an amphibian. Evidence for only one class I locus in the *Xenopus* MHC. J Immunol 1993; 151:5376–5386.

74. Sato K, Flajnik MF, Pasquier LD, Katagiri M, Kasahara M. Evolution of the MHC: isolation of class II β-chain cDNA clones from the amphibian *Xenopus laevis*. J Immunol 1993; 150:2831–2843.

75. Namikawa C, Salter-Cid L, Flajnik MF, Kato Y, Nonaka M, Sasaki M. Isolation of *Xenopus LMP-7* homologues. Striking allelic diversity and linkage to MHC. J Immunol 1995; 155:1964–1971.

10

Regulation of Complement Protein Gene Expression

HARVEY R. COLTEN
Northwestern University Medical School, Chicago, Illinois

GÉRARD GARNIER
Washington University School of Medicine, St. Louis, Missouri

I. INTRODUCTION

During the late 19th century with the emergence of immunology and microbiology as separate disciplines, the distinction between acquired and innate host defenses against infectious agents was soon appreciated. As a result, two parallel lines of investigation developed: exploration of mechanisms that generate the diversity of humoral and cellular systems induced by and specifically recognizing foreign antigens; definition of the systems that allow disposal of toxins, microbes, and tissue debris in the absence of a specific immune response. By the early 1930s it was clear that these nonspecific host defenses were *also* modulated in response to microbial infection or tissue injury (1). This modulation was designated the acute-phase response, a physiological alteration that includes marked changes in hepatic protein synthesis and an overall change in nitrogen balance, fever, leukocytosis, changes in energy balance, and mineral metabolism (2). More recently, the scope of the changes accompanying an acute-phase response and the proximate mediators have been elucidated. In aggregate, all of these changes provide a rapid response to noxious stimuli and may also facilitate acquisition of specific immunity.

Among the acute-phase proteins that are important in both nonspecific and specific host defenses are members of the complement system. The increase in complement proteins is neither quantitatively nor kinetically the most impressive among the acute-phase plasma proteins. For example, serum concentrations of C3 protein rise only about twofold over baseline within a week following an acute-phase stimulus, whereas serum levels of two other positive acute-phase proteins, C-reactive protein and serum amyloid A, increase 100–1000 fold within hours. The serum complement proteins are almost entirely of hepatic origin (3–5). Recent data provide minimal estimates of 0.1–2.6% and 3.1–5.7% of serum complement that are from marrow derived and all extrahepatic sources, respectively (6). These studies of in vivo complement metabolism and allotypic changes posttransplantation confirmed evidence derived from tissue culture studies that extrahepatic sources of complement are important (7–10, reviewed in 11). However, the in vivo studies (6) no doubt still underestimate the contribution of extrahepatic complement production to the content of these proteins outside the vascular space. Neither precise measures of constitutive expression nor the kinetics of extrahepatic induction of complement genes in vivo are known because all of these estimates are derived from cell cultures. However, acute-phase-induced changes in complement gene expression in fibroblasts and other cell types are quantitatively much greater than in hepatocytes (12,13). Some studies suggest that this is true in vivo as well. For example, the increase in extrahepatic complement expression in kidney, lung, and heart exceeds by severalfold the increase in expression of the corresponding genes in liver during evolution of systemic lupus erythematosus and inflammatory bowel disease (14–17). Moreover, some of the complement proteins (e.g., C2) are *only* acute-phase-responsive in extrahepatic sites and therefore do not satisfy classic criteria as acute-phase reactants (i.e., plasma concentration changes during an acute-phase reaction). These observations have focused interest on the mechanisms regulating complement gene expression. A recent review has compiled data on transcriptional regulation of complement (18). This chapter will briefly summarize recent studies of transcriptional control but focus in more depth on posttranscriptional control of complement protein production.

II. GENERAL

The various cell types that express complement proteins are listed in Tables 1 and 2. For the most part, the data on which these tables are based depend on study of primary cell culture, but for some measurement of specific mRNA by *in situ* hybridization provides in vivo confirmation. For a few cell types, transplantation has offered another approach by demonstrating changes in allotypic variants of complement proteins in the recipient following transplant from a donor with a different genetic allotype (4,6,10,19). While considerable insights have been attained in studies of complement gene expression in permanent cell lines (mostly of malignant origin), these cannot be used as sole evidence

Table 1 Complement Receptors/Regulatory Proteins Expressed on Membranes

CR1 (CD35)	Hematopoietic cells including erythrocytes; glomerular podocytes; mast cells, PMN (186), Schwann cells in (fetal) peripheral nerve (187); HSV-infected epidermal and endothelial cells (188).
CR2 (CD21)	Some T-cell tumors, mature and late pre-B cells not on others in B-cell lineage, follicular dendritic cells (186).
CR3 (CD11b/18)	PMNs (not on granulocyte precursors), monocytes; natural killer cells (186,189).
CR4 (CD11c/18)	Polymorphonuclear leukocytes, platelets, B+T cells (186,190).
C5a receptor	Bronchial epithelium, smooth muscle cells, endothelium, hepatocytes, hematopoietic cells, mast cells (191).
DAF (CD55)	Hematopoietic cells (192–195) but not precursors (196), endothelium (197), adult epithelium (198), trophoblast (196), endometrium (199).
MCP (CD46)	Hematopoietic cells (except erythrocytes) (200,201); fibroblast, epithelium, endothelium (202), sperm, trophoblasts (203), endometrium (199).
HRF$_{20}$ (CD59)	Erythrocytes (204,205), endothelium (206), platelets (207), endometrium (199).

Table 2 Sites of Complement Protein Synthesis

	Classic Pathway	Alternative Pathway	Terminal Components	References
Liver	+	+	+	5,208,209
Mononuclear phagocytes	+	+	+	Reviewed in 210
Lymphocytes		+	+	211,212
Polymorphonuclear leukocytes			+	58,213
Fibroblasts	+	+	+	12
Epithelial cells				
Gastrointestinal	+	+		9,39
Genitourinary	+	+		214,215
Lung	+	+		216
Endothelial cells		+		60,95
Adipocytes		+		217
Synovium	+	+		218
Myoblast/myocyte		+		219,220
Central nervous system	+	+		178

for that cell as a locus of complement expression because even the most differentiated of these cell lines differ from the normal cell of origin in important ways. However, these cell lines have been extremely useful as models for elucidating transcriptional and posttranscriptional mechanisms for constitutive and regulated complement gene expression, once the authentic cell of origin is known.

Newly synthesized proteins destined for secretion or insertion into cell membranes are transported to the cell surface by different subcellular pathways (20) and with different kinetics (21–23). In addition, not all cell-associated complement proteins are integral membrane constituents since some (e.g., decay-accelerating factor (DAF]) are anchored via a phosphoglycerolinositol linkage. These complexities and space limitations for this chapter will require restriction of the discussion for the most part to a few of the secreted proteins, for which intensive study has been undertaken.

III. DEVELOPMENT

Most of the complement effector proteins are synthesized early in fetal life. The placenta is an effective barrier to passage of complement either from or to the fetal circulation in humans, mice, and ungulates. This makes it possible to establish with in vivo studies, for components with allotypic variants and/or genetic deficiency, that the fetus is capable of synthesizing several complement proteins (24–27). In general, the soluble complement proteins are synthesized by the fetus at or shortly before the onset of immunoglobulin synthesis. For example, C1, C4, and C2 are expressed early in gestation (~8 weeks in humans) (28–32). In the fetal liver, C2 is synthesized at a constant rate throughout gestation but in mononuclear cells a marked developmental change has been observed in postnatal extrahepatic C2 expression (33). That is, in marrow no functional C2 production is detected. The proportion of tissue macrophages that synthesize C2 elsewhere varies between ~45%

at most sites (34) and ~2% in bronchoalveolar macrophages. Fetal liver is a hematopoietic organ. It is not known, therefore, whether C2 production in fetal liver is entirely derived from hepatocytes, from hematopoietic precursors, or from both. By contrast, C4 expression in fetal liver changes dramatically with gestation but in postnatal life is relatively uniform in marrow derived cells in many extrahepatic tissues. Rates of C4 synthesis in the first trimester are only 20–25% that observed in later (>20 weeks) fetal life (30). Expression of C3 in fetal liver can be detected at a stage in gestation (~4 weeks) coincident with the appearance of hepatic cells in the primitive liver (29). These studies of the ontogeny of human complement are based on incomplete data because systematic sampling is difficult and/or unethical. Application of ontogenetic data across species is of uncertain value, so that large gaps remain in current understanding of the developmental regulation of complement. Recent advances in methods for exploring stem cell biology should make it possible to address several of these phenomena in more depth (35).

One area that has received some attention, however, is the example of C3 and Bf expression in which extrahepatic tissues undergo important developmental changes in the transition from fetal through adult life. In adult human peripheral blood monocytes and macrophages or in murine fibroblasts, lipopolysaccharide (LPS) induces a 5–30-fold increase in C3 and Bf synthesis and secretion (12,36–38). This effect is mediated both transcriptionally and translationally. However, LPS does not upregulate C3 and Bf protein synthesis in newborn blood monocytes. This effect is specific for the complement genes (e.g., LPS-induced superoxide generation is equally inducible in neonatal and adult cells). Further exploration of this phenomenon in fibroblasts permitted evaluation of transcriptional/translational regulation and extension to fetal cells. LPS induces specific C3 and Bf mRNA in newborn fibroblasts but C3 or Bf protein synthesis does not increase and in fetal cells LPS does not even induce C3 or Bf mRNA (38). In adult hepatocytes and intestinal epithelium, a similar LPS unresponsiveness is observed (39,40). The failure of LPS to upregulate complement effector proteins in tissues "constitutively" exposed to bacteria has an obvious biological advantage.

Expression of complement regulatory proteins (CD46, CD55) has been detected in 19–24-week fetal tissue (32), but the earliest onset of synthesis for either has not been established. CD59 (homologous restriction factor, HRF) and CD46 (membrane cofactor protein, MCP) are expressed on fetal epithelium, hepatocytes, and hematopoietic cells in liver as early as 6 weeks of gestation and CD55 (decay accelerating factor, DAF) expression is restricted to the hematopoietic cells (41).

IV. CONSTITUTIVE AND REGULATED EXPRESSION

For a few of the complement genes, C3, factor B, and C4 (and its analogue in mouse SLP), structural and functional mapping of important *cis* elements and corresponding *trans* factors governing constitutive and regulated expression have been defined. These investigations were prompted by studies extending over several years that uncovered significant intraspecies and tissue specific variation in constitutive expression as well as marked changes induced by chemical and physical stimuli.

A. Complement Protein C3

C3 is encoded by an approximately 41 Kb gene that generates a 5.1 Kb poly A+ mature mRNA (42,43). This transcript yields a prepro C3 protein of ~190 kD (44,45) that undergoes co- and postsynthetic processing to yield the two chain disulfide bridged mature C3 protein. Cleavage of the pro-C3 linker peptide is mediated by furin (46). Generation of the critical thiolester bond results from isomerization of a lactam to a thiolactone (47), perhaps facilitated by a specific enzyme (48). However, other work suggests that an enzymatic step is not essential (49). C3 is regulated by acute-phase stimuli mediated via the cytokines interleukin I (IL-1) (13), IL-6 (50–52), and tumor necrosis factor (TNF)-α (53). The effect of interferon-γ on C3 expression is variable among species and even within a species appears to be genetically variable. For example, IFN-γ has a limited upregulatory effect on C3 expression in several cell types including glial cells (54), glomerular epithelial (55) and mesangial cells (56), alveolar epithelium (57), blood leukocytes (58,59), and endothelium (60). It downregulates or has no effect on C3 in monocytes and macrophages (61; Cole and Colten, unpublished) but shows a marked synergistic effect, upregulating C3 in the presence of other inflammatory cytokines or lipopolysaccharide in several cell types (59,62). The effect of IFN-γ on C3 expression is probably indirect and complex. It requires de novo protein synthesis in at least one cell type (astroglia) (54) and involves increased mRNA stability in several cell types (63). This is similar to the effect of IFN-γ on expression of human C4, but the mechanisms governing this phenomenon for either C4 or C3 are not clear. This has been demonstrated most clearly in the hepatoma-derived cell line HepG2 (63). In this cell, C3 transcription is actually decreased to about 30% of constitutive following IFN-γ. Because the impact on mRNA stability is greater than on transcription, net C3 protein production is increased by exposure to IFN-γ. The increase in C3 synthesis and the synergistic effect of costimulation by IL-1 and IL-6 are exerted in part at the transcriptional level (64,65). The effects of these inflammatory cytokines and even constitutive C3 expression are counterregulated by growth factors like TGF-β in astrocytes (66) or GM-CSF in monocytes (67). In contrast, MCSF increases C3 expression in monocytes/macrophages (68).

Glucocorticoids downregulate C3 synthesis in human monocytes/macrophages at the transcriptional level (69,70), although the opposite effect of corticosteroids has been observed in endothelial (71) and alveolar epithelial cells (57,72). In two rat hepatoma cell lines hydrocortisone markedly increases (>ninefold) C3 synthesis at concentrations $<10^{-6}$ (73). These data suggest either a species- or cell-specific effect of this mediator. Other hormones also regulate C3 expression (74) (e.g., estrogen and progesterone, especially in tissues highly responsive to female sex hormones such as uterine epithelium [75–77]). Many other factors have been shown to modulate C3 expression. Lipopolysaccharide in many cell types (36,58), C5a and FMLP in hepatocytes (78), immune complexes (79) and IgG2a and IgG2b (through Fc gamma R II receptor) (80) in macrophages, IL-2 in renal epithelium (81), IL-4 in pulmonary epithelium (82), heparin (83), dihydroxyvitamin D3 in osteoblasts (84,85), and histamine (through H1 receptor) in macrophages (86), have strong stimulatory effects on C3 synthesis. Histamine apparently has the opposite effect when mediated via receptor H2. Where studied in detail, the effects of these mediators on C3 expression are tissue specific. Like several other acute-phase proteins, C3 is also regulated by hypoxia (87) in the cell line HepG2. Incubation of the cells in an atmosphere containing 1% O_2 leads to an increase in C3 mRNA of three- to five fold over normoxic conditions. Induction of C3 mRNA by hypoxia required new protein synthesis but otherwise little is known about any of the mechanisms accounting for this interesting effect.

For most of these mediators the precise level(s) of C3 regulation are not known but for IL-1/IL-6-regulated expression considerable effort has yielded information on the critical *cis* and *trans* elements governing transcription of this gene Detailed studies of the murine and human C3 promoter reveal a high degree of structural and functional similarity (64,65). Primer extension analyses of HepG2 and liver tissue C3 mRNA identified the transcriptional initiation site in the human (42,43) and murine (64,88) genes 61 bp and 56 bp upstream of the ATG initiation codon, respectively. TATA box motifs GATAAA in humans (43,65) and TATAAA in mice (88) are located at $-31/-26$ and $-30/-25$, respectively, from the transcription start site. This position was confirmed functionally by mutational analysis of the murine gene (64).

In the human C3 gene a genomic segment extending 199 bp upstream of the cap site was sufficient to drive constitutive expression of a reporter gene in transfected human hepatoma-derived Hep3B2 cells and 5' extension to -237 further increased transcription (65). A shorter 87 bp segment $(-127/-75)$ from this region dramatically enhanced constitutive transcription driven by a heterologous albumin promoter, suggesting cooperative effects between C3 and albumin *cis* elements, since minimal effects on the heterologous TK promoter were observed. Gel shift and footprinting analyses identified several sites of interaction with Hep3B2 nuclear proteins within a short region $(-134/-82)$ containing two C/EBPdirect repeats. Mutational analysis involving short sequence substitutions showed that the proximal repeat and an adjacent sequence are important for C3-promoted transcription (65,89). Antibody supershift analysis showed that the protein that constitutively binds to the repeat is C/EBPα (89). The minimal region conferring IL-1 and IL-6 responsiveness $(-114/-71)$ includes the proximal repeat and the adjacent sequence; the response is abolished by nucleotide substitutions within either site. However, nuclear extracts from untreated and IL-1 stimulated cells show identical footprinting patterns because one DNA-binding protein is substituted for the other. That is, IL-1-mediated upregulation results from replacement of constitutively bound C/EBPα by C/EBPδ (89). The response is coincident with a decrease in C/EBPα mRNA level and an increase of C/EBPδ mRNA. Enhancement of the IL-1 response by exogenous C/EBPδ and an increase in nuclear expression of C/EBPδ following stimulation established directly the relative importance of C/EBPδ in IL-1-regulated expression of the C3 gene (89). A more distal region $(-199/-156)$ for IL-1 and IL-6 upregulation was also identified functionally using 5' deletion mutants (65), but the precise *cis* elements and nuclear factors involved have not yet been isolated and characterized. In contrast to the proximal enhancer, deletion of this region does not affect constitutive expression

In the murine gene, a proximal 5'-flanking segment $(-110/+43)$, highly homologous to the human sequence (including the two C/EBP repeats and adjacent sequence), also confers high constitutive expression to a reporter gene when transfected in another hepatoma derived line, HepG2 (64). Addition of distal sequences $(-1457/-800$ and/or $-280/-110)$ markedly reduced transcription, indicating the presence of negative regulatory elements upstream of the enhancer. Footprinting analysis of the proximal 5' region identified a large protected area $(-69/-89)$ containing the proximal C/EBP repeat and an adjacent sequence similar to, but not competed by, the NFκB cognate site. Mutations at either site abrogated constitutive expression and enhancement of reporter gene expression driven by a heterologous promoter. As for the human gene, the C/EBP repeat was required for IL-1 and IL-6 responsiveness. However, mutation of the adjacent site did not affect the murine response to IL-6, although it may have altered IL-1-regulated expression. These observations require further study to separate mechanisms involved in IL-1 and IL-6 regulated C3 expression. That the two cytokines can separately upregulate C3 expression has been demonstrated in several hepatoma-derived cell lines including Hep3B, where IL-1 and IL-6 have an additive effect on C3 expression (90). Among several inbred mice, tissue and strain-specific differences in the effect of IL-1 on C3 expression have been observed (13). For example, in B10.P1 (H-2^u) IL-1 increases C3 expression in liver, spleen, kidney, lung, and peritoneal macrophages but the magnitude of the response varies considerably. In the B10.AKM (H-2^k) strain the direction of the effect of IL-1 on C3 expression in different tissues differs. That is, IL-1 upregulates C3 expression in kidney and lung but downregulates C3 expression in liver, spleen, and peritoneal macrophages. At least for the macrophage this is not a characteristic of all H-2^k strains because in AKR/ J (H-2^k) macrophages C3 expression is stimulated by IL-1. These observations are of particular interest in view of the recent discovery of an alternative promoter driving C3 expression at nonhepatocellular sites (see below).

Preliminary evidence has recently been obtained that identifies a tissue-specific promoter of full-length C3 expression that differs from the hepatocyte specific promoter. A strain of C3 null mice has been generated by replacing the hepatocyte specific C3 promoter with a neomycin resistance gene. No detectable C3 is expressed in liver as assessed by RNA blot protein biosynthethic studies or C3 in plasma, but expression of C3 mRNA in extrahepatic tissues such as lung and kidney is indistinguishable in the knockout and wild type (Colten et al., unpublished). Characterization of this heretofore unrecognized C3 promoter is underway.

Alternative C3 transcripts, shorter (4.2 and 1.8 Kb) than the 5.1 Kb liver C3 mRNA have been detected in murine T-cell- and macrophage-derived cell lines (91) coincident with the expression of a B-cell growth factor activity, termed alpha factor, initially found in macrophage cell line-conditioned media. Translation of size-fractionated RNA showed a correlation between the alternate C3 transcripts and alpha-type BCGF activity. The 5′ end of the 1.8 Kb mRNA has been localized within the sequences encoding the C3 alpha chain, 1.8 Kb upstream of the polyadenylation site of the liver transcript (92). An alternative promoter believed to be driving transcription of the 1.8 Kb C3 transcript was functionally identified within the preceding intron [intron 25 of the human gene (intron 8 of the alpha' chain)]. However, *cis* elements, cell-type specificity, and conditions for enhanced expression remain to be defined, since this promoter activity in myeloma cells required the addition of a heterologous enhancer to effect reporter gene transcription. It is not known if these alternative transcripts are expressed in vivo and which tissues or cell types produce them, but transfection of an expression plasmid encoding the 1.8 Kb transcript generated alpha-type BCGF activity (92), confirming the initial suggestion that the truncated C3 protein was functional.

B. Factor B

Constitutive and regulated expression of factor B (Bf), a key component of the alternative pathway of complement activation, are in many respects similar to that outlined for C3. That is, a broad array of proinflammatory cytokines (IL-1β, IL-6, TNFα, IFN-γ) (53,93–95) and hormones (96) increase Bf expression and several growth factors (IL-4, PDGF, EGF, and FGF) are counterregulatory (97,98). Hepatic and extrahepatic expression of Bf are likewise under independent control. The mechanisms governing tissue-specific regulation of Bf have been more fully elucidated than for C3 so far. These studies have demonstrated multiple mechanisms controlling Bf protein production as a function of tissue and cell type.

Human (99–101) and murine (102,103) factor B cDNAs have been cloned and sequenced. The Bf gene is located in the major histocompatibility complex gene cluster (HLA in humans, H-2 in mice), on chromosome 6 in humans (104,105) and 17 in mice

(106,107), immediately 3′ to the C2 gene (108,109). In *Xenopus* the Bf gene is duplicated (110) but in other species there is only a single copy/haploid. The human (111) and murine (103) Bf genes each consist of 18 exons spanning 6 Kb of genomic DNA and have exon/intron organizations similar to each other and to the human and mouse C2 genes (103,112). Similarities in the coding region generate 85% amino acid identity between human and mouse. The product of human Bf gene transcription is a ∼2.5 Kb mature mRNA (99). The sequence flanking the 5′ end of Bf, corresponding to the C2-Bf intergenic region, is also highly conserved between the two species (108,109). Analysis of this region allowed mapping of the transcriptional start sites for liver in the human (108) and mouse (109) genes at 129 bp and 105 bp, respectively, from the putative initiation codon, only a little more than 400 bp from the C2 polyadenylation site. TATA box elements, TATAAA (−28/−23) in humans and CATAAA (−31/−26) in mice, are present at ∼30 bp from the transcription start sites. An additional transcriptional initiation site for a tissue-specific long mRNA has been identified in the mouse gene, 302 bp upstream of the other start site (113).

Deletion analysis of the human Bf gene 5′-flanking region in transfected HepG2 cells showed the presence of a functional enhancer between −496 and −260 from the transcription start site (108). A binding site for HNF-4 was identified in this segment and functionally established in the corresponding murine sequence (114). The minimal promoter was localized between −260 and +20. Cell-type specificity of expression in the human hepatoma HepG2 requires both promoter and enhancer. Extension to −1050 further increased expression, suggesting the presence of other sequences for constitutively enhanced transcription of Bf that are within the C2 gene. Whether these are active in vivo is unknown.

Minimal boundaries for cytokine responses have been defined in the human gene for IFNγ (−496 to +19) (108,109), IL-6 (−496 to +20) (115), and IL-1 (−640 to −463) (109). Responsiveness to IL-1 correlates with a human DNA segment (−734 to −496) homologous to the mouse sequence where an NFκB site was shown to mediate the response (116). Evidence that posttranscriptional mechanisms also affect regulation of Bf by IL-1 and IL-6 have been obtained in studies of the hepatoma-derived Hep3B cell line (90,117). In contrast to IL-1 and IL-6 regulation, responsiveness of the human gene to IFNγ did not correlate well with sequences matching other IFN response consensus sequences (i.e., the response required an additional segment). For the murine gene, an analysis of reporter gene expression using a series of 5′ deletion constructs in fibroblasts showed a better correlation between IFNγ responsiveness and IFN response consensus elements (109). However, the amplitude of the response was less than with the human gene in HepG2. This difference might reflect the combined effects of constitutive and inducible enhancers in HepG2, which cannot be separated using 5′-deletion constructs. In other cell types IFN-γ regulation of Bf expression is complex because it is dependent on transcriptional and posttranscriptional mechanisms (118–120).

Robust extrahepatic factor B expression has been noted in several species and the kidney appears to be quantitatively the most important site (13,14,121,122). In murine kidney and intestine, two Bf transcripts (2.4 Kb and 2.7 Kb) are generated in about equal amounts. The long Bf mRNA is generated by transcription initiated at a site 302 bp upstream of the transcriptional start site that predominates in liver, where 95% of Bf mRNA is 2.4 Kb (113,121). Transcription of Bf long is driven by an upstream promoter that does not require any downstream sequences (114) and is independently regulated. For instance, LPS upregulates Bf short mRNA with little or no effect on Bf long (113).

On the other hand, constitutive and regulated expression of both transcripts in kidney and intestine vary considerably among different mouse strains (121). There is little or no difference in hepatic Bf as a function of these strain differences. The mechanisms accounting for this tissue specificity have recently been elucidated. Among different mouse strains polymorphisms in the 5′ flanking sequences correlated well with marked differences in constitutive extrahepatic factor B expression. For example, mice with H-2^d and H-2^u haplotypes express high amounts of Bf mRNA in kidney, whereas expression of kidney Bf mRNA in mice bearing H-2^f and H-2^z is low or undetectable. Six point substitutions and a six bp deletion in the C2-Bf intergenic region have been recognized as differentiating high- from low-expressor strains (121). However, nearly all of the differences in Bf expression can be accounted for by a single bp substitution T → C, three nucleotides from the upstream transcriptional initiation site. This substitution markedly decreases affinity for the DNA-binding protein HNF-4 (114) and decreases expression of a reporter gene in either human or murine hepatoma cells. Cotransfection of HNF-4 and Bf-reporter constructs into cells that do not express HNF-4 allowed a semiquantitative estimate of the change in affinity that results from the T → C substitution. This in turn suggested that differences in Bf expression among mouse strains were more profound in extrahepatic sites than in liver because at high HNF-4 input, for example, in hepatocytes this difference in affinity is largely overcome. Hence, constitutive transcription is driven rather well, even by the "low-affinity" promoter.

Posttranscriptional mechanisms further amplify the differences between hepatic and extrahepatic Bf expression For example, the constitutive expression of Bf long mRNA in kidney and intestine in an amount approximately equal to Bf short decreases the net amount of factor B protein produced under nonstimulated conditions. That is, the presence of the 5′ untranslated extension in Bf long results in a translation rate half of that programmed by Bf short in a cell-free system or in cells transfected with the corresponding cDNAs. Of the four putative translational start sites in this 5′ extension, deletion of only one accounted for the majority of the effect (122). Similar impairment of translation by out-of-frame AUG start sites has been observed for other genes (123–125) in which tissue specific alternative transcripts including C2 (see below) are generated.

C. C4 and C2

The genes encoding the C4 and C2 proteins of the classic complement activation pathway, like factor B, are within the class III region of the major histocompatibility complex. In contrast to the broad array of cytokines that regulate C3 and Bf expression, C4 and C2 are regulated following an acute-phase stimulus only by IFN-γ. In mice, one of the C4-like genes (Slp) is also under hormonal control but the mechanisms accounting for this interesting phenomenon are incompletely understood (see below).

Variable numbers of C4 genes are observed among different species. For example, only a single copy of C4 is found in the haploid guinea pig genome, whereas, although most humans have two highly homologous (>99%) C4 genes (C4A and C4B), many individuals with deletions or duplications of C4 have been recognized. Mice and cattle also generally express two C4 genes. The evolution of the gene duplications leading to this variability among species has apparently arisen at different independent times (126,127).

1. Complement Protein C4

In humans, the C4 genes reside within modules (RP, C4, 21 hydroxylase [CYP21] and gene X) that duplicate or delete as a unit (128–130). In the first module the C4A gene is nearly always 21 Kb whereas in the second module, the C4B gene is either 21 Kb or 14.6 Kb (131). This size polymorphism is due primarily to the presence of a retroposon, HERV-K (C4) (human endogenous retrovirus) in intron 9 (132) an element that is also observed in the C4 genes of several other non-human primates (133).

Each of the C4 genes encodes a ~5.5. Kb mRNA that programs translation of a 185 Kd prepro C4 protein (134,135) that undergoes extensive co- and postsynthetic processing, including cleavage of signal peptide, excision of two interchain linking peptides, generation of a critical thiolester bridge, glycosylation, sulfation and carboxyterminal modification by a metalloproteinase (136–139), and secretion with a half-time of 60–90 min (5). Sulfation of the C4 protein makes it more susceptible to activation by the C1 enzyme, thereby increasing its biological activity (139) Thus far, evidence for in vivo modulation of C4 function via sulfation or other posttranslational modifications has not been investigated but the possibility of any or several functioning as control points cannot be excluded.

Mechanisms governing constitutive and regulated C4 expression have been examined primarily in mice and, to a much lesser extent, in humans. The emphasis on murine C4 expression is the result of genetically determined variations in C4 plasma concentration among different inbred mouse strains (140) and the novel effect of testosterone in vivo on expression of the C4-like Slp gene in almost all mice (141). These large differences in C4 expression seemed 15 years ago to be ideal targets for studies that might have broad biological significance. Unfortunately, even today these mechanisms have not been fully elucidated and controversy surrounds many of the conclusions that have been derived.

Analysis of *cis* elements important in C4 expression have defined several important regulatory elements in this "TATA-less" gene required for basal expression (142,143). One of these, 3' to the transcriptional initiation site and two others including an E box motif and a consensus sequence for NF1 binding, have been evaluated with footprint and functional analytic methods (144,145). A typical IFN response element has not been identified. Some evidence has suggested that, in fact, the effect of IFN-γ on C4 expression is mediated posttranscriptionally (63). These studies of human C4 expression in monocyte- and hepatocyte-derived cell lines and in primary fibroblast cultures attempted to resolve some differences from earlier work that suggested variable upregulation (146–151) of C4 by IFN-γ in different cell types. A dose-dependent increase in C4 mRNA stability (baseline T 1/2 ~2 h to 5–12 h) was observed accompanied by a *decrease* in transcription rate in the presence of the cytokine (63) in the hepatoma-derived cell line HepG2. The observations by Mitchell et al. might help to explain an earlier finding that the magnitude and duration of the response of the C4A and C4B genes differ considerably (146). A direct comparison of mRNA stability of C4A and C4B would test this hypothesis. Some evidence has been advanced that posttranscriptional mechanisms also account for the 20-fold difference in expression of C4 among different mouse strains (152, 153). In this study of high- and low-expressor mouse strains minimal differences in nuclear C4 mRNA and marked differences in cytoplasmic C4 mRNA were observed. In vitro transcription (nuclear run on) and expression of chimeric reporter genes also suggested that the differences observed with these assays were substantially less than the 10–20-fold differences in C4 mRNA and protein that differentiate the high- and low-expressor mouse strains. Finally, in at least some C4 low strains (e.g., H-2^k), posttranscriptional mechanisms involving alternative splicing also contribute to the relatively low steady-state C4 level (153).

Sex-limited regulation of the C4-like Slp gene expression is complex, involving multiple mechanisms at several levels. The 5'-flanking sequences of C4 and Slp genes are highly conserved, including the position for transcriptional initiation (154). However, the Slp gene lacks a 31 bp segment at -1.6 Kb and a 60 bp segment at $--0.2$ Kb. Analysis of C4/Slp hybrid promoter constructs showed that sequences responsible for low-constitutive (in the absence of hormonal regulation) Slp gene expression reside in a 400 bp segment immediately 5′ of the transcriptional initiation site (155). This segment contains sequences that interact with a nuclear factor similar to that of the transcription factors H2TF1 and NFκB (156). The binding site GGGAAGTCCC at $-259/-250$ is absent from the Slp gene due to the missing 60 bp segment.

Slp expression is high in adult males or testosterone-injected females in most murine strains. A testosterone-responsive element was localized by DNAse hypersensitivity (157) and transfection experiments (158,159) about 2 Kb upstream of the Slp transcriptional start site, a region where C4 and Slp sequences start to diverge. Footprint analysis revealed a set of four protected areas centered at positions -2290, -2230, -2040, and -1955 (159). This complex enhancer appeared to be the 5′ LTR of an endogenous provirus inserted 2 Kb upstream of the Slp gene (160). A 160 bp fragment of this region confers testosterone responsiveness to a reporter gene in cells expressing the androgen receptor or in nonexpressing cells cotransfected with an expression plasmid for the receptor. The element at -2230 shows androgen receptor binding and confers some androgen responsiveness by itself (160). However, the same site can also interact with the glucocorticoid receptor and the specificity and high amplitude of the response to androgens requires adjacent accessory sequences (160,161). The view that sexual dimorphism in Slp expression directly results from transcriptional regulation by testosterone was challenged by in vivo studies of nuclear hepatic RNA (162) showing that growth hormone (GH), not testosterone, regulates hepatic Slp expression. Hypophysectomized males lose Slp expression, which can be restored by GH injection, but not by testosterone. In addition, androgen receptor-defective males initially Slp deficient have their hepatic Slp expression level induced to the level of control males after GH treatment. Although in these studies the effect of GH in hypophysectomized females is not analyzed, the slow (20 days) kinetics of testosterone induction in females compared to the time (6 days) for restoration by GH in hypophysectomized males suggests that testosterone acts indirectly through GH. Intermittent GH production seems to be the factor determining Slp production in the males, since transgenic animals of both sexes overexpressing GH constitutively and ubiquitously lack Slp expression (162).

Another point of controversy (163) was derived from relatively modest (five- to sixfold) differences in C4 and Slp promoter efficiency (155) and in androgen inducibility (159) observed in transient transfection experiments using relatively small promoters linked to reporter genes. These contrast with the dramatic differences (several hundred-fold) observed in vivo. Stable and transient transfection in L cells of various cosmid clones bearing the entire C4 or Slp gene including 1–18 Kb of 5′-flanking sequences, on the other hand, showed a very high expression of C4 transcript whereas Slp mRNA was undetectable (163). Nevertheless, in the same study, cell-free transcription assays using a series of 5′ deletion templates (up to -2.6 Kb) in nuclear extracts from L cells and liver (male and female) showed about equal transcription levels for C4 and Slp. It was suggested that sex-limited regulation of Slp may be exerted transcriptionally at a postinitiation level and/or that it requires nuclear structures lacking in cell-free assays.

A different approach to elucidating the mechanism of sex-limited expression of the Slp gene established sex-determined, gene-specific DNA methylation of homologous proximal sites in Slp and C4 genes (164); TTCCGGGC ($-124/-117$) in Slp and

TTCCCGGC (−123/−116) in C4. Mutational analysis in transfection assays suggested a role for this element in Slp expression. The site in Slp is markedly more methylated at −121 in female than in male liver genomic DNA, whereas the C4 element is comparatively poorly methylated in both sexes. Evidence for nuclear factor interaction was found with both forms of the Slp site but involving different proteins. In contrast, protein interaction was detected only on the methylated form of the C4 site and with a different binding pattern and tissue distribution than with either form of the Slp site. The nuclear factor that binds to the nonmethylated Slp element originally identified in the Cyp 2d-9 promoter was purified and sequenced (165) and is composed of GABPα and GABPβ1 transcription factors. Additional studies will no doubt resolve the confusion that remains in this interesting and important area.

2. Complement Protein C2

The 18 Kb C2 gene (112) is highly homologous to Bf in overall structure and sequence but differs in size because of the size of a few of its introns (103,111). One of these introns contains a retroposon of the SINE type (166) As for Bf, several start sites initiate transcription of C2 mRNA (167). At least three of these sites (−240, −180 and −27 from the translational start site) are utilized in liver but in U937 (a monocyte cell line) only the −27 site is active. Studies mapping these promoter regions and elucidation of the nucleoproteins that govern constitutive and regulated tissue-specific C2 expression have been few (168) but this would clearly be a fruitful area for further investigation. Termination of C2 transcription depends on binding of the myc-associated zinc finger (MAZ) protein (169,170) to a site of the C2 polyadenylation signal, apparently protecting the closely approximated Bf promoter from interference. As indicated above, however, important regulatory sequences in murine Bf for regulated expression reside upstream of the C2 polyadenylation signal. The functional significance of this observation has not yet been explored.

Additional transcripts are generated from the C2 gene by alternative splicing. Several of these transcripts have important effects on production of C2 protein. Volanakis and colleagues (171) have identified at least six transcripts arising from the single human C2 gene. Three of these acount for the previously recognized (172) C2 primary translation products of which only one (the largest) is secreted. The smallest of the three polypeptides is derived from a transcript (173) from which exon 2 and 3 are deleted (C2$\Delta_{2,3}$). Though it lacks a carboxyterminal segment of the signal peptide, the C2 polypeptide derived from this transcript enters and remains within the endoplasmic reticulum (ER). Its failure to exit this compartment may be the result of aberrant processing by the signal peptidase. The function of this retained protein is unknown. The intermediate size C2 polypeptide is apparently derived from another alternative transcript, a transcript from which exon 17 is deleted. The C2Δ_{17} is also retained in the ER and has a significant inhibitory effect on secretion of full-length C2 (174). All cells that express C2 produce the three size isoforms and each is upregulated by IFN-γ. An effect of C2Δ_{17} and possibly C2$\Delta_{2,3}$ on C2 secretion does not appear, therefore, to be modulated or tissue specific. Hence, additional study will be required to establish the importance of these findings. Murine C2 mRNA also undergoes alternative splicing to generate two mature transcripts (103). One encodes full-length C2; a 21 bp segment at the 5′ end of exon 14 that encodes a seven-residue sequence within the binding pocket of the C2 serine proteinase active site. This latter transcript is expressed in high amounts (50% of total C2 mRNA) in heart. The function of the protein encoded by this transcript and its fate are not known. Finally, alternative splicing is important in expression of many other complement genes (175–177).

V. OTHER COMPLEMENT GENES

Extensive studies of the structure and regulation of other complement genes have been published. The reader is referred to recent reviews and to the original articles (11,18,178–185). Unfortunately, space does not permit a discussion of either these or of the molecular genetic studies that have revealed from natural and experimental deficiencies insight into the molecular and cellular biology of complement gene expression.

REFERENCES

1. Tillett WS, Francis T Jr. Serological reactions in pneumonia with non-protein somatic fraction of Pneumococcus. J Exp Med 1930; 52:561–571.
2. Kushner I. The phenomenon of the acute phase response. Ann NY Acad Sci 1982; 389:39–48.
3. Ehrlich P, Morgenroth J. Ueber haemolysine. Berl Klin Wochenschr 1900; 37:453–458.
4. Alper CA, Raum D, Awdeh Z, Petersen BH, Taylor PD, Starzl TE. Studies of hepatic synthesis in vivo of plasma proteins including orosomucoid, transferrin, alpha-l-antitrypsin, C8 and factor B. Clin Immunol Immunopathol 1980; 16:84–89.
5. Morris KM, Aden DP, Knowles BB, Colten HR. Complement biosynthesis by the human hepatoma derived cell line HepG2. J Clin Invest 1982; 70:906–913.
6. Naughton MA, Botto M, Carter MJ, Alexander GJM, Goldman JM, Walport MJ. Extrahepatic secreted complement C3 contributes to circulating C3 levels in humans. J Immunol 1996; 156:3051–3056.
7. Thorbecke GJ, Hochwald GM, Van Furth LK, Muller-Eberhard HJ, Jacobson EB. Problems in determining the sites of synthesis of complement components. In: Wolstenholme GEW, Knight J, eds. Complement. London: Churchill, 1965:99–119.
8. Andrews PA, Finn JE, Lloyd CM, Zhou W, Mathieson PW, Sacks SH. Expression and tissue localization of donor-specific complement C3 synthesized in human renal allografts. Eur J Immunol 1995; 25:1087–1093.
9. Molmenti EP, Ziambaras T, Perlmutter DH. Evidence for an acute phase response in human intestinal epithelial cells. J Biol Chem 1993; 268:14116–14124.
10. Wurzner R, Joysey VC, Lachmann PJ. Complement component C7. Assessment of in vivo synthesis after liver transplantation reveals that hepatocytes do not synthesize the majority of human C7. J Immunol 1994; 152:4624–4629.
11. Colten HR. Extrahepatic complement gene expression. In: Erdei A, ed. New Aspects of Complement Structure and Function. Austin, TX: RG Landes Co., 1994:1–13.
12. Katz Y, Cole FS, Strunk RC. Synergism between interferon-gamma and lipopolysaccharide for synthesis of factor B, but not C2, in human fibroblasts. J Exp Med 1988; 167:1–14.
13. Falus A, Beuscher HU, Auerbach HS, Colten HR. Constitutive and IL-1 regulated murine complement gene expression is strain and tissue specific. J Immunol 1987; 138:856–860.
14. Passwell J, Schreiner GF, Nonaka M, Beuscher HU, Colten HR. Local extrahepatic expression of complement genes C3, factor B, C2 and C4 is increased in murine lupus nephritis. J Clin Invest 1988; 82:1676–1684.
15. Ahrenstedt O, Knutson L, Nilsson B, Nilsson-Ekdahl K, Odlind B, Hallgren R. Enhanced local production of complement components in the small intestines of patients with Crohn's disease. N Engl J Med 1990; 322:1345–1349.

16. Passwell JH, Schreiner GF, Wetsel RA, Colten HR. Complement gene expression in hepatic and extrahepatic tissues of NZB and NZBxW (F1) mouse strains. Immunology 1990; 71:290–294.

17. Ault BH, Colten HR. Cellular specificity of murine renal C3 expression in two models of inflammation. Immunology 1994; 81:655–660.

18. Volanakis JE. Transcriptional regulation of complement genes. Annu Rev Immunol 1995; 13:277–305.

19. Alper CA, Johnson AM, Birtch AG, Moore FD. Human C3: evidence for the liver as the primary site of synthesis. Science 1969; 163:286–288.

20. Saucan L, Palade GE. Membrane and secretory proteins are transported from the Golgi complex to the sinusoidal plasmalemma of hepatocytes by distinct vesicular carriers. J Cell Biol 1994; 125:733–741.

21. Boll W, Partin JS, Katz AI, Caplan MJ, Jamieson JD. Distinct pathways for basolateral targeting of membrane and secretory proteins in polarized epithelial cells. Proc Natl Acad Sci USA 1991; 88:8592–8596.

22. Green R, Shields D. Somatostatin discriminates between the intracellular pathways of secretory and membrane proteins. J Cell Biol 1984; 99:97–104.

23. Saucan L, Palade GE. Differential colchicine effects on the transport of membrane and secretory proteins in rat hepatocytes in vivo: bipolar secretion of albumin. Hepatology 1992; 15:714–721.

24. Bach S, Ruddy S, MacLaren JA, Austen KF. Electrophoretic polymorphism of the fourth component of human complement (C4) in paired maternal and fetal plasmas. Immunology 1971; 21:869–78.

25. Propp RP, Alper CA. C3 synthesis in the human fetus and lack of transplacental passage. Science 1968; 162:672–673.

26. Alper CA, Boenisch T, Watson L. Genetic polymorphism in human glycine-rich beta glycoprotein. J Exp Med 1972; 135:68–80.

27. Ruddy S, Klemperer MR, Rosen FS, Austen KF, Kumate J. Hereditary deficiency of the second component of complement (C2) in man. Immunology 1970; 18:943–954.

28. Adinolfi M, Gardner B, Wood CBS. Ontogenesis of two components of human complement: beta 1E and beta 1C-1A globulins. Nature 1968; 219:189–191.

29. Gitlin D, Biasucci A. Development of gamma-G, gamma-A, gamma-M, beta 1c, beta 1a′C′1 esterase inhibitor, ceruloplasmin, transferrin, hemopexin, haptoglobin, fibrinogen, plasminogen, alpha-1-antitrypsin, orosomucoid, beta-lipoprotein, alpha-2-macroglobulin and prealbumin in the human conceptus. J Clin Invest 1969; 48:1433–1446.

30. Colten HR. Ontogeny of the human complement system: in vitro biosynthesis of individual complement components by fetal tissue J Clin Invest 1972; 51:725–750.

31. Colten HR, Silverstein AM, Borsos T, Rapp HF. Ontogeny of the first component of sheep complement. Immunology 1968; 15:459–461.

32. Gorelick A, Oglesby T, Rashbaum W. Ontogeny of complement regulatory proteins: varied expression in different fetal tissues. Arthritis Rheumatol 1993; 36:S257.

33. Alpert SE, Auerbach HS, Cole FS, Colten HR. Macrophage maturation: differences in complement secretion by marrow, monocyte and tissue macrophages detected with an improved hemolytic plaque assay. J Immunol 1983; 130:102–107.

34. Cole FS, Auerbach HS, Goldberger G, Colten HR. Tissue specific pretranslational regulation of complement production in human mononuclear phagocytes. J Immunol 1985; 134:2610–2616.

35. Kohchi C, Oshima H, Mizuno D, Soma G. Expression of transcripts of complement components and their receptors during differentiation of embryonal carcinoma cell lines. Biochem Biophys Res 1992; 189:863–868.

36. Strunk RC, Whitehead AS, Cole FS. Pretranslational regulation of the synthesis of the third component of complement in human mononuclear phagocytes by the lipid A portion of lipopolysaccharide. J Clin Invest 1985; 76:985–990.

37. St John Sutton MB, Strunk RC, Cole FS. Regulation of the synthesis of the third component of complement and factor B in cord blood monocytes by lipopolysaccharide. J Immunol 1986; 136:1366–1372.

38. Strunk RC, Fleischer JA, Katz Y, Cole FS. Developmentally regulated effects of lipopolysaccharide on biosynthesis of the third component of complement and factor B in human fibroblasts and monocytes. Immunology 1994; 82:314–320.

39. Andoh A, Fujiyama Y, Bamba T, et al. Differential cytokine regulation of complement C3, C4 and factor B synthesis in human intestinal epithelial cell line, Caco-2. J Immunol 1993; 151:4239–4247.

40. Perlmutter DH, Colten HR. Complement: Molecular Genetics. In: Gallin JI, Goldstein IM, Snyderman R, eds. Inflammation, 2d ed. New York: Raven Press, 1992:81–102.

41. Simpson KL, Houlihan JM, Holmes CH. Complement regulatory proteins in early human fetal life: CD59, membrane cofactor protein (MCP) and decay-accelerating factor (DAF) are differentially expressed in the developing liver. Immunology 1993; 80:183–190.

42. Vik DP, Amiguet P, Moffat GJ, Fey M, Amiguet-Barras F, Wetsel RA, Tack BF. Structural features of the human C3 gene: intron/exon organization, transcriptional start site, and promoter region sequence. Biochemistry 1991; 30:1080–1085.

43. Fong KY, Botto M, Walport MJ, So AK. Genomic organization of human complement component C3. Genomics 1990; 7:579–586.

44. Brade V, Hall RE, Colten HR. Biosynthesis of pro-C3, a precursor of the third component of complement. J Exp Med 1977; 146:759–765.

45. de Bruijn MHL, Fey GH. Human complement component C3: cDNA coding sequence and derived primary structure. Proc Natl Acad Sci USA 1985; 82:708–712.

46. Misumi Y, Oda K, Fujiwara T, Takami N, Tashiro K, Ikehara Y. Functional expression of furin demonstrating its intracellular localization and endoprotease activity for processing of proalbumin and complement pro-C3. J Biol Chem 1991; 266:16954–16959.

47. Khan SA, Erickson BW. An equilibrium model of the metastable binding sites of alpha 2 macroglobulin and complement proteins C3 and C4. J Biol Chem 1982; 257:11864–11867.

48. Iijima M, Tobe T, Sakamoto T, Tomita M. Biosynthesis of the internal thioester bond of the third component of complement. J Biochem 1984; 96:1539–1546.

49. Pangburn MK. Spontaneous reformation of the intramolecular thioester in complement protein C3 and low temperature capture of a conformational intermediate capable of reformation. J Biol Chem 1992; 267:8584–8590.

50. Ramadori G, van Damme J, Rieder H, Meyer zum Buschenfelde KH. Interleukin 6, the third mediator of acute-phase reaction, modulates hepatic protein synthesis in human and mouse. Comparison with interleukin 1 beta and tumor necrosis factor -alpha. Eur J Immunol 1988; 18:1259–1264.

51. Katz Y, Revel M, Strunk RC. Interleukin 6 stimulates synthesis of complement proteins factor B and C3 in human skin fibroblasts. Eur J Immunol 1989; 19:983–988.

52. Baumann H, Prowse KR, Won KA, Marinkovic S, Jahreis GP. Regulation of acute phase protein genes by hepatocyte-stimulating factors, monokines and glucocorticoids. Tokai J Exp Clin Med 1988; 13:277–292.

53. Perlmutter DH, Dinarello CA, Punsal PI, Colten HR. Cachectin/tumor necrosis factor regulates hepatic acute-phase gene expression. J Clin Invest 1986; 78:1349–1354.

54. Barnum SR, Jones JL. Differential regulation of C3 gene expression in human astroglioma cells by interferon-gamma and interleukin-1 beta. Neurosci Lett 1995; 197:121–124.

55. Sacks SH, Zhou W, Pani A, Campbell RD, Martin J. Complement C3 gene expression and regulation in human glomerular epithelial cells. Immunology 1993; 79:348–354.

56. Sacks S, Zhou W, Campbell RD, Martin J. C3 and C4 gene expression and interferon-gamma-mediated regulation in human glomerular mesangial cells. Clin Exp Immunol 1993; 93:411–417.

57. Hill LD, Sun L, Leuschen MP, Zach TL. C3 synthesis by A549 alveolar epithelial cells is increased by interferon gamma and dexamethasone. Immunology 1993; 79:236–240.

58. Botto M, Lissandrini D, Sorio C, Walport MJ. Biosynthesis and secretion of complement component (C3) by activated human polymorphonuclear leukocytes. J Immunol 1992; 149:1348–1355.

59. Tsukamoto H, Nagasawa K, Yoshizawa S, Tada Y, Ueda A, Ueda Y, Niho Y. Synthesis and regulation of the fourth component of complement (C4) in the human monocytic cell line U937: comparison with that of the third component of complement (C3). Immunology 1992; 75:565–569.

60. Brooimans RA, van der Ark AA, Buurman WA, van Es LA, Daha MR. Differential regulation of complement factor H and C3 production in human umbilical vein endothelial cells by IFN-gamma and IL-1. J Immunol 1990; 144:3835–3840.

61. Lappin DF, Birnie GD, Whaley K. Modulation by interferons of the expression of monocyte complement genes. Biochem J 1990; 268:387–392.

62. Garnier G, Circolo A, Colten HR. TNF-alpha regulation of murine factor B and C3 differs in skin and kidney fibroblasts. Mol Immunol 1996 33(suppl 1):63 (abstr).

63. Mitchell TJ, Naughton M, Norsworthy P, Davies KA, Walport MJ, Morley BJ. IFN-gamma upregulates expression of the complement components C3 and C4 by stabilization of mRNA. J Immunol 1996; 156:4429–4434.

64. Kawamura N, Singer L, Wetsel RA, Colten HR. Cis- and trans-acting elements required for constitutive and cytokine-regulated expression of the mouse complement C3 gene. Biochem J 1992; 283:705–712.

65. Wilson DR, Juan TS, Wilde MD, Fey GH, Darlington GJ. A 58-base-pair region of the human C3 gene confers synergistic inducibility by interleukin-1 and interleukin-6. Mol Cell Biol 1990; 10:6181–6191.

66. Barnum SR, Jones JL. Transforming growth factor-beta 1 inhibits inflammatory cytokine-induced C3 gene expression in astrocytes. J Immunol 1994; 152:765–773.

67. Hogasen AK, Hestdal K, Abrahamsen TG. Granulocyte-macrophage colony stimulating factor, but not macrophage colony-stimulating factor, suppresses basal and lipopolysaccharide-stimulated complement factor production in human monocytes. J Immunol 1993; 151:3215–3224.

68. Andoh A, Fujiyama Y, Kitoh K, Niwakawa M, Hodohara K, Bamba T, Hosoda S. Macrophage colony-stimulating factor (M-CSF) enhances complement component C3 production by human monocytes/macrophages. Int J Hematol 1993; 57:53–59.

69. Lemercier C, Julen N, Coulpier M, Dauchel H, Ozanne D, Fontaine M, Ripoche J. Differential modulation by glucocorticoids of alternative complement protein secretion in cells of the monocyte/macrophage lineage. Eur J Immunol 1992; 22:909–915.

70. Lappin DF, Whaley K. Modulation of complement gene expression by glucocorticoids. Biochem J 1991; 280:117–123.

71. Coulpier M, Andreev S, Lemercier C, Dauchel H, Lees O, Fontaine M, Ripoche J. Activation of the endothelium by IL-1 alpha and glucocorticoids results in major increase of complement C3 and factor B production and generation of C3a. Clin Exp Immunol 1995; 101:142–149.

72. Zach TL, Hill LD, Herrman VA, Leuschen MP, Hostetter MK. Effect of glucocorticoids on C3 gene expression by the A549 human pulmonary epithelial cell line. J Immunol 1992; 148:3964–3969.

73. Strunk RS, Tashjian AH, Colten HR. Complement biosynthesis in vitro by rat hepatoma cell strains. J Immunol 1975; 114:331–335.

74. Churchill WH, Weintraub RM, Borsos T, Rapp HJ. Mouse complement: the effect of sex hormones and castration on two of the late-acting components. J Exp Med 1967; 125:657–672.

75. Isaacson KB, Coutifaris C, Garcia C-R, Lyttle CR Production and secretion of complement component 3 by endometriotic tissue. J Clin Endocrinol Metab 1989; 69:1003–1009.

76. Sundstrom SA, Komm BS, Xu Q. The stimulation of uterine complement component C3 gene expression by anti-estrogens. Endocrinology 1990; 126:1449–1456.

77. Sayegh RA, Tao XJ, Awwad JT, Isaacson KB. Localization of the expression of complement component 3 in the human endometrium by in situ hybridization. J Clin Endocrinol Metab 1996; 81:1641–1649.

78. McCoy R, Haviland DL, Molmenti EP, Ziambaras T, Wetsel RA, Perlmutter DH. N-formylpeptide and complement C5a receptors are expressed in liver cells and mediate hepatic acute phase gene regulation. J Exp Med 1995; 182:207–217.

79. Laufer J, Boichis H, Farzam N, Passwell JH. IgA and IgG immune complexes increase human macrophage C3 biosynthesis. Immunology 1995; 84:207–212.

80. Bajtay Z, Falus A, Erdei A, Gergely J. Fc gamma R-dependent regulation of the biosynthesis of complement C3 by murine macrophages: the modulatory effect of IL-6. Scand J Immunol 1992; 35:195–201.

81. Brooimans RA, Stegmann AP, van Dorp WT, van der Ark AA, van der Woude FJ, van Es LA, Daha MR. Interleukin 2 mediates stimulation of complement C3 biosynthesis in human proximal tubular epithelial cells. J Clin Invest 1991; 88:379–384.

82. Christian-Ritter KK, Hill LD, Hoie EB, Zach TL. Effect of interleukin-4 on the synthesis of the third component of complement by pulmonary epithelial cells. Am J Pathol 1994; 144:171–176.

83. Hogasen AK, Abrahamsen TG. Heparin suppresses lipopolysaccharide-induced monocyte production of several cytokines, but simultaneously stimulates C3 production. Thromb Res 1995; 80:179–184.

84. Hong MH, Jin CH, Sato T, Ishimi Y, Abe E, Suda T. Transcriptional regulation of the production of the third component of complement (C3) by 1 alpha, 25-dihydroxyvitamin D3 in mouse marrow-derived stromal cells (ST2) and primary osteoblastic cells. Endocrinology 1991; 129:2774–2779.

85. Sato T, Hong MH, Jin CH, Ishimi Y, Udagawa N, Shinki T, Abe E, Suda T. The specific production of the third component of complement by osteoblastic cells treated with 1 alpha,25-dihydroxyvitamin D3. FEBS Lett 1991; 285:21–24.

86. Falus A, Meretey K. Effect of histamine on the gene expression and secretion of complement components C2, factor B and C3 in murine macrophages-an opposite signal processing via H1 and H2 receptors. Mol Immunol 1988; 25:1093–1097.

87. Wenger RH, Rolfs A, Marti HH, Bauer C, Gassmann M. Hypoxia, a novel inducer of acute phase gene expression in a human hepatoma cell line. J Biol Chem 1995; 270:27865–27870.

88. Wiebauer K, Domdey H, Diggelmann F, Fey G. Isolation and analysis of genomic clones encoding the third component of mouse complement. Proc Natl Acad Sci USA 1982; 79:7077–7081.

89. Juan TS, Wilson DR, Wilde MD, Darlington GJ. Participation of the transcription factor C/EBP delta in the acute-phase regulation of the human gene for complement component C3. Proc Natl Acad Sci USA 1993; 90:2584–2588.

90. Jiang S-L, Lozanski G, Samols D, Kushner I. Induction of human serum amyloid A in Hep3B cells by IL-6 and IL-1 beta involves both transcriptional and post-transcriptional mechanisms. J Immunol 1995; 154:825–831.

91. Lernhardt W, Raschke WC, Melchers F. Alpha-type B cell growth factor and complement component C3: their possible structural relationship. Curr Top Microbiol Immunol 1986; 132:98–104.

92. Cahen-Kramer Y, Martensson IL, Melchers F. The structure of an alternate form of complement C3 that displays costimulatory growth factor activity for B lymphocytes. J Exp Med 1994; 180:2079–2088.

93. Perlmutter DH, Goldberger G, Dinarello CA, Mizel SB, Colten HR. Regulation of class III major histocompatibility complex gene products by interleukin-1. Science 1986; 232:850–852.

94. Perlmutter DH, Colten HR, Adams SP, May LT, Sehgal PB, Fallon RJ. A cytokine-selective defect in interleukin-1 beta mediated acute phase gene expression in a subclone of the human hepatoma cell line (HepG2). J Biol Chem 1989; 164:7669–7674.

95. Ripoche J, Mitchell A, Erdei A, Madin C, Moffatt B, Mokoena T, Gordon S, Sim RB. Interferon gamma induces synthesis of complement alternative pathway proteins by human endothelial cells in cultures. J Exp Med 1988; 168:1917–1922.

96. Hasty LA, Brockman WW, Lambris JD, Lyttle CR. Hormonal regulation of complement factor B in human endometrium. Am J Reprod Immunol 1993; 30:63–67.

97. Circolo A, Pierce GF, Katz Y, Strunk RC. Antiinflammtory effects of polypeptide growth factors. Platelet-derived growth factor, epidermal growth factor and fibroblast growth factor inhibit the cytokine-induced expression of the alternative complement pathway activator factor B in human fibroblasts. J Biol Chem 1990; 265:5066–5071.

98. Circolo A, Welgus HG, Pierce GF, Kramer J, Strunk RC. Differential regulation of the expression of proteinases/antiproteinases in fibroblasts. Effects of interleukin-1 and platelet-derived growth factor. J Biol Chem 1991; 266:12283–12288.

99. Woods DE, Markham AF, Ricker AT, Goldberger G, Colten HR. Isolation of cDNA clones for the human complement protein factor B, a class III major histocompatibility complex gene product. Proc Natl Acad Sci USA 1982; 79:5661–5665.

100. Mole JE, Anderson JK, Davison EA, Woods DE. Complete primary structure for the zymogen of human complement factor B. J Biol Chem 1984; 259:3407–3412.

101. Christie DL, Gagnon J, Porter RR. Partial sequence of human complement component factor B: novel type of serine protease. Proc Natl Acad Sci USA 1980; 77:4923–4927.

102. Sackstein R, Colten HR, Woods DE. Phylogenetic conservation of a class III major histocompatibility complex antigen, factor B. Isolation and nucleotide sequencing of mouse factor B cDNA clones. J Biol Chem 1983; 258:14693–14697

103. Ishikawa N, Nonaka M, Wetsel RA, Colten HR. Murine complement C2 and factor B genomic and cDNA cloning reveals different mechanisms for multiple transcripts of C2 and B. J Biol Chem 1990; 265:19040–19046.

104. Carroll MC, Campbell RD, Bentley DR, Porter RR. A molecular map of the human major histocompatibility complex class III region linking complement genes C4, C2 and factor B. Nature 1984; 307:237–241.

105. Dunham I, Sargent CA, Trowsdale J, Campbell RD. Molecular mapping of the human major histocompatibility complex by pulsed-field gel electrophoresis. Proc Natl Acad Sci USA 1987; 84:7237–7241.

106. Chaplin DD, Woods DE, Whitehead AS, Goldberger G, Colten HR, Seidman JG. Molecular map of the murine S region. Proc Natl Acad Sci USA 1983; 80:6947–6951.

107. Muller U, Stephan D, Philippsen P, Steinmetz M. Orientation and molecular map position of the complement genes in the mouse MHC. EMBO J 1987; 6:369–373.

108. Wu LC, Morley BJ, Campbell RD. Cell-specific expression of the human complement protein factor B gene: Evidence for the role of two distinct 5'-flanking elements. Cell 1987; 48:331–342.

109. Nonaka M, Gitlin JD, Colten HR. Regulation of human and murine complement: comparison of 5' structural and functional elements regulating human and murine complement factor B gene expression. Mol Cell Biochem 1989; 89:1–14.

110. Kato Y, Salter-Cid L, Flajnik MF, Namikawa C, Sasaki M, Nonaka M. Duplication of the MHC-linked xenopus complement factor B gene. Immunogenetics 1995; 42:196–203.

111. Campbell RD, Bentley DR. The structure and genetics of the C2 and factor B genes. Immunol Rev 1985; 87:19–37.

112. Ishii Y, Zhu ZB, Macon KJ, Volanakis JE. Structure of the human C2 gene. J Immunol 1993; 151:170–174.

113. Nonaka M, Ishikawa N, Passwell J, Natsuume-Sakai S, Colten HR. Tissue-specific initiation of murine complement factor B mRNA transcription. J Immunol 1989; 142:1377–1382.

114. Garnier G, Circolo A, Colten HR. Constitutive expression of murine complement factor B gene is regulated by the interaction of its upstream promoter with hepatocyte nuclear factor 4. J Biol Chem 1996; 271:30205–30211.

115. Morrone G, Ciliberto G, Oliviero S, Arcone R, Dente L, Content J, Cortese R. Recombinant interleukin 6 regulates the transcriptional activation of a set of human acute phase genes. J Biol Chem 1988; 263:12554–12558.

116. Nonaka M, Huang ZM. Interleukin-1-mediated enhancement of mouse factor B gene expression via NF kappa B-like hepatoma nuclear factor. Mol Cell Biol 1990; 10:6283–6289.

117. Jiang S-L, Samols D, Rzewnicki D, Macintyre SS, Greber I, Sipe J, Kushner I. Kinetic modeling and mathematical analysis indicate that acute phase gene expression in Hep3B cells is regulated by both transcriptional and posttranscriptional mechanisms. J Clin Invest 1995; 95:1253–1261.

118. Lappin DF, Birnie GD, Whaley K. Interferon-mediated transcriptional and post-transcriptional modulation of complement gene expression in human monocytes. Eur J Biochem 1990; 194:177–184.

119. Lappin DF, Guc D, Hill A, McShane T, Whaley K. Effect of interferon-gamma on complement gene expression in different cell types. Biochem J 1992; 281:437–442.

120. Lappin DF, Guc D, Hill A, McShane T, Whaley K. Effect of interferon-gamma on complement gene expression in different cell types. Biochem J 1992; 281:437–442.

121. Garnier G, Ault B, Kramer M, Colten HR. cis and trans elements differ among mouse strains with high and low extrahepatic complement factor B gene expression. J Exp Med 1992; 175:471–479.

122. Garnier G, Circolo A, Colten HR. Translational regulation of murine complement factor B alternative transcripts by upstream AUG codons. J Immunol 1995; 154:3275–3282.

123. Kew D, Jin DF, Kim F, Laddis T, Kilpatrick DL. Translational status of proenkephalin mRNA in the rat reproductive system. Mol Endocrinol 1989; 3:1191–1196.

124. Iwaki A, Iwaki T, Goldman JE, Liem RKH. Multiple mRNAs of rat brain alpha-crystallin B chain result from alternative transcriptional initiation. J Biol Chem 1990; 265:22197–22203.

125. Teruya JH, Kutsunai SY, Spear DH, Edwards PA, Clarke CF. Testis-specific transcription initiation sites of rat farnesyl pyrophosphate synthetase mRNA. Mol Cell Biol 1990; 10:2315–2326.

126. Tosi M, Levi-Strauss M, Georgatsou E, Amor M, Meo T. Duplications of complement and non-complement genes of the H-2S region: evolutionary aspects of the C4 isotypes and molecular analysis of their expression variants. Immunol Rev 1985; 87:151–183.

127. Gitelman SE, Bristow J, Miller WL. Mechanism and consequences of the duplication of the human C4/P450c21/gene X locus Mol Cell Biol 1992; 12:2124–2134.

128. Shen LM, Wu LC, Sanlioglu S, Chen R, Mendoza AR, Dangel A, Carroll MC, Zipf W, Yu CY. Structure and genetics of the partially duplicated gene RP located immediately upstream of the complement C4A and C4B genes in the HLA class III region. J Biol Chem 1994; 269:8466–8476.

129. Morel Y, Bristow J, Gitelman SE, Miller WL. Transcript encoded on the opposite strand of the human steroid 21-hydroxylase/complement component C4 gene locus. Proc Natl Acad Sci 1989; 86:6582–6586.

130. Bristow J, Tee M, Gitelman S, Mellon S, Miller W. Tenascin-X: a novel cellular matrix protein encoded by the human XB gene overlapping P450c21B. J Cell Biol 1993; 122:265–278.

131. Carroll MC, Belt T, Palsdottir A, Porter RR. Structure and organization of the C4 genes. Philos Trans R Soc Lond [Biol] 1984; 306:379–388.

132. Dangel AW, Mendoza AR, Baker BJ, Daniel CM, Carroll MC, Wu L-C, Yu CY. The dichotomous size variation of human complement C4 genes is mediated by a novel family of endogenous retroviruses, which also establishes species-specific genomic patterns among Old World primates. Immunogenetics 1994; 40:425–436.

133. Dangel AW, Baker BJ, Mendoza AR, Yu CY. Complement component C4gene intron 9 as a phylogenetic marker for primates: long terminal repeats of the endogenous retrovirus ERV-K(C4) are a molecular clock of evolution. Immunogenetics 1995; 42:41–52.

134. Hall RE, Colten HR. Cell-free synthesis of the fourth component of guinea pig complement (C4): identification of a precursor of serum C4 (pro-C4). Proc Natl Acad Sci USA 1977; 74:1707–1710.

135. Whitehead AS, Goldberger G, Woods DE, Markham AF, Colten HR. Use of a cDNA clone for the fourth component of human complement for analysis of a genetic deficiency of C4 in guinea pig. Proc Natl Acad Sci USA 1983; 80:5387–5391.

136. Goldberger G, Colten HR. Precursor complement protein (pro-C4) is converted in vitro to native C4 by plasmin. Nature Lond 1980; 286:514–516.

137. Karp DR. Post-translational modification of the fourth component of complement. Sulfation of the alpha chain. J Biol Chem 1983; 258:12745–12748.

138. Karp DR. Post-translational modification of the fourth component of complement: effect of tunicamycin and amino acid analogs on the formation of the internal thiol ester and disulfide bonds. J Biol Chem 1983; 258:14490–14495.

139. Hortin GL, Farries TC, Graham JP, Atkinson JP. Sulfation of tyrosine residues increases activity of the fourth component of complement. Proc Natl Acad Sci USA 1989; 86:1338–1342.

140. Shreffler DC, David CS. The H-2 major histocompatibility complex and the I immune response region: genetic variation, function and organization. Adv Immunol 1975; 20:125–195.

141. Passmore HC, Shreffler DC. A sex-limited serum protein variant in the mouse: hormonal control of phenotypic expression. Biochem Genet 1971; 5:201–209.

142. Miyagoe Y, Galibert MD, Georgatsou E, Fourel G, Meo T. Promoter elements of the mouse complement C4 gene critical for transcription activation and start site location. J Biol Chem 1994; 269: 8268–8279.

143. Vaishnaw AK, Hargreaves R, Campbell RD, Morley BJ, Walport MJ. Dnase I hypersensitivity mapping and promoter polymorphism analysis of human C4. Immunogenetics 1995; 41:354–358.

144. Huang ZM, Zeng JH, Mo RR, Takahashi M, Nonaka M. Differential binding of NF-1-like nuclear factor to the mouse C4 and SLP promoters as a major determinant of basal transcriptional activity. Mol Immunol 1993; 30(Suppl 1):18 (abstr).

145. Galibert MD, Miyagoe Y, Meo T. E-box activator of the C4 promoter is related to but distinct from the transcription factor upstream stimulating factor. J Immunol 1993; 151:6099–6109.

146. Miura N, Prentice HL, Schneider PM, Perlmutter DH. Synthesis and regulation of the two human C4 genes in stable transfected mouse fibroblasts. J Biol Chem 1987; 262:7298–7305.

147. Kulics J, Circolo A, Strunk RC, Colten HR. Regulation of synthesis of complement component C4 in human fibroblasts: cell- and gene-specific effects of cytokines and lipopolysaccharide. Immunology 1994; 82:509–515.

148. Kulics J, Colten HR, Perlmutter DH. Counter-regulatory effects of interferon-gamma and endotoxin on expression of the human C4 genes. J Clin Invest 1990; 85:943–949.

149. Andoh A, Fujiyama Y, Sumiyoshi K, Hodohara K, Okabe H, Ochi Y, Bamba T, Brown WR. Modulation of complement C3, C4 and factor B production in human intestinal epithelial cells: differential effects of TNF-alpha, IFN-gamma and IL-4. Pathophysiology 1995; 2:251–259.

150. Zhou W, Campbell RD, Martin J, Sacks SH. Interferon-gamma regulation of C4 gene expression in cultured human glomerular epithelial cells. Eur J Immunol 1993; 23:2477–2481.

151. Seelen MA, Brooimans RA, van der Woude FJ, van Es LA, Daha MR. IFN-gamma mediates stimulation of complement C4 biosynthesis in human proximal tubular epithelial cells. Kidney Intl 1993; 44:50–57.

152. Nakayama K, Pattanakitsakul S, Yokoyama S, Kimur H, Nonaka M, Takahashi M. Post-transcriptional regulation of complement C4 in low C4-producing strains of mouse. Immunogenetics 1990; 31:361–367.

153. Zheng J-H, Takahashi M, Nonaka M. Tissue-specific RNA processing for the complement C4 gene transcript in the H-2^x mouse strain. Immunogenetics 1993; 37:390–393.

154. Nonaka M, Kimura H, Yeul YD, Yokoyama S, Nakayama K, Takahashi M. Identification of the 5'-flanking regulatory region responsible for the difference in transcriptional control between mouse complement C4 and Slp genes. Proc Natl Acad Sci USA 1986; 83:7883–7887.

155. Yu DY, Nonaka M, Takahashi M. Mapping of the transcriptional regulatory domains responsible for the difference in the promoter activity between mouse C4 and Slp (sex-limited protein) genes. J Immunol 1988; 141:4381–4387.

156. Yu DY, Huang ZM, Murakami S, Takahashi M, Nonaka M. Specific binding of a hepatoma nuclear factor to the NF kappa B/H2TF1 recognition motif found in the C4 promoter, but not in the Slp promoter. J Immunol 1989; 143:2395–2400.

157. Hemenway C, Robins DM. Dnase I-hypersensitive sites associated with expression and hormonal regulation of mouse C4 and Slp genes. Proc Natl Acad Sci USA 1987; 84:4816–4820.

158. Stavenhagen J, Loreni F, Hemenway C, Kalff M, Robins DM. Molecular genetics of androgen-dependent and independent expression of mouse sex-limited protein. Mol Cell Biol 1987; 7:1716–1724.

159. Loreni F, Stavenhagen J, Kalff M, Robins DM. A complex androgen-responsive enhancer resides 2 kilobases upstream of the mouse Slp gene. Mol Cell Biol 1988; 8:2350–2360.

160. Stavenhagen JB, Robins DM. An ancient provirus has imposed androgen regulation on the adjacent mouse sex-limited protein gene. Cell 1988; 55:247–254.

161. Adler AJ, Danielsen M, Robins DM. Androgen-specific gene activation via a consensus glucocorticoid response element is determined by interaction with nonreceptor factors. Proc Natl Acad Sci USA 1992; 89:11660–11663.

162. Georgatsou E, Bourgarel P, Meo T. Male-specific expression of mouse sex-limited protein requires growth hormone, not testosterone. Proc Natl Acad Sci USA 1993; 90:3626–3630.

163. Miyagoe Y, Georgatsou E, Varin-Blank N, Meo T. The androgen-dependent C4-Slp gene is driven by a constitutively competent promoter. Proc Natl Acad Sci USA 1993; 90:5786–5790.

164. Yokomori N, Moore R, Negishi M. Sexually dimorphic DNA demethylation in the promoter of the Slp (sex-limited protein) gene in mouse liver. Proc Natl Acad Sci USA 1995; 92:1302–1306.

165. Yokomori N, Kobayashi R, Moore R, Sueyoshi T, Negishi M. A DNA methylation site in the male-specific P450 (Cyp 2d-9) promoter and binding of the heteromeric transcription factor GABP. Mol Cell Biol 1995; 15:5355–5362.

166. Zhu ZB, Hsieh SL, Bentley DR, Campbell RD, Volanakis JE. A variable number of tandem repeats (VNTR) locus within the human complement C2 gene is associated with a retroposon derived from a human endogenous retrovirus. J Exp Med 1992; 175:1783–1787.

167. Horiuchi T, Macon KJ, Kidd VJ, Volanakis JE. Translational regulation of complement protein C2 expression by differential utilization of the 5' untranslated region of mRNA. J Biol Chem 1990; 265:6521–6524.

168. Sullivan KE, Wu LC, Campbell RD, Valle D, Winkelstein JA. Transcriptional regulation of the gene for the second component of human complement: promoter analysis. Eur J Immunol 1994; 24:393–400.

169. Ashfield R, Enriquez-Harris P, Proudfoot NJ. Transcriptional termination between the closely linked human complement genes C2 and factor B: common termination factor for C2 and c-myc? EMBO J 1991; 10:4197–4207.

170. Bossone SA, Asselin C, Patel AJ, Marcu KB. MAZ, a zinc finger protein, binds to c-MYC and C2 gene sequences regulating transcriptional initiation and termination. Proc Natl Acad Sci USA 1992; 89:7452–7456.

171. Cheng J, Volanakis JE. Alternatively spliced transcripts of the human complement C2 gene. J Immunol 1994; 152:1774–1782.

172. Perlmutter DH, Cole FS, Goldberger G, Colten HR. Distinct primary translation products from human liver mRNA give rise to secreted and cell-associateed forms of complement protein C2. J Biol Chem 1984; 259:10380–10385.

173. Akama H, Johnson CA, Colten HR. Human complement protein C2. Alternative splicing generates templates for secreted and intracellular C2 proteins. J Biol Chem 1995; 270:2674–2678.

174. Tsukamoto H, Tousson A, Marchase RB, Volanakis JE. Down-regulation of secretion of human complement component C2 by the product of an alternatively spliced C2 messenger RNA. J Immunol 1996; 156:4901–4908.

175. Hara T, Suzuki Y, Semba T, Hatanaka M, Matsumoto M, Seya T. High expression of membrane cofactor protein of complement (CD46) in human leukemia cell lines: implication of an alternatively spliced form containing the STA domain in CD46 upregulation. Scand J Immunol 1995; 42:581–590.

176. Nonaka M, Miwa T, Okada N, Nonaka M, Okada H. Multiple isoforms of guinea pig decay-accelerating factor (DAF) generated by alternative splicing. J Immunol 1995; 155:3037–3048.

177. Liszewski MK, Tedja I, Atkinson JP. Membrane cofactor protein (CD46) of complement. Processing differences related to alternatively spliced cytoplasmic domains. J Biol Chem 1994; 269:10776–10779.

178. Barnum SR. Complement biosynthesis in the central nervous system [Review]. Crit Rev Oral Biol 1995; 6:132–146.

179. Wetsel RA. Structure, function and cellular expression of complement anaphylatoxin receptors [Review]. Curr Opin Immunol 1995; 7:48–53.

180. Gerard C, Gerard NP. C5A anaphylatoxin and its seven transmembrane-segment receptor [Review]. Annu Rev Immunol 1994; 12:775–808.

181. Gulati P, Lemercier C, Guc D, Lappin D, Whaley K. Regulatrion of the synthesis of C1 subcomponents and C1-inhibitor. Behring Inst Mitt 1993; 93:196–203.

182. Hasty LA, Lambris JD, Lessey BA, Pruksananonda K, Lyttle CR. Hormonal regulation of complement components and receptors throughout the menstrual cycle. Am J Obstet Gynecol 1994; 170:168–175.

183. Cui W, Hourcade D, Post T, Greenlund AC, Atkinson JP, Kumar V. Characterization of the promoter region of the membrane cofactor protein (CD46) gene of the human complement system and comparison to a membrane cofactor protein-like genetic element. J Immunol 1993; 151:4137–4146.

184. Whaley K, Guc D, Gulati P, Lappin D Synthesis of complement components by synovial membrane [Review]. Immunopharmacology 1992; 24:83–89.

185. Thomas DJ, Lublin DM. Identification of 5′-flanking regions affecting the expression of the human decay accelerating factor gene and their role in tissue-specific expression. J Immunol 1993; 1560:151–160.

186. Ross GD, Medof ME. Membrane complement receptors specific for bound fragments of C3. Adv Immunol 1985; 37:217–267.

187. Vedeler CA, Scarpini E, Beretta S, Doronzo R, Matre R. The ontogenesis of Fc gamma receptors and complement receptor CR1 in human peripheral nerve. Acta Neuropathol 1990; 80:35–40.

188. Kubota Y, Gaither TA, Cason J, O'Shea JJ, Lawley TJ. Characterization of the C3 receptor induced by herpes simplex virus type 1 infection of human epidermal, endothelial and A431 cells. J Immunol 1987; 138:1137–1142.

189. Todd RF, Schlossman SF. Differential antigens on human monocytes and macrophages defined by monocloncal antibodies. In: Volkman A, ed. Mononuclear Phagocyte Biology. New York: Marcel Dekker, 1984: 129–149.

190. LeBien TW, Kersey JH. A monoclonal antibody (TA-1) reactive with human T lymphocytes and monocytes. J Immunol 1980; 125:2208–2214.

191. Haviland DL, McCoy RL, Whitehead WT, Akama H, Molmenti EP, Brown A, Haviland JC, Parks WC, Perlmutter DH, Wetsel RA. Cellular expression of the C5a anaphylatoxin receptor (C5aR): demonstration of C5aR on nonmyeloid cells of the liver and lung. J Immunol 1995; 154:1861–1869.

192. Nicholson-Weller A, Burge J, Fearon DT, Weller PF, Austen KF. Isolation of a human erythrocyte membrane glycoprotein with activity for C3 convertases of the complement system. J Immunol 1982; 129:184–189.

193. Pangburn MK, Schreiber RD, Muller-Eberhard HJ. Deficiency of an erythrocyte membrane protein with complement regulatory activity in paroxysmal nocturnal hemoglobinuria. Proc Natl Acad Sci USA 1983; 80:56430–5434.

194. Kinoshita T, Medof ME, Silber R, Nussenzweig V. Distribution of decay accelerating factor in the peripheral blood of normal individuals and patients with paroxysmal nocturnal hemoglobinuria. J Exp Med 1985; 162:75–92.

195. Nicholson-Weller A, March JP, Rosen CE, Spicer DB, Austen KF. Surface membrane expression by human blood leukocytes and platelets of decay accelerating factor, a regulatory protein of the complement system. Blood 1985; 65:1237–1244.

196. Holmes CH, Simpson KL, Wainwright SD, Tate CG, Houlihan JM, Sawyer IH, Rogers IP, Spring FA, Anstee DJ, Tanner MJ. Preferential expression of complement regulatory protein decay accelerating factor at the fetomaternal interface during human pregnancy. J Immunol 1990; 144:3099–3105.

197. Asch AS, Kinoshita T, Jaffe EA, Nussenzweig V. Decay accelerating factor is present on cultured human umbilical vein endothelial cells. J Exp Med 1986; 163:221–226.

198. Medof ME, Walter EI, Rutgers JL, Knowles DM, Nussenzweig V. Identification of the complement decay accelerating factor on epithelium and glandular cells and in body fluids. J Exp Med 1987; 165:848–864.

199. Jensen TS, Bjorge L, Wollen AL, Ulstein M. Identification of the complement regulatory proteins CD46, CD55, and CD59 in human fallopian tube, endometrium, and cervical mucosa and secretion. Am J Reprod Immunol 1995; 34:1–9.

200. Cole JL, Housley GA, Dykman TR, MacDermott RP, Atkinson JP. Identification of an additional class of C3-binding membrane proteins of human peripheral blood leukocytes and cell lines. Proc Natl Acad Sci USA 1985; 82:856–863.

201. Seya T, Ballard LL, Bora NS, Kumar V, Cui W, Atkinson JP. Distribution of membrane cofactor protein of complement on human peripheral blood cells. An altered form is found on granulocytes. Eur J Immunol 1988; 18:1289–1294.

202. McNearney T, Ballard L, Seya T, Atkinson JP. Membrane cofactor protein of complement is present on human fibroblasts, epithelial and endothelial cells. J Clin Invest 1989; 84:538–545.

203. McIntyre JA, Faulk WP, Verhulst SJ, Colliver JA. Human trophoblast-lymphocyte cross-reactive (TLX) antigens define a new alloantigen system. Science 1983; 222:1135–1137.

204. Sugita Y, Nakano Y, Tomita M. Isolation from human erythrocytes of a new membrane protein which inhibits the formation of complement transmembrane channels. J Biochem 1988; 104:633–637.

205. Rollins SA, Sims PJ. The complement inhibitory activity of CD59 resides in its capacity to block incorporation of C9 into membrane C5b-9-1. J Immunol 1990; 144:3478–3483.

206. Nose M, Katoh M, Okada N, Kyogoku M, Okada H. Tissue distribution of HRF20, a novel factor preventing the membrane attack of homologous complement and its predominant expression on endothelial cells in vivo. Immunology 1990; 70:145–149.

207. Sims PJ, Rollins SA, Wiedmer T. Regulatory control of complement on blood platelets. Modulation of platelet procoagulant responses by a membrane inhibitor of the C5b-9 complex. J Biol Chem 1989; 264:19228–19235.

208. Brauer RB, Baldwin WM 3rd, Wang D, Horwitz LR, Hess AD, Klein AS, Sanfilippo F. Hepatic and extrahepatic biosynthesis of complement factor C6 in the rat. J Immunol 1994; 153:3168–3176.

209. Armbrust T, Schwogler S, Zohrens G, Ramadori G. C1 esterase inhibitor gene expression in rat Kupffer cells, peritoneal macrophages and blood monocytes: modulation by interferon gamma. J Exp Med 1993; 178:373–380.

210. McPhaden AR, Whaley K. Complement biosynthesis by mononuclear phagocytes [Review[. Immunol Res 1993; 12:213–232.

211. Schwaeble W, Dippold WG, Schafer MK, Pohla H, Jonas D, Luttig B, Weihe E, Huemer HP, Dierich MP, Reid KB. Properdin, a positive regulator of complement activation, is expressed in human T cell lines and peripheral blood T cells J Immunol 1993; 151:2521–2528.

212. Reed W, Roubey RA, Dalzell JG, Matteucci BM, Myones BL, Hunt SW 3d, Kolb WP, Ross GD. Synthesis of complement component C5 by human B and T lymphoblastoid cell lines. Immunogenetics 1990; 31:145–151.

213. Hogasen AK, Wurzner R, Abrahamsen TG, Dierich MP. Human polymorphonuclear leukocytes store large amounts of terminal complement components C7 and C6, which may be released on stimulation. J Immunol 1995; 154:4734–4740.

214. Timmerman JJ, Verweij CL, van Gijlswijk-Janssen DJ, van der Woude FJ, van Es LA, Daha MR. Cytokine-regulated production of the major histocompatibility complex class III encoded complement proteins factor B and C4 by human glomerular mesangial cells. Hum Immunol 1995; 43:19–28.

215. Moutabarrik A, Nakanishi I, Matsumoto M, Zaid D, Seya T. Human glomerular epithelial cells synthesize and secrete the third component of complement. Nephron 1995; 70:55–61.

216. Strunk RC, Eidlen DM, Mason RJ. Pulmonary alveolar type II epithelial cells synthesize and secrete proteins of the classical and alternative complement pathways. J Clin Invest 1988; 81:1419–1426.

217. Choy LN, Rosen BS, Spiegelman BM. Adipsin and an endogenous pathway of complement from adipose cells. J Biol Chem 1992; 267:12736–12741.

218. Guc D, Gulati P, Lemercier C, Lappin D, Birnie GD, Whaley K. Expression of the components and regulatory proteins of the alternative complement pathway and the membrane attack complex in normal and diseased synovium. Rheumatol Int 1993; 13:139–146.

219. Legoedec J, Gasque P, Jeanne JF, Fontaine M. Expression of the complement alternative pathway by human myoblasts in vitro: biosynthesis of C3, factor B, factor H and factor I. Eur J Immunol 1995; 25:3460–3466.

220. Lang TJ, Shin ML. Activation of the alternative complement pathway and production of factor H by skeletal myotubes. J Neuroimmunol 1993; 44:185–192.

11

Characterization of Complement Anaphylatoxins and Their Biological Responses

JULIA A. EMBER, MARK A. JAGELS, and TONY E. HUGLI
The Scripps Research Institute, La Jolla, California

I. INTRODUCTION

Elucidating the physiological role of complement (C) components in immune and inflammatory responses has a long and rich history. Recent development of more sophisticated molecular and biochemical technologies has made it possible to explore and identify new biological phenomena and confirm known functions associated with the various complement factors. It has been an exciting time to observe the recent discovery of novel functions and actions being attributed to components derived from this complex humoral system, whose role in host defense gains stature with each new finding. Biological functions, such as the involvement of C3 and C4 products (i.e., C3b and C4b) in opsonization and phagocytosis and promotion of cellular lytic and activation events by a complex composed of the "late" C5b to C9 components, are now well documented in the literature. Many of the mechanisms underlying these functions have also been described in detail thanks to the "molecular revolution" of the past decade.

A similar list of associated functions have been assigned over the years to the smaller bioactive fragments released from C3, C4, and C5 during complement activation, and these fragments are known as the anaphylatoxins. The term *anaphylatoxin* was coined nearly 90 years ago by Friedberger (1). It is a descriptive label for an activity found in complement-activated serum, that produced rapid anaphylactoid-like death when injected into laboratory animals. It has remained the generic name for molecules now chemically identified as C3a, C4a, and C5a. We will use the chemical names primarily to differentiate these factors from one another. Since the anaphylatoxins are derived from three components of the complement system that are genetically and structurally related, it is not surprising that chemical similarities exist between C3a, C4a, and C5a, and yet there are significant structural differences that result in these three factors having unique functional characteristics. One must understand the chemical nature of these relatively small factors to appreciate their functional diversity and to be able to elucidate the mechanisms of action for the numerous and sometimes unique cellular responses elicited by each of these molecules.

As a group, the anaphylatoxins are humoral mediators mainly recognized for their proinflammatory and immunoregulatory functions that act as bioactive sentinels in host defense. It was known by the late 1960s that these factors possessed a potent ability to contract smooth muscle tissues and to both enhance vascular permeability and recruit white blood cells when injected into the skin of animals (2,3) or humans (4–6). Many other actions have been attributed to one or another of the anaphylatoxins, including a host of cellular effects that imply important physiological functions, as well as a number of tissue-specific effects. However, assignment of specific physiological or pathophysiological effects attributed solely to the anaphylatoxins remains difficult because a multitude of mediators have overlapping functions that exist to protect the host. The biological consequences of these mediators are highly redundant and complex. Therefore, even total removal or inhibition of a given mediator does not necessarily alter the *in vivo* condition or response. This means that mediators as a group may regulate or promote an essential function, but elimination of a single member of that group may not alter a physiological response. Experimental models must be carefully chosen in order to assign roles correctly to individual mediators, a concept rapidly being recognized by investigators using "knockout" animals as an approach to understanding biology.

There is renewed excitement and interest in the area of anaphylatoxin research because of recent advances in the field. New molecular data has been recently provided, such as cloning of the C5a receptor (C5aR) (7,8) and the C3a receptor (C3aR) (9–11). For example, we learned that the C3aR has novel and unique structural characteristics compared with most other G-protein coupled receptors, including the C5aR. Recent evidence that C5a plays an important role in immune injury in the lung (12–14) and in postischemic vascular and tissue injury (15–17) supports the contention that regulation of selected complement activation products may be of therapeutic value. The discovery that both C3a and C5a receptors may exist on numerous cell types other than circulating white cells, such as hepatocytes, lung epithelial cells (18), endothelial cells (19), or the astrocytes and microglial cells in brain tissue (20,21), has serious implications for anaphylatoxins playing a role in vascular, pulmonary, and degenerative neurological diseases. As we learn more about the impact of complement fragments on cellular and tissue functions, it will be apparent when and to what extent these humoral factors integrate into normal host defense mechanisms vs. promoting or exacerbating pathological conditions.

This chapter will describe the chemical nature of the anaphylatoxins and their receptors, as well as the diverse biology associated with these humoral factors. We will attempt to interpret the meaning of the various functions of C3a and C5a in terms of physiological processes and suggest ways in which the activities of these factors might contribute to specific elements or to the overall immune response in the host.

II. STRUCTURES OF THE ANAPHYLATOXINS

A. Primary Structures of the Molecules

Numerous reviews dating back to the late 1970s have summarized the biochemical nature of the anaphylatoxin molecules (22–27). With the advent of conventional chromatographic purification schemes for isolation of the human factors C3a, C4a, and C5a from complement-activated serum, it was possible to obtain these molecules in homogeneous form and in milligram quantities (28–30). Anaphylatoxins were isolated from 1–4 L of complement-activated human serum in yields of approximately 20% recovery for C3a (10–12 mg/L), 15% for C4a (3 mg/L), and 10–12% for C5a (0.25–0.4 mg/L). This represents a 1000-fold purification for C3a to approximately a 20,000-fold purification for C5a, with proportionate loses at each step in the isolation procedure. Immunoaffinity columns have also been designed to successfully recover the anaphylatoxins from the activated serum. An alternative isolation scheme can be designed that relies on purification of the parent components C3, C4, and C5 followed by a selective cleavage of each component to generate the corresponding anaphylatoxin. Except for C1s that selectively cleaves C4 into C4a and C4b, it is difficult to prepare active stable forms of the C3 or C5 convertases (31,32) and so this method has not been widely used. Limited cleavage of C3 or C5 by trypsin can generate C3a and C5a, but multiple other products are formed, including degradation products of the C3a and C5a, which reduces efficiency of the method and complicates purification. A chromatographic purification scheme was later developed that yields all three of the anaphylatoxins from the same batch of C-activated serum (33). This approach has also proved successful for the isolation of anaphylatoxins from C-activated sera from various animal species. Once the purified anaphylatoxins became available, extensive biochemical and biological characterizations were possible. In fact, the greatest advancement in our knowledge and understanding of both the biochemistry and function of these potent factors could only occur after the chromatographic purification schemes were perfected. It is also true that identification, characterization, and the eventual cloning of receptors for these factors were made possible only by the availability of milligram quantities of the anaphylatoxins themselves.

One important influence on the ability to isolate intact anaphylatoxins from serum relates to an enzyme in serum previously termed serum carboxypeptidase B, kininase I, or anaphylatoxin inactivator (34). This active circulating B-type carboxypeptidase, now known as serum carboxypeptidase N or SCPN (35), must be inhibited during complement activation if intact anaphylatoxins are to be recovered directly from serum. Inhibition of SCPN was originally accomplished using epsilon-aminocaproic acid (36) and later by more potent carboxypeptidase B-type inhibitors such as Ondetti's inhibitor (2-mercaptomethyl-5-guanidinopentanoic acid) (37) or Plummer's inhibitor (2-mercaptomethyl-3-guanidinoethylthiopropanoic acid) (38). The multisubunit, zinc-containing serum enzyme is much larger than the pancreatic carboxypeptidase B, having a Mr of 280,000–300,000 and a specificity for C-terminal basic residues. The specificity preference of SCPN for lysyl residues over arginine is a paradox because most of the known potential substrates for SCPN in blood have C-terminal arginyl groups. Although the enzyme is believed primarily to control anaphylatoxins, by reducing or eliminating proinflammatory functions of these factors by rapidly converting them to their respective des Arg forms, SCPN can also efficiently remove the C-terminal arginine from bradykinin, kallidin, fibrinopeptides, and other plasma protein fragments generated by any of the trypsin-like coagulation or complement enzymes. SCPN appears to be a critically important plasma enzyme. As a consequence, it is not surprising that individuals with total deficiencies in this enzyme have never been reported. A case report of a familial SCPN deficiency has been described and a male patient in this study had chronic, recurrent angioedema and urticaria. The plasma level of circulating SCPN in this patient was only 21% of normal (39).

Certain physical properties of the anaphylatoxins were considered unusual, such as their highly cationic nature and stability to extremes of heat, pH, and denaturing salt concentrations. Once the primary structures of the three human anaphylatoxins were determined (40–42), and the secondary structures were characterized as containing high levels of helical conformation (42,43), it became apparent why they were so resistant to denaturation and why they had the ability to renature after being totally unfolded. The alpha helical content of these three molecules in solution was estimated to be relatively high (e.g., 41–43% for C3a; 54% for C4a; and 48–50% for C5a based on circular dichroism measurements). The helical content of crystalline C3a was estimated to be 54% from x-ray diffraction analysis, which also demonstrated that the N- and C-terminal ends of the molecule assume irregular conformations (i.e., nonhelical). The three intrachain disulfide bonds form covalent linkages that anchor the helical regions together to form a tightly packed "core." Because of the high helical content of native C3a, C4a, and C5a, and the covalent disulfide bridges, the anaphylatoxins assume a compact conformation and exhibit remarkable stability.

The primary structures of human C3a, C4a, and C5a were each determined using classical protein sequence analysis techniques. The amino acid compositional data and electrophoretic behavior provided evidence of purity for these three molecules. The mass spectral analysis of C3a and C4a not only helped to confirm the primary structures but also provided evidence that no posttranslational modifications had occurred. The mass spectral estimation of molecular weights for C3a and C3a$_{desArg}$ were virtually the same as that calculated from the sequence analyses (see Fig. 1). The mass spectral analysis of human C5a was not as useful as that for C3a and C4a in confirming the protein sequence data because of glycosylation. The oligosaccharide unit in human C5a was partially degraded during isolation, and therefore products of various sizes were detected by this technique. Since the oligosaccharide unit attached to glutamine 64 apparently plays no role in the function of intact human C5a (44), this heterogeneity of structure did not adversely influence further biological characterizations of the molecule. However, in the case of the less potent C5a$_{desArg}$ derivative, the oligosaccharide unit apparently exhibits a negative effect on function. Removal of the oligosaccharide from C5a$_{desArg}$ resulted in enhanced neutrophil chemotactic potency by some 10–15-fold and C5aR binding affinity was enhanced (44).

The comparison of C3a, C4a, and C5a primary structures indicated that although these molecules had common genetic ancestry they now vary markedly in composition. Only 13 residue positions have been totally conserved between C3a, C4a, and C5a in the various species analyzed, with 6 of these positions being the immutable cysteinyl residues (see Fig. 2). When comparing the primary structures of C3a, C4a, or C5a from various species, a significant lack of homology among species is recognized. This level of sequence diversity is clearly manifest in the failure of antibody to a given anaphylatoxin from one species to cross-react fully with the same anaphylatoxin from another species. The greatest homology in structure exists adjacent to the two Cys-Cys sequences in all of these molecules. The relatively conserved C-terminal portion of each anaphylatoxin defines a unique effector site in each of these molecules. The C-terminal pentatapeptide sequence -L-G-L-A-R is characteristic for all known C3a molecules, -A/V-G/H-L-A/Q-R is characteristic for C4a, and -M/I/V-Q-L-G-R represent a relatively conserved effector sequence in C5a. Studies based on limited proteolytic degradation of the natural factors (45,46), and using the bioactive synthetic analogues that mimic the sequences of these C-terminal regions (as described in Section C.), provided further evidence that the C-terminal portion of these molecules represented essential effector sites. Thus the primary structural data for these molecules contributed the foundation for structure/function analyses, as well as the opportunity for mapping the ligand/receptor interactions.

B. Architecture of the Folded Anaphylatoxins

When the anaphylatoxin molecule is folded, as represented by crystallographic (47) and by nuclear magnetic resonance (48) analyses of human C3a, the majority of the variable residues are surface exposed. The folded conformation of all the anaphylatoxins can be

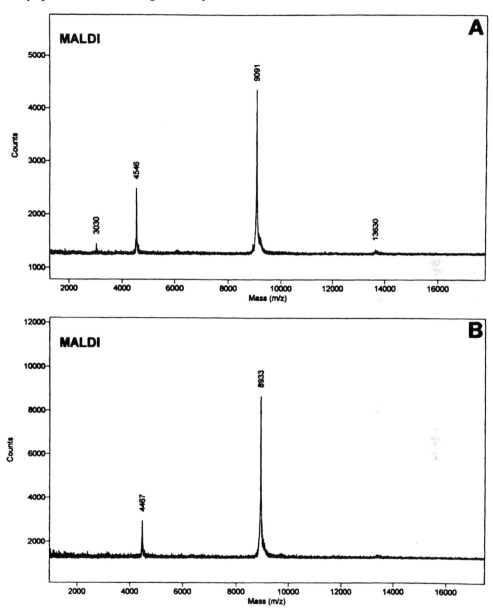

Figure 1 The mass spectral analysis of human C3a and C3a$_{desArg}$ is shown in panels A and B, respectively. The calculated molecular weight for C3a was 9094 and for C3a$_{desArg}$ was 8932 based on the amino acid sequence. The estimated weights by mass spectral analysis match almost exactly the predicted molecular weight of these factors. The analysis was performed using the matrix-assisted laser desorption ionization (MALDI) technique. The main peaks represent the purified protein ionized with one charge and the lower molecular weight peaks represent the C3a (C3a$_{desArg}$) molecule having two or more charges.

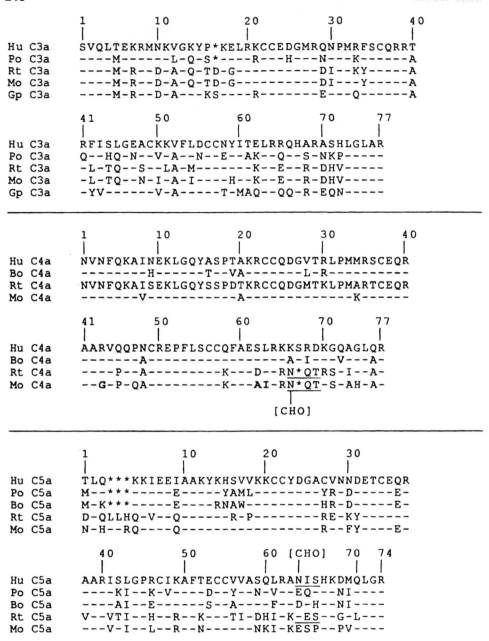

```
            1          10          20          30          40
            |          |           |           |           |
Hu C3a    SVQLTEKRMNKVGKYP*KELRKCCEDGMRQNPMRFSCQRRT
Po C3a    ----M------L-Q-S*----R---H---N---K------A
Rt C3a    ----M-R--D-A-Q-TD-G----------DI--KY-----A
Mo C3a    ----M-R--D-A-Q-TD-G----------DI---Y-----A
Gp C3a    ----M-R--D-A---KS----R-------E---Q------A

            41         50          60          70          77
            |          |           |           |           |
Hu C3a    RFISLGEACKKVFLDCCNYITELRRQHARASHLGLAR
Po C3a    Q--HQ-N--V-A--N--E--AK--Q--S-NKP-----
Rt C3a    -L-TQ--S--LA-M-------K--E--R-DHV-----
Mo C3a    -L-TQ--N-I-A-I----H--K--E--R-DHV-----
Gp C3a    -YV------V-A-----T-MAQ--QQ-R-EQN-----

            1          10          20          30          40
            |          |           |           |           |
Hu C4a    NVNFQKAINEKLGQYASPTAKRCCQDGVTRLPMMRSCEQR
Bo C4a    ---------H------T--VA-------L-R----------
Rt C4a    NVNFQKAISEKLGQYSSPDTKRCCQDGMTKLPMARTCEQR
Mo C4a    -------V-----------A-------------K------

            41         50          60          70          77
            |          |           |           |           |
Hu C4a    AARVQQPNCREPFLSCCQFAESLRKKSRDKGQAGLQR
Bo C4a    -------A-----------------A-I---V---A-
Rt C4a    ----P--A---------K---D--RN*QTRS-I--A-
Mo C4a    --G-P-QA---------K---AI-RN*QT-S-AH-A-
                                        |
                                     [CHO]

            1          10          20          30
            |          |           |           |
Hu C5a    TLQ***KKIEEIAAKYKHSVVKKCCYDGACVNNDETCEQR
Po C5a    M--***-----E-----YAML--------YR-D-----E-
Bo C5a    M-K***-----E----RNAW--------HR-D-----E-
Rt C5a    D-QLLHQ-V--Q------R-P--------RE-KY------
Mo C5a    N-H--RQ----Q---------------R--FY----E-

            40         50          60 [CHO]    70    74
            |          |           |           |     |
Hu C5a    AARISLGPRCIKAFTECCVVASQLRANISHKDMQLGR
Po C5a    ----KI--K-V----D--Y--N-V--EQ---NI----
Bo C5a    ----AI--E------S--A----F--D-H--NI----
Rt C5a    V--VTI--H--R--K---TI-DHI-K-ES--G-L---
Mo C5a    ---V-I--L--R--N------NKI-KESP--PV----
```

Figure 2 The complete amino acid sequences for the C3a, C4a, and C5a molecules from various species are presented. The human factors have been used as the reference sequence in each case and identity is signified by a dash (-). A gap (i.e., insertion or deletion) is designated by (*) and the glycosylation sites have been underlined. The abbreviations used were human (Hu), pig (Po), cow (Bo), rat (Rt), mouse (Mo), and guinea pig (Gp). The bold residues in mouse C4a indicate sites where variations were detected for different inbred strains of mice. The C3a sequences were taken from (26), the C4a sequences from (246), and C5a from (136).

generally modeled after this C3a folded structure. The N-terminal helical region is mobile both in the crystal structure and in solution, but it tends to dock onto the "disulfide-linked core" portion of the molecule in an antiparallel orientation. The three remaining helices of the "core" are also folded in an antiparallel arrangement, with each being anchored by covalent disulfide bonds. The longer C-terminal helix extends beyond the globular body of the "core" and terminates as the effector site of the molecule. Therefore, the central core portion of the folded anaphylatoxin molecule is rigid with the N- and C-terminal ends having flexibility and freedom of movement. The C-terminal residues in human C3a up to position 69–70 assume no regular conformation (i.e., are nonhelical) and may either remain flexible or fold back onto the helical portion in a pseudo-beta turn conformation. The synthetic analogue peptide studies suggest that a portion of the long helix attached to the irregular C-terminal effector region in C3a is important for optimal potency of these factors (49,50). A model of the folded C5a molecule is presented to illustrate that the conformation of these molecules is very similar, having four helices and three disulfide bonds (Fig 3).

A number of studies were performed to characterize the stability of the anaphylatoxins and to explore denaturation/renaturation of the folded structure. It was surprising to

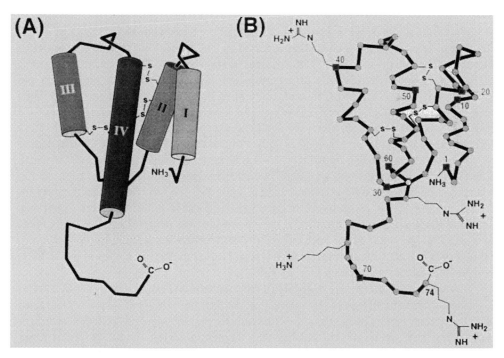

Figure 3 The model of human C5a indicates four antiparallel helical regions (I–IV) and the essential C-terminal effector site at the end of helix IV that make up the folded C5a structure (view A). The folded C5a has three disulfide bonds that stabilize the "core" portion of the molecule. The backbone architecture, disulfide bond arrangements, and the irregular C-terminal loop appears to be similar for each of the anaphylatoxins as portrayed here for human C5a (view B). C3a, C4a, and C5a each have four antiparallel helices folded into a compact globular form with the C-terminal end containing the effector sites. In this model we show several conserved cationic side chains that have been implicated in secondary binding interactions for C5a with the C5a receptor.

learn that these molecules could withstand temperatures in excess of 80–90° C and pH extremes of 2–12 without measurable losses in activity (43). Both C3a and C5a will spontaneously refold and return to a conformation indistinguishable from the native structure after being fully unfolded by exposure to reducing agents and denaturing salts such as guanidine HCl. This ability of anaphylatoxins to reversibly assume a native conformation predicted success in recovery of active forms of the cloned anaphylatoxins from cellular expression systems. In fact, this property of the anaphylatoxins to renature reversibly was exploited in designing techniques to recover cloned C3a (51) and C5a (52–55) from cell lysates. It is important to note that although the C-terminal portion of these molecules contains the effector sites, the intact folded structures are required for optimal potency. This behavior indicates that secondary contacts exist on the anaphylatoxin surface for binding to their receptors and that affinity of binding depends on both the molecular conformation and the C-terminal sequence of the molecule. The secondary contacts and their distributions and special arrangements help define potency of the native factors and are presumed to hold the key for designing agonists and antagonists of these molecules that might find utility as both research and clinical tools.

C. Synthetic Analogues of the Anaphylatoxins

Recognition that one could synthesize fragments of the anaphylatoxins capable of exhibiting a full range of activities was first reported in 1977 (56). This report provided clear evidence of bioactivity associated with synthetic peptides based on the C-terminal sequence of the human anaphylatoxin C3a. In recent years, numerous synthetic homologues and analogues of C3a, C4a, and C5a molecules have been designed and many exhibited relatively high levels of potency. These peptides have generally been full agonists of the respective anaphylatoxin on which the analogue structure was based. C3a peptides have been designed with potencies ranging as high or higher than 100% of native C3a depending on the assay, but potencies up to only 0.1–1.0% were obtained for analogues of native C5a (Table 1). Selected synthetic C3a/C5a analogues have been successfully utilized in searching for new biologic activities and in analyzing the structural requirements for ligand binding to the respective C3a or C5a receptors. In addition to the significant advances made in designing agonists of the anaphylatoxins, major efforts are being made to design analogue antagonists. Such molecules could perhaps be used clinically as effective inhibitors of cell activation during various types of inflammatory processes in which these complement factors may play a primary role.

Numerous advantages are realized in using synthetic analogues of the anaphylatoxins in place of the natural factors. In addition to confirming biological responses obtained with the natural factors, large quantities of synthetic peptides can be produced with high purity, they have greater overall stability than the natural factors, and they have a lesser potential for contamination by endotoxins. It is known that the effector site at the C-terminal end of C5a, unlike the C-terminal portion of C3a (which contains most of the binding sites for interactions with the receptor), represents only one of several sites required for optimal C5a–receptor interaction (45). Therefore, it is important to understand which regions of the ligand participate in receptor binding and whether various cellular responses are triggered by different types of interaction with the C3a/C5a molecules. As a consequence, synthetic analogues of these molecules provide ideal tools for analyzing these detailed ligand–receptor interactions.

Table 1 Examples of Potent Synthetic Analogues and Potential Antagonists of Human C3a and C5a

Peptide	Potency	References
C3a and C3a Analogues:		
Intact human C3a	2.0–4.3 nM[a]	50
	3 nM ED$_{50}$[b]	88
C-N-Y-I-T-E-L-R-R-Q-H-A-R-A-S-H-L-G-L-A-R (native sequence)	1.9–4.1 nM[a]	50
	92 nM[c]	85
Fmoc-Ahx-Y-R-R-G-R-A-A-A-L-G-L-A-R	3 nM ED$_{50}$[a]	80,81
W-W-G-K-K-Y-R-A-S-K-L-G-L-A-R	6 nM[c]	85
C3a Antagonists		
Y-R-R-G-R-Ahx-C̄-G-G-L-C̄-L-A-R*	0.5, K$_i$/ED$_{50}$[d]	88
Y-R-R-G-R-Ahx-C̄-G-A-L-C̄-L-A-R*	0.4, K$_i$/ED$_{50}$[d]	88
C5a and C5a Analogues		
Intact human C5a	0.03 nM, K$_i$[e]	60
H-K-D-M-Q-L-G-R (native sequence)	300 μM, K$_i$[e]	65
F-K-D-M-Q-L-G-R	0.2 μM, K$_i$[e]	60
H-K-D-Cha-Cha-L-(dA)-R	1.6 μM, K$_i$[e]	64
Y-F-K-A-Cha-Cha-L-(dF)-R	8 nM, K$_i$[e]	67
F-L-A-Cha-Cha-(dA)-R	90 nM, K$_i$[e]	68
Y-S-F-K-P-M-P-L-(dA)-R	7.1 μM, K$_i$[f]	74
C5a Antagonists		
NMe-F-L-P-dCha-W-(dR)	60 nM, IC$_{50}$[g]	89
	100 nM, IC$_{50}$[h]	
F-L-A-Cha-G-L-(dA)-R	8.9 nM, K$_i$[i]	91
[N,N'-bis(4-amino-2 methyl-6-quinolyl)urea]**	3 μM, IC$_{50}$[j]	90
	8 μM, EC$_{50}$[k]	67

Fmoc-, fluorenyl methoxycarbonyl; Ahx-, aminohexyl; Cha-, cyclohexylalanine; NMe-, N-methyl; (dA), (dF) and (dR) are D-amino acids.

[a] Guinea pig ileal strip contraction.

[b] ED$_{50}$, half maximal concentration inducing ATP release from guinea pig platelets.

[c] Threshold concentration for inducing aggregation of guinea pig platelets.

[d] K$_i$/ED$_{50}$ ratio: nM K$_i$ determined by competition of human ^{125}I-C3a binding to guinea pig platelets; nM ED$_{50}$, half maximal concentration inducing ATP release from guinea pig platelets.

[e] K$_i$ determined by competition of human ^{125}I-C5a binding to human PMN membranes.

[f] K$_i$ determined by competition of human ^{125}I-C5a binding to human PMNs.

[g] IC$_{50}$ determined by competition of 20 pM human ^{125}I-C5a binding to human PMN membranes.

[h] IC$_{50}$ to inhibit C5a-induced PMN degranulation.

[i] K$_i$ determined by competition of human ^{125}I-C5a binding to human PMN membranes, combined with low chemokinetic activity.

[j] IC$_{50}$ determined by competition of human ^{125}I-C5a binding to human PMN membranes.

[k] EC$_{50}$ to inhibit C5a-induced PMN degranulation.

* Cyclic peptides.

** Substituted 4,6-diamino-quinolines. Has no inhibitory effect on binding or functional activity of C-terminal C5a peptides.

a. Synthetic Analogues of C5a

Recent biological studies performed using synthetic C-terminal fragments of both human C5a (57–60) and rat C5a (61,62) provided evidence that the C-terminal portion of C5a indeed contains the effector site of this molecule. Synthetic C-terminal analogues were prepared as models of the effector site in human C5a and were shown to exhibit the full spectrum of biological activities expressed by the parent protein (see Table 1). Active C5a analogues provided an opportunity to examine those parameters responsible for functional expression, including both the steric and conformational properties required of the effector portion of the ligand (58). Removal of the C-terminal arginine from human C5a reduces spasmogenic potency by approximately 1000-fold, but only reduces the chemotactic activity by approximately 10-fold (44,46,63). The C-terminal pentapeptide MQLGR (46,59) and the C-terminal octapeptide HKDMQLGR (60,64) express the same effector functions as does human C5a, with the exception that the synthetic fragments exhibit significantly less potency (e.g., 0.01–0.1%) than the natural molecule. Efforts to design analogues with greater potency than those based on the natural C5a sequence resulted in highly modified C5a peptides of 8–10 residues in length (58,64–66). Major developments in these efforts were achieved by single residue replacements in the sequence of the octamer HKDMQLGR, such as His 68 $\rightarrow$ Phe 68 (60), that resulted in a 1000–1500-fold increase in receptor binding affinity. A systematic effort to increase hydrophobicity and change chirality at selected positions resulted in modified C5a peptides with as much as a 20-fold increase in receptor affinity and biological potency (64,67,68). Various decapeptide analogues of C5a were synthesized containing prolyl substitutions to restrict flexibility of the C-terminal peptide. One particular series of analogues having Gln 71 replaced by proline exhibited significantly greater potency than either the natural C5a decapeptide or some of the other substituted analogues, and these analogues remained full agonists of natural C5a (69,70). It was concluded that the proline at this position would force residues 71–74 to adopt a beta turn-like structure that may mimic the preferred conformation for the effector site residues in the natural factor.

It has been suggested that regions other than the C-terminal portion of C5a, such as the N-terminal helical portion, either participate directly in receptor binding or in stabilizing the native C5a conformation (71,72). If dependence on secondary binding sites distant from the C-terminal region explains why the intact factor is considerably more potent than the synthetic C-terminal C5a analogues, optimization of potency will require a more complex peptide design than simply constructing mimics of the C-terminal region. Recent synthetic studies have extended on the C-terminal effector site by adding portions of the core region of C5a to the C-terminal decapeptide. Receptor affinity of C5a peptides that contain portions of the core region (i.e., residues 40–64) linked as an extension of the C-terminal octapeptide was enhanced and potency increased by 1000-fold (73). The core portion that was added did include the Arg 40 and Arg 46, residues that have been implicated as functionally important from mutagenesis studies. However, even these much bulkier peptides that represent a greater proportion of the C5a structure remain disappointingly low in potency compared with the natural factor. These studies further suggest that multiple contacts on the three-dimensional conformation of the intact C5a molecule are very important for optimal potency.

There are few examples of synthetic anaphylatoxin analogues being used in vivo, because they are so rapidly degraded by the serum carboxypeptidase N. One of the conformationally restricted C-terminal analogue of C5a mentioned above, YSFKPM-

PL(dA)R, was designed to resist carboxypeptidase digestion by introducing a d-alanine in the penultimate C-terminal position (74). This modified C5a peptide was tested as a molecular adjuvant in both a mouse and rabbit model, based on the known immunostimulatory properties of C5a (75). This synthetic C5a analogue was used to stimulate an in vivo antibody response against a peptide epitope (YKQGGFLGL) in human MUCl glycoprotein used as the antigen. A high-titer antibody response was only observed when the mice were immunized with a covalent conjugate of the C5a fragment and the MUCl peptide (YKQGGFLGL-YSFKPMPL(dA)R), but not when the individual peptides were used. These results provide preliminary evidence that peptides with C5a-like activity may be useful adjuvants in enhancing the antigen-specific antibody response.

b. Synthetic Analogues of C3a

Although no more than five to eight residues of the C-terminal portion of C3a were shown to be essential for biological (spasmogenic) activity (56), potency is markedly enhanced as the length of the C-terminal C3a peptides is increased (76). C3a analogues of the C-terminal pentapeptide, LGLAR, were shown to exhibit measurable biological potency. However, substitution of either Leu-75, Ala-76 or Arg-77 resulted in major reductions in potency (77). A synthetic 21-residue C-terminal fragment of C3a (i.e., C3a 57–77; see Table 1) expresses approximately equipotent spasmogenic activity on guinea pig tissue to that of the natural human C3a molecule (50,76). This 21-residue fragment of C3a was shown to assume a partial helical conformation in trifluoroethanol, a helix-inducing solvent (50). Analogues of the 21-residue C3a peptide, (C3a 57–77), containing various substituted residues that disrupt helix formation exhibited less potency than C3a 57–77, while incorporation of helix promoting residues in the 21-mer enhanced potency above that of C3a 57–77 (49). Synthetic C-terminal C3a peptides that were shorter than the tridecapeptide C3a 65–77 assumed irregular and/or beta-turn-like conformations in trifluoroethanol, while the 21-residue analogue C3a 57–77 assumed a partially helical conformation (50). It was concluded that a helical conformation contributes to the higher potency of the 21-residue analogue of C3a (C3a 57–77). Circular dichroism (CD) was used to evaluate the conformations of these various peptides. More recently, NMR studies of human C3a suggested that the long C-terminal helix extends from residues 49 to 65 or 66 and that the remaining 11–12 residues at the C-terminal end assume no regular structure (78). A combination of the five–eight residues in the effector site and the adjacent helical portion of the C-terminal region appears to provide most of the contacts in C3a required for receptor binding. These data suggest that the longer and more potent synthetic analogues of C3a may be able to mimic the conformation of the C-terminal region of the native molecule. In a more hydrophobic environment than water, such as at the surface of the membrane or the C3a receptor, the longer (i.e., 21-residue) synthetic C3a peptides may readily assume a helical structure like that in the natural factor, thus promoting their effectiveness.

Substituted C3a analogue peptides have recently been designed that are shorter than the 21-residue peptide C3a 57–77, but are considerably more potent in some of the biological assay systems tested (79–83). This enhanced activity was achieved simply by attaching a hydrophobic fluorenyl-methoxycarbonyl (Fmoc) or 2-nitro-4-azidophenyl (Nap) group to the N-terminus of a 5–13-residue C-terminal C3a peptide. Two to 10-fold increases in biological potency for the Fmoc-and Nap-modified C3a peptides over C3a 57–77 were obtained using a guinea pig platelet ATP-release assay. The potency-enhancing effect from attaching hydrophobic groups to the N-termini of C3a peptides was interpreted as promoting uptake of the ligand by the platelet membrane. These authors suggest that the hydrophobic group inserts into the lipid bilayer, thereby increasing the effective peptide concentration and thus enhancing receptor-ligand binding. A 13-residue C3a analogue with a N-terminal Nap group attached via a 6-aminohexanoic acid spacer (Nap-Ahx-Y-R-R-G-R-A-A-A-L-G-L-A-R) exhibited sixfold greater potency than that of natural C3a when assayed by guinea pig platelet ATP-release (80). This remarkable increase in potency (100-fold over the unmodified 13-residue C3a peptide) suggested that the hydrophobic

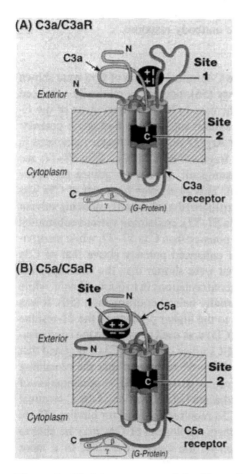

Figure 4 Models are proposed for illustrating the interactions between C3a or C5a and their respective receptors. The design for this model was adapted from the C5a/C5aR model proposed by Siciliano et al. (67). Both C3aR and C5aR are G-protein coupled transmembrane receptors of the rhodopsin family. The C3a molecule has at least two major binding sites. A noneffector binding site (Site 1) exists on C3a along the C-terminal helical region and either makes contact with the large extracellular loop (as shown here) or with other exposed regions of the receptor, including the N-terminal region (see A). Site 2 contains the C-terminal effector region of C3a, including the sequence LGLAR, which is shown penetrating into the "pore" formed by the seven transmembrane regions of C3aR. This model for C3a/C3aR interaction corresponds to a model originally proposed for multisite binding of C5a with its receptor (45). The model for C5a interaction with C5aR indicates that the noneffector site (site 1) on C5a binds to the N-terminal region of the C5a receptor, while the C-terminal effector site (site 2) of C5a penetrates the "pore" (see B).

group on the C3a peptide may be interacting specifically with the C3a receptor. When these (Nap-Ahx-Y-R-R-G-R-A-A-A-L-G-L-A-R) same peptides were cross-linked to guinea pig platelets they identified a protein of 86–115 kDa (79). This size for the C3a receptor is in agreement with similar studies in which native C3a was crosslinked to guinea pig platelets (84).

A systematic study was conducted to determine the optimal distance for placing a hydrophobic group adjacent to the C-terminal effector site in the C3a peptide. Analogue C3a peptides of 10–18 residues in length were evaluated using guinea pig platelet aggregation and vascular permeability assays. The natural amino acid tryptophan was used as the N-terminal hydrophobic group in a series of peptides of 10–18 residues in length, and the 13-residue analogue exhibited the highest potency. This peptide (WWGKKYRA-SKLGLAR) was approximately 16 times more potent than the 21-residue peptide C3a 57–77 (50,85). Based on these sequence and structural requirements for optimal biological potency of a highly substituted C3a analogue, it appears that a bulky hydrophobic unit can specifically interact with a secondary binding site on the receptor. These results helped to formulate a conceptual model for the C3a receptor–ligand interaction as shown in Figure 4, based on current knowledge of the folded natural C3a and structural requirements for the synthetic analogues (86).

Antagonist studies of C3a or C5a analogues have been relatively rare and it has been difficult to make progress in this area. Although the pharmacological value of such analogues could be great, the actual design of antagonists based on the C-terminal peptides has been disappointing. Cyclic disulfide analogues of C3a were reported as weak antagonists of C3a (87,88), while only two different structures have been reported as antagonists of C5a (89–91) see Table 1. In general, most analogues of C5a that mimic the C-terminal effector site have exhibited weak C5a agonist effects (89,91,92), presumably because interaction with the receptor site is sufficient to trigger signaling events. A recently designed antagonist (67,90) seems to avoid the activation events while still binding to the receptor and blocking C5a action. The antagonist is structurally quite different from the C-terminal peptide of C5a and apparently binds to the receptor at a site distant from the effector binding site. Binding studies demonstrated that this antagonist is able to inhibit binding and cell activation by C5a, but unable to prevent binding of potent, synthetic C-terminal analogues of C5a (67), (see Table 1). With detailed molecular analysis and a deeper understanding of the respective ligand and receptor binding interactions for these inflammatory molecules, it should be possible to design even more potent agonists and effective antagonist molecules in the near future. Table 1 summarizes several of the more promising designs for C3a and C5a analogue peptides exhibiting either agonist and antagonist behavior.

III. C3a AND C5a RECEPTORS

A. Protein and Gene Structures for the Anaphylatoxin Receptors

Early characterizations of the C5a receptor (CD88) C5aR on human neutrophils clearly established three facts that later played a prominent role in elucidation of the C5a/C5aR interaction and the isolation of the receptor gene. It was determined that C5a (^{125}I-labeled) binds to a receptor on the neutrophil with nanomolar affinity; that there are as many as 100,000 thousand copies of the receptor per cell; and that certain degradation products of C5a (i.e., C5a des Arg and C5a 1–69) compete with binding of the intact factor (93). The observation that a C5a fragment, devoid of the C-terminal effector site (i.e., C5a 1–69), could still bind to the receptor led to the hypothesis that both a primary effector and secondary binding sites exist on the C5a ligand and each is important for optimal interaction with the receptor (45,46,93). Characterization of the binding affinity and numbers of receptors on neutrophils, later estimated to average 80,000 copies with an affinity of approximately 2 nM (94,95), provided the critical information that indicated a differentiated leukocytic cell line would be an appropriate source from which to isolate and clone the C5a receptor gene.

The gene structure for the human C5a receptor was reported by two separate groups in 1991. One group used a library obtained from dibutyryl-cAMP-induced human myeloid U937 cells (7) and the other group used a dibutyryl-cAMP-induced human myeloid HL-60 cell library (8). Both groups obtained cDNA clones with open reading frames of 1050 base pairs coding for an identical protein of 350 amino acid residues with a calculated Mr of 39,320. A single glycosylation site was located at Asn 5 of the first extracellular domain of C5aR. The presence of a N-linked oligosaccharide group is presumed to explain the difference in size between the nude protein of 39 k Da and the 40–48 kDa estimated for C5aR expressed on human leukocytes. The size of the natural C5a receptor was estimated using a variety of chemical cross-linking techniques to attach $[^{125}I]$C5a to the receptor on neutrophils (94,96,97). The effects of glycosylation of C5aR on binding of the ligand were explored by replacing Asn 5 with an Ala residue (98). When both the Ala 5-C5aR mutant molecule and wild type C5aR were expressed on CHO cells and compared, the dissociation constants were 20 nM and 13 nM, respectively. These results suggest that glycosylation of the C5aR has little influence on ligand binding and hence on C5a-induced functions.

The cloned C5aR was expressed in COS-7 cells and high-affinity C5a binding was demonstrated. The Boulay group (8) concluded that there were both high-affinity (Kd=1.7 nM) and low-affinity (Kd=20–25 nM) C5a receptors expressed on these COS cells, while the Gerard group (7) described only the high-affinity receptors (i.e., Kd = 1.4 nM) and demonstrated G-protein-dependent phosphorylation for phosphatidylinositols in response to C5a. The genes encoding C5aR, along with two structurally related formyl peptide receptors (FPRH1 and FPRH2), have been mapped to band position q13.2 in human chromosome 19 (99).

The C5aR protein deduced from the cDNA clones identified the characteristic structure of a member of the rhodopsin superfamily of receptors. Biological responses of leukocytes are initiated when C5a binds to C5aR, a seven membrane-spanning receptor coupled to a regulatory heterodimeric guaninine nucleotide-binding protein (G_i proteins) (7,100,101). Despite the persistent presence of the activating ligand, the cellular responses are transient and the cells rapidly become refractory to further stimulation, termed homologous desensitization. Receptor phosphorylation appears to be the key mechanism by which many G-protein-coupled receptors are regulated. It has been shown that C5aR is phosphorylated exclusively at serine residues localized on its carboxyl tail, by a member of the G-protein-coupled receptor kinase family (102). Despite the fact that a putative PKC consensus motif is present in the third cytoplasmic loop of C5aR, C5a-dependent phosphorylation is mainly resistant to PKC inhibitors. Therefore, PKC is not the main enzyme involved in agonist-dependent phosphorylation.

Several neutrophil signal transduction pathways are regulated by G_i-coupled C5aR, one involving the activation of phospholipase C (PLC). The ligand-bound receptor interacts with pertussis toxin (PTx)-sensitive G-proteins, such as the G_i proteins, and releases the $\beta\gamma$ subunits, which then stimulate PLC-β and phosphatidylinositol 3-kinase (PI-3) activities, followed by activation of phospholipase A_2 (PLA_2) and phospholipase D (103). The PLC/PKC limb of postreceptor events modulates intracellular calcium fluxes, which may be important for degranulation of neutrophils. Another pathway involves activation of PI-3 kinase and the generation of phosphatidylinositol (3–5) triphosphate (PIP_3) which may be critical for cytoskeletal reorganization and the chemotactic response. Reports show that PTx-insensitive $G\alpha_{16}$ subunits coupled to C5aR are also able to activate PLC, but the PTx-sensitive pathways may be predominant in mature leukocytes, since neutrophil responses to C5a were found to be largely PTx sensitive (104,105).

C5aR and other seven transmembrane receptors coupled to G_i are capable of activating the Ras/Raf/MAP kinase pathway (100,105). The $\beta\gamma$ subunits can activate the mitogen-activated protein kinase (MAP) pathway in a Ras-dependent manner. Raf-1 binds to Ras-GTP, which activates Raf-1 kinase activity. Activated Raf-1 phosphorylates and activates mitogen-activated protein kinase/Erk kinase(MEK-1), which in turn phosphorylates and activates MAP kinase. The MAP kinase cascade could contribute to the functional assembly of the NADPH oxidase responsible for oxygen radical generation.

Sequence comparisons between C5aR and other members of the rhodopsin superfamily indicated that a relatively close homology exists only with human neurokinin A (substance K) and formyl peptide receptors (7). Even these receptors, having the highest degree of sequence identity, exhibit only 25% (substance K) and 35% (formyl peptide) structural identity to C5aR. More recently, the cDNA sequences for mouse C5aR (106), guinea pig (107), rat (108), canine, and a partial sequence for bovine C5aR have been determined (109). Figure 5A contains the sequences for human, guinea pig, dog, rat, and mouse C5aR and the conserved sites have been identified (*), as well as the seven transmembrane segments (I–VII). It is interesting to note that the extracellular N-terminal region, which is believed to contain one of the ligand-binding sites, is poorly conserved between species while the transmembrane regions and the intracellular C-terminal region which binds the G-protein are highly conserved.

An interesting difference between the animal and human C5aR clones is the origin of the genetic materials. The mouse gene was obtained from a genomic DNA library, the guinea pig clones were from a megakaryrocyte cDNA library, rat C5a clones were from a lung cDNA library, the canine cDNA clone for C5aR was originally an orphan clone from a thyroid cDNA library, while the human cDNA clones were from leukocytic cell lines. This indicates a widely diverse distribution of the C5aR gene throughout many tissues of the body. Identity between the C5aR protein sequences from these various species was only 65–76%, which is considered relatively low for rhodopsin family receptors in cross-species comparisons.

The C3a receptor was first demonstrated on guinea pig platelets using cross-linking techniques and was estimated to be 95–105 kDa (84). A later report confirmed the unusually large size for this receptor (i.e., 83–114 kDa) that exhibits a diffuse band in gels, suggesting a highly glycosylated protein (79). These data raised the question of whether the C3aR was also a G-protein-coupled receptor, and how the C3a receptor could be related to the C5a receptor and yet be so much larger in size. Part of the mystery was solved when it was determined that the amino acid portion of human C3aR had a Mr of 53,864 Da and contained 144 additional residues in the second extracellular domain when compared to C5aR. Sensitivity of C3a-dependent mobilization of intracellular calcium to pertussis toxin in differentiated U937 cells and in human neutrophils indicated that the

```
                                                              I
Hu C5aR   1:MNSFNYTTPDYGHYDDKDTLDLNTPVDKTSNT--LRVPDILALVIFAVVFLVGVLGNALV 58
Dg C5aR   1:MASMNFSPPEYPDY-GTATLDPNIFVDESLNTPKLSVPDMIALVIFVMVFLVGVPGNFLV 59
Gp C5aR   1:----MMVTVSY-DYD-YNSTFLPDGFVDNYVE-RLSFGDLVAVVIMVVVFLVGVPGNALV 53
Rt C5aR   1:MDPISNDSSE-ITYDYSDGTPNPDMPADGVYIPKMEPGDIAALIIYLAVFLVGVTGNALV 59
Mo C5aR   1:MDPIDNSSFE-INYDHY-GTMDPNIPADGIHLPKRQPGDVAALIIYSVVFLVGVPGNALV 58
            *            * * *   ****** ** **


                          II
Hu C5aR  59:VWVTAFEAKRTINAIWFLNLAVADFLSCLALPILFTSIVQHHHWPFGGAACSILPSLILL 118
Dg C5aR  60:VWVTGFEVRRTINAIWFLNLAVADLLSCLALPILFSSIVQQGYWPFGNAACRILPSLILL 119
Gp C5aR  54:VWVTACEARRHINAIWFLNLAAADLLSCLALPILLVSTVHLNHWYFGNTACKVLPSLILL 113
Rt C5aR  60:VWVTAFEAKRTVNAIWFLNLAVADLLSCLALPILFTSIVKHNHWPFGDQACIVLPSLILL 119
Mo C5aR  59:VWVTAFEPDGPSNAIWFLNLAVADLLSCLAMPVLFTTVLNHNYWYFDATACIVLPSLILL 118
            ****  *   ********* ** ***** *  *    *  *   **   *******


              III                              IV
Hu C5aR 119:NMYASILLLATISADRFLLVFKPIWCQNFRGAGLAWIACAVAWGLALLLTIPSFLYRVVR 178
Dg C5aR 120:NMYASILLLTTISADRFVLVFNPIWCQNYRGPQLAWAACSVAWAVALLLTVPSFIFRGVH 179
Gp C5aR 114:NMYTSILLLATISADRLLLVLSPIWCQRFRGGCLAWTACGVAWVLALLLSSPSFLYRRTH 173
Rt C5aR 120:NMYSSILLLATISADRFLLVFKPIWCQKFRPGLAWMACGVTWVLALLLTIPSFVFRRIH 179
Mo C5aR 119:NMYASILLLATISADRFLLVFKPIWCQKVRGTGLAWMACGVAWVLALLLTIPSFVYREAY 178
            ***  ***** ****** **    ***** *    * **  ** *    **** *** *


                                        V
Hu C5aR 179:EEYFPPKVLCGVDYS-HDKRRERAVAIVRLVLGFLWPLLTLTICYTFILLRTWSRRATRS 237
Dg C5aR 180:TEYFPFWMTCGVDYSGVGVLVERGVAILRLLMGFLGPLVILSICYTFLLIRTWSRKATRS 239
Gp C5aR 174:NEHFSFKVYCVTDY-GRDISKERAVALVRLVVGFIVPLITLTACYTFLLLRTWSRKATRS 232
Rt C5aR 180:KDPYSDSILCNIDYSKGPFFIEKAIAILRLMVGFVLPLLTLNICYTFLLIRTWSRKATRS 239
Mo C5aR 179:KDFYSEHTVCGINYGGGSFPKEKAVAILRLMVGFVLPLLTLNICYTFLLLRTWSRKATRS 238
              *  *       *   *  **  **  **  *    **** * ***** ****


                   VI                               VII
Hu C5aR 238:TKTLKVVVAVVASFFIFWLPYQVTGIMMSFLEPSSPTFLLLNKLDSLCVSFAYINCCINP 297
Dg C5aR 240:TKTLKVVVAVVSFFVLWLPYQVTGMMMALFYKHSESFRRVSRLDSLCVAVAYINCCINP 299
Gp C5aR 233:AKTVKVVVAVVSNFFVFWLPYQVTGILLAWHSPNSATYRNTKALDAVCVAFAYINCCINP 292
Rt C5aR 240:TKTLKVVMAVVTCFFVFWLPYQVTGVILAWLPRSSSTFQSVERLNSLCVSLAYINCCVNP 299
Mo C5aR 239:TKTLKVVMAVVICFFIFWLPYQVTGVMIAWLPPSSPTLKRVEKLNSLCVSLAYINCCVNP 298
            ** *** ***  **  ********      *        *   **  ****** **


             
Hu C5aR 298:IIYVVAGQGFQGRLRKSLPSLLRNVLTEESVVRESKSFTRSTVDTMAQKTQAV     350
Dg C5aR 300:IIYVLAAQGFHSRFLKSLPARLRQVLAEESVGRDSKSITLSTVDTPAQKSQGV     352
Gp C5aR 293:IIYVVAGHGFQGRLLKSLPSVLRNVLTEESLNRDTRSFTRSTVDTMPQKSESV     345
Rt C5aR 300:IIYVMAGQGFHGRLRRSLPSIIRNVLSEDSLGRDSKSFTRSTMDTSTQKSQAV     352
Mo C5aR 299:IIYVMAGQGFHGRLLRSLPSIIRNALSEDSVGRDSKTFTPSTDDTSPRKSQAV     351
            ****  *  **    ** *   ***  *  *  *    * ** **    *  *
```

Figure 5A The complete protein sequences for the C5a receptor from human (Hu), dog (Dg), guinea pig (Gp), rat (Rt), and mouse (Mo) are presented. The alignments were optimized to obtain maximal identity and the seven transmembrane regions have been identified by a line and roman numerals. The residue positions that have been conserved in all species are denoted by an (*). The C5a receptors from various species are similar in size and each molecule has a potential glycosylation site near the N-terminus.

C3aR was a G-protein coupled receptor (110,111). Cloning of the human C3a receptor was recently reported by three different laboratories (9–11). As with the C5aR, the known biological effects of C3a and evidence that C3a stimulates or binds to only selected cell types led investigators to use expression libraries from human neutrophils or from differentiated leukocytic cells lines (i.e., HL-60 and U937) for isolating C3aR cDNA. Since there are glycosylation sites at the N-terminal end and in the large second extracellular loop of the human C3aR molecule, it is proposed that C3aR may have both a higher

```
                                  I
           _____
Hu C3aR   1:MASFSAETNSTDLLSQPWNEPPVILSMVILSLTFLLGLPGNGLVLWVAGLKMQRTVNTIW 60
Gp C3aR   1:MDSSSAETNSTGLHLEPQYQPETILAMAILGLTFVLGLPGNGLVLWVAGLKMRRTVNTVW 60
Rt C3aR   1:MESFTADTNSTDLHSRPLFKPQDIASMVILSLTCLLGLPGNGLVLWVAGVKMKRTVNTVW 60
Mo C3aR   1:MESFDADTNSTDLHSRPLFQPQDIASMVILGLTCLLGLLANGLVLWVAGVKMKTTVNTVW 60
            *  *  * **** **    *    *  *  ** **   *** ********* **   **** *

                    II                              III
           _____                _____
Hu C3aR  61:FLHLTLADLLCCLSLPFSLAHLALQGQWPYGRFLCKLIPSIIVLNMFASVFLLTAISLDR 120
Gp C3aR  61:FLHLTVADFVCCLSLPFSMAHLALRGYWPYGEILCKFIPTVIIFNMFASVFLLTAISLDR 120
Rt C3aR  61:FLHLTLADFLCCLSLPFSVAHLILRGHWPYGLFLCKLIPSVIILNMFASVFLLTAISLDR 120
Mo C3aR  61:FLHLTLADFLCCLSLPFSLAHLILQGHWPYGLFLCKLIPSIIILNMFASVFLLTAISLDR 120
            *****  **  ******** ***  *  ****   *** *  * *  **************

                                  IV
            _____
Hu C3aR 121:CLVVFKPIWCQNHRNVGMACSICGCIWVVAFVMCIPVFVYREIFTTDNHNRCGYKFGLSS 180
Gp C3aR 121:CLMVLKPIWCQNHRNVRTACIICGCIWLVAFVLCIPVFVYRETFTLENHTICTYNFS-PG 179
Rt C3aR 121:CLMVHKPIWCQNHRSVRTAFAVCGCVWVVTFVMCIPVFVYRDLLVVDDYSVCGYNFDSSR 180
Mo C3aR 121:CLIVHKPIWCQNHRNVRTAFAICGCVWVVAFVMCVPVFVYRDLFIMDNRSICRYNFDSSR 180
            **  * ********* *   *   *** * * **  ******           *  *

Hu C3aR 181:SLDYPDF-YG-D-PLENRSLENIVQRPGEMNDRLDP-SSFQTNDHPWTVPTVFQPQTFQRPS 238
Gp C3aR 180:SFDYLDYAYDRD-AWGYGTPDPIVQLPGEMEHRSDP-SSFQTQDGPWSVTTTLYSQTSQRPS 239
Rt C3aR 181:AYDYWDYMYNSHLPEINPPDNS----TGHVDDRTAPSSSVPARD-LWTATTALQSQTFHTSP 237
Mo C3aR 181:SYDYWDYVYKLSLPESNSTDNSTAQLTGHMNDRSAP-SSVQARDYFWTVTTALQSQPFLTSP 241
             ** *  *         *         *   *  **    *  *  *

Hu C3aR 239:ADSLPRGSARLTSQNLYSNVFKPADVVSPKIPSGFPIEDHETSPLDNSDAFLSTHLKLFPSA 300
Gp C3aR 240:EDSFHMDSAKLSGQGKYVDV-----VLPTNL-CGLPMEENRTNTLHNA-AFLSSDLDV-SNA 294
Rt C3aR 238:EDPFSQDSA--SQQPHYGG--KPPTVLIATIPGGFPVEDHKSNTL-NTGAFLSAH-TEPSLT 293
Mo C3aR 242:EDSFSLDSA--NQQPHYGG--KPPNVLTAAVPSGFPVEDRKSNTL-NADAFLSAH-TELFPT 297
             *  **      *             *  *   *   *  ****

                                         V
                              _____
Hu C3aR 301:SSNSFYESELPQGFQDYYNLGQFTDDDQVPTPLVAITITRLVVGFLLPSVIMIACYSFIVFR 362
Gp C3aR 295:TQKCLSTPEPPQDFWD--DLSPFTHEYRTPRLLKVITFTRLVVGFLLPMIIMVACYTLIIFR 353
Rt C3aR 294:-ASSSPLY-AHDFPDDYFDQLMYGNHAWTP--QVAITISRLVVGFLVPFFIMITCYSLIVFR 351
Mo C3aR 298:-ASSGHLY-PYDFQGDYVDQFTYDNHVPTP--LMAITITRLVVGFLVPFFIMVICYSLIVFR 355
                  *          *     **  ****** *  ** ** * **

                               VI
                  _____
Hu C3aR 363:MQRGRFAKSQSKTFRVAVVVVAVFLVCWTPYHIFGVLSLLTDPETPLGKTLMSWDHVCIAL 423
Gp C3aR 354:MRRARVVKSWNKALHLAMVVVTIFLICWAPYHVFGVLILFINPESRVGAALLSWDHVSIAL 414
Rt C3aR 352:MRKTNLTKSRNKTLRVAVAVVTVFFVCWIPYHIVGILLVITDQESALREVVLPWDHMSIAL 412
Mo C3aR 356:MRKTNFTKSRNKTFRVAVAVVTVFFICWTPYHLVGVLLLITDPESSLGEAVMSWDHMSIAL 416
             *     **  *    *  **  * ** ***  * *       *      *** ***

            VII
           _____
Hu C3aR 424:ASANSCFNPFLYALLGKDFRKKARQSIQGILEAAFSEELTRSTHCPSNNVISERNS-TT-V 482
Gp C3aR 415:ASANSCFNPFLYALLGRDLRKRVRQSMKGILEAAFSEDISKSTSFIQAKAFSEKHSLSTNV 475
Rt C3aR 413:ASANSCFNPFLYALLGKDFRKKARQSVKGILEAAFSEELTHSTSCTQDKAPSKRNHMSTDV 473
Mo C3aR 417:ASANSCFNPFLYALLGKDFRKKARQSIKGILETAFSEELTHSTNCTQDKASSKRNNMSTDV 477
            **************** * ** *** **** ****  **       *    *   *
```

Figure 5B The complete protein sequences for the C3a receptor from human (Hu), guinea pig (Gp), rat (Rt), and mouse (Mo) are presented. The alignments were optimized for maximal identity and the seven transmembrane regions have been identified by a line and roman numerals. The residue positions that have been conserved in all species are denoted by an (*). These C3a receptors are similar to each other in size, but are considerably larger than the C5aR. The identifying feature between the C3aR and C5aR is the large second extracellular loop region comprised of approximately 170 residues. The expressed C3aR receptor on guinea pig cells has been estimated to be much larger than the 54 kDa nude protein reported here (84). This difference may be accounted for by glycosylation, since multiple oligosaccharide groups could be attached at several potential sites in the C3aR.

oligosaccharide content and a larger protein size than C5aR and most other known rhodopsin receptors. When the C3aR sequence is compared with that of C5aR or fMLP receptors there was 37.5% and 34.3% identity, respectively. Human C3aR has been expressed in HEK-293 and RBL-2H3 cells in which competitive binding with hC3a was demonstrated. C3aR expressed in CHO cells exhibited C3a-induced hydrolysis of phosphoinositides, which confirms that the expressed C3aR exhibits functional activity.

The C3aR has now been cloned from several animals including mouse (112,113), guinea pig, and rat (114,115), and the sequences of these receptor molecules are compared in Figure 5B. The patterns of identity between C3aR obtained from different species show relatively high levels in the N-terminal extracellular region and for the transmembrane segments. The second intracellular loop is also highly conserved, perhaps because the two cysteinyl residues participate in critical disulfide bonds. The large second extracellular loop has only modest homology while the C-terminal intracellular region, which contains the G-protein binding site, is highly conserved. Because the major unique feature for C3aR compared to other rhodopsin receptors is the unusually large second extracellular loop, this region may prove to be particularly important for binding the C3a molecule (see Fig. 4).

B. Distribution of the Anaphylatoxin Receptors

Early functional and chemical cross-linking studies using purified factors indicated that C5a receptors (CD88) exist on neutrophils (93), monocytes (macrophages) (116,117), basophils (118,119) and eosinophils (120), as well as platelets (121,122) and mast cells (123,124) from certain species. C5aR is expressed on myeloid cell lines, such as U937 and HL-60, but only after these cells are induced to differentiate to a more mature stage of development. Recently, evidence has been presented that C5aR is expressed on liver parenchymal cells, lung vascular smooth muscle, lung and umbilical vascular endothelial cells, bronchial and alveolar epithelial cells, as well as astrocytes and microglial cells (18,21,125). Tissue distribution of C5aR was most predominant in human heart, lung, spleen, spinal cord, and in many regions of the brain. The C5a receptors are distributed much more widely than previously believed in terms of both cell and tissue type, and it is now clear that these receptors are present not just on myeloid inflammatory cells but on a variety of tissue cells. Distribution of CD88 on mast cells and macrophages in skin, digestive, vascular, and pulmonary tissue, along with numerous receptor-bearing organ cells, suggest that particular tissues are more highly responsive to C5a stimulation than others.

The C3a receptor has been demonstrated on guinea pig platelets (121), rat mast cells (124), human alveolar macrophages, neutrophils, basophils (126), and eosinophils (127) by either functional assays or using chemical cross-linking techniques. Flow cytometry was used to identify C3aR on peripheral monocytes and umbilical vein endothelial cells, as well as the Raji cell line and differentiated HL-60 and U-937 monocytic cell lines (11). Northern blot analysis showed high levels of mRNA for C3aR in human lung and spleen, with lower levels in heart, placenta, kidney, thymus, testis, ovaries, small intestine, colon, and several regions of the brain (10). This wide distribution of message for the C3aR is surprising since C3a was believed to have a more limited functional and physiological role than C5a. Observations of C3a as a chemotactic factor for eosinophils and perhaps basophils, but not neutrophils, suggests a specialized role for C3a in inflammatory responses involving these cell types (127). There is new biology to be learned from the recent discovery that C3a receptors are as widely distributed as receptors for cytokines and a host of other important mediators.

C. Mapping of the Anaphylatoxin/Receptor-Binding Sites

1. Mapping the C5a and C3a Molecule.

Peptide modeling of the C-terminal effector site of C5a (128) demonstrated that even synthetic analogues as large as 21-residues exhibit only low levels of activity. These results further suggested that interactions in addition to the C-terminal region are required for full potency of C5a. When the 74-residue C5a molecule was truncated at the C-terminus by limited enzymatic cleavage to form the fragment C5a 1–69, this degradation product retained an ability to bind to the C5a receptor (45,46). Together, these studies indicated that the C-terminus of the molecule plays a major role in receptor binding and is essential for function, while establishing that multiple sites exist on C5a for binding to the receptor. Epitope-specific antibodies that interact with either the "core" 1–69 region or the C-terminal portion, and block C5a binding to the receptor, also support the concept of multiple binding sites on C5a (129,130). Further investigations to elucidate the exact location of the receptor binding sites on C5a were made possible by isolation of a molecular clone of C5a (52–55) and expression of the recombinant product.

Site-directed mutagenesis studies confirmed earlier enzymatic cleavage studies indicating that the C-terminal arginine is crucial for obtaining maximal receptor binding and biological potency (72,131,132). Additional residues having a significant effect on receptor binding of C5a within the C-terminal region are Gly 73, Leu 72, Met 70, Lys 68, His 67 and Ser 66, based on residue replacement studies (132,133). These studies also identified a number of residues in the core and N-terminal regions of the molecule that appear to be involved directly or indirectly in receptor interaction. Regions identified in the mutagenesis studies either have direct interaction with the receptor or stabilize conformation of the active molecule. Mollison et al. (72) identified three discontinuous binding regions of the molecule involved in receptor interaction, suggesting that C5a achieves high-affinity binding with the receptor through interaction of its C-terminus in concert with residues on the disulfide-linked core and possibly side chains on a turn connecting the core portion to the N-terminal helix. Substitution of Arg 40 → Gly or Lys reduces receptor binding and biological activity without causing detectable conformation changes as evaluated by NMR (72). This result indicates that Arg 40 and perhaps several nearby residues on the folded C5a molecule interact directly with the receptor. Another group was unable to reproduce these results (131), while the potential role of Arg 40 was confirmed by Toth et al. (132). Additional sites on the surface of the core and at the N-terminal region of C5a molecule were identified as participating in the receptor interaction including residues centered around Tyr 15 (72,132), residues Ile 6 and Tyr 13 (62), and residues Lys 19 and Lys 20 (131,134). Studies exploring the binding requirements for C5a sometimes used C3a/C5a chimeras, utilizing structural elements of C3a to provide a framework for selecting regions of C5a for mutation. These studies identified helix III (C5a 34–41) and loop 3 (C5a 41–47) of the C5a core as potential sites for receptor interaction, in addition to the C-terminal region (131,132). Conserved residues such as Arg 62 and Lys 67 (see Fig. 3B), are likely candidates for charge-charge interactions.

Primary structure comparisons revealed that rat C5a contains three additional residues (LLH, residues 4–6) near the N-terminus of the molecule, compared to human C5a (see Fig 2). It was suggested that this insertion is responsible for the 5–25 times greater potency of rat C5a and C5a$_{desArg}$ in biological assays, compared to human C5a and C5a$_{desArg}$ (135). When recombinant human C5a was engineered with this three-residue insert, the mutant hu C5a (LLH) failed to show enhanced potency, indicating that other sequence/ conformational differences were responsible for the markedly enhanced potency of rat C5a and C5a$_{desArg}$ (136). These data indicate that the many sequence differences between rat and human C5a in the C-terminal region may account for much of the potency variation between C5a from these two species.

A unique site-directed mutagenesis study was carried out in which a C3a/C5a hybrid molecule was generated by substituting three of the five residues at the C-terminal end of C5a (MQLGR) to create the C-terminal sequence (LGLAR) of native C3a (137). This hybrid anaphylatoxin molecule exhibited both C3a and C5a characteristics as detected by receptor binding and functional assays. This biological characterization took advantage of two specific guinea pig strains, one deficient for C3aR and the other for C5aR. The results of this study indicated that the C3a/C5a hybrid molecule interacts with both of the receptors, but with different affinities. Affinity of the C3a/C5a hybrid molecule for C3aR was 100–1000-fold less than that of native C3a, confirming that more than five C-terminal residues of C3a are required for optimal interaction with its receptor and that the additional sub-site interactions are specific for the C3a structure. Affinity of the hybrid molecule for C5aR decreased less dramatically than it did for C3aR, being only 10-fold less than native C5a. These effects on receptor binding indicated that structural elements in the core portion of C5a, which were conserved in this hybrid molecule, play a significant role in receptor recognition for C5a, while the exact sequence of C-terminal residues appear to be less crucial for C5a, as long as Leu 72 and Arg 74 remains intact (137).

Current knowledge regarding receptor interaction sites of C3a is based on the previously discussed synthetic analogue studies. These studies identified the C-terminal pentamer LGLAR as the minimal structural element required for C3a function (56). Unlike C5a, for which intensive efforts largely failed to generate analogues equipotent with the natural factor, the 21-residue C-terminal analogue of C3a (C3a 57–77) is nearly equipotent to the intact factor in some assay systems (50,76), and several modified shorter analogues actually exceeded potency of the natural C3a (79,80,85). A common feature of the modified analogues of C3a is the addition of a bulky hydrophobic moiety. One study determined that an optimal distance exists between the C-terminal arginyl residue and the hydrophobic group. This result indicated that a specific, multisite interaction exists between the C3a receptor and the synthetic analogues (85,86). One can therefore hypothesize that both primary and secondary binding sites exists on the C3a molecule, as in C5a, but that the sites are contiguous and in close proximity on the C-terminal helix (86). These characteristics of the C3a binding site identify a clear difference between the nature of C3a and C5a binding with their respective receptors (see Fig. 4A, B).

The C3a/C5a hybrid studies are the only mutagenesis studies, to our knowledge, aimed at investigating the C3a receptor binding sites (137). The conclusion from these studies confirmed that a secondary binding site is also required for optimal binding affinity of C3a to its receptor.

2. Mapping the C5a and C3a Receptor

Cloning of the C5a receptor (7,8) provided new opportunities for elucidating the requirements for ligand–receptor interactions between C5a and its receptor. Antibodies generated against peptides based on the extracellular loops of C5aR were used to confirm receptor expression and to investigate ligand binding to the C5a receptor. Antibodies generated to peptides that mimic portions of the N-terminal extracellular region of C5aR are not only excellent markers of cells and tissues expressing the receptor (18,20,21,138), but block binding and cellular activation by the intact ligand C5a (139,140). Surprising was that neither cell binding nor cellular activation by the synthetic C-terminal analogues of C5a was blocked by these antibodies (139,141). These results strongly suggested that the N-terminal region of the receptor is not the primary effector binding site for C5a, but defines a secondary non-effector binding site (139). Based on epitope mapping, using a panel of blocking monoclonal antibodies specific for defined sequences in the N-terminal region of C5aR, regions representing aspartic acid-rich sequences of the N-terminus (i.e., residues C5aR [16–23] or residues C5aR [19–29]) were identified as the secondary ligand-binding domain in C5aR (140,142). Antibodies raised to peptides representing other extracellular regions of C5aR either bound very weakly to the receptor and/or failed to interfere with ligand binding (140). To date, the primary or effector binding site on C5aR for C5a has not been identified using these immunological mapping techniques.

The importance of the N-terminal region of C5aR in ligand binding was further confirmed in a series of mutagenesis studies. Truncation of the N-terminal 1–22 residues in C5aR (67,143) abrogated C5a binding, but had no effect on binding of the bioactive C-terminal analogues of C5a (67,143). Point mutations were used to convert the five aspartic acid residues present in the N-terminal region to alanines (i.e., Asp 10, 15, 16, 21, 27 → Ala), resulting in significant loss in binding affinity of C5a. These data indicated the critical role of aspartic acid residues in C5aR for ligand/receptor interactions (143,144).

The existence of at least two separate binding sites on the receptor for C5a was further confirmed by a study utilizing proteolytic cleavage of the receptor (67). A specific spider venom protease from *Plectruerys tristes* cleaves C5aR between the second and third transmembrane helices (i.e., first extracellular loop), which abrogates C5a binding without interfering with binding of synthetic C5a C-terminal analogues (67). These effects are indistinguishable from effects obtained by removal of a portion of the N-terminal region by chymotrypsin digestion (140,145,146), or by receptor N-terminal truncation by mutagenesis (67,143,144). Additional studies creating receptor chimeras between portions of the formyl-peptide receptor (FPR) and C5aR confirmed the role of the N-terminal region for ligand-binding (144) and localized the second binding site of C5aR to the region containing the second and third extracellular loops (147). These results indicate that the primary, effector-binding site of C5a is located on the C-terminal half of C5aR.

Based on all of these results, a model was designed that proposes that one interaction occurs between the aspartic acid side chains in the N-terminal portion of the C5a receptor and the conserved, cationic residue side chain of Arg 40 (and possibly Arg 37 and Lys 12) in human C5a. A second interaction must occur between another anionic site on C5aR, presumably located on one of the extracellular loop or transmembrane regions, and conserved basic residues Arg 62, His 66, Lys 67, and Arg 74 of the human C5a molecule. Based on this model (see Fig 4B), contact between C5a and the N-terminal site on the receptor would raise the effective C5a concentration, thereby promoting interaction with the primary effector-binding site and resulting in receptor activation (67).

Studies focusing on localizing the primary effector-binding site on C5aR have used point-mutation techniques. Replacement of residues Asp 82, Glu 179 and Glu 180 by alanine had no effect on C5a binding (148). Replacement of Glu199 and Arg206 by alanine caused a major depression in binding and identified these residues as part of the effector binding site in C5aR (148a,148b). These results concluded that specific residues of the second intracellular loop and residues on the fifth intramembrane helix may participate in formation of the primary effector-binding site of C5aR (see Fig. 4). Truncation of the C-terminal, intracellular tail of C5aR revealed that deletion of residues 314–350 disrupts expression, while deletion of the last 26 residues (i.e., 326–350) does not affect expression or ligand binding of the receptor (149).

Similar studies are in progress to determine the architecture and to localize binding sites on the C3a receptor. As described earlier, the recently cloned human C3aR contains an unusually large extracellular loop (between transmembrane helices 4 and 5), a feature unique among G-protein-coupled receptors (9–11). Since it has been postulated that the large extracellular loop might contain some or all the structural determinants for C3a binding, this region will be the focus of future studies. Generation of loop-deletion mutants and chimeric C3aR/C5aR receptors are in progress in several laboratories, and it is hoped that these techniques will provide answers for these questions.

IV. BIOLOGICAL CHARACTERISTICS OF THE ANAPHYLATOXINS

A. Effects of Anaphylatoxins on Myeloid Cells

The discussion in the following sections will be primarily limited to effects of the C3a and C5a anaphylatoxins on myeloid cells. Since there is minimal evidence for specific bioactivities associated with C4a, we will address the known functions of the two better-characterized factors C3a and C5a. This does not exclude the possibility that C4a may have yet undiscovered activities or be physiologically active through nonspecific cationic effects, as will be outlined in the later sections.

Cellular responses to the anaphylatoxin C5a reflect the prominent pro-inflammatory character of the molecule (see Table 2). Perhaps the property most closely identified with C5a is the potent chemotactic activity for granulocytes, particularly neutrophils and eosinophils. C5a induces chemotactic migration for either of these cell types in vitro at an EC_{50} of between 0.5 and 2.0 nM (127,150,151). C5a is also a potent activator of inflammatory mediator release from all granulocytes. In neutrophils and eosinophils, C5a induces release of all known classes of secretory granules, leading to extracellular liberation of a wide range of inflammatory mediators including elastase, peroxidase, glucuronidase, and lactoferrin in neutrophils. Peroxidase, major basic protein (MBP), eosinophil-derived neurotoxin (EDN), and eosinophil cationic protein (ECP) are released from eosinophils (152–154) and arachidonate and vasoamines from basophils by C5a (119,155,156). C5a also activates the NADPH-oxidase pathway in granulocytes, leading to an oxidative burst (153,157). Many of these responses to C5a have been well characterized and described in detail in previous articles and reviews (25). Treatment of granulocytes with cytochalasin B or an equivalent microfilament-disrupting agent is required to elicit these responses *in vitro* at a maximal level, with the exception of chemotaxis. This same requirement is shared by other granulocyte-activating factors including f-MLF and IL-8. Experimental evidence suggests that phagocytosis or adhesive interactions with other cell types or with the extracellular matrix replaces the effect of cytochalasin B for the in vivo cellular response to C5a (158–160). Consistent with this hypothesis, C5a has been shown to act as a proadhesive stimulus for granulocytes. C5a leads to an activated phenotype in both neutrophils and eosinophils, as reflected by an increased expression of β_2 integrins and concurrent shedding of L-selectin (161–163). C5a has also been shown to increase adher-

Table 2 Cellular Effects of the Anaphylatoxins C3a and C5a

Inflammatory effects	Effects	Known responding cells
C5a	Chemotaxis	Neutrophils, eosinophils, basophils monocytes/macrophages, microglial cells (?), astroctyes (?) dendritic cells
	Degranulation	Neutrophils, eosinophils, platelets[a], mast cells
	NADPH Oxidase (O_2^-)	Neutrophils, eosinophils
	Promotes adhesion	Neutrophils, eosinophils, platelets
	Arachidonic acid metabolism	Neutrophils, eosinophils, basophils, monocytes/macrophages, mast cells
C3a	Chemotaxis	Eosinophils
	Degranulation	Eosinophils, mast cells, platelets[a]
	NADPH oxidase (O_2^-)	Eosinophils
	Promotes adhesion	Eosinophils, platelets[a]
Immunoregulatory effects		
C5a	Induces acute phase proteins	Hepatocyte cell lines
	Induces cytokine production	Monocytes (IL-6, IL-8, IL-1)
	Enhances antibody production	PBMC
C3a	Inhibits antibody production	PBMC, B cells
	Alters cytokine production	PBMC, Monocytes, B cells

[a] Guinea pig only; not human.

ence of neutrophils and eosinophils to cultured endothelial cells (164,165; M. Jagels, unpublished observation), indicating the dynamic adhesive events stimulated by this factor.

As observed in neutrophils and eosinophils, C5a also leads to activation of tissue mast cells and circulating basophils. C5a causes mast cell degranulation, leading to release of potent vasoactive mediators such as histamine and serotonin (2,3,166). C5a has also been reported to promote chemotactic movement of mast cells (167). There is also strong evidence that C5a induces arachidonate mobilization and metabolism in many granulocytic cells, leading to a variety of eicosanoid products, depending on the activated cell type. In addition to inducing histamine release, C5a appears to induce production of thromboxane TxA_2 and cysteinyl-leukotrienes in mast cells (135,168). In basophils, C5a may lead to production of LTB_4, which may lead to further amplification of the humoral immune response (169). There is compelling evidence that these arachidonate products play an important role in many pathological effects of C5a as discussed below. Removal of the C-terminal arginine in human C5a by serum carboxypeptidase N leads to a measurably diminished cellular responsiveness to this factor, thereby leading to the nomenclature $C5a_i$ (inactive) or $C5a_{desArg}$.

In human monocytes, C5a also acts primarily as a proinflammatory mediator. C5a is chemotactic for human monocytes (170,171) and upregulates expression of monocyte β_2 integrin expression and enhances monocyte adhesion to cultured endothelium (172,173). In addition, C5a is capable of either directly inducing or synergistically enhancing LPS-induced production of inflammatory cytokines, including IL-1, IL-6 and IL-8 (174–176). C5a augments specific and polyclonal antibody responses by PBMC in vitro, apparently through an induction of monocyte-derived cytokines (177). C5a increased production of

IL-6 in human and mouse mixed lymphocyte response as an in vitro assay of the cellular immune response and enhanced the proliferative T cell responses in these assays (178). Mitogen induced T- or B-cell responses were found to be unaffected by C5a. It is interesting that $C5a_{desArg}$ was found to be nearly equipotent to C5a in these assays, suggesting that receptor expression and/or signaling may differ between mononuclear cells and cells of granulocytic lineage.

In contrast to the broad, proinflammatory effects of C5a, the effects of C3a appear to be much more selective in terms of cellular responsiveness, and less specifically proinflammatory, depending on cell type. Despite an awareness that C3a exerts a multitude of effects on several cell types, the cellular C3a receptor has only recently been identified. Studies thus far, based on molecular data and antibody-binding studies, suggest that the C3a receptor is broadly expressed on myeloid cells including neutrophils, eosinophils, monocytes, and B lymphocytes (9–11,179). The effects of C3a on eosinophils are qualitatively similar to those of C5a. C3a is chemotactic for eosinophils, and can induce both granule release and an oxidative burst (127,154,157). It is known that C3a, like C5a, also upregulates expression of β_2 integrins and induces shedding of L-selectin on eosinophils, observations consistent with the profile of C3a as a selective activating factor for eosinophils. C3a is at least 10-fold less potent than C5a in inducing these responses, a differential potency compensated in part by the potential plasma levels of each factor that can be generated (180). Despite the molecular data strongly suggesting that neutrophils bear the C3a receptor, these cells appear to be essentially devoid of responsiveness to C3a, with the exception of being capable of inducing an intracellular calcium flux (110,154). This selective activity of C3a on eosinophils has led to considerable interest in this molecule as a potential participant in allergic diseases. C3a is also an effective activator of mast cells, leading to a full profile of mediator release (2,3,166). In fact, most of the immediate tissue and in vivo effects of C3a are consistent with its role as a mast cell activator.

While the effects of C3a and C5a on granulocytes appear quite similar, their effects on mononuclear cells are more divergent. Studies conducted over a decade ago demonstrated that while C5a enhanced in vitro humoral responses in mixed PBMC, C3a effectively suppressed these responses at physiologically relevant concentrations (178,181,182). These early studies concluded that C3a could lead to induction of a suppressor cell population, which was then responsible for the diminished antibody production. More recent studies have suggested not only that highly purified and resting tonsilar B cells may bear receptors for C3a, but that they respond directly to C3a in terms of diminished antibody and cytokine production after costimulation with a combination of *Staphylococcus aureus cowan* and IL-2 (179).

Recent reports suggest that C3a may induce differing responses from mixed PBMCs exposed to LPS, depending on the adhesive state of these cells. It was reported that C3a suppressed cytokine production when these cells were cultured in polypropylene tubes, which prevents cell-matrix adhesion. However, C3a enhanced LPS-induced cytokine production when cultures were carried out in standard polystyrene tissue culture plates (183). Recent studies in our laboratory, using purified monocytes, have demonstrated a clear suppressive effect of C3a on LPS-induced production of inflammatory cytokines. In contrast, C3a enhances LPS-induced production of the immunosuppressive cytokine IL-10. One interesting observation common to each of the above three studies is that $C3a_{desArg}$ retains biological activity in each of these assays. The fact that these actions of $C3a_{desArg}$ occur through specific receptor interactions is still highly contentious. Most functional responses of myeloid cells, including essentially all eosinophil responses, and the immunosuppressive effects of C3a on humoral immune responses in mixed PBMC populations, are not elicited by $C3a_{desArg}$ at submicromolar concentrations. On the other hand, in the systems just mentioned above, as well as in mast cell activation, the potency of $C3a_{desArg}$ ranges from being equipotent with C3a to having approximately 10% of the activity of the parent molecule. The residual activity of $C3a_{desArg}$ has frequently been attributed to the nonspecific polycation effects as defined originally by Mousli et al. (184). At the biochemical level, C3a (and $C3a_{desArg}$) is a highly charged cationic protein at physiological pH. It was found that in rat peritoneal mast cells, C3a and $C3a_{desArg}$ were nearly equipotent in inducing histamine release (123). It was further found that a number of otherwise unrelated cationic molecules also induced histamine release, and that their potency correlated with their charge to mass ratio. Based primarily on these data, it was concluded that rat mast cells do not bear specific C3a receptors and that the activating effects of C3a were essentially nonspecific, but related to the cationic nature of the molecule. This property has also been used to explain mast cell-activating capabilities of the anaphylatoxin C4a. C4a is a comparably charged molecule to C3a, and has been found to activate mast cells at concentrations roughly equivalent to those of $C3a_{desArg}$, approximately 2–10 micromolar (24). It is unknown if a similar polycation effect occurs with nonmast cells, including monocytes or B lymphocytes. Therefore, the controversy continues concerning receptor-specific activity for $C3a_{desArg}$. This does not belie the potential physiological significance of the circulating forms of C3a and C4a (i.e., $C3a_{desArg}$ and $C4a_{desArg}$) forms, since micromolar levels of C4a and/or C3a may be generated in vivo.

B. Effects of the Anaphylatoxins on Nonmyeloid Cells

On a historical basis, biological responsiveness to anaphylatoxins has been thought to be restricted to cells of a myeloid lineage. This concept resulted principally from a lack of tissue effects implicating nonmyeloid cells, and a failure to demonstrate anaphylatoxin receptors on nonmyeloid cells. Recent studies, partly fueled by the recent identification and characterization of the C3a receptor, demonstrate that the anaphylatoxins have a broader spectrum of actions than originally recognized. Some of the most exciting findings in this area have been reports from Ward's laboratory demonstrating that endothelial cells are directly activated by C5a. In 1992, Murphy et al. reported that cultured rat pulmonary vascular endothelial cells produce oxygen free radical upon stimulation by C5a or TNF-α (185). Although the authors cautioned that superoxide production by endothelial cells is not a response that may be generalized across species, human C5a was found to be active in this model. These findings were extended in 1994 by Foreman et. al. (19) who demonstrated that cultures of human umbilical vein endothelial cells (HUVEC) exhibited upregulation of P-selectin and released von Wildebrand factor when stimulated by C5a. Since this important adhesion molecule is involved in leukocyte homing to inflamed tissue, and von Wildebrand factor is an important component in the coagulation cascade, the role of C5a in vasoactivity was expanded. Concentrations of C5a required to elicit these responses were on the order of 100 nM, approximately 100 times the Kd for C5a receptors on the granulocytes. Unfortunately, no further characterizations of the specificity (i.e., $C5a_{desArg}$, synthetic C5a agonists, receptor blocking antibodies, Scatchard analysis, or signal transduction) were presented with these studies. It remains unclear whether endothelial activation relies on a novel signaling mechanism for C5a. Although there have not been reports from other groups demonstrating a direct effect of C5a on endothelial cells, these findings were supported by studies by Haviland et al., showing staining of pulmonary vascular endothelial cells with anti-C5a receptor antibodies (18). A more complete pharmacological and biochemical characterization of the endothelial response to C5a is certainly needed and will undoubtedly help establish this exciting area of research.

Another tissue that appears to have a unique and specific responsiveness to C5a is the liver. Buchner et al. demonstrated that C5a directly stimulates synthesis and release of acute phase proteins from HepG2 cells, a hepatoma cell line (138). These studies demonstrated C5a receptor expression by RT-PCR and antibody binding, and functional responsiveness of these cells by transcriptional and protein expression upregulation of alpha-1-antitrypsin and alpha-1-antichymotrypsin. This report was immediately followed by studies by McCoy et al., confirming the expression of functional receptors for both C5a and formyl peptides on HepG2 cells (186). In addition to alpha-1 antichymotrypsin, these authors reported increased production of complement C3 and factor B, as well as decreases in albumin and transferrin synthesis. Dose–response and binding studies in these two reports suggest that C5a is effective at concentrations comparable to those necessary for granulocyte activation, and binding studies suggest a comparable affinity (Kd = 1-2 nM) and a receptor density of approximately 28,000/cell, a level somewhat lower than that observed on neutrophils (187). Using in situ hybridization and immunohistochemistry, the same group provided evidence that the C5a receptor is expressed on normal liver parenchymal cells, suggesting that their observations with the HepG2 cell line were not an artifact from using transformed cells (18). In addition, work by Jaeschke et al. suggests that cells in the liver (hypothesized by the authors to be Kupfer cells, which are of myeloid lineage) produced cysteinyl leukotrienes in response to C5a (188). It was suggested that the arachidonate products may contribute to liver injury in endotoxin-induced shock. The cellular source of these arachidonate products has not yet been firmly assigned and could derive from vascular endothelial cells, mast cells, tissue macrophages, and/or hepatocytes.

The C5a receptor has also been identified on cultured human fetal astrocytes and astrocyte cell lines (189). Although there is growing evidence for a role of complement in demyelinating diseases, neurodegeneration, and other central nervous system diseases, the potential effects of C5a in these disorders have remained a topic of extensive controversy (190). When injected into the rat brain, C5a induces specific identifiable behavioral changes (191). There is also evidence of specific cellular C5a binding in brain slices, and reports that C5a is chemotactic for rat microglial cells and astrocytes (125,192,193). By RT-PCR, Western blotting and immunolocalization, Gasque et al. demonstrated receptor expression on cultured human astrocytes (189). The receptors appear to be functionally coupled, because an intracellular calcium flux was induced by C5a at concentrations as low as 1 nM. The potential role of C5a in CNS disease is strongly implicated by the present data and therefore remains a topic worthy of further study.

Reports of C5a receptor expression and/or responsiveness for cell types other than those described above remain inconclusive. Although Haviland et al. detected mRNA for C5a receptor in a broad spectrum of tissues (18), it is difficult to assign a nonmyeloid source for this mRNA. Using antibodies generated against the C5a receptor, this group also demonstrated staining of bronchial epithelium and vascular smooth muscle in the lung. As a caution, Werfel et al., reported that many antibodies generated against the C5a receptor molecule cross-react with antigen(s) present on the surface of many epithelial cell types, which appears unrelated to the C5a receptor (194). Identification of receptor expression solely by antibody binding must therefore be interpreted with this reservation in mind. To our knowledge there are no reports of functional responses of isolated or cultured epithelial or smooth muscle cells to C5a.

The potential effects of C3a on nonmyeloid cells have not been explored in great detail, partly due to a lack of information concerning this receptor. Since the receptor to C3a has recently been identified and cloned, and antibodies generated to the molecule, it is only a matter of time until the biological manifestations associated with this receptor have been identified. Although Northern blot analysis has suggested a wide distribution of the C3a receptor, evidence for direct C3a stimulation on nonmyeloid cells has not been reported. Again, the presence of mast cells and myeloid cells in these tissues prevents conclusive assignment of receptor expression to a particular cell type. It is anticipated that the new molecular tools available will accelerate characterization of the cellular distribution of the C3a receptor, which will considerably expand our knowledge of this ligand/receptor system in the next few years.

C. Tissue Effects of the Anaphylatoxins

Effects of the anaphylatoxins on isolated tissues are consistent with their known role as spasmogens. C5a and C3a induce smooth muscle contraction in virtually all tissue types tested including ileal, uterine, bronchial, and vascular smooth muscle (24,135). This contractile effect is prominent in tissues obtained from various species, although the extent or magnitude of the effect differs from species to species because the secondary mediators responsible for contraction varies. Ileal contraction in virtually all species tested, except for the rat, appears to be histamine-dependent, consistent with the hypothesis that mast cell stimulation is largely responsible for these effects. In many rat tissues and in bronchial smooth muscle of most species, constriction appears to depend on formation of cysteinyl leukotrienes (LTC_4, LTD_4, and LTE_4; also known as SRS-A) and not on histamine. Contractile effects on vascular tissue appear to involve both cysteinyl leukotrienes and TxA_2. The cellular source of anaphylatoxin-induced leukotrienes and prostanoids remains undefined, but the findings suggest that mast cells, resident macrophages, and perhaps endothelial cells play a prominent role in both pulmonary and vascular effects of C3a and C5a.

When injected intradermally, C5a elicits an immediate inflammatory response characterized by redness, edema, and eventual infiltration of leukocytes (150). Granulocytes are elicited into the skin rapidly, within 30 mins. Monocytes also appear, approximately 2–4 h after injection of C5a (195). The redness (vasodilation) and swelling are most likely consequences of mast cell activation by C5a, while neutrophil recruitment is presumably due to the chemotactic properties of the molecule. Mast cell activation may also contribute to cellular recruitment through elaboration of additional chemotactic factors or through de novo generation of C3a and/or C5a by granular proteinases (196). The release of mast cell products may augment cellular infiltration in the Arthus reaction by increasing vascular permeability, thereby increasing availability of C5 at the injury site for conversion to C5a (197). Monocyte recruitment is probably augmented by tissue injury and activation of the endothelium through neutrophil degranulation. Activated neutrophils and mast cells generate monocyte-directed chemotactic factors that are combined with the direct chemotactic effects of C5a on monocytes.

Many tissue effects of C3a are virtually identical to those of C5a and this supports the notion that mast cells are again prominent players at the tissue level. Intradermal injection of C3a leads to a classical wheal and flare response, but without a significant leukocyte infiltration, suggesting that the chemotactic properties of C3a for eosinophils may be insufficient at these levels to induce eosinophil recruitment (150). As an alternative, C3a may be converted to the chemotactically inactive des Arg form before eosinophil recruitment can occur. The lack of neutrophil or monocyte recruitment suggests that local mast cell activation *per se* is insufficient to generate chemotactic signals for either of these circulating cell types.

It has also been reported that C5a has a contractile effect on porcine myocardium (198). Both histamine and thromboxane were detected in the tissue perfusate, although inhibitor studies demonstrated that histamine was principally responsible for the contractile effect. Both C3a and C5a contract guinea pig airway smooth muscle (199,200) and this effect has been shown to be largely histamine independent (201). C5a was shown to contract this airway tissue mainly by releasing arachidonate products and it appears that the cysteinyl-leukotrienes are involved along with histamine. In the case of C3a, the prostaglandins appear to be more prominently involved than the leukotrienes in mediating the contraction of airway tissue (i.e., lung strips).

D. In Vivo Effects of Anaphylatoxins

The effects of intrapulmonary instillation of C5a are dramatic, although they are in part difficult to rationalize. Instillation of intact C5a into guinea pig airway leads to rapid pulmonary distress, with evidence of bronchoconstriction, vasoconstriction, and increased capillary permeability (202). Leukocyte aggregates in the vasculature are evident, as is focal hemorrhage. Tachypnea continues for approximately 20 mins before respiration gradually returns to normal. It is surprising that although C5a alone fails to induce lethality in guinea pigs over a 30 min period in this model, the same dose of $C5a_{desArg}$ was lethal in 50% of the animals tested. These results suggest that the des Arg form of C5a retains bioactivity at the tissue level. An acceptable explanation of why $C5a_{desArg}$ would be more toxic that intact C5a remains to be determined. It is noteworthy that porcine C5a and $C5a_{desArg}$ were used in these studies, and that porcine $C5a_{desArg}$ retains a greater degree of spasmogenic activity than does its human counterpart. C3a induced essentially the same profile of effects as C5a when instilled into the guinea pig lung, except that greater quantities of C3a were required to obtain a comparable effect (202). In contrast to $C5a_{desArg}$, $C3a_{desArg}$ was inactive in this system. It should be noted that these factors appear to be more toxic when instilled into the lungs than when injected into the bloodstream. This indicates that the larger effects of the factors occur extravascularly and so once they escape the vasculature they may become a significant threat to the host animal.

Systemic intravenous administration of C5a demonstrates many of the same pathophysiological effects as intratracheal administration (203). C5a is not generally lethal when injected into a number of animal models excluding the guinea pig. However, complement activation with cobra venom factor, which can rapidly convert the entire C3 and C5 pool, or coadministration of C5a with an inhibitor of carboxypeptidase N, leads to a potentially lethal systemic response in many animal models (12,203,204). Therefore, rapid conversion of C5a to $C5a_{desArg}$ probably accounts for the protective effect of SCPN. However, this mechanism may be overwhelmed by massive complement activation. Depending on the dose and the type of animal being tested, C5a may lead to respiratory distress, characterized by rapid, shallow breathing, presumably resulting from the spasmogenic effects of C5a. This effect is transient, and generally there is no evidence of leukocyte infiltration into the lung or damage to the vascular endothelium. Intravascular administration of C5a also leads to a transient peripheral hypotension. Evidence suggests that this response is caused primarily from pulmonary vasoconstriction, leading to a reduced cardiac output, rather than through a peripheral vasodilation (205). There is some evidence that peripheral vasodilation, secondary to production of PGI_2 and PGE_2, may make a minor contribution (206). The cellular source of these prostanoids has been hypothesized to include circulating leukocytes, tissue mast cells, or vascular endothelial cells (207,208). Plugging of pulmonary vascular beds by activated and aggregated leukocytes may also contribute to the diminished venous return from the lungs.

Intravascular C5a leads to other important hemodynamic effects that may contribute to concurrent pathophysiological conditions (i.e., ischemia, sepsis, immune complex disease). C5a leads to an immediate leukopenia upon intravenous administration, which results primarily from depletion of the granulocyte pool (209). The lung appears to be a primary site for the localization of noncirculating neutrophils, although they also localize prominently in the liver, spleen, and kidneys (210). The neutropenic event appears to be almost entirely dependent on the C5a (or $C5a_{desArg}$), because it rapidly reverses upon termination of C5a infusion. This process was recognized by physiologists decades ago in response to a variety of injected stimuli, and was termed "margination" (211). An attractive hypothesis, which has unfortunately become somewhat dogmatic, is that cells activated by C5a become adherent to the vasculature in the lung, leading to depletion of the circulating pool. This would have important consequences in terms of lung injury, since adhesion of leukocytes to the vasculature is a key first step in the inflammatory process. Unfortunately, a number of lines of evidence strongly suggest that margination is not an adhesion-dependent process. Important is that the neutropenia reverses rapidly upon removal of the activating stimulus, whereas firm adhesion has been shown to be slowly reversible, even under sheer stress (212). In addition, blocking antibodies to either integrin or selectin molecules fail to prevent the leukopenia induced by C5a (213,214). Using intravital microcopy techniques, Von Andrian conclusively demonstrated that leukocyte rolling and the physiological phenomenon of imargination are independent responses (212). It therefore appears that leukopenia results from cell stiffening and deformation (i.e., polarization) caused by actin filament assembly within the granulocytes as a response to C5a stimulation (215,216). Activated cells then become trapped in the small vasculature, resulting in plugged vessels. C5a-induced leukocyte trapping in the lung is not entirely without pathological effects, however. There is significant evidence that once these cells become trapped, in some instances they may form adhesive interactions with the endothelium, especially at higher concentrations of C5a (217). The process of trapping or margination therefore may supplant the need for upregulation of E- or P-selectins on the endothelium. Selectins are normally required for rolling, the first step in leukocyte transendothelial migration, but leukocyte aggregation and vasular plugging may replace this requirement.

A second major hemodynamic consequence of intravascular exposure to C5a is leukocytosis, a response resulting from bone marrow leukocyte mobilization. The cellular interactions involved in this process remain undefined, but it is known that C5a induces granulocyte release specifically, without inducing release of platelets, erythrocytes, or other myeloid cells (209). This effect is not specific to C5a, but is induced by a number of neutrophil chemoattractants. An increased circulating pool of neutrophils could potentially enhance any inflammatory response in which neutrophils play a role. C5a may therefore also act indirectly as a proinflammatory mediator simply by its ability to increase the number of cells capable of participating in the inflammatory response.

E. Pathophysiological Role of the Anaphylatoxins

Although the proinflammatory effects of anaphylatoxins are indisputably beneficial in the context of localized infections or injuries, there are a number of noninfectious diseases and syndromes in which anaphylatoxins appear to play a deleterious role. Perhaps the most direct link between complement activation and a pathological response results from extracorporeal circulation of the blood, either during hemodialysis or in coronary bypass surgery (218–220). This "postpump syndrome" is characterized by mild respiratory distress, pulmonary hypertension, occasional vascular leakage. The cause of these physiologic changes appears to be identical to those responses observed in experimental animal studies. The responses to intravenous administration of C3a or C5a (i.e., increased capillary permeability and edema, bronchoconstriction, pulmonary vasoconstriction, leukocyte aggregation in the lung vasculature, and possibly peripheral vasodilation), mimic this syndrome in humans. This syndrome appears to be an entirely complement-driven process, subsequent to complement activation through contact with nonbiocompatible materials making up the blood contact surfaces of dialysis and perfusion apparatus. Although the short-term consequences of these effects appear to result in minimal morbidity, there is concern that repeated intravascular complement activation, as occurs in patients undergoing chronic dialysis, may lead to long-term pathology of the lung (220). Furthermore, in the setting of cardiopulmonary bypass, the leukocyte aggregation in the lung and impaired pulmonary blood flow may detrimentally affect perfusion of the heart and other organs following surgery, and may contribute to a syndrome like acute respiratory distress syndrome (ARDS), which develops in a small percentage of bypass patients (218,219). The length of time a patient requires ventillatory support following surgery has been correlated with C3a levels in the blood following reperfusion (221).

ARDS and multiple system organ failure (MSOF) are two related syndromes that develop most frequently as a consequence of severe polytrauma or septicemia (222–224). The progression of ARDS and MSOF are similar and are characterized in the early stages by increased vascular permeability, impaired organ perfusion, and, in the case of ARDS, respiratory insufficiency. Later stages are characterized by a continuation of the early malfunctions, with progressive damage to endothelium, necrosis, leukocyte infiltration, and tissue necrosis and remodeling (225,226). In ARDS the damage is localized primarily to the lung, whereas in MSOF damage is disseminated not only to the lung but also to the liver, kidneys, and digestive tract. Several studies have suggested that complement activation, and particularly generation of C3a and C5a, may play an important role in the initiation of these syndromes, as well as their progression (227–229). Complement activation can be extensive following severe trauma, presumably secondary to tissue injury and activation by enzymes of the coagulation cascade. In cases of severe trauma, C3a levels suggesting conversion of virtually the entire C3 pool can be measured (230). The generation of these high levels of anaphylatoxins presumably lead to pathophysiology reminiscent of infusion of cobra venom factor or high levels of C3a or C5a in animals: bronchoconstriction, vascular permeability, peripheral hypotension and leukocyte plugging in the vasculature. As opposed to animal models, however, complement activation may be prolonged and continuous, as a consequence of continued production of C3 and C5 without resolution of the activating events. It is hypothesized that extended complement activation leads to activation of leukocytes trapped in the vasculature, causing production of superoxide and release of proteinases, which damage the endothelium and further contribute to vascular leakage. Studies have demonstrated that in victims of severe trauma anaphylatoxin levels are uniformly elevated. However, in those patients who develop ARDS or MSOF levels of C3a remain elevated, whereas in those patients who recover normally, C3a levels drop rapidly following the initial insult (230). Generation of C5a may also augment monocyte production of TNF-α and IL-1, two cytokines also implicated in the development of ARDS, particularly secondary to sepsis or infection.

C5a has also been shown to play an important role in the development of tissue injury, and particularly pulmonary injury, in animal models of septic shock. Treatment of either rats or pigs with antibodies directed against C5a before treatment with either endotoxin or *E. coli* bacteria resulted in decreased tissue injury, as well as decreased production of IL-6 (231,232). Furthermore, depletion of complement with cobra venom factor prior to infusion of endotoxin resulted in decreased liver production of cysteinyl-leukotrienes and reduced injury to the liver (188). Antibodies against C5a were also protective in cobra venom factor model of lung injury in rats, and in immune complex-induced lung injury (12). In the immune complex injury model, anti-C5a therapy also reduced intrapulmonary TNF-α levels and the upregulation of ICAM-1 in the vasculature. The importance of C5a in immune complex-mediated lung injury was confirmed in mice by Bozic et. al (233). Studies carried out with C5a receptor knockout mice established that increases in lung permeability and leukocyte infiltration induced by immune complexes were almost completely reversed compared to the wild type control. Using the same C5aR-deficient strain, this group could also demonstrate that C5a is essential for antibacterial host defense mechanisms in the lung (234). Although neutrophil influx in response to intratracheally administered *P. aeruginosa* was equivalent in the deletion mutants and in wild type controls, the C5aR-deficient mice were unable to clear the organism, resulting in essentially 100% mortality in the knockouts. It remains unclear if the importance of C5a can be generalized to all immune complex diseases and mucosal host defense, or if it is in some way selective for the lung. In either case, this appears to be a definitive example of an important new role and function for this humoral factor.

C5a has also been implicated as a major mediator in myocardial ischemia–reperfusion injury. Complement depletion and inhibition with anti-C5a antibodies has been shown to reduce infarct size significantly (235,236). These effects appear to be mediated by both neutrophil-dependent and independent mechanisms. Neutrophil activation and plugging in the coronary vessels lead to a capillary no-reflow phenomenon, and neutrophil inhibition or depletion has been shown to have a protective effect (237). Complement activation also appears to lead to myocardial ischemia by inducing production of the coronary vasoconstrictors TxA_2 and cysteinyl-leukotrienes, apparently via activation of coronary mast cells (238,239). Generation of C3a and C4a could presumably contributes to this effect as well.

It is likely that complement activation contributes to the pathogenesis of several other diseases, although the direct role of C3a or C5a may not be as clearly established. Inhibition of complement activation through administration of soluble CR1 has a protective effect in reversed passive Arthus reactions, glycogen-induced peritoneal inflammation, thermal injury, and in xenograft and allograft rejection. (240–242). Complement levels are elevated in patients with rheumatoid arthritis and systemic lupus erythematosus, and plasma C3a and C5a levels correlate with severity of the disease state (243–245). The effects of complement activation, and particularly generation of anaphylatoxins, must therefore be considered in any acute or chronic inflammatory condition. The findings that C5a blockade effectively inhibits or eliminates a number of *in vivo* responses, including the mucosal host response to *P. aeruginosa*, suggests that redundant pathways for C5a-mediated effects either do not exist under all conditions or are not always sufficient to replace critical or essential anaphylatoxin-mediated functions in inflammation and in selective mechanisms of host defense.

REFERENCES

1. Friedberger E. Weitere Untersuchungen uber Eisissanaphylaxie: IV. Mitteilung. Immunitaetaforsch Exp Ther 1910; 4:636–690.
2. Cochrane CG, Müller-Eberhard HJ. The derivation of two distinct anaphylatoxin activities from the third and fifth components of human complement. J Exp Med 1968; 127:368–371.
3. Dias da Silva W, Lepow IH. Complement as a mediator of inflammation. II. Biological properties of anaphylatoxin prepared with purified components of human complement. J Exp Med 1967; 125:921–946.
4. Lepow IH, Willms-Kretschmer RA, Patrick RA, Rosen FS. Gross and ultrastructural observations of lesions produced by intradermal injection of human C3a in man. Am J Pathol 1970; 61:13–20.
5. Wuepper KD, Bokisch VA, Müller-Eberhard HJ, Stoughton RB. Cutaneous responses to human C3 anaphylatoxin in man. Clin Exp Immunol 1972; 11:13–20.
6. Vallota EH, Müller-Eberhard HJ. Isolation and characterization of a new and highly active form of C5a anaphylatoxin from epsilon-aminocaproic acid-containing porcine serum. J Exp Med 1973; 137:1109–1123.
7. Gerard NP, Gerard C. The chemotactic receptor for human C5a anaphylatoxin. Nature 1991; 349:614–617.
8. Boulay F, Mery L, Tardif M, Brouchon L, Vignalis P. Expression cloning of a receptor for C5a anaphylatoxin on differentiated HL-60 cells. Biochemistry 1991; 30:2993–2999.
9. Crass T, Raffetseder U, Martin U, Grove M, Klos A, Köhl J, Bautsch W. Expression cloning of the human C3a anaphylatoxin receptor (C3aR) from differentiated U-937 cells. Eur J Immunol 1996; 26:1944–1950.
10. Ames RS, Li Y, Sarau HM, Nuthulaganti P, Foley JJ, Ellis C, Zeng Z, Su K, et al. Molecular cloning and characterization of the human anaphylatoxin C3a receptor. J Biol Chem 1996; 271:20231–20234.
11. Roglic A, Prossnitz ER, Cavanagh SL, Pan Z, Zou A, Ye RD. cDNA cloning of a novel G protein-coupled receptor with a large extracellular loop structure. Biochim Biophys Acta 1996; 1305:39–43.
12. Mulligan MS, Schmid E, Till GO, Friedl HP, Hugli TE, Johnson KJ, Ward PA. Requirement and role of C5a in acute lung inflammatory injury in rats. J Clin Invest 1996; 98:503–512.
13. Mulligan MS, Schmid E, Till GO, Hugli TE, Friedl HP, Roth RA, Ward PA. C5a-dependent upregulation in vivo of lung vascular P-selectin. J Immunol 1997; 158:1857–1861.
14. Schmid E, Warner RL, Crouch LD, Friedl HP, Till GO, Hugli TE, Ward PA. Neutrophil chemotactic activity and C5a following systemic activation of complement in rats. Inflammation 1997; 21:325–333.
15. Ito BR, Del Balzo U. Effect of platelet depletion and inhibition of platelet cyclooxygenase on C5a-mediated myocardial ischemia. Am J Physiol 1994; 267:H1288–H1294.
16. Ivey CL, Williams FM, Collins PD, Jose PJ, Williams TJ. Neutrophil chemoattractaants generated in two phases during reperfusion of ischemic myocardium in the rabbit. Evidence for a role for C5a and interleukin-8 (comment). J Clin Invest 1995; 95:2720–2728.
17. Amsterdam EA, Stahl GL, Pan HL, Rendig SV, Fletcher MP, Longhurst JC. Limitation of reperfusion injury by a monoclonal antibody to C5a during myocardial infarction in pigs. Am J Physiol 1995; 268:H448–H457.

18. Haviland DL, McCoy RL, Whitehead WT, Akama H, Molmenti EP, Brown A, Haviland JC, Parks WC. Cellular expression of the C5a anaphylatoxin receptor (C5aR): demonstration of C5aR on nonmyeloid cells of the liver and lung. J Immunol 1995; 154:1861–1869.

19. Foreman KE, Vaporciyan AA, Bonish BK, Jones ML, Glovsky MM, Eddy SM, Ward PA. C5a-induced expression of P-selectin in endothelial cells. J Clin Invest 1994; 94:1147–1155.

20. Gasque P, Chan P, Fontaine M, Ischenko A, Lamacz M, Götze O, Morgan BP. Identification and characterization of the complement C5a anaphylatoxin receptor on human astrocytes. Relevance to inflammation in the brain. J Immunol 1995; 155:4882–4889.

21. Gasque P, Singhrao SK, Neal JW, Götze O, Morgan BP. Expression of the receptor for C5a (CD88) is upregulated on reactive astrocytes, microglia and endothelial cells in inflammed human CNS. Am J Pathol 1997; 150:31–41.

22. Hugli TE, Müller-Eberhard HJ. Anaphylatoxins: C3a and C5a. Advances in Immunology. Dixon FJ, Kunkel HG (ed.). New York: Academic Press, 1978: 1–53.

23. Hugli TE. Chemical aspects of the serum anaphylatoxins. Contemp Top Mol Immunol 1978; 7:181–214.

24. Hugli TE. The structural basis for anaphylatoxin and chemotactic functions of C3a, C4a, and C5a. CRC Crit Rev Immunol 1981; 1:321–366.

25. Hugli TE. Structure and function of the anaphylatoxins. Semin Immunopathol 1984; 7:193–219.

26. Hugli TE. Structure and function of C3a anaphylatoxin. Curr Top Micribiol Immunol 1989; 153:181–208.

27. Goldstein IM. Inflammation: Basic Principles and Clinical Correlates, 2nd ed.; Gallin JI, Goldstein IM, Snyderman R. (ed.) New York: Raven Press, 1992: 63–80.

28. Hugli TE, Vallota EH, Müller-Eberhard HJ. Purification and partial characterization of human and porcine C3a anaphylatoxin. J Biol Chem 1975; 250:1472–1478.

29. Gorski JP, Hugli TE, Müller-Eberhard HJ. Characterization of human C4a anaphylatoxin. J Biol Chem 1981; 256:2707–2711.

30. Fernandez HN, Hugli TE. Partial characterization of human C5a anaphylatoxin. I. Chemical description of the carbohydrate and polypeptide portions of human C5a. J Immunol 1976; 117:1688–1694.

31. Budzko DB, Bokisch VA, Müller-Eberhard HJ. A fragment of the third component of human complememnt with anaphylatoxin activity. Biochemistry 1971; 10:1166–1172.

32. Meuer S, Becker S, Hadding U, Bitter-Suermann D. The anaphylatoxic peptide C3a of guinea pig complement, in purification, physiochemical and antigenic properties. Z Immunotatsforch 1978; 154:135.

33. Hugli TE, Gerard C, Kawahara M, Scheetz, II, Barton R, Briggs S, Koppel G, Russell S. Isolation of three separate anaphylatoxins from complement-activated human serum. Mol Cell Biochem 1981; 41:59–66.

34. Bokisch VA, Müller-Eberhard HJ. Anaphylatoxin inactivator of human plasma: Its isolation and characterization as a carboxypeptidase. J Clin Invest 1970; 49:2427–2436.

35. Plummer TH, Jr., Hurwitz NY. Human plasma carboxypeptidase N. J Biol Chem 1978; 253:3907–3912.

36. Vallota EH. Inhibition of C5 conversion by epsilon amino caproic acid (EACA): a limiting factor in the generation of C5a anaphylatoxin. Immunology 1978; 34:439–447.

37. Ondetti MA, Condon ME, Reid J, Sabo EF, Cheung HS, Cushman DW. Design of potent and specific inhibitors of carboxypeptidase A and B. Biochemistry 1979; 18:1427–1430.

38. Plummer TH, Jr., Ryan TJ. A potent mercapto bi-product analogue inhibitor for human carboxypeptidase N. Biochem Biophys Res Commun 1981; 98:448–454.

39. Mathews KP, Pan PM, Gardner NJ, Hugli TE. Familial carboxypeptidase N deficiency. Ann Intern Med 1980; 93:443–445.

40. Hugli TE. Human anaphylatoxin (C3a) from the third component of complement. Primary structure. J Biol Chem 1975; 250:8293–8301.

41. Moon KE, Gorski JP, Hugli TE. Complete primary structure of human C4a anaphylatoxin. J Biol Chem 1981; 256:8685–8692.

42. Fernandez HN, Hugli TE. Primary structural analysis of the polypeptide portion of human C5a anaphylatoxin. Polypeptide sequence determination and assignment of the oligosaccharide attachment site in C5a. J Biol Chem 1978; 253:6955–6964.

43. Hugli TE, Morgan WT, Müller-Eberhard HJ. Circular dichroism of C3a anaphylatoxin. Effects of pH, heat, guanidinium chloride, and mercaptoethanol on conformation and function. J Biol Chem 1975; 250:1479–1483.

44. Gerard C, Chenoweth DE, Hugli TE. Response of human neutrophils to C5a: a role for the oligosaccharide moiety of human C5a desArg-74 but not of C5a in biologic activity. J Immunol 1981; 127:1978–1982.

45. Chenoweth DE, Hugli TE. Human C5a and C5a analogs as probes of the neutrophil C5a receptor. Mol Immunol 1980; 17:151–161.

46. Gerard C, Chenoweth DE, Hugli TE. Molecular aspects of the serum chemotactic factors. J Reticuloendothel Soc 1979; 26:711–718.

47. Huber R, Scholze H, Paques EP, Deisenhofer J. Crystal structure analysis and molecular model of human C3a anaphylatoxin. Hoppe Seylers Z Physiol Chem 1980; 361:1389–1399.

48. Chazin WJ, Hugli TE, Wright PE. 1H NMR studies of human C3a anaphylatoxin in solution: sequential resonance assignments, secondary structure, and global fold. Biochemistry 1988; 27:9139–9148.

49. Hoeprich PD, Jr., Hugli TE. Helical conformation at the carboxy-terminal portion of human C3a is required for full activity. Biochemistry 1986; 25:1945–1950.

50. Lu ZX, Fok K-F, Erickson BW, Hugli TE. Conformational analysis of COOH-terminal segments of human C3a. Evidence of ordered conformation in an active 21-residue peptide. J Biol Chem 1984; 259:7367–7370.

51. Fukuoka Y, Yasui A, Tachibana T. Active recombinant C3a of human anaphylatoxin produced in *Escherichia coli*. Biochem Biophys Res Commun 1991; 175:1131–1138.

52. Kan C-C, Fukuoka Y, Hugli TE, Fey GH. Expression of recombinant human C5a in E. coli. [abstract]. Fed Proc 1986; 45:1941

53. Mandecki W, Mollison KW, Bolling TJ, Powell BS, Carter GW, Fox JL. Chemical synthesis of a gene encoding the human complement fragment C5a and its expression in *Escherichia coli*. Proc Natl Acad Sci USA 1985; 82:3543–3547.

54. Mollison KW, Fey TA, Krause RA, Mandecki W, Fox JL, Carter GW. High-level C5a gene expression and recovery of recombinant human C5a from *Escherichia coli*. Agents Actions 1987; 21:366–371.

55. Bautsch W, Emde M, Kretzschmar T, Köhl J, Suckau D, Bitter-Suermann D. Human C3a anaphylatoxin: gene cloning and expression in *Escherichia coli*. Immunobiology 1992; 185:41–52.

56. Hugli TE, Erickson BW. Synthetic peptides with the biological activities and specificity of human C3a anaphylatoxin. Proc Natl Acad Sci USA 1977; 74:1826–1830.

57. Morgan EL, Sanderson S, Scholz W, Noonan DJ, Weigle WO, Hugli TE. Identification and characterization of the effector region within human C5a responsible for stimulation of IL-6 synthesis. J Immunol 1992; 148:3937–3942.

58. Ember JA, Sanderson SD, Taylor SM, Kawahara M, Hugli TE. Biologic activity of synthetic analogues of C5a anaphylatoxin. J Immunol 1992; 148:3165–3173.

59. Chenoweth DE, Erickson BW, Hugli TE. Human C5a-related synthetic peptides as neutrophil chemotactic factors. Biochem Biophys Res Commun 1979; 86:227–234.

60. Or YS, Clark B, Lane B, Mollison KW, Carter GW, Luly JR. Improvements in the minimum binding sequence of C5a: examination of His 67. J Med Chem 1992; 35:402–406.

61. Ember JA, Cui L, Carney DF, Pettis RJ, Erickson BW, Hugli TE. Molecular and functional characterization of superpotent rat C5a. [abstract]. Protein Sci 1993; 2 (supplement 1):159.

62. Carney DF, Hugli TE. Site-specific mutations in the N-terminal region of human C5a that affect interactions of C5a with neutrophil C5a receptor. Protein Sci 1993; 2:1391–1399.

63. Gerard C, Hugli TE. Identification of classical anaphylatoxin as the des-Arg form of the C5a molecule: evidence of a modulator role for the oligosaccharide unit in human des-Arg74-C5a. Proc Natl Acad Sci USA 1981; 78:1833–1837.

64. Kawai M, Quincy DA, Lane B, Mollison KW, Or YS, Luly JR, Carter GW. Structure-function studies in a series of carboxyl-terminal octapeptide analogues of anaphylatoxin C5a. J Med Chem 1992; 35:220–223.

65. Kawai M, Quincy DA, Lane B, Mollison KW, Luly JR, Carter GW. Identification and synthesis of a receptor binding site of human anaphylatoxin C5a. J Med Chem 1991; 34:2068–2071.

66. Köhl J, Lübbers B, Klos A, Bautsch W, Casaretto M. Evaluation of the C-terminal C5a effector site with short synthetic C5a analog peptides. Eur J Immunol 1993; 23:646–652.

67. Siciliano SJ, Rollins TE, DeMartino J, Konteatis Z, Malkowitz L, Van Riper G, Bondy S, Rosen H, et al. Two-site binding of C5a by its receptor: an alternative binding paradigm for G protein-coupled receptors. Proc Natl Acad Sci USA 1994; 91:1214–1218.

68. Kawai M, Lane B, Mollison KW, Luly JR, Carter GW. Improved binding potency of a C5a related octapeptide by incorporation of N-methyl amino acids [abstract]. 12th American Peptide Symposium 1991, Cambridge, MA, 525.

69. Sanderson SD, Kirnarsky L, Sherman SA, Ember JA, Finch AM, Taylor SM. Decapeptide agonists of human C5a: the relationship between conformation and spasmogenic and platelet aggregatory activities. J Med Chem 1994; 37:3171–3180.

70. Sanderson SD, Kirnarsky L, Sherman SA, Vogen SM, Prakash O, Ember JA, Finch AM, Taylor SM. Decapeptide agonist of human C5a: the relationship between conformation and neutrophil response. J Med Chem 1995; 38:3669–3675.

71. Gerard C, Showell HJ, Hoeprich PD, Hugli TE, Stimler NP. Evidence for a role of the amino terminal region in the biological activity of the classical anaphylatoxin porcine C5a des Arg-74. J Biol Chem 1985; 260:2613–2616.

72. Mollison KW, Mandecki W, Zuiderweg ERP, Fayer L, Fey TA, Krause RA, Conway RG, Miller RG, et al. Identification of receptor-binding residues in the inflammatory complement protein C5a site-directed mutagenesis. Proc Natl Acad Sci USA 1989; 86:292.

73. Vlattas I, Sytwu II, Dellureficio J, Stanton J, Braunwalder AF, Galakatos N, Kramer R, Seligmann B, et al. Identification of a receptor-binding region in the core segment of the human anaphylatoxin C5a. J Med Chem 1994; 37:2783–2790.

74. Tempero RM, Hollingsworth MA, Burdick MD, Finch AM, Taylor SM, Vogen SM, Morgan EL, Sanderson SD. Molecular adjuvant effects of a conformationally biased agonist of human C5a anaphylatoxin. J Immunol 1997; 158:1377–1382.

75. Morgan EL. Complement fragment C5a and immunoregulation. Compl Today 1993; 1:56–75.

76. Caporale LH, Tippett PS, Erickson BW, Hugli TE. The active site of C3a anaphylatoxin. J Biol Chem 1980; 255:10758–10763.

77. Unson CG, Erickson BW, Hugli TE. Active site of C3a anaphylatoxin: contributions of the lipophilic and orienting residues. Biochemistry 1984; 23:585–589.

78. Kalnik MW, Chazin WJ, Wright PE. The three-dimensional solution structure of human anaphylatoxin C3a. In: Techniques in Protein Chemistry II. Villafranca JJ (ed). San Diego, CA: Academic Press, 1991; 37:393–400.

79. Gerardy-Schahn R, Ambrosius D, Saunders D, Casaretto M, Mittler C, Karwarth G, Goergen S, Bitter-Suermann D. Characterization of C3a receptor-proteins on guinea pig platelets and human polymorphonuclear leukocytes. Eur J Immunol 1989; 19:1095–1102.

80. Gerardy-Schahn R, Ambrosius D, Casaretto M, Grötzinger J, Saunders D, Wollmer A, Brandenburg DM, Bitter-Suermann D. Design and biological activity of a new generation of synthetic C3a analogues by combination of peptidic and non-peptidic elements. Biochem J 1988; 255:209–216.

81. Ambrosius D, Casaretto M, Gerardy-Schahn R, Saunders D, Brandenburg D, Zahn H. Peptide analogues of the anaphylatoxin C3a; syntheses and properties. Biol Chem Hoppe-Seyler 1989; 370:217–227.

82. Köhl J, Casaretto M, Gier M, Karwath G, Gietz C, Bautsch W, Saunders D, Bitter-Suermann D. Reevaluation of the C3a active site using short synthetic C3a analogues. Eur J Immunol 1990; 20:1463–1468.

83. Kola A, Klos A, Bautsch W, Kretzschmar T, Köhl J. Functional activities of synthetic anaphylatoxic peptides in widely used biological assays. Clin Exp Immunol 1992; 88:368–372.

84. Fukuoka Y, Hugli TE. Demonstration of a specific C3a receptor on guinea pig platelets. J Immunol 1988; 140:3496–3501.

85. Ember JA, Johansen NL, Hugli TE. Designing synthetic superagonists of C3a anaphylatoxin. Biochemistry 1991; 30:3603–3612.

86. Ember JA, Johansen NL, Hugli TE. A new approach to designing active analogues of proteins. Biochem Soc Trans 1990; 18:1154–1155.

87. Pohl M, Ambrosius D, Grötzinger J, Kretzschmar T, Saunders D, Wollmer A, Brandenburg D, Bitter-Suermann D, et al. Cyclic disulfide analogues of the complement component C3a: Synthesis and conformational investigations. Int J Pept Res 1993; 41:362–375.

88. Kretzschmar T, Pohl M, Casaretto M, Przewosny M, Bautsch W, Klos A, Saunders D, Köhl J. Synthetic peptides as antagonists of the anaphylatoxin C3a. Eur J Biochem 1992; 210:185–191.

89. Konteatis ZD, Siciliano SJ, Van Riper G, Molineaux CJ, Pandya S, Fischer P, Rosen H, Mumford RA, et al. Development of C5a receptor antagonist: differential loss of functional responses. J Immunol 1994; 153:4200–4205.

90. Lanza TJ, Durette PL, Rollins T, Siciliano S, Cianciarulo DN, Kobayashi SV, Caldwell CG, Springer MS, et al. Substituted 4,6-diaminoquinolines as inhibitors of C5a receptor binding. J Med Chem 1992; 35:252–258.

91. Kawai M, Lane B, Mollison KW, Luly JR, Carter GW. Potent C5a peptide analogues with diminished chemokinetic activity [abstract]. 12th American Peptide Symposium 1991, Cambridge, MA, 526.

92. Mollison KW, Krause RA, Fey TA, Miller L, Wiedeman PE, Kawai M, Lane B, Luly JR, et al. Hexapeptide analogs of C5a anaphylatoxin reveal heterogeneous neutrophil agonism/antagonism [abstract]. FASEB J 1992; 5:(5-#6502) A2058.

93. Chenoweth DE, Hugli TE. Demonstration of specific C5a receptor on intact human polymorphonuclear leukocytes. Proc Natl Acad Sci USA 1978; 75:3943–3947.

94. Huey R, Hugli TE. Characterization of a C5a receptor on human polymorphonuclear leukocytes (PMN). J Immunol 1985; 135:2063–2068.

95. Huey R, Fukuoka Y, Hoeprich PD, Jr., Hugli TE. Cellular receptors to the anaphylatoxins C3a and C5a. Biochem Soc Symp 1986; 51:69–81.

96. Rollins TE, Springer MS. Identification of the polymorphonuclear leukocyte C5a receptor. J Biol Chem 1985; 260:7157–7160.

97. Johnson RJ, Chenoweth DE. Labeling the granulocyte C5a receptor with a unique photoreactive probe. J Biol Chem 1985; 260:7161–7164.

98. Pease JE, Barker MD. N-linked glycosylation of the C5a receptor. Biochemistry 1993; 31:719–726.

99. Bao L, Gerard NP, Eddy RL, Jr., Shows TB, Gerard C. Mapping of genes for the human C5a receptor (C5aR), human FMLP receptor (FPR), and two FMLP receptor homologue orphan receptors (FPRH1, FPRH2) to chromosome 19. Genomics 1992; 13:437–440.

100. Gerard C, Gerard NP. The pro-inflammatory seven-transmembrane segment receptors of the leukocyte. Curr Opin Immunol 1994; 6:140–145.

101. Rollins TE, Siciliano S, Kobayashi S, Cianciarulo DN, Bonilla Argudo V, Collier K, Springer MS. Purification of the active C5a receptor from human polymorphonuclear leukocytes as a receptor-Gi complex. Proc Natl Acad Sci USA 1991; 88:971–975.

102. Giannini E, Brouchon L, Boulay F. Identification of the major phosphorylation sites in human C5a anaphylatoxin receptor in vivo. J Biol Chem 1995; 270:19166–19172.

103. Jiang H, Kuang Y, Wu Y, Smrcka A, Simon MI, Wu D. Pertussis toxin-sensitive activation of phospholipase C by the C5a and fMet-Leu-Phe receptors. J Biol Chem 1996; 271:13430–13434.

104. Buhl AM, Osawa S, Johnson GL. Mitogen-activated protein kinase activation requires two signal inputs from the human anaphylatoxin C5a receptor. J Biol Chem 1995; 270:19828–19832.

105. Buhl AM, Avdi N, Worthen GS, Johnson GL. Mapping of the C5a receptor signal transduction network in human neutrophils. Proc Natl Acad Sci USA 1994; 91:9190–9194.

106. Gerard C, Bao L, Orozco O, Pearson M, Kunz D, Gerard NP. Structural diversity in the extracellular faces of peptidergic G-protein-coupled receptors. J Immunol 1992; 149:2600–2606.

107. Fukuoka Y, Ember JA, Yasui A, Hugli TE. Molecular cloning of guinea pig C5a anaphylatoxin receptor: further evidence of interspecies diversity in the extracellular domain of C5a receptor. Int Immunol 1997; submitted.

108. Akatsu H, Miwa T, Sakurada C, Fukuoka Y, Ember JA, Yamamoto T, Hugli TE, Okada H. cDNA cloning and characterization of rat C5a anaphylatoxin receptor. Microbiol Immunol 1997; 41:575–580.

109. Perret JJ, Raspe E, Vassart G, Parmentier M. Cloning and functional expression of the canine anaphylatoxin C5a receptor. Biochemistry 1992; 288:911–917.

110. Norgauer J, Dobos G, Kownatzki E, Dahinden C, Burger R, Kupper R, Gierschik P. Complement fragment C3a stimulates Ca^{2+} influx in neutrophils via a pertussis-toxin-sensitive G protein. Eur J Biochem 1993; 217:289–294.

111. Klos A, Bank S, Gietz C, Bautsch W, Köhl J, Burg M, Kretzschmar T. C3a receptor on dibutyryl-cAMP-differentiated U937 cells and human neutrophils: the human C3a receptor characterized by functional responses and ^{125}I-C3a binding. Biochemistry 1992; 31:11274–11282.

112. Tornetta MA, Foley JJ, Sarau HM, Ames RS. The mouse anaphylatoxin C3a receptor: molecular cloning, genomic organization and functional expression. J Immunol 1997; 158:5227–5282.

113. Hsu MH, Ember JA, Wang M, Prossnitz ER, Hugli TE, Ye RD. Cloning and functional characterization of the mouse C3a anaphylatoxin receptor gene. Immunogenetics 1997; in press.

114. Fukuoka Y, Hugli TE. Molecular characterization of the guinea pig and rat C3a receptor [abstract]. Microcirculation 1997; 4:121.

115. Fukuoka Y, Ember JA, Hugli TE. Molecular cloning and characterization of guinea pig C3a receptor. J Biol Chem 1997; submitted.

116. Chenoweth DE, Soderberg CS, von Wedel R. Dibutyryl cAMP induced expression of C5a receptors on U937 cells [abstract]. J Leukocyte Biol 1984; 36:241.

117. Chenoweth DE, Goodman MG, Weigle WO. Demonstration of a specific receptor for human C5a anaphylatoxins on murine macrophages. J Exp Med 1982; 156:67–78.

118. Schulman ES, Post TJ, Henson PM, Giclas PC. Differential effects of the complement peptides, C5a and C5a desArg on human basophils and lung mast cell histamine release. J Clin Invest 1988; 81:918–923.

119. MacGlashan DW, Jr., Hubbard WC. IL-3 alters free arachidonic acid generation in C5a-stimulated human basophils. J Immunol 1993; 151:6358–6369.

120. Gerard NP, Hodges MK, Drazen JM, Weller PF, Gerard C. Characterization of a receptor for C5a anaphylatoxin on human eosinophils. J Biol Chem 1989; 264:1760–1766.

121. Fukuoka Y, Hugli TE. C5a receptors on guinea pig platelets [abstract]. Fed Proc 1988; 2:A1007.

122. Kretzschmar T, Kahl K, Rech K, Bautsch W, Köhl J, Bitter-Suermann D. Characterization of the C5a receptor on guinea pig platelets. Immunobiology 1991; 183:418–432.

123. Johnson AR, Hugli TE, Müller-Eberhard HJ. Release of histamine from rat mast cells by the complement peptides C3a and C5a. Immunology 1975; 28:1067–1080.

124. Fukuoka Y, Hugli TE. Anaphylatoxin binding and degradation by rat peritoneal mast cells. Mechanisms of degranulation and control. J Immunol 1990; 145:1851–1858.

125. Lacy M, Jones J, Whittemore SR, Haviland DL, Wetsel RA, Barnum SR. Expression of the receptors for the C5a anaphylatoxin, interleukin-8 and FMLP by human astrocytes and microglia. J Neuroimmunol 1995; 61:71–78.

126. Glovsky MM, Hugli TE, Ishizaka T, Lichtenstein LM, Erickson BW. Anaphylatoxin-induced histamine release with human leukocytes: Studies of C3a leukocyte binding and histamine release. J Clin Invest 1979; 64:804–811.

127. Daffern PJ, Pfeifer PH, Ember JA, Hugli TE. C3a is a chemotaxin for human eosinophils but not for neutrophils. I. C3a stimulation of neutrophils is secondary to eosinophil activation. J Exp Med 1995; 181:2119–2127.

128. Khan SA, Erickson BW, Kawahara MS, Hugli TE. A synthetic analogue of human C5a with spasmogenic activity [abstract]. XIth International Complement Workshop, Miami, FL, 1985; 2:(118) 42.

129. Oppermann M, Schulze M, Götze O. A sensitive enzyme immunoassay for the quantitation of human C5a/C5a(desArg) anaphylatoxin using a monoclonal antibody with specificity for a neoepitope. Comp Inflamm 1991; 8:13

130. Johnson RJ, Tamerius JD, Chenoweth DE. Identification of an antigenic epitope and receptor binding domain of human C5a. J Immunol 1987; 138:3856–3862.

131. Bubeck P, Grötzinger J, Winkler M, Köhl J, Wollmer A, Klos A, Bautsch W. Site-specific mutagenesis of residues in the human C5a anaphylatoxin which are involved in possible interaction with the C5a receptor. Eur J Biochem 1994; 219:897–904.

132. Toth MJ, Huwyler L, Boyar WC, Braunwalder AF, Yarwood D, Hadala J, Haston WO, Sills MA, et al. The pharmacophore of the human C5a anaphylatoxin. Protein Sci 1994; 3:1159–1168.

133. Zuiderweg ERP, Nettesheim DG, Mollison KW, Carter GW. Tertiary structure of human complement component C5a in solution from nuclear magnetic resonance data. Biochemistry 1989; 28:172–185.

134. Mollison KW, Fey TA, Krause RA, Miller L, Edalji L, Conway RG, Mandecki W, Shallcross MA, et al. C5a structural requirements for neutrophil receptor interaction. Prog Inflamm Res Ther 1991; 17–21.

135. Hugli TE, Marceau F, Lundberg C. Effects of complement fragments on pulmonary and vascular smooth muscle. Am Rev Respir Dis 1987; 135:S9–13.

136. Cui L, Carney DF, Hugli TE. Primary structure and functional characterization of rat C5a: an anaphylatoxin with unusually high potency among C5a. Protein Science 1994; 3:1169–1177.

137. Bautsch W, Kretzschmar T, Stühmer T, Kola A, Emde M, Köhl J, Klos A, Bitter-Suermann D. A recombinant hybrid anaphylatoxin with dual C3a/C5a activity. Biochem J 1992; 288:261–266.

138. Buchner RR, Hugli TE, Ember JA, Morgan EL. Expression of functional receptors for human C5a anaphylatoxin (CD88) on the human hepatocellular carcinoma cell line HepG2. Stimulation of acute-phase protein-specific mRNA and protein synthesis by human C5a anaphylatoxin. J Immunol 1995; 155:308–315.

139. Morgan EL, Ember JA, Sanderson SD, Scholz W, Buchner R, Ye RD, Hugli TE. Anti-C5a Receptor Antibodies. Characterization of neutralizing antibodies specific for a peptide, C5aR-(9-29), derived from the predicted amino-terminal sequence of the human C5a receptor. J Immunol 1993; 151:377–388.

140. Oppermann M, Raedt U, Hebell T, Schmidt B, Zimmermann B, Götze O. Probing the human receptor for C5a anaphylatoxin with site-directed antibodies: Identification of a potential ligand binding site on the NH-2-terminal domain. J Immunol 1993; 151:3785–3794.

141. Ember JA, Morgan EL, Sanderson SD, Hugli TE. Anti-C5a receptor antibody inhibits biologic activity of C5a but not synthetic C5a analogues [abstract]. FASEB J 1994; 8:A500

142. Ember JA, Morgan EL, Hugli TE. Epitope mapping of neutralizing anti-C5a receptor (CD88) antibodies [abstract]. FASEB J 1996; 10:(A1293)-Abs #1693.

143. DeMartino JA, Van Riper G, Siciliano SJ, Molineaux CJ, Konteastis ZD, Rosen H, Springer MS. The amino terminus of the human C5a receptor is required for high affinity C5a binding and for receptor activation by C5a but not C5a analogs. J Biol Chem 1994; 269:14446–14450.

144. Mery L, Boulay F. The NH2-terminal region of C5aR but not that of FPR is critical for both protein transport and ligand binding. J Biol Chem 1994; 269:3457–3463.

145. Jagels MA, Travis J, Potempa J, Pike R, Hugli TE. The leukocyte C5a receptor is cleaved by proteinases derived from *Porphyromonas gingivalis*. Infect Immun 1995; 64:1984–1991.

146. Jagels MA, Ember JA, Travis J, Potempa J, Pike R, Hugli TE. Cleavage of the human C5a receptor by proteinases derived from *Porphyromonas gingivalis*. In: Intracellular Protein Catabolism. Suzuki K, Bond J, (eds) New York: Plenum Press, 1996; 19:155–164.

147. Pease JE, Burton DR, Barker MD. Generation of chimeric C5a/formyl peptide receptors: towards the identication of the human C5a receptor binding site. Eur J Immunol 1994; 24:211–215.

148. Pease JE, Burton DR, Barker MD. Site directed mutagenesis of the complement C5a receptor-examination of a model for its interaction with the ligand C5a. Mol Immunol 1994; 31:733–737.

148a. Monk PN, Barker MD, Partridge LJ, Pease JE. Mutation of glutamate 199 of the human C5a receptor defines a binding site for ligand distinct from the receptor N terminus. J Biol Chem 1995; 270:16625–16629.

148b. DeMartino JA, Konteatis ZD, Siciliano SJ, Van Riper G, Underwood DJ, Fischer PA, Springer MS. Arginine 206 of the C5a receptor is critical for ligand recognition and receptor activation by C-terminal hexapeptide analogs. J Biol Chem 1995; 270:15966–15969.

149. Klos A, Matje C, Rheinheimer C, Bautsch W, Köhl J, Martin U, Burg M. Amino acids 327–350 of the human C5a-receptor are not essential for [^{125}I]C5a binding in COS cells and signal transduction in Xenopus oocytes. FEBS Lett 1994; 344:79–82.

150. Fernandez HN, Henson PM, Otani A, Hugli TE. Chemotactic response to human C3a and C5a anaphylatoxins. I. Evaluation of C3a and C5a leukotaxis in vitro and under stimulated in vivo conditions. J Immunol 1978; 120:109–115.

151. Morita E, Schröder J-M, Christophers E. Differential sensitivities of purified human eosinophils and neutrophils to defined chemotaxins. Scand J Immunol 1989; 29:709–716.

152. Henson PM. The immunologic release of constituents from neutrophil leukocytes. I. The role of antibody and complement on nonphagocytosable surfaces or phagocytosable particles. J Immunol 1971; 107:1535–1546.

153. Goetzl EJ, Austen KF. Stimulation of human neutrophil leukocyte aerobic glucose metabolism by purified chemotactic factors. J Clin Invest 1974; 53:591–599.

154. Takafuji S, Tadokoro K, Ito K, Dahinden CA. Degranulation from human eosinophils stimulated with C3a and C5a. Int Arch Allergy Immunol 1994; 104:27–29.

155. Hartman CT, Jr., Glovsky MM. Complement activation requirements for histamine release from human leukocytes: influence of purified C3a hu and C5a hu on histamine release. Int Arch Allergy Appl Immunol 1981; 66:274–281.

156. Siraganian RP, Hook WA. Complement induced histamine release from human basophils. II. Mechanism of the histamine reaction. J Immunol 1976; 116:639–646.

157. Elsner J, Oppermann M, Czech W, Dobos G, Schopf E, Norgauer J, Kapp A. C3a activates reactive oxygen radical species production and intracellular calcium transients in human eosinophils. Eur J Immunol 1994; 24:518–522.

158. Laurent F, Benoliel AM, Capo C, Bongrand P. Oxidative metabolism of polymorphonuclear leukocytes: modulation by adhesive stimuli. J Leukocyte Biol 1991; 49:217–226.

159. Henson PM, Zanolari B, Schwartzman NA, Hong SR. Intracellular control of human neutrophil secretion. I. C5a-induced stimulus-specific desensitization and the effects of cytochalasin B. J Immunol 1978; 121:851–855.
160. Becker EL, Showell HJ, Henson PM, Hsu LS. The ability of chemotactic factors to induce lysosomal enzyme release. 1. The characteristics of the release, the importance of surfaces, and the relation of enzyme release to chemotactic responsiveness. J Immunol 1974; 112:2047–2054.
161. Kishimoto TK, Jutila MA, Berg EL, Butcher EC. Neutrophil Mac-1 and MEL-14 adhesion proteins inversely regulated by chemotactic factors. Science 1989; 245:1238–1241.
162. Neeley SP, Hamann KJ, White SR, Baranowski SL, Burch RA, Leff AR. Selective regulation of expression of surface adhesion molecules Mac-1, L-selectin, and VLA-4 on human eosinophils and neutrophils. Am J Respir Cell Mol Biol 1993; 8:633–639.
163. Lundahl J, Hallden G, Hed J. Differences in intracellular pool and receptor-dependent mobilization of the adhesion-promoting glycoprotein Mac-1 between eosinophils and neutrophils. J Leukocyte Biol 1993; 53:336–341.
164. Tonnesen MG, Smedly LA, Henson PM. Neutrophil-endothelial cell interactions. J Clin Invest 1984; 74:1581–1592.
165. Weber C, Katayama J, Springer TA. Differential regulation of $\beta1$ and $\beta2$ integrin activity by chemoattractants in eosinophils. Proc Natl Acad Sci USA 1996; 93:10939–10944.
166. Cochrane CG, Müller-Eberhard HJ. The derivation of two distinct anaphylatoxin activities from the third and fifth components of human complement. J Exp Med 1968; 127:371–386.
167. Nilsson G, Johnell M, Hammer CH, Tiffany HL, Nilsson K, Metcalfe DD, Siegbahn A, Murphy PM. C3a and C5a are chemotaxins for human mast cells and act through distinct receptors via a pertussis toxin-sensitive signal transduction pathway. J Immunol 1996; 157:1693–1698.
168. Clancy RM, Hugli TE. Role of complement anaphylatoxins in neutrophil arachidonic acid metabolism. *In*: Leukotrienes in cardiovascular and pulmonary function. Alan R. Liss, Inc. New York, 1985; 173–184.
169. Hilger RA, Koller M, Konig W. Inhibition of leukotriene formation and IL-8 release by the PAF-receptor antagonist SM-12502. Inflammation 1996; 20:57–70.
170. Pieters WR, Houghten RA, Koenderman L, Raaijmakers JA. C5a-induced migration of human monocytes is primed by dexamethasone. Am J Respir Cell Mol Biol 1995; 12:691–696.
171. Snyderman R, Shin HS, Hausman MH. A chemotactic factor for mononuclear leukocytes. Proc Soc Exp Biol Med 1971; 138:387–390.
172. Issekutz AC, Chuluyan HE, Lopes N. CD11/CD18-independent transendothelial migration of human polymorphonuclear leukocytes and monocytes: involvement of distinct and unique mechanisms. J Leukocyte Biol 1995; 57:553–561.
173. Monk PN, Barker MD, Partridge LJ. Multiple signalling pathways in the C5a-induced expression of adhesion receptor Mac-1. Biochim Biophys Acta 1994; 1221:323–329.
174. Ember JA, Sanderson SD, Hugli TE, Morgan EL. Induction of interleukin-8 synthesis from monocytes by human C5a anaphylatoxin. Am J Pathol 1994; 144:393–403.
175. Okusawa S, Dinarello CA, Yancy KB, Endres S, Lawley TJ, Frank MM, Burke JF, Gelfand JA. C5a induction of human interleukin 1. Synergistic-effect with endotoxin or interferon-gamma. J Immunol 1987; 139:2635–2639.
176. Scholz W, McClurg MR, Cardenas GJ, Smith M, Noonan DJ, Hugli TE, Morgan EL. C5a-mediated release of interleukin 6 by human monocytes. Clin Immunol Immunopathol 1990; 57:297–307.
177. Morgan EL, Thoman ML, Weigle WO, Hugli TE. Anaphylatoxin-mediated regulation of the immune response. II. C5a-mediated enhancement of human humoral and T cell-mediated immune responses. J Immunol 1983; 130:1257–1261.
178. Morgan EL, Weigle WO, Hugli TE. Anaphylatoxin-mediated regulation of human and murine immune responses. Fed Proc 1984; 43:2543–2547.

179. Fischer WH, Hugli TE. Regulation of B cell functions by C3a and C3adesArg: Suppression of TNF-α, IL-6, and the polyclonal immune response. J Immunol 1997; in press.
180. Wagner JL, Hugli TE. Radioimmunoassay for anaphylatoxins: A sensitive method for determining complement activation products in biological fluids. Anal Biochem 1984; 136:75–88.
181. Morgan EL, Thoman ML, Weigle WO, Hugli TE. Human C3a-mediated suppression of the immune response. I. Suppression of murine in vitro antibody responses occurs through the generation of nonspecific Lyt-2+ suppressor T cell. J Immunol 1985; 134:51–57.
182. Morgan EL, Weigle WO, Hugli TE. Anaphylatoxin-mediated regulation of the immune response. I. C3a-mediated suppression of human and murine humoral immune responses. J Exp Med 1982; 155:1412–1426.
183. Takabayashi T, Vannier E, Clark BD, Margolis NH, Dinarello CA, Burke JF, Gelfand JA. A new biologic role for C3a and C3a desArg. J Immunol 1996; 156:3455–3460.
184. Mousli M, Hugli TE, Landry Y, Bronner C. A mechanism of action for anaphylatoxin C3a stimulation of mast cells. J Immunol 1992; 148:2456–2461.
185. Murphy HS, Shayman JA, Till GO, Mahrougui M, Owens CB, Ryan US, Ward PA. Superoxide responses of endothelial cells to C5a and TNF-α: divergent signal transduction pathways. Am J Physiol 1992; 263:L51–L59.
186. McCoy R, Haviland DL, Molmenti EP, Ziambaras T, Wetsel RA, Perlmutter DH. N-formylpeptide and complement C5a receptors are expressed in liver cells and mediate hepatic acute phase gene regulation. J Exp Med 1995; 182:207–217.
187. Wetsel RA. Structure, function and cellular expression of complement anaphylatoxin receptors. Curr Opin Immunol 1995; 7:48–53.
188. Jaeschke H, Raftery MJ, Justesen U, Gaskell S, J. Serum complement mediates endotoxin-induced cysteinyl leukotriene formation in rats in vivo. Am J Physiol 1992; 263:G947–G952.
189. Gasque P, Fontaine M, Morgan BP. Complement expression in human brain. J Immunol 1995; 154:4726–4733.
190. Morgan BP. Complement in Health and Disease. Whaley K, Loos M, Weiler JM (eds). Dordrecht, The Netherlands: Kluwer Academic, 1993:353.
191. Williams CA, Schupf N, Hugli TE. Anaphylatoxin C5a modulation of an alpha-adrenergic receptor system in the rat hypothalamus. J Neuroimmunol 1985; 9:29–40.
192. Armstrong RC, Harvath L, Dubois-Dalcq ME. Type I astrocytes and oligodendrocyte-type 2 astrocyte glial progenitors migrate toward distinct molecules. J Neurosci Res 1990; 27:400–407.
193. Yao J, Harvath L, Gilbert DL, Colton CA. Chemotaxis by a CNS macrophage, the microglia. J Neurosci Res 1990; 27:30–36.
194. Werfel T, Zwirner J, Oppermann M, Sieber A, Begemann G, Drommer W, Kapp A, Götze O. CD88 antibodies specifically bind to C5aR on dermal CD117+ and CD14+ cells and react with a desmosomal antigen in human skin. J Immunol 1996; 157:1729–1735.
195. Issekutz AC, Issekutz TB. Quantitation and kinetics of blood monocyte migration to acute inflammatory reactions, and IL-1 α, tumor necrosis factor-α, and IFN-gamma. J Immunol 1993; 151:2105–2115.
196. Schwartz LB, Kawahara MS, Hugli TE, Vik D, Fearon DT, Austen KF. Generation of C3a anaphylatoxin from human C3 by human mast cell tryptase. J Immunol 1983; 130:1891–1895.
197. Ramos BF, Zhang Y, Jakschik BA. Neutrophil elicitation in the reverse passive Arthus reaction. J Immunol 1994; 152:1380–1384.
198. Amsterdam EA, Rendig SV, Longhurst JC. Contractile actions of C5a on isolated porcine myocardium. Am J Physiol 1992; 263:H740–H745.
199. Stimler NP, Brocklehurst WE, Bloor CM, Hugli TE. Anaphylatoxin-mediated contraction of guinea pig lung strips: a nonhistamine tissue response. J Immunol 1981; 126:2258–2261.
200. Stimler NP, Bloor CM, Hugli TE. C3a-induced contraction of guinea pig lung parenchyma: role of cyclooxygenase metabolites. Immunopharmacology 1983; 5:251–257.

201. Regal JF, Eastman AY, Pickering RJ. C5a-induced tracheal contraction: a histamine independent mechanism. J Immunol 1980; 124:2876–2878.
202. Stimler NP, Hugli TE, Bloor CM. Pulmonary injury induced by C3a and C5a anaphylatoxins. Am J Pathol 1980; 100:327–348.
203. Huey R, Bloor CM, Kawahara MS, Hugli TE. Potentiation of the anaphylatoxins in vivo using an inhibitor of serum carboxypeptidase N (SCPN). I. Lethality and pathologic effects on pulmonary tissue. Am J Pathol 1983; 112:48–60.
204. Kubo H, Morgenstern D, Quinian WM, Ward PA, Dinauer MD, Doerschuk CM. Preservation of complement-induced lung injury in mice with deficiency of NADPH oxidase. J Clin Invest 1996; 97:2680–2684.
205. Lundberg C, Marceau F, Hugli TE. C5a-induced hemodynamic and hematologic changes in the rabbit. Role of cyclooxygenase products and polymorphonuclear leukocytes. Am J Pathol 1987; 128:471–483.
206. Rampart M, Bult H, Herman AG. Activated complement and anaphylatoxins increase the in vitro production of prostacyclin by rabbit aorta endothelium. Naunyn-Schmiedebergs Arch Pharmacol 1983; 322:158–165.
207. Marceau F, Lundberg C, Hugli TE. Effects of the anaphylatoxins on circulation. Immunopharmacology 1987; 14:67–84.
208. Bult H, Herman AG, Laekeman GM, Rampart M. Formation of prostanoids during intravascular complement activation in the rabbit. Br J Pharmacol 1985; 84:329–336.
209. Kajita T, Hugli TE. C5a-induced neutrophilia: a primary humoral mechanism for recruitment of neutrophils. Am J Pathol 1990; 137:467–477.
210. Hangen DH, Segall GM, Harney EW, Stevens JH, McDougall IR, Raffin TA. Kinetics of leukocyte sequestration in the lungs of acutely septic primates. A study using ^{111}In-labelled autologous leukocytes. J Surg Res 1990; 48:196–203.
211. Athens JW, Haab OP, Raab SO, Mauer AM, Ashenbucker GE, Cartwright GE, Wintrobe MM. Leukokinetic studies. IV. The total blood, circulating and marginal granulocyte pool and the granulocyte turnover rate in normal subjects. J Clin Invest 1961; 40:989–995.
212. von Andrian UH, Hansell P, Chambers JD, Berger EM, Filho IT, Butcher EC, Arfors K-E. L-selectin function is required for β-2 integrin-mediated neutrophil adhesion at physiologic shear rates in vivo. Am J Physiol 1992; 263:H1034–H1044.
213. Jagels MA, Chambers JD, Arfors K-E, Hugli TE. C5a and TNF-α-induced leukocytosis occurs independently of β integrins and L-selectin. Differential effects on neutrophil adhesion molecule expression in vivo. Blood 1995; 85:2900–2909.
214. Lundberg C, Wright SD. Relation of the CD11/CD18 family of leukocyte antigens to the transient neutropenia caused by chemoattractants. Blood 1990; 76:1240–1245.
215. Worthen GS, Schwab B, III, Elson EL, Downey GP. Mechanics of stimulated neutrophils: cell stiffening induces retention in capillaries. Science 1991; 245:183–245.
216. Erzurum SC, Downey GP, Doherty DE, Schwab B, III, Elson EL, Worthen GS. Mechanisms of lipopolysaccharide-induced neutrophil retention. J Immunol 1992; 149:154–162.
217. Albelda SM, Smith CW, Ward PA. Adhesion molecules and inflammatory injury. FASEB J 1994; 8:504–512.
218. Howard RJ, Crain C, Franzini DA, Hood CI, Hugli TE. Effects of cardiopulmonary bypass on pulmonary leukostasis and complement activation. Arch Surg 1988; 123:1496–1501.
219. Kirklin JK, Westaby S, Blackstone EH, et al. Complement and the damaging effects of cardiopulmonary by pass. J Cardiovasc Surg 1983; 86:845–857.
220. Craddock PR, Fehr J, Brigham KL, et al. Complement and leukocyte-mediated pulmonary dysfunction in hemodialysis. N Engl J Med 1977; 296:769–774.
221. Moore FD, Jr., Warner KG, Assousa S, Valeri CR, Khuri SF. The effects of complement activation during cardiopulmonary bypass. Ann Surg 1988; 208:95–103.
222. Faist E, Baue AE, Dittmer H, Heberer G. Multiple organ failure in polytrauma patients. J Trauma 1983; 23:775–787.

223. Parsons PE, Worthen GS, Moore EE, Tate RM, Henson PM. The association of circulating endotoxin with the development of the adult respiratory distress syndrome. Am Respir Dis 1989; 140:294–301.

224. Murray JF, Matthay MA, Luce J, Flick MR. An expanded definition of the adult respiratory distress syndrome. Am Rev Respir Dis 1988; 138:720–723.

225. Herndon DN, Traber DL. Pulmonary failure and acute respiratory distress syndrome. Multiple organ failure. In: Pathophysiology and Basic Concepts of Therapy. Deitch EA (ed). New York: Thieme, 1990: 192–214.

226. Shoemaker WC, Appel PL, Czer SC, Bland R, Schwartz S, Hopkins JA. Pathogenesis of respiratory failure (ARDS) after hemorrhage and trauma. Crit Care Med 1980; 8:504–512.

227. Hack CE, Nuijens JH, Felt-Bersma RJF, Schreuder WO, Eerenberg-Belmer AJM, Paardekooper J, Bronsveld W, Thijs LG. Elevated plasma levels of the anaphylatoxins C3a and C4a are associated with fatal outcome in sepsis. Am J Med 1989; 86:20–26.

228. Hammerschmidt DE, Weaver LJ, Hudson LD, Craddock PR, Jacob HS. Association of complement activation and elevated plasma-C5a with adult respiratory distress syndrome. Lancet 1980; 1:947–949.

229. Heideman M, Hugli TE. Anaphylatoxin generation in multisystem organ failure. J Trauma 1984; 24:1038–1043.

230. Meade P, Shoemaker WC, Donnelly TJ, Abraham E, Jagels MA, Cryer HG, Hugli TE, Bishop MH, et al. Temporal patterns of hemodynamics, oxygen transport, cytokine activity, and complement activity in the development of adult respiratory distress syndrome after severe injury. J Trauma 1994; 36:651–657.

231. Smedegard G, Cui L-X, Hugli TE. Endotoxin-induced shock in the rat. A role for C5a. Am J Pathol 1989; 135:489–497.

232. Hopken U, Mohr M, Struber A, Montz H, Burchardi H, Götze O, Oppermann M. Inhibition of interleukin-6 synthesis in an animal model of septic shock by anti-C5a monoclonal antibodies. Eur J Immunol 1996; 26:1103–1109.

233. Bozic CR, Lu B, Hopken UE, Gerard C, Gerard NP. Neurogenic amplification of immune complex inflammation. Science 1996; 273:1722–1725.

234. Hopken UE, Lu B, Gerard NP, Gerard C. The C5a chemoattractant receptor mediates mucosal defence to infection. Nature 1996; 383:86–89.

235. Maroko PR, Carpenter CB, Chiariello M, Fishbein MC, Radvany P, Kostman JD, Hale SL. Reduction by cobra venom factor of myocardial necrosis after coronary artery occulsion. J Natl Cancer Inst 1978; 61:661–670.

236. Weisman HF, Bartow T, Leppo MK, Marsh HC, Jr., Carson GR, Concino MF, Boyle MP, Roux KH, et al. Soluble complement receptor type 1: in vivo inhibitor of complement suppressing post-ischemic myocardinal inflammation and necrosis. Science 1990; 249:146–151.

237. Del Balzo U, Engler RL, Ito BR. Complement C5a-mediated myocardial ischemia and neutrophil sequestration: two independent phenomena. Am J Physiol 1993; 264:H336–H344.

238. Ito BR, Engler RL, Del Balzo U. Role of cardiac mast cells in complement C5a-induced myocardial ischemia. Am J Physiol 1993; 264:H1346–H1354.

239. Ito BR, Roth DR, Engler RL. Thromboxane A_2 and peptidoleukotrienes contribute to the myocardial ischemia and contractile dysfunction in response to intracoronary infusion of complement C5a. Circ Res 1990; 66:596–607.

240. Mulligan MS, Yeh CG, Rudolph AR, Ward PA. Protective effects of soluble CR1 in complement- and neutrophil-mediated tissue injury. J Immunol 1992; 148:1479–1485.

241. Yeh CG, Marsh HC, Jr., Carson GR, Berman L, Concino MF, Scesney SM, Kuestner RE, Skibbens R, et al. Recombinant soluble human complement receptor type 1 inhibits inflammation in the reversed passive Arthus reaction in rats. J Immunol 1991; 146:250.

242. Pruitt SK, Bollinger RR. The effect of soluble complement receptor type 1 on hyperacute allograft rejection. J Surg Res 1991; 50:350.

243. Belmont HM, Buyon J, Giorno R, Abramson S. Up-regulation of endothelial cell adhesion molecules characterizes disease activity in systemic lupus erythematosus. The Shwartzman phenomenon revisited. Arthritis Rheum 1994; 37:376–383.

244. Porcel JM, Ordi J, Castro-Salomo A, Vilardell M, Rodrigo MJ, Gene T, Warburton F, Kraus M, et al. The value of complement activation products in the assessment of systemic lupus erythematosus flares. Clin Immunol Immunopathol 1995; 74:283–288.

245. Jose PJ, Moss IK, Maini RN, Williams TJ. Measurement of the chemotactic complement fragment C5a in rheumatoid synovial fluids by radioimmunoassay: role of C5a in the acute inflammatory phase. Ann Rheum Dis 1989; 49:747–752.

246. Cui L, Ferreri K, Hugli TE. Structural characterization of the C4a anaphylatoxin from rat. Mol Immunol 1988; 25:663–671.

12

Complement-Mediated Phagocytosis

MELVIN BERGER

Case Western Reserve University School of Medicine, and
Rainbow Babies and Childrens Hospital, Cleveland, Ohio

Enhancement of phagocytosis is arguably the most important contribution of complement to the body's host defense mechanisms, as evidenced by the severity of infections with a broad range of bacteria in patients deficient in the early components and C3, compared to the more restricted spectrum of infections in patients deficient in C5 and later components. C3 is well suited to serve as the source of the major opsonins of the complement system, since its concentration in plasma is higher than any other component. Although C3 fragments and their receptors most commonly come to mind when one is discussing the participation of complement in phagocytosis, it is important to recognize the critical role of C5a and C5a des Arg in attracting and activating the phagocytes and the participation of C1q as an activator and/or opsonin as well. All of these effects are mediated by specific receptors on the plasma membrane of the phagocytic cell. The structures of the receptors are reviewed in Chapters 8 and 11. The physiology of the interactions of complement-derived activators and opsonins with these receptors and their roles in the host defense against infection and in immunologic homeostasis will be discussed here.

I. OVERVIEW OF PHAGOCYTOSIS

The process of phagocytosis itself initially involves the specific attachment of a particulate target to the phagocytic cell (Fig. 1). After the initial binding of the target, a sequential series of attachments is formed as the cell extends pseudopods around the target. Evidence that these attachments represent the continued formation of receptor-opsonin bonds is provided by studies using as targets B lymphocytes whose surface IgG was partially capped vs. uniformly distributed, with IgG antibody as the opsonin. With the former, the phagocytic machinery extended only as far as the cap. They were not completely ingested, as were the targets on which the surface antigen (and opsonins) were fully circumferential (1). Thus, phagocytosis is most often visualized as a "zipper" mechanism with sequential formation of receptor–opsonin complexes "pulling" extensions of the cell membrane around the target (reviewed in 2). Although usually illustrated in two dimensions, this is really a three-dimensional process and a phagocytic "cup" is formed. The extension of the cell membrane around the target thus involves flexibility of the plasma membrane, focal activation of receptors, and repeated reorganization of the cytoskeleton, with actin

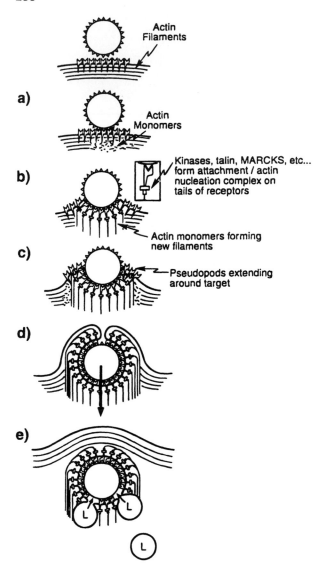

Figure 1 Hypothetical scheme for phagocytosis. (a) Upon binding of opsonin to receptor, local increase in free Ca^{2+} disrupts submembranous microfilaments by depolymerizing actin, perhaps through activation of gelsolin. Tail of receptor becomes phosphorylated. (b) Assembly of intracellular attachment/actin nucleation complex containing talin, kinases, MARCKS, etc. on phosphorylated tail of receptor leads to formation of new actin filaments perpendicular to original plane of membrane, thus deforming membrane around target. (c) Continued formation of opsonin-receptor bonds leads to assembly of additional attachment/actin polymerization complexes. New and lengthening actin filaments propel extension of plasma membrane around target. (d) Phagocytic cup engulfs target completely and seals. (e) Phagocytic vacuole is internalized into cell and fuses with lysosomes, whose contents are delivered into vacuole.

polymerization at the site of newly occupied receptors serving as the primary driving force for pseudopod extension (2). If the opsonins are present on a large surface rather than a particle that is small relative to the overall size of the cell, a similar process of sequential receptor binding will occur and the cell will spread, becoming tightly adherent to the opsonized surface rather than ingesting the small target. This process has been termed "frustrated phagocytosis" and may occur in vivo if large surfaces (i.e., basement membranes) are targets of autoantibodies or become covered with immune complexes or C3 fragments deposited by alternative pathway activation. Similar phenomena may occur when phagocytes attack a multicellular parasite.

Phagocytosis involves two types of membrane fusion events. The first involves fusion of the opposing edges of the plasma membrane of the phagocytic cup as it closes, completing engulfment of the target into a phagocytic vacuole. The second involves the subsequent fusion of lysosomes and other intracellular granules with that vacuole to form a mature phagolysosome containing an activated oxidase complex and digestive enzymes that can kill and degrade the target. In physiological terms, killing would be most efficient and damage to bystander cells and tissues would be minimized if the phagocyte secreted its digestive enzymes and oxidative products only into the phagocytic vacuole. If the cell ingested only a few small particles, enzyme secretion and oxidase activation would therefore be limited, and extracellular release of injurious enzymes and metabolites would not occur. If the vacuole fails to seal, and/or if "frustrated phagocytosis" is occurring on a surface, enzymes and toxic oxygen metabolites may be released, causing local tissue damage.

The relationships between focal activation of the cell's phagocytic machinery and the generalized metabolic activation that might be induced by strong soluble stimuli may be difficult to determine. Most opsonin receptors that provide signals for phagocytosis employ a series of protein tyrosine kinases, in contrast to chemoattractant receptors that generally employ heterotrimeric G-proteins to mediate signals that activate phospholipase C, releasing Ca^{2+} and diacyl glycerol. Chemoattractant receptors can function as monomers, whereas phagocytosis generally requires aggregation of opsonin receptors at focal points of contact with the target. This causes focal accumulation of receptor-associated tyrosine kinases, serine/threonine kinases, and phosphorylated substrates that promote local actin polymerization (2). However, occupancy and/or cross-linking of opsonin receptors may simultaneously activate multiple signaling pathways that may converge with those activated by chemoattractants and other soluble stimuli. Phagocytosis is frequently accompanied by activation of phospholipases, liberating diacylglycerol and arachidonic acid and that can stimulate intracellular enzymes and/or serve as a source of mediators such as LTB_4, These can then activate other cells, even though the phospholipase activity may not be necessary for the process of ingestion per se. Although small local increases in free Ca^{2+} that facilitate local cytoskeletal reorganization may be sufficient for engulfment without generally activating the cell, if enough receptors are cross-linked by opsonins on a surface and/or if there is a high target to two phagocyte ratio, the total increase in free intracellular Ca^{2+} may be sufficient to cause generalized cellular activation mimicking that caused by ionophores or chemoattractants. An important situation in which activation of the oxidase and/or secretory machinery can be dissociated from the process of phagocytosis per se is in the presence of cytochalasin B, which causes depolymerization of actin filaments. Release of O_2^- or granular enzymes upon cross-linking of opsonin receptors in cytochalasin-treated cells demonstrates that phagocytosis per se is not necessary for secretion. It is not clear to what extent these processes may occur independently in vivo, and/or whether individual receptors use the same or different signal transduction pathways to initiate ingestion and/or secretory responses.

Many investigators use assays of O_2^- or H_2O_2 production as surrogate markers in phagocytosis assays. In this situation it is not always clear how much of the total production of oxygen metabolites is being measured and whether they are being produced and/or measured intracellularly or extracellularly. If the cells have been "primed," it is possible that increased oxidative metabolism may accompany the same amount of ingestion as observed with unprimed cells. In experimental situations in which this might be a critical result, the ingestion of the particles should be measured directly, independently of the respiratory burst.

Since the intimate details of the focal signaling necessary to accomplish the task of ingestion per se are only partially understood, it is difficult to explain all of the mechanisms by which general activation and/or "priming" of the cell facilitate those focal activation events and/or lead to an overall increase in the phagocytic activity of the cell. One of the most notable ways in which this can occur is the increase in surface expression of CR1 and CR3 induced by stimulating PMN with chemoattractants or other soluble activators (see below and Table 1). Other ways in which this can occur involve changing the functional status of the receptors by increasing the affinity of their ligand-binding sites, as in the case of CR3, by causing the receptors to aggregate within the membrane, and/or by promoting their linkage to signal-transducing elements. Since phagocytosis involves rearrangement and attachment of cytoskeletal elements to plasma membrane structures at sites at which receptors are binding opsonins, many investigators have used measurements of detergent insolubility of receptors (presumably caused by attachment to insoluble cytoskeletal elements), ability of receptors to move within the plane of the membrane, and/or cocapping experiments to indicate states of activation of the receptors. These are all complex phenomena that may be manifestations of different molecular effects, and may or may not directly correlate with steps in the ingestion process per se. Furthermore, although frequently considered analogous, spreading of cells on opsonins bound to microtiter plates may not always be the functional equivalent of ingesting particles coated with the same opsonins.

II. ROLE OF C5a AND C5a des arg IN ACTIVATING PHAGOCYTES

C5a is a 74 residue cationic glycopeptide released from the α-chain of C5 during its cleavage by the C5 convertases of the classical and alternative pathway. C5a and/or other

Table 1 Mechanisms of Increasing Complement Receptor Function in Human Neutrophils

	CR1	CR3
Increased surface expression	+	+
Clustering of receptors in membrane	+	+
Attachment to cytoskeleton	+	+
Phosphorylation of tail	+	+
Increased affinity of binding site for ligand	−	+

active C5 fragments containing this region can also be cleaved by other noncomplement proteases of both host and bacterial origin (3) that may be found at physiologically significant concentrations in inflammatory exudates. C5a is highly homologous with C4a and C3a, which share its anaphylotoxin activity on mast cells, but the other anaphylotoxins lack chemotactic activity for neutrophils. Cloning of the receptors strongly suggests that C3a and C3a des Arg bind to a different receptor on granulocytes than C5a and C5a des Arg (4,5). The C5a receptor has been designated CD88, but the C3a receptor has not yet been assigned a CD designation. The cloning results are consistent with previous studies demonstrating the lack of cross-desensitization of either receptor by the ligand (i.e., C3a or C5a) for the other and with studies showing that antireceptor monoclonal antibodies that completely abrogate the effect of one ligand fail to affect the other (6–9). Daffern et al. recently attempted to resolve the issue of C3a activation of neutrophils by using highly purified preparations of neutrophils and eosinophils, and combinations of the two types of cells (9). Eosinophils responded to C3a even in the presence of antibody to the C5a receptor. In contrast, neutrophils failed to respond to natural or recombinant human C3a, whereas mixtures of the two types of cells responded to both C3a and C5a. It was thus concluded that the reported activation of neutrophil preparations by C3a probably involves direct activation of the eosinophils present in most neutrophil preparations by C3a and subsequent secondary activation of the neutrophils by mediators (such as PAF) released from the eosinophils (9). This sequence of events could certainly explain many previous observations on differences between the kinetics and extent of activation of neutrophils by the two different fragments.

Although the C5a receptor has an affinity for C5a in the nanomolar range (4), the chemotactic activity of low concentrations of C5a, and particularly C5a des Arg, can be enhanced by the abundant plasma protein Gc globulin (vitamin D-binding protein), which is referred to as a cochemotaxin. Recent studies (10, 11) suggest that the Gc globulin may bind to sialic acid on the carbohydrate chain of the C5a des Arg. This complex may bind through the Gc globulin to the neutrophil plasma membrane in a conformation that more readily "presents" the protein core of the C5a des Arg to its receptor. The binding of the Gc globulin and or its complex with C5a/C5a des Arg to the neutrophil may involve proteolytic processing of the Gc globulin by the neutrophil (11).

Approximately 200,000 C5a receptors are expressed constitutively on the neutrophil plasma membrane (4). This constitutive expression differs from that of the receptors for formyl peptides and other chemoattractants, whose expression is lower and/or must be upregulated by translocation from intracellular pools when the cells are activated (4,12,13). The circulating neutrophil may thus be particularly sensitive to C5a. The importance of this chemoattractant in vivo has recently been emphasized by the demonstration that C5a receptor "knockout" mice are extremely sensitive to pulmonary infection with bacterial inocula that were readily cleared by their wild-type counterparts (14).

The C5a receptor (CD88) is a member of the "seven membrane spanner" family of receptors. Together with other chemoattractant receptors, however, it exhibits some structural differences from the β-adrenergic receptors and other archetypical members of this family (4,12). Upon binding its ligand, the C5a receptor primarily employs a pertussis toxin-sensitive heterotrimeric G protein (containing Gi2) to activate the MAP kinase pathway via RAS and RAF (15), although Gα16 has been shown to mediate C5a receptor signal transduction in some myeloid cell lines (16). Ultimately, the effects of C5a receptor occupancy are mediated by activation of phosphatidyl inositol phospholipase C (PIPLC), production of inositol triphosphate, and the release of intracellular Ca^{2+} stores (4,17).

Diacylglycerols that can activate protein kinase C are also liberated by PIPLC. The liberation of these intracellular mediators can lead to a number of functional responses by the cell including actin polymerization, shape change, chemotaxis per se, initiation of the oxidative respiratory burst, and secretion. At lower concentrations of C5a or C5a des Arg, below the threshold for activation of the cells, this full-blown response may not be seen, but the phenomenon of priming can occur. Priming refers to an effect of low doses of activators at which oxidative and/or secretory responses are not induced, but that result in greater responses upon subsequent exposure to higher doses of the same or heterologous stimuli than would be seen with the higher dose alone (17). The mechanisms of this state of increased responsiveness have not been clearly delineated but may involve preassociation of signaling molecules with the receptors, partial intracellular assembly of the oxidase and/or other multisubunit enzymes, and/or translocation of other receptors to the plasma membrane. Neutrophils arriving at sites of infection are almost certainly primed and/or activated as a result of the chemoattractants that drew them to that site in the first place. This phenomenon is likely to be of major physiologic importance in vivo. The phenomenon of priming also has important implications for in vitro assays of "opsonophagocytosis" in which bacteria, antibodies, serum, and phagocytes are all mixed together. Generation of C5a may prime the phagocytes and increase the expression of CR1 and CR3 (see below), resulting in greater phagocytosis per se and/or an enhanced oxidative response to any given degree of phagocytosis. This phenomenon is not always taken into consideration, however, and results of such assays are often considered indicative of the number of C3 fragments bound to the bacteria, although this might not correlate directly. Effects of differential production of C5a in such assays can be avoided by first washing the opsonized bacteria before adding them to the phagocytes and/or by using C5-depleted sera.

In addition to initiating signal transduction, binding of C5a to its receptor also leads to phosphorylation of the receptor itself. This causes internalization of the receptor and desensitization of the cell to the effects of C5a. Unoccupied receptors are subsequently recycled to the plasma membrane, restoring the cell's responsiveness (13).

Several species of bacteria secrete proteases capable of cleaving C5 and releasing fragments with C5a activity. In addition, some organisms produce proteases that inactivate C5a and/or its receptor, thus providing them some protection against this potent neutrophil activator. In particular, enzymes from *Entamoeba histolytica* (18) and some strains of streptococci (19) can degrade C5a, while a "gingipain" from *Porphyromonas gingivalis* can cleave and inactivate the neutrophil C5a receptor (20).

III. C1q, COLLECTINS, AND C1q RECEPTORS

C1q has been reported to enhance both phagocytosis and production of reactive oxygen intermediates by neutrophils, monocytes, and macrophages. However, there continues to be controversy about the identity of the receptors involved, the signaling pathways employed, and the physiological significance of the phenomena described in vitro. Part of this controversey undoubtedly arises from the apparent low affinity of C1q binding and the use of different assays and antibodies in different laboratories.

Tenner and Cooper showed that the oxidative response of PMN to aggregated IgG could be enhanced by addition of C1q to the assay mixtures (21). This effect was much greater if the C1q was preincubated with the aggregated IgG, presumably because this allowed increased binding of C1q to the aggregates before the complexes interacted with the PMN. They also reported that C1q bound to latex beads in the absence of IgG could induce oxidative responses as well, but no response was induced by free C1q itself. The response to C1q-coated latex beads could be blocked by free C1q, but only partial inhibition was achieved even with very large excesses. Intact macromolecular C1 was not capable of inducing this response (21). Sorvillo et al. showed that addition of C1q promoted the attachment of EIgM to monocytes and that this could be further enhanced by treating the E or the monocytes with fibronectin (22). C1q itself was unable to induce phagocytosis of EIgM, but if there were also C3 fragments on the EIgM, C1q enhanced their ingestion (22). This effect was most dramatic if the monocytes were first allowed to adhere to fibronectin-coated plates (22). Subsequently, Tenner et al. showed that adherence of cultured macrophages to plates coated with C1q or surfactant protein A (SP-A, see below), enhanced phagocytosis of IgG or C4b coated E, but effects of C1q or SP-A bound to the targets themselves were not demonstrated (23). More recently, Ohkuro et al. showed that treatment of tetanus toxoid–antitetanus IgG complexes with C1q enhanced the binding and uptake of these complexes by PMN, and that this enhancement could, in turn, be inhibited by excess fluid-phase C1q (24).

The phagocytosis-enhancing effect of bound C1q is teleologically appealing, since after binding and activation of macromolecular C1 by IgG or IgM on the surface of a particulate activator such as a bacterium or in a multivalent complex, C1INH would cause dissociation of C1r and C1s, leaving the C1q still bound by its globular heads, but with its collagen-like tail exposed. Interaction of this tail with its own receptor would then be expected to increase the overall binding avidity of the target with the phagocyte and/or to activate additional signaling pathways that could augment the effects of the interactions of IgG and C4/C3 fragments with their respective receptors. In the case of IgM, this mechanism might be even more important, since phagocytes lack receptors for the Fc of that class of antibodies. The relatively modest effects of target-bound C1q compared to the effects of adherence to C1q-coated surfaces are consistent with a low-affinity receptor, however, and suggest that its true physiological role may be to enhance phagocytosis mediated by other opsonins rather than to initiate cellular responses by itself.

Guan et al used affinity chromatography with the collagenlike region of C1q to isolate a protein from extracts of the U937 cell line with molecular weight of 100,000, which increased to 126,00 upon reduction (25,26). Monoclonal antibodies to this protein inhibited the C1q-mediated enhancement of phagocytosis of EIgMC4b by monocytes, but not the enhancement of O_2^- production, suggesting that these two effects were mediated by different receptors (26). Jack et al. isolated a protein with similar properties from neutrophil extracts using C1q-Sepharose, and showed that the binding of C1q to PMN increased upon activation of the cells, presumably by translocation of an intracellular pool of stored receptors (27). Tenner et al. subsequently showed that neutrophils from a patient with leukocyte adhesion deficiency, which lack CD18-containing integrins, failed to produce O_2^- when incubated in microtiter plates coated with the collagenlike regions of C1q. The response of normal neutrophils to this stimulus was inhibited by antibodies to CD11b/CD18 (28). This suggests that CD11b/CD18 might participate in signaling by C1q and its receptor(s), perhaps via a mechanism analogous to the participation of integrins in signaling by IgG and CD16 (FcγRIII) on PMN (see below).

In contrast to the 126 kDa protein studied by Tenner et al. (25,26), Ghebrehiwet and his colleagues have isolated a 60–70 kDa protein from Raji cells and PMN (29) and have reported that this protein is expressed on many other diverse types of cells as well. The surface expression of this protein does not appear to be upregulated upon PMN activation and there does not appear to be any intracellular storage of additional receptors not present on the plasma membrane (30). These workers have reported that organisms opsonized with C1q as well as soluble C1q itself are capable of inducing superoxide responses, although 10–100-fold higher concentrations of free C1q were necessary to achieve the same response as for particle bound ligand (30). An additional, distinct 33 kDa PMN surface protein, which binds to the globular heads of C1q, has also been described (31,32), but its function and significance are not known.

C1q shares several structural features with other proteins such as conglutinnin, pulmonary surfactant protein-A (SP-A), and mannose-binding protein (formerly MBP, now MBL).* All of these proteins are multimers whose structural domains are similar to that of C1q (33). They all have a collagenlike domain and a lectinlike carbohydrate recognition domain capable of Ca^{2+}-dependent binding to a variety of glycans, hence these proteins are referred to as collagenlike lectins, or "collectins" (33). MBL and SP-A have been reported to have opsonic activity for bacteria and viruses (34–36).

MBL has also been reported to associate with a serine protease, termed MASP, which is capable of activating the classical pathway of complement (37). Since all collecting, including C1q, appear to have similar capabilities in enhancing phagocytosis, and all have similar collagenlike regions, it seems reasonable to hypothesize that at least some of their functions are mediated by a common receptor for their collagen-like regions (33,38,39). Indeed, Geertsma et al. have demonstrated that C1q inhibited binding of SP-A opsonized *S. aureus* to monocytes (35). In addition, Tenner et al. demonstrated that one of the monoclonal antibodies they developed against the 126 kDa C1qR also inhibited the enhancement of phagocytosis induced by MBL (40) and that surface-bound SP-A had effects similar to C1q in enhancing phagocytosis (23). Taken together, these data argue that there is a single receptor for all of these proteins and that the 126 kDa protein is, at least, a functionally important part of that receptor. However, most attention in the literature has focussed on a 50–60 kDa "collectin receptor" protein with a high degree of sequence similarity to the Ro/SS-A antigen recognized by autoantibodies in the sera of patients with Sjögren's syndrome, and also with calreticulin (39). There is not yet sufficient data in the literature to determine the exact relationship between the 68 kDa protein described by Ghebrehiwet and the "collectin receptor". It is likewise not known whether either or both of these associate with the 126 kDa protein described by Tenner's group into a single functional complex, or whether these groups are studying separate phenomena mediated by independent receptors. It is interesting, however, that the collectin receptor has been identified on lymphoblasts and many other nonphagocytic cell types, while the larger C1qR identified by Tenner's group has been found only on "professional phagocytes."

Mutations in MBL have been described in patients with recurrent infections, establishing the physiological importance of this protein in the host defense (41,42). In particular, mutations in residue 54 cause functional defects as well as decreased concentrations of this protein in plasma (41–43), but the relative importance of MBL in activating the classical pathway without antibody (37,43) vs. serving as an opsonin, or both, have not been delineated. It seems likely that SP-A plays an important role in phagocytic defense in the lung, since several groups have demonstrated that it enhances phagocytosis of pathogenic bacteria by alveolar macrophages (44–46). It has recently been reported that

---

* It has been suggested that this protein should be termed mannose-binding lectin and abbreviated MBL to avoid confusion with other proteins that have been abbreviated MBP.

SP-A "knockout" mice are extremely sensitive to pulmonary infection with group B *Streptococcus* (47).

IV. ROLE OF OPSONIC FRAGMENTS OF C3

The basic tenets of the role of C3 in phagocytosis were established by experiments in several laboratories about 20 years ago, before complement or Fc receptors had been identified or characterized, and remain true today. Building on the earlier descriptions of the role of bound C3 in promoting immune adherence, several groups used sheep erythrocyte intermediates to define the relative contributions of complement and IgM and IgG antibodies to the enhancement of phagocytosis by neutrophils and macrophages. With this test particle, it was found that bound C3b promoted avid binding of the sensitized erythrocyte to the phagocyte, forming impressive rosettes, but that this was insufficient to cause ingestion per se (48–55). In contrast, opsonization with small amounts of IgG, which by themselves were insufficient to promote much binding or ingestion, readily induced phagocytosis if the targets were also coated with C3b (48–55). A classic illustration of this is shown in the results of Ehlenberger and Nussenzweig (54), reproduced here as Figure 2. These experiments established the basic paradigm that C3 fragments can promote adherence but that an activating or "second" signal, such as that provided by IgG interacting

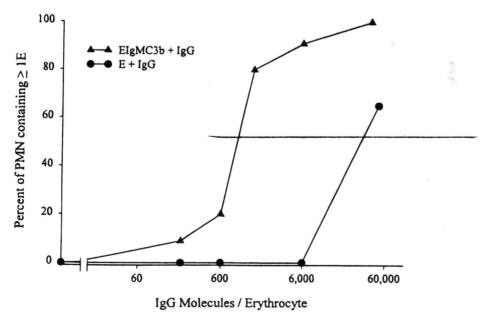

Figure 2 Role of C3b and IgG in phagocytosis of sheep erythrocytes by human PMN. Sheep erythrocytes (E) were incubated alone or sensitized with rabbit IgM and purified classical pathway components, then with control buffer or rabbit IgG containing [^{125}I]IgG to allow quantitation of the amount of IgG per erythrocyte. Coverslips bearing PMN were overlaid with E and incubated at 37°C for 30–45 min. Extracellular E were removed by washing and lysis, coverslips were stained, and ingested E were counted. Results are expressed as the percentage of PMN containing one or more E. (From Ref. 54.)

with Fcγ receptors, is necessary to initiate the process of ingestion. IgM does not provide this signal because there are no Fc receptors for μ chains on phagocytes. Under some circumstances, this "second signal" can be provided independently of the opsonized target, leading to a state of "activation" of the complement receptor itself. In other situations, especially when the C3b is bound to a carbohydrate-rich particle such as zymosan, which is a good activator of the alternative pathway, the surface of the particle itself may provide the second signal by interacting with lectinlike receptors on the phagocyte (52,56–59). It is interesting that C3 fragments, together with IgG and/or the surface of the target cells, can play analogous roles in the cytolytic activity of large granular lymphocytes. Thus, C3b and iC3b promote adherence but not cytotoxicity. If IgG is also present, and/or if the surface carbohydrates on the target cell can activate the killer cell, marked cytolysis will occur, even if the latter interaction by itself does not provide sufficient adhesion (60–64). Identification and analysis of the structures of the receptors for each of the different opsonins has provided insights that explain many of the phenomena described earlier, but several questions still remain under active investigation.

A. Role of C3b and CR1

CR1 (CD35) is primarily stored inside circulating monocytes and PMN and undergoes a complex trafficking pattern that includes translocation to the plasma membrane as well as ligand-independent internalization and degradation when the cells are activated. The intracellular receptors are stored in small, low-density "secretory" vesicles quite distinct from the traditional PMN granules (65,66). These storage vesicles resemble the small vesicles in which transporters and other important membrane proteins whose functions must be rapidly upregulated in response to hormones are stored in other types of cells. Examples of this type of regulation include the translocation of glucose transporters in response to insulin in fat cells and the translocation of water channels in response to antidiuretic hormone in renal tubular cells (67,68). The translocation of these vesicles is an early event in PMN activation and occurs very rapidly. Upon priming or activation of the cells by a chemoattractant or other activator, the surface expression of CR1 (and CR3, see below) can increase as much as 10-fold within minutes, reaching a maximum of about 50,000 molecules per cell (69,70). Although this requires an increase in the concentration of free intracellular Ca^{2+} (71), the concentrations required are much lower than necessary for exocytosis of traditional primary or secondary granules (66,72). It is thus possible to upregulate surface CR1 expression maximally without significant secretion of granular enzymes or O_2^- (66,73). Apparently, some of the intracellular Ca^{2+} stores are physically released during purification of PMN as a result of mechanical stress during centrifugation and vortexing (71). This leads to a "spontaneous" increase in the amount of CR1 and CR3 on the plasma membrane as soon as isolated cells are warmed to 37°C (69). Thus, isolated PMN frequently have more CR1 and CR3 on their surface than do cells stained in whole blood before vortexing or centrifugation (69).

Once on the cell surface, CR1 remains predominantly in a clustered distribution (65,74–78), which may reflect the addition to the plasmalemma of the small patch of membrane of the vesicle in which the CR1 molecules were stored intracellularly (65). Clustering may also be due to linkage of CR1 to cytoskeletal or signal-transducing elements. This clustered distribution likely facilitates interaction of multiple CR1 molecules with multiple C3b fragments deposited in close proximity to a convertase site when particulate complement activators are being used as the targets (75,76). Upon activation, the endocytic activity of the phagocytes also increases dramatically and some of the CR1 is internalized even in the absence of ligand (79). Electron microscopic studies suggest that this may occur through coated pits as well as "uncoated" regions of the plasma membrane (80). The internalized CR1 may then be recycled to the plasma membrane or degraded, although the regulation of these two processes, which likely compete, has not yet been determined.

The relationship between this complex trafficking pattern and the participation of CR1 in phagocytosis under different conditions has not yet been elucidated. Examination of the sequence of CR1 shows that its cytoplasmic tail lacks tyrosines and any of the activation motifs or protein kinase-binding domains that are characteristic of other receptors involved in immunological effector mechanisms (81). This likely explains the lack of signaling by CR1 upon ligation and, therefore, the inability of C3b to induce phagocytosis in the absence of other opsonins. Indeed, the only recognizable motif in the tail of CR1 is the amino acid sequence VHPRTL (81), which is highly homologous to a protein kinase C phosphorylation site in the epidermal growth factor receptor (82). It has been reported from several laboratories that CR1 becomes phosphorylated during PMN activation and that its phosphorylation and internalization are increased by PMA and other activators of protein kinase C (79,83–86), implicating this site. PMA has also been reported to increase the association of CR1 with the detergent-insoluble cytoskeleton (84,86) and to activate CR1 transiently, enabling them to induce phagocytosis without an independent second signal (85,87,88). However, the relations between phosphorylation, internalization, and "activation" of CR1 for phagocytosis have not been defined. It seems likely that the phenomena of adsorptive endocytosis of CR1 cross-linked by antireceptor antibodies or small C3b oligomers (77,78,88) may represent an acceleration of the phenomenon of ligand-independent internalization, perhaps caused by concentrating more of the receptors in coated pits. However, as Okada and Brown showed, this phenomenon is most likely distinct from "activated" phagocytosis by CR1, since the latter, but not the former, is inhibitable by NaF (88).

If PMN or monocytes are allowed to adhere to certain connective tissue proteins such as fibronectin or laminin (89–92), to surfaces coated with C1q (23), or have been pretreated with PMA (85), E(IgM)C3b can be ingested in the absence of other opsonins (Reviewed in 92 and 93). The signals for this "activation" by connective tissue proteins are transmitted into the cell by integrins including members of the $\beta2$ family as well as $\alpha v \beta3$ and a unique "leukocyte response integrin," which is distinct from but shares some epitopes with the $\beta3$ class (94,95). The actual alterations in CR1 that accompany this change in function have not been completely defined, but current ideas are summarized in Table 1. The observations that phorbol esters mimic this effect suggest that protein kinase C is involved, but it is not clear that its actual effect is on CR1 per se rather than another molecule that may serve as a bridge between CR1 and intracellular signaling mechanisms. There are no reports in the literature that PMA treatment or adherence increases the intrinsic affinity of CR1 for C3b. Although Fallman et al, have shown that cross-linking by $F(ab')_2$ fragments of anti-CR1 can lead to phospholipase-D activation (96), the relationship of this to phagocytosis and the possible involvement of coreceptors such as CR3 have not been defined. It is possible that the phenomenon of "activation" of CR1 really represents an effect on CR3. This would increase the affinity of its lectinlike site for carbohydrate side chains on CR1 and thus recruit this multifunctional protein as a signal transducer, much in the same way that it is employed for signaling by the glycolipid anchored form of FcγRIII. FcγRIII is incapable of intracellular signaling by itself since it has no cytoplasmic tail at all (reviewed in 97). Other possible mechanisms of activation of CR1 could involve interactions of its cytoplasmic tail with intermediate molecules that could facilitate its linkage to the cytoskeleton and/or segregation into specialized lipid domains within the plasma membrane, but these remain only speculations at this point. The phenomenon of activation of phagocytic receptors by adherence of the cells to connective tissue proteins is likely of major physiological importance since it provides a convenient mechanism by which phagocytes can remain quiescent while circulating intravascularly, yet rapidly transform into activated killers at sites of infection or inflammation in the tissues (93).

The inability of CR1 to induce phagocytosis without other signals observed under most conditions in vitro correlates with in vivo observations on the clearance of IgM-sensitized erythrocytes (reviewed in Chap. 20). In guinea pig models, E(IgM) injected intravenously are initially sequestered in the liver and/or spleen but is not ingested, and is then released after the fixed C3b has been cleaved to C3d. If the animals have been treated with BCG however, many of the cells will be phagocytosed during the initial sequestration, suggesting that the BCG treatment of the animals has resulted in an in vivo state that corresponds to the activated state discussed above.

CR2 (CD21) is not constitutively expressed on PMN or circulating monocytes, and is not generally considered to be an important phagocytic receptor. Expression of CR2 can be induced on macrophages under some conditions in vitro (98), and its participation in phagocytosis parallels that of CR1. The fact that EIgMC3d are not rapidly cleared from the circulation in patients with autoimmune hemolytic anemia suggests that CR2 is not expressed at high levels on fixed phagocytes of the reticuloendothelial system, and confirms that this receptor has little phagocytic activity in vivo.

B. iC3b-Dependent and -Independent Activities of CR3

Although in some ways the actions of CR3 in complement-mediated phagocytosis are similar to those of CR1, the total spectrum of activity of CR3 is much more complex. CR3 is the archetypical member of the leukocyte $\beta2$ integrin family (99–102) and can transmit signals not only from the outside of the cell to the inside when it binds ligands but also from the "inside out," which can change its binding avidity and phagocytic activity when the cell is primed. With EIgMC3bi as the test particles, and with resting phagocytes, the interaction will be like that of EC3b with CR1: There will be avid rosette formation but no ingestion. With primed cells, however, EC3bi can be ingested without additional opsonins. As with CR1, there are intracellular stores of CR3 in the "secretory vesicles" in PMN and monocytes, and surface expression of CR3 is upregulated along with that of CR1 (103–106). However, there are additional stores of CR3 in the membranes of a subset of PMN specific granules. More complete cellular activation, with greater increases of the $[Ca^{2+}]i$, is associated with additional increases in surface expression of CR3 (66,71,72,107,108). Maximal expression of CR3 on PMN is 4–10 times higher than that of CR1 (100,103,106). Besides this mechanism of increasing the number of CR3 molecules on the cell surface, it has been clearly documented that CR3 can also be activated into a state with enhanced binding and functional activity (Table 1). For example, in a study by Wright and Meyer, phorbol ester treatment increased plasma membrane expression of CR3 4fold, but attachment of EIgMC3bi increased 10-fold and phagocytosis increased 40-fold (85). Monoclonal antibodies that specifically recognize neoepitopes associated with this activated state (109–113) have been produced in several laboratories.

CR3 is a multifunctional molecule with binding sites for many ligands in addition to iC3b. These confer additional properties and roles in phagocytosis quite distinct from those of CR1. Most notably, CR3 also serves as the neutrophils' major adherence protein. Also known as Mac-1 or CD11b/CD18, CR3 is a member of the β2 family of leukocyte integrins, which also includes CD11a/CD18 (LFA-1) and CD11c/CD18 (CR4). Mutations in the common CD18 chain lead to absence of all three of these molecules from the cell surface and to the clinical syndrome recognized as leukocyte adherence deficiency (LAD), marked by recurrent severe infections despite elevated numbers of circulating white blood cells (104,114–116). Two major ligand-binding domains in CR3 have been characterized. The "I" or "inserted" domain is so named because it is a ~200 amino acid sequence found in the α chains of the β2 and a few β1 integrins but not in the α chains of other integrin families (100,101,117,118). This domain has also been referred to as the "A" domain because of homology with the type A domain of von Willebrand's factor (VWFA) (117,119). This domain is responsible for cation-dependent binding to iC3b, ICAM-1, fibrinogen, and other proteins, although it is not exactly clear how many different binding sites per se exist within this domain (111,117,118). It was originally thought that this domain bound to the sequence RGD within its ligands, but more recent evidence suggests that the actual binding to this domain is through other sequences (120), and that the RGD binds to a different integrin referred to as the "leukocyte response integrin (LRI)" (94). Ligation of this LRI then transmits a signal through an "integrin-associated protein" that somehow induces conformational changes in CR3 that promote binding of its various protein ligands (95). Studies with CR3 truncation mutants show that the cytoplasmic tails of both chains play roles in determining the affinity of the extracellular ligand-binding sites (121). Thus, "inside-out" signaling is likely mediated, at least in part, by changes in the phosphorylation of the cytoplasmic tails (113,121–123).

In addition, CR3 contains a lectin-like site that can bind a variety of polysaccharides including β-glucans (59,124). It has recently been shown that binding of certain soluble glucans to this site can activate PMN for cytotoxic activity towards iC3b-bearing targets such as sheep erythrocytes that would otherwise rosette with the PMN but would not be lysed (125). This activation likely represents the process that occurs with iC3b on a zymosan particle. Binding of the polysaccharides to the lectin site provides the "second" signal that activates the cell, but the iC3b plays a major role in promoting the binding of the particle in the first place (59,125). Thus, unopsonized zymosan is not a good activator (59,125). CR3 has been reported to have lectinlike interactions that are important for the entry of leishmania and histoplasma into macrophages (126–129). More recent results suggest that the binding of leishmania is not independent of iC3b (130). The "activation" of CR3 induced by the leukocyte response integrin and its integrin-associated protein (94,95) seems analogous to that induced by binding of β-glucans to the lectin-binding site of CR3: Two different interactions, with different ligands frequently on the same target, cooperate to promote the overall effect of CR3 binding. Activation of CR3 for phagocytosis can also be induced by PMA (85) and by cytokines including TNF and GM-CSF, which also induce alterations of the phosphorylation of the cytoplasmic tails of the CD11b and CD18 chains (122,123).

The lectin site on CR3 can also mediate binding of CR3 to the carbohydrate side chains of molecules such as FcγRIIIB and CD14 (the LPS-LPS binding protein receptor), which are anchored in the plasma membrane by phosphatidyl inositol glycolipids and have no cytoplasmic tails. This binding then allows CR3 to function as a signal transducer for the glycolipid anchored proteins (97). A linkage between CR3 and FcγR was initially suggested by the observations that patients with LAD have partial defects in IgG-mediated phagocytosis (131) and that monoclonal antibodies against CR3 blocked phagocytosis but not binding of IgG-coated erythrocytes to PMN (132). Recent experiments have shown that cotransfection with CR3 is necessary for phagocytosis by transfected FcγRIIIB in fibroblasts that do not constitutively express complement or Fcγ receptors (133). It has likewise been reported that a soluble fragment of FcγRIII could bind to CR3 or CR4 by a mechanism inhibitable by soluble glucans or zymosan and that this interaction could induce cytokine production by PMN and monocytes (134). These observations confirm the likely physiological importance of this phenomenon. It is not known if CR1 and/or other traditional transmembrane proteins can also recruit CR3 to participate in this kind of interaction, perhaps through their carbohydrate side chains, which might explain their increased phagocytic activity observed under certain conditions such as following PMA stimulation and/or adherence. It is possible in this regard that early reports of cocapping of CR1 with FcγR on PMN (135) might be due to linkage of both of those receptors to clustered CR3 molecules. Zhou and Brown have shown that the respiratory burst induced by the simultaneous binding of antibodies to FcγRIII and CR3 is inhibited by Fab of anti-FcγRII. This finding suggests that linkage or aggregation of all three receptors is necessary for optimal intracellular signal transduction and activation of tyrosine kinase pathways (136). Such linkages of complement receptors and Fcγ receptors might thus explain the increased opsonic efficacy of C3b-IgG conjugates (137), which are likely to be good physiological models for the binding of C3 fragments to antibody molecules on the surface of bacteria (138) in vivo.

Many investigators have used adherence to ligands on plastic plates as a model for the interactions of receptors with opsonins during phagocytosis. Adherence of PMN to surfaces coated with ligands for CR3 is accompanied by phosphorylation of multiple proteins including the src family tyrosine kinase fgr (139), which is also activated during this process; the myristoylated protein kinase C substrate MARCKS (140), which is believed to have a role in remodeling the cytoskeleton and linking it to the plasma membrane (141); and the cytoskeletal protein paxillin (142). Since these proteins are also phosphorylated during FcγR mediated phagocytosis, this is likely indicative of a role for these proteins in CR3-mediated signaling and/or in the mechanical processes of CR3-mediated phagocytosis as well. Electron microscopic examination of macrophages ingesting zymosan has shown that MARCKS, protein kinase C-α, myosin I, F-actin, and talin all colocalize in the cortical cytoplasm adjacent to the newly forming phagocytic cup (141). Inhibitors of protein kinase C reduced binding and phagocytosis of zymosan, and also reduced the focal accumulation of these proteins below those particles that did attach (141). Cross-linking of CR3 causes release of inositol phosphates (143), localized release of Ca^{2+} stores (144), and association of the receptors with talin (145), a protein that provides transmembrane linkages with the cytoskeleton and initiates actin assembly. It may also be involved in movement of the phagocytic cup around the particle being ingested (Fig. 1). It is interesting that the phosphorylation of several of these proteins upon ligation of CR3 is enhanced in cells that have been pretreated with TNF, fMLP, or PMA (139,146). This suggests that the "activated" state of the receptor, which has also been reported to correlate with clustering of receptors within the plane of the membrane (147), may also involve aggregation of receptor cytoplasmic tails and downstream substrates in the protein tyrosine kinase and C-kinase cascades. Upon ligand binding, phosphorylation and overall cellular stimulation could then proceed more efficiently and rapidly. It is important to note that while phagocytosis is frequently accompanied by activation of the microbicidal oxidase, signaling for the engulfment process per se may employ pathways for focal actin polymerization that differ from those involved in generalized cell activation. For example, engulfment can occur without observable whole-cell Ca^{2+} transients, and is not inhibited by pertussis toxin to nearly the same extent as is activation of the oxidase or secretion (143).

When considering the activation of CR3's phagocytic activity by adherence of the cell to CR3 ligands, it is apparent that both "outside-in" and "inside-out" signaling are occurring at the same time. It is likely that different subsets of CR3 molecules at different sites on the plasma membrane serve different functions at the same time (110,148). This may be analogous to the controlled sequence of activation and inactivation of CR3 during cell movement. In this sequence, CR3 molecules are first translocated from intracellular stores to the surface at the leading edge of the plasma membrane of a moving cell, their binding sites are transiently activated and then inactivated, and then they move backwards in the plane of the membrane to become internalized and repeat the cycle (149,150). A similar sequence of transient activation and inactivation could be involved in the movement of the leading edges of the forming phagocytic cup.

C. CR4

CR4, also known as p150,95 and CD11c/CD18, remains less well characterized than other members of the leukocyte β2 integrin family. Although it has been suggested that this protein might be responsible for the reported binding of C3dg to neutrophils (151), the true binding specificity of CR4 remains incompletely defined. Recent studies suggest that, as in CR3, interactions between the cytoplasmic tails of the β and α chains regulate CR4's binding activity, such that in its native state in resting cells the affinity for iC3b-coated particles is relatively low (152). CR4 is expressed on human neutrophils, and its expression is upregulated during neutrophil activation, but maximal CR4 expression on circulating cells is much less than that of CR1 or CR3 (106,153,154). In contrast, CR4 is the major C3 receptor on tissue macrophages, including alveolar macrophages (153–155). The interaction of iC3b on some bacteria and other test particles with CR4 on alveolar macrophages is not sufficient to induce phagocytosis (155). However, on other bacteria, such as *Mycobacterium tuberculosis*, C3 fragments and CR4 seem to play a major role in phagocytosis (156). It thus seems possible that the binding avidity and/or functional activity of CR4 is regulated in a manner analogous to that of CR3, and that lectin-like interactions with certain bacterial polysaccharides may have an activating effect. This requires further investigation. CR4 expression has been reported on NK cells and cytotoxic T-lymphocytes and it likely plays a role in cell-mediated cytotoxicity analogous to that discussed earlier for CR3 (157).

V. CONCLUSIONS

Phagocytosis plays a critically important role in the host's defenses against infectious disease. Complement facilitates phagocytosis by providing C5a, which serves as a potent chemoattractant and neutrophil activator; and C3b and iC3b fragments, which serve as the major opsonins derived from the complement system. C1q also likely plays a role in enhancing phagocytosis of particles opsonized with C3b and iC3b. With resting phagocytes and sheep erythrocytes as targets, C3b and iC3b serve mainly to promote adherence of the erythrocytes, to the phagocytes, CR1 (CD35) and CR3 (CD11b/CD18) do not provide signals to activate the phagocyte machinery. Classic studies showed that these signals could be provided by IgG, even at concentrations too low to cause adherence. This synergism of complement and IgG acting together exemplifies the amplification of the effects of antibody by complement. Under certain circumstances, with "primed" or adherent phagocytes, C3 fragments and their receptors alone are sufficient to induce phagocytosis. The physiology of the activation of and signaling by CR1 and CR3 is just beginning to be understood at a molecular level. Further investigation of these receptors should not only yield important insights into the molecular mechanisms of signal transduction and engulfment but may also suggest therapeutically useful means to "stimulate the phagocytes."

ACKNOWLEDGMENTS

This work was supported by NIH grant AI22687. The author wishes to thank Dr. Andrea Tenner for helpful discussions and Ms. Pat Ortez for assistance in preparing the manuscript.

REFERENCES

1. Griffin FM Jr, Griffin JA, Silverstein SC. Studies on the mechanisms of phagocytosis II. The interaction of macrophages with anti-IgG coated bone marrow-derived lymphocytes. J Exp Med 1976; 144:788–809.
2. Greenberg S, Silverstein SC. Phagocytosis. In: Paul WE, ed. Fundamental Immunology, 3rd ed. New York: Raven Press, 1993; 941–964.
3. Wetsel RA, Kolb WP. Expression of C5a-like biological activities by the fifth component of human complement (C5) upon limited digestion with noncomplement enzymes without release of polypeptide fragments. J Exp Med; 1983; 157:2029–2048.
4. Gerard C, Gerard NP. C5a anaphylatoxin and its seven transmembrane-segment receptor. Annu Rev Immunol 1994; 12:775–808.
5. Ames RS, Li Y, Sarau HM, Nuthulaganti P, Foley JJ, Ellis C, Zeng Z, Su K, Jurewicz AJ, Hertzberg RP, Bergsma DJ, Kumar C. Molecular cloning and characterization of the human anaphylatoxin C3a receptor. J Biol Chem 1996; 271:20231–20234.
6. Norgauer J, Dobos G, Kownatzki E, Dahinden C, Burger R, Kupper R, Gierschik P. Complement fragment C3a stimulates Ca2+ influx in neutrophils via a pertussis-toxin-sensitive G protein. Eur J Biochem 1993; 217:289–294.
7. Ehrengruber MU, Geiser T, Deranleau DA. Activation of human neutrophils by C3a and C5a. Comparison of the effects of shape changes, chemotaxis, secretion, and respiratory burst. FEBS Lett 1994; 346:181–1844.
8. Elsner J, Oppermann M, Czech W, Kappa A. C3a activates the respiratory burst in human polymorphonuclear neutrophilic leukocytes via pertussis toxin-sensitive G-proteins. Blood 1994; 83:3324–3331.
9. Daffern PJ, Pfeifer PH, Ember JA, Hugli TE. C3a is a chemotaxin for human eosinophils but not for neutrophils. I. C3a stimulation of neutrophils is secondary to eosinophil activation. J Exp Med 1995; 181:2119–2127.
10. Perez, HD. Gc globulin (vitamin D-binding protein) increases binding of low concentrations of C5a des Arg to human polymorphonuclear leukocytes: an explanation for its cochemotaxin activity. Inflammation 1994; 18:215–220.
11. Kew RR, Fisher JA, Webster RO. Co-chemotactic effect of Gc-globulin (vitamin D binding protein) for C5a. Transient conversion into an active co-chemotaxin by neutrophils. J Immunol 1995; 155:5369–5374.

12. Murphy, PW. The molecular biology of leukocyte chemoattractant receptors. Annu Rev Immunol 1994; 12:593–633.

13. Van Epps DE, Simpson S, Bender JG, Chenoweth C. Regulation of C5a and formyl peptide receptor expression on human polymorphonuclear leukocytes. J Immunol 1990; 144:1062–1068.

14. Hopken UE, Lu B, Gerard NP, Gerard C. The C5a chemoattractant receptor mediates mucosal defence to infection. Nature 1996; 383:86–89.

15. Buhl AM, Avdi N, Worthen GS, Johnson GL. Mapping of the C5a receptor signal transduction network in human neutrophils. Proc Natl Acad Sci 1994; 91:9190–9194.

16. Burg M, Raffetseder U, Grove M, Klos A, Kohl J, Bautsch W. G alpha-16 complements the signal transduction cascade of chemotactic receptors for complement factor C5a (C5a-R) and N-formylated peptides (fMLF-R) in *Xenopus laevis* oocytes. FEBS Lett 1995; 377:426–428.

17. Snyderman R, Uhing RJ. Chemoattractant stimulus–response coupling. In: Gallin JI, Goldstein IM, Snyderman R, eds. Inflammation: Basic Principles and Clinical Correlates, 2nd ed. New York: Raven Press, 1992:421–439.

18. Reed SL, Ember JA, Herdman DS, DiScipio RG, Hugli TE, Gigli I. The extracellular neutral cysteine proteinase of *Entamoeba histolytica* degrades anaphylatoxins C3a and C5a. J Immunol 1995; 155:266–274.

19. Takahashi S, Nagano Y, Nagano N, Hayashi O, Taguchi F, Okawaki Y. Role of C5a-ase in group B streptococcal resistance to opsonophagocytic killing. Infect Immun 1995; 63:4764–4769.

20. Jagels MA, Travis J, Potempa J, Pike R, Hugli TE. Proteolytic inactivation of the leukocyte C5a receptor by proteinases derived from *Porphyromonas gingivalis*. Infect Immun 1996; 64:1984–1991.

21. Tenner AJ, Cooper NR. Stimulation of a human polymorphonuclear leukocyte oxidative response by the C1q subunit of the first complement component. J Immunol 1982; 128:2547–2552.

22. Sorvillo JM, Gigli I, Pearlstein E. The effect of fibronectin on the processing of C1q- and C3b/bi-coated immune complexes by peripheral blood monocytes. J Immunol 1986; 136:1023–1026.

23. Tenner AJ, Robinson SL, Borchelt J, Wright JR. Human pulmonary surfactant protein (SP-A), a protein structurally homologous to C1q, can enhance FcR- and CR1-mediated phagocytosis. J Biol Chem 1989; 264:13923–13928.

24. Ohkuro M, Kobayashi K, Takahashi K, Nagasawa S. Effect of C1q on the processing of immune complexes by human neutrophils. Immunology 1994; 83:507–511.

25. Guan EN, Burgess WH, Robinson SL, Goodman EB, McTigue KJ, Tenner AJ. Phagocytic cell molecules that bind the collagen-like region of C1q. Involvement in the C1q-mediated enhancement of phagocytosis. J Biol Chem 1991; 266:20345–20355.

26. Guan E, Robinson SL, Goodman EB, Tenner AJ. Cell-surface protein identified on phagocytic cells modulates the C1q-mediated enhancement of phagocytosis. J Immunol 1994; 152:4005–4016.

27. Jack RM, Lowenstein BA, Nicholson-Weller A. Regulation of C1q receptor expression on human polymorphonuclear leukocytes. J Immunol 1994; 153:262–269.

28. Goodman EB, Anderson DC, Tenner AJ. C1q triggers neutrophil superoxide production by a unique CD18-dependent mechanism. J Leukocyte Biol 1995; 58:168–176.

29. Ghebrehiwet B, Silvestri L, McDevitt C. Identification of the raji cell membrane-derived C1q inhibitor as a receptor for human C1q. J Exp Med 1984; 160:1373–1389.

30. Eggleton P, Ghebrehiwet B, Coburn JP, Sastry KN, Zaner KS, Tauber AI. Characterization of the human neutrophil C1q receptor and functional effects of free ligand on activated neutrophils. Blood 1994; 84:1640–1649.

31. Ghebrehiwet B, Lim BL, Peerschke, EIB, Willis AC, Reid KB. Isolation cDNA cloning and over expression of a 33-kD cell surface glycoprotein which binds to the globular "heads" of C1q. J Exp Med 1994; 179:1809–1821.

32. Eggleton P, Ghebrehiwet B, Sastry KN, Coburn JP, Zaner KS, Reid KB. Identification of a gC1q-binding protein (gC1q-R) on the surface of human neutrophils. J Clin Invest 1995; 95:1569–1578.

33. Malhotra R, Thiel S, Reid KBM, Reid KB, Sim RB. Human leukocyte C1q receptor binds other soluble proteins with collagen domains. J Exp Med 1990; 172:955–959.

34. Turner, MW. Mannose binding protein. Biochem Soc Trans 1994; 22:88–94.

35. Geertsma MF, Nibbering PH, Haagsman HP, Daha MR, van Furth R. Binding of surfactant protein A to C1q receptors mediates phagocytosis of *Staphylococcus aureus* by monocytes. Am J Physiol 1994; 267:L578–L584.

36. Hartshorn KL, Sastry K, White MR, Tauber AI, Anders EM, Super M, Ezekowitz RA. Human mannose-binding protein functions as an opsonin for influenza A viruses. J Clin Invest 1993; 91:1414–1420.

37. Sato T, Endo Y, Matsushita M, Fujita T. Molecular characterization of a novel serine protease involved in activation of the complement system by mannose-binding protein. Int Immunol 1994; 6:665–669.

38. Malhotra R, Sim RB. Chemical and hydrodynamic characterization of the human leucocyte receptor for complement subcomponent C1q. Biochem J 1989; 262:625–631.

39. Malhotra R, Willis AC, Jensenius JC, Jackson J, Sim RB. Structure and homology of human C1q receptor (collectin receptor). Immunology 1993; 78:341–348.

40. Tenner AJ, Robinson SL, Ezekowitz RA. Mannose binding protein (MBP) enhances mononuclear phagocyte function via a receptor that contains the 126,000 M(r) component of the C1q receptor. Immunity 1995; 3:485–493.

41. Lipscombe RJ, Sumiya M, Summerfield JA, Turner MW. Distinct physicochemical characteristics of human mannose binding protein expressed by individuals of differing genotype. Immunology 1995; 85:660–667.

42. Summerfield JA, Ryder S, Sumiya M, Thursz M, Gorchein A, Monteil MA, Turner MW. Mannose binding protein gene mutations associated with unusual and severe infections in adults. Lancet 1995; 345:886–889.

43. Matsushita M, Ezekowitz RA, Fujita T. The gly-54→Asp allelic form of human mannose binding protein (MBP) fails to bind MBP-associated serine protease. Biochem J 1995; 311:1021–1023.

44. van Iwaarden F, Welmers B, Verhoef J, Haagsman HP, van Golde LM. Pulmonary surfactant protein A enhances the host-defense mechanism of rat alveolar macrophages. Am J Respir Cell Mol Biol 1990; 2:91–98.

45. Manz-Keinke H, Plattner H, Schlepper-Schafer J. Lung surfactant protein A (SP-A) enhances serum-independent phagocytosis of bacteria by alveolar macrophages. Eur J Cell Biol 1992; 57:95–100.

46. Tino MJ, Wright JR. Surfactant protein A stimulates phagocytosis of specific pulmonary pathogens by alveolar macrophages. Am J Physiol 1996; 270:L677–L688.

47. LeVine AM, Bruno MD, Whitsett JA, Korfhagen TR. Group B streptococal infection in SP-A deficient mice. Pediatr Pulmonol 1996; Suppl 13:330.

48. Huber H, Polley MJ, Linscott WD, Fudenberg HH, Muller-Eberhard HJ. Human monocytes: distinct receptors for the third component of complement and for IgG. Science 1968; 162:1281–1283.

49. Bianco C, Griffin FM, Silverstein SC. Studies of the macrophage complement receptor: Alteration of receptor function upon macrophage activation. J Exp Med 1975; 141:1278–1290.

50. Griffin FR Jr, Bianco C, Silverstein SC. Characterization of the macrophage receptor for complement and demonstration of its functional independence from the receptor for the Fc portion of immunoglobulin G. J Exp Med 1975, 141:1269–1277.

51. Mantovani, B. Different roles of IgG and complement receptors in phagocytosis by polymorphonuclear leukocytes. J Immunol 1975; 115:15–17.

52. Goldstein IM, Kaplan HB, Radin A, Frosch M. Independent effects of IgG and complement upon human polymorphonuclear leukocyte function. J Immunol 1976; 117:1282–1287.

53. Scribner DJ, Fahrney D. Neutrophil receptors for IgG and complement: Their roles in the attachment and ingestion phases of phagocytosis. J Immunol 1976; 116:892–897.

54. Ehlenberger AG, Nussenzweig V. The role of membrane receptors for C3b and C3d in phagocytosis. J Exp Med 1977; 145:357–371.

55. Newman SL, Johnston RB Jr. Role of binding through C3b and IgG in polymorphonuclear neutrophil function: studies with Trypsin-generated C3b. J Immunol 1979; 123:1839–1846.

56. Stossel TP, Alper CA, Rosen FS. Serum-dependent phagocytosis of paraffin oil emulsified with bacterial lipopolysaccharide. J Exp Med 1973; 137:690–705.

57. Henson, PM. The immunologic release of constituents from neutrophil leukocytes. The role of antibody and complement on nonphagocytosable surfaces or phagocytosable particles. J Immunol 1971; 107:1535–1546.

58. Czop JK, Austen KF. Functional discrimination by human monocytes between their C3b receptors and their recognition units for particulate activators of the alternative complement pathway. J Immunol 1980; 125:124–128.

59. Ross GD, Cain JA, Lachmann PJ. Membrane complement receptor type three (CR_3) has lectin-like properties analogous to bovine conglutinin and functions as a receptor for zymosan and rabbit erythrocytes as well as a receptor for iC3b. J Immunol 1985; 135:3307–3315.

60. Van Boxel JA, Paul WE, Frank MM, Green I. Antibody-dependent lymphoid cell-mediated cytotoxicity: role of lymphocytes bearing a receptor for complement. J Immunol 1973; 110:1027–1036.

61. Perlmann P, Perlmann H, Müller-Eberhard HJ. Cytolytic lymphocytic cells with complement receptor in human blood. Induction of cytolysis by IgG antibody but not by target cell-bound C3 . J Exp Med 1975; 141:287–296.

62. Ghebrehiwet B, Medicus RG, Müller-Eberhard HJ. Potentiation of antibody-dependent cell-mediated cytotoxicity by target cell-bound C3b[1]. J Immunol 1979; 123:1285–1288.

63. Perlmann H, Perlmann P, Schreiber RD, Muller-Eberhard HJ. Interaction of target cell-bound C3bi and C3d with human lymphocyte receptors. Enhancement of antibody-mediated cellular cytoxicity. J Exp Med 1981; 153:1592–1603.

64. Klein E, DiRenzo L, Yefenof E. Contribution of CR3, CD11b/CD18 to cytolysis by human NK cells. Mol Immunol 1990; 27:1343–1347.

65. Berger M, Wetzler E, Welter EM, Turner JR, Tartakoff AM. Unique intracellular sites for storage and recycling of C3b receptors in human neutrophils. Proc Nat Acad Sci (USA) 1991; 88:3019–3023.

66. Sengelov H, Kjeldsen L, Kroeze W, Berger M, Borregaard N. Secretory vesicles are the intracellular reservoir of complement receptor 1 in human neutrophils. J Immunol 1994; 153:804–810.

67. Al-Aqwati, Q. Rapid insertion and retrieval of pumps and channels into membranes by exocytosis and endocytosis. In: Graves JS, ed. Regulation and Development of Membrane Transport Processes. New York: John Wiley & Sons, 1985:149–157.

68. Nielson S, Marples D, Birn H, Mohtashami M, Dalby NO, Trimble M, Knepper M. Expression of VAMP2-like protein in kidney collecting duct intracellular vesicles. J Clin Invest 1995; 96:1834–1844.

69. Fearon DT, Collins LA. Increased expression of C3b receptors on PMN leukocytes induced by chemotactic factors and by purification procedures. J Immunol 1983; 130:370–375.

70. Berger M, Cross AS. Lymphoblastoid cell supernatants increase expression of C3b receptors on human polymorphonuclear leukocytes—direct binding studies with ^{125}I-C3b. Immunology 1984; 51:431–440.

71. Berger M, Birx DL, Wetzler EM, O'Shea JJ, Brown EJ, Cross AS. Calcium requirements for increased complement receptor expression during neutrophil activation. J Immunol 1985; 135:1342–1348.

72. Sengelov H, Kjeldsen L, Borregaard N. Control of exocytosis in early neutrophil activation. J Immunol 1993; 150:1535–1543.

73. Berger M, Wetzler E, Wallis RS. Tumor necrosis factor is the major monocyte product that increases complement receptor expression on mature human neutrophils. Blood 1988; 71:151–158.

74. Petty HR, Smith LM, Fearon DT, McConnell HM. Lateral distribution and peripheral distribution of the C3b receptors of complement, HLA antigens and lipid probes in peripheral blood leukocytes. Proc Nat Acad Sci (USA) 1980; 77:6587–6591.

75. Paccaud JP, Carpentier JL, Schifferli JA. Difference in the clustering of complement receptor type 1 (CR1) on polymorphonuclear leukocytes and erythrocytes: effect on immune adherence. Eur J Immunol 1990; 20:283–289.

76. Dierich MP, Reisfeld RA. C3-mediated cytoadherence. Formation of C3 receptor aggregates as prerequisite for cell attachment. J Exp Med 1975; 142:242–247.

77. Fearon DT, Kaneko I, Thomson GG. Membrane distribution and adsorptive endocytosis by C3b receptors on human polymorphonuclear leukocytes. J Exp Med 1981; 153:1615–1628.

78. Abrahamson DR, Fearon DT. Endocytosis of the C3b receptor of complement within coated pits in human polymorphonuclear leukocytes and monocytes. Lab Invest 1983; 48:162–168.

79. Turner JR, Tartakoff AM, Berger M. Intracellular degradation of the C3b/C4b receptor in the absence of ligand. J Biol Chem 1988; 263:4914–4920.

80. Berger M, Sieverding E, August JT, Tartakoff AM. Internalization of type I complement receptors and de novo multivesicular body formation during chemoattractant induced endocytosis in human neutrophils. J Clin Invest 1994; 94:1113–1125.

81. Klickstein LB, Wong WW, Smith JA, Weis JH, Wilson JG, Fearon DT. Human C3b/C4b receptor (CR1). Demonstration of long homologous repeating domains that are composed of the short consensus repeats characteristic of C3/C4 binding proteins. J Exp Med 1987; 165:1095–1112.

82. Hunter T, Ling N, Cooper JA. Protein kinase C phosphorylation of the EGF receptor at a threonine residue close to the cytoplasmic face of the plasma membrane. Nature 1984; 311:480–483.

83. Changelian PS, Fearon DT. Tissue-specific phosphorylation of complement receptors CR1 and CR2. J Exp Med 1986; 163:101–115.

84. Changelian PS, Jack RM, Collins LA, Fearon DT. PMA induces the ligand-independent internalization of CR1 on human neutrophils. J Immunol 1985; 134:1851–1858.

85. Wright SD, Meyer BC. Phorbol esters cause sequential activation and deactivation of complement receptors on polymorphonuclear leukocytes. J Immunol 1986; 136:1759–1764.

86. O'Shea JJ, Brown EJ, Gaither TA, Takahashi T, Frank MM. Tumor-promoting phorbol esters induce rapid internalization of the C3b receptor via a cytoskeleton-dependent mechanism. J Immunol 1985; 135:1325–1330.

87. Bussouno F, Fischer E, Turrini F, Kazatchkine MD, Arese P. Platelet-activating factor enhances complement-dependent phagocytosis of diamide-treated erythrocytes by human monocytes through activation of protein kinase C and phosphorylation of complement receptor type one (CR-1). J Biol Chem 1989; 264:21711–21719.

88. Okada K, Brown EJ. Sodium fluoride reveals multiple pathways for regulation of surface expression of the C3b/C4b receptor (CR1) on human polymorphonuclear leukocytes. J Immunol 1988; 140:878–884.

89. Pommier CG, Inada S, Fries LF, Takahashi T, Frank MM, Brown EJ. Plasma fibronectin enhances phagocytosis of opsonized particles by human peripheral blood monocytes. J Exp Med 1983; 157:1844–1856.

90. Wright SD, Craigmyle LS, Silverstein SC. Fibronectin and serum amyloid P component stimulate C3b- and C3bi-mediated phagocytosis in human monocytes. J Exp Med 1983; 158:1338–1343.

91. Bohnsack JF, Kleinman HK, Takahashi T, O'Shea JJ, Brown EJ. Connective tissue proteins and phagocytic cell function: laminin enhances complement- and Fc-mediated phagocytosis by cultured human macrophages. J Exp Med 1985; 161:912–923.

92. Wright SD, Griffin FM Jr. Activation of phagocytic cells' C3 receptors for phagocytosis. J Leukocyte Biol 1985; 38:327–339.

93. Brown EJ. Phagocytosis. BioEssays 1995; 17:109–117.

94. Gresham HD, Goodwin JL, Allen PM, Anderson DC, Brown EJ. A novel member of the integrin receptor family mediates Arg-Gly-Asp-stimulated neutrophil phagocytosis. J Cell Biol 1989; 108:1935–1943.

95. Zhou M, Brown EJ. Leukocyte response integrin and integrin-associated protein act as a signal transduction unit in generation of a phagocyte respiratory burst. J Exp Med 1993; 178:1165–1174.

96. Fällman M, Andersson R, Andersson T. Signaling properties of CR3 (CD11b/CD18) and CR1 (CD35) in relation to phagocytosis of complement-opsonized particles. J Immunol 1993; 151:330–338.

97. Petty HR, Todd RF III. Receptor-receptor interactions of complement receptor type 3 in neutrophil membranes. J Leukocyte Biol 1993; 54:492–494.

98. Inada S, Brown EJ, Gaither TA, Hammer CH, Takahashi T, Frank MM. C3d receptors are expressed on human monocytes after in vitro cultivation. Proc Natl Acad Sci 1983; 80:2351–2355.

99. Kishimoto TK, Larson RS, Corbi AL, Dustin ML, Staunton DE, Springer TA. The leukocyte integrins. Adv Immunol 1989; 46:149–182.

100. Arnaout, MA. Structure and function of the leukocyte adhesion molecules CD11/CD18. Blood 1990; 75:1037–1050.

101. Springer, TA. Adhesion receptors of the immune system. Science 1990; 346:425–434.

102. Edwards, SW. Cell signalling by integrins and immunoglobulin receptors in primed neutrophils. TIBS 1995; 20:362–367.

103. Todd RF III, Arnaout MA, Rosin RE, Crowley CA, Peters WA, Babior BM. Subcellular localization of the large subunit of Mol, a surface glycoprotein associated with neutrophil adhesion. J Clin Invest 1984; 74:1280–1290.

104. Arnaout MA, Spits H, Terhorst C, Pitt J, Todd RF III. Deficiency of a leukocyte surface glycoprotein (LFA-1) in two patients with Mol deficiency. Effects of cell activation on Mol/LFA-1 surface expression in normal and deficient leukocytes. J Clin Invest 1984; 74:1291–1300.

105. Berger M, O'Shea J, Cross AS, Folks TM, Chused TM, Brown EJ, Frank MM. Human neutrophils increase expression of C3bi as well as C3b receptors upon activation. J Clin Invest 1984; 74:1566–1571.

106. Miller LJ, Bainton DF, Borregaard N, Springer TA. Stimulated mobilization of monocyte Mac-1 and p150,95 adhesion proteins from an intracellular vesicular compartment to the cell surface. J Clin Invest 1987; 80:535–544.

107. O'Shea JJ, Brown EJ, Seligmann BE, Metcalf JA, Frank MM, Gallin JI. Evidence for distinct intracellular pools of receptors for C3b and C3bi in human neutrophils. J Immunol 1985; 134:2580–2587.

108. Sengelov H, Kjeldsen L, Diamond MS, Springer TA, Anderson HC, Kishimoto TK, Bainton DF. Subcellular localization and dynamics of Mac-1 ($\alpha m \ \beta_2$) in human neutrophils. J Clin Invest 1993; 92:1467–1476.

109. Altieri DC, Edgington TS. A monoclonal antibody reacting with distinct adhesion molecules defines a transition in the functional state of the receptor C11b/CD18 (Mac-1). J Immunol 1988; 141:2656–2660.

110. Diamond MS, Springer TA. A subpopulation of Mac-1 (CD11b/CD18) molecules mediates neutrophil adhesion to ICAM-1 and fibrinogen. J Cell Biol 1993; 120:545–556.

111. Diamond MS, Springer TA, Garcia-Aguilar J, Bickford JK, Corbi AL. The I domain is a major recognition site on the leukocyte integrin Mac-1 (CD11b/CD18) for four distinct adhesion ligands. J Cell Biol 1993; 120:1031–1043.

112. Frelinger AL III, Cohen I, Plow EF, Smith MA, Roberts J, Lam SC, Ginsberg MH. Selective inhibition of integrin function by antibodies specific for ligand-occupied receptor conformers. J Biol Chem 1990; 265:6346–6352.

113. Diamond MS, Springer TA. The dynamic regulation of integrin adhesiveness. Curr Biol 1994; 4:506–517.

114. Anderson DC, Schmalsteig FC, Finegold MJ, Hughes BJ, Rothlein R, Miller LJ, Kohl S, Tosi MF, Jacobs RL, Waldrop TC. The severe and moderate phenotypes of heritable Mac-1, LFA-1 deficiency: their quantitative definition and relation to leukocyte dysfunction and clinical features. J Infect Dis 1985; 152:668–689.

115. Todd, RF, Freyer DR. The CD11/CD18 leukocyte glycoprotein deficiency. Hematol Oncol Clin North Am 1988; 2:13–31.

116. Anderson DC, Springer TA. Leukocyte adhesion defiency: an inherited defect in the Mac-1, LFA-1, and p150,95 glycoproteins. Annu Rev Med 1987; 38:175–194.

117. Arnaout MA, Gupta SK, Pierce, MW, Tenen DG. Amino acid sequence of the alpha subunit of human leukocyte adhesion receptor Mol (complement receptor type 3). J Cell Biol 1988; 106:2153–2158.

118. Zhou L, Lee DH, Plescia J, Lau CY, Altieri, DC. Differential ligand binding specificities of recombinant CD11b/CD18 integrin I-domain. J Biol Chem 1994; 269:17075–17079.

119. Colombatti A, Bonaldo P. The superfamily of proteins with von Willebrand factor type A-like domains: one theme common to components of extracellular matrix, homeostasis, cellular adhesion and defense mechanisms. Blood 1991; 77:2305–2315.

120. VanStrijp JA, Russell DG, Tuomanen E, Brown EJ, Wright SD. Ligand specificity of purified complement receptor type three (CD11b/CD18, alpha m beta 2, Mac-1). Indirect effects of an Arg-Gly-Asp (RGD) sequence. J Immunol 1993; 151:3324–3326.

121. Rabb H, Michishita M, Sharma CP, Brown D, Arnaout MA. Cytoplasmic tails of human complement receptor type 3 (CR3, CD11b/CD18) regulate ligand avidity and the internalization of occupied receptors. J Immunol 1993; 151:990–1002.

122. Chatila T, Geha RS, Arnaout MA. Constitutive and stimulus-induced phosphorylation of CD11/CD18 leukocyte adhesion molecules. J Cell Biol 1989; 109:3435–3444.

123. Buyon JP, Slade SG, Reibman J, Abramson SB, Philips MR, Weissmann G, Winchester R. Constitutive and induced phosphorylation of the α- and β-chains of the CD11/CD18 leukocyte integrin family-relationship to adhesion-dependent functions. J Immunol 1990; 144:191–197.

124. Thornton BP, Vetvicka V, Pitman M, Goldman RC, Ross GD. Analysis of the sugar specificity and molecular location of the beta-glucan-binding lectin site of complement receptor type 3 (CD11b/CD18). J Immunol 1996; 156:1235–1246.

125. Vetvicka V, Thornton BP, Ross GD. Soluble β-glucan polysaccharide binding to the lectin site of neutrophil or natural killer cell complement receptor type 3 (CD11b/CD18) generates a primed state of the receptor capable of mediating cytotoxicity of iC3b-Opsonized target cells. J Clin Invest 1996; 98:50–61.

126. Mosser DM and Edelson PJ. The mouse macrophage receptor for C3bi (CR3) is a major mechanism in the phagocytosis of leishmania promastigotes. J Immunol 1985; 135:2785–2789.

127. Blackwell JM, Ezekowitz RAB, Roberts MB, Channon JY, Sim RB, Gordon S. Macrophage complement and lectin-like receptors bind leishmania in the absence of serum. J Exp Med 1985; 162:324–331.

128. Bullock WE, Wright SD. Role of the adherence-promoting receptors CR3, LFA-1, and p150,95, in binding of *Histoplasma capsulatum* by human macrophages. J Exp Med 1987; 165:195–210.

129. Wilson ME, Pearson RD. Roles of CR3 and mannose receptors in the attachment and ingestion of *Leishmania donovani* by human mononuclear phagocytes. Infect Immun 1988; 56:363–369.

130. Mosser DM, Springer TA, Diamond MS. Leishmania promastigotes require opsonic complement to bind to the human leukocyte integrin mac-1 (CD11b/CD18). J Cell Biol 1992; 116:511–520.

131. Arnaout MA, Pitt J, Cohen HJ, Melamed J, Rosen FS, Colten HR. Deficiency of a granulocyte membrane glycoprotein (p 150) in a boy with recurrent bacterial infections. N Engl J Med 1983; 306:693–699.

132. Arnaout MA, Todd RF III, Dana N, Melamed J, Schlossman SF, Colten HR. Inhibition of phagocytosis of complement C3- or IgG-coated particles and of iC3b binding by monoclonal antibodies to a monocyte–granulocyte membrane glycoprotein (Mol). J Clin Invest 1983; 72:171–179.

133. Krauss JC, Poo H, Xue W, Mayo-Bond L, Todd RF III, Petty HR. Reconstitution of antibody-dependent phagocytosis in fibroblasts expressing Fcγ receptor IIIB and the complement receptor Type 3. J Immunol 1994; 153:1769–1777.

134. Galon J, Gauchat J, Mazieres N. Soluble Fcγ receptor type III (FcγRIII, CD16) triggers cell activation through interaction with complement receptors. J Immunol 1996; 157:1184–1192.

135. Jack RM, Fearon DT. Altered surface distribution of both C3b receptors and Fc receptors on neutrophils induced by anti-C3b receptor or aggregated IgG. J Immunol 1984; 132:3028–3033.

136. Zhou MJ, Brown EJ. CR3 (Mac-1, αM β2, CD11b/CD18) and Fc gamma RIII cooperate in generation of a neutrophil respiratory burst: requirement for Fc gamma RIII and tyrosine phosphorylation. J Cell Biol 1994; 125:1407–1416.

137. Fries LF, Siwik SA, Malbran A, Frank MM. Phagocytosis of target particles bearing C3b-IgG covalent complexes by human monocytes and polymorphonuclear leucocytes. Immunology 1987; 62:45–51.

138. Brown E, Berger M, Joiner K, Frank MM. Classical complement pathway activation by antipneumococcal antibodies leads to covalent binding of C3b to antibody molecules. Infect Immun 1983; 42:594–598.

139. Berton G, Fumagalli L, Laudanna C, Sorio C. β2 Integrin-dependent protein tyrosine phosphorylation and activation of the FGr protein tyrosine kinase in human neutrophils. J Cell biol 1994; 126:1111–1121.

140. Fallman M, Gallberg M, Hellberg C, Anderson T. Complement receptor-mediated phagocytosis is associated with accumulation of phosphatidylcholine-derived diglyceride in human neutrophils. J Biol Chem 1992; 267:2656–2663.

141. Allen LH, Aderem A. A role for MARCKS, the α isozyme of protein kinase C and myosin I in zymosan phagocytosis by macrophages. J Exp Med 1995; 182:829–840.

142. Graham IL, Anderson DC, Holers VM, Brown EJ. Complement receptor 3 is required for tyrosine phosphorylation in adherent and non-adherent neutrophils. J Cell Biol 1994; 127:1139–1147.

143. Fallman M, Lew DP, Stendahl O, Andersson T. Receptor-mediated phagocytosis in human neutrophils is associated with increased formation of inositol phosphates and diacylglycerol. J Clin Invest 1989; 84:886–891.

144. Petersen M, Williams JD, Hallett MB. Cross-linking of CD11b or CD18 signals localized release of Ca^{2+} from intracelular stores in neutrophils. Immunology 1993; 80:157–159.

145. Horwitz A, Duggan K, Bret C, Beckerle MC, Burridge K. Interaction of plasma membrane fibronectin receptors with talin-a transmembrane linkage. Nature 1986; 320:531–533.

146. Fuortes M, Jen W, Nathan C. β-Integrin-dependent tyrosine phosphorylation of paxillin in human neutrophils treated with tumor necrosis factor. J Cell Biol 1994; 127:1477–1483.

147. Detmers PA, Wright SD, Olsen E, Kimball B, Cohn ZA. Aggregation of complement receptors on human neutrophils in the absence of ligand. J Cell Biol 1987; 105:1137–1145.

148. Graham I, Gresham HD, Brown E. An immobile subset of plasma membrane CD11b/CD18 (Mac-1) is involved in phagocytosis of targets recognized by multiple receptors. J Immunol 1989; 142:2352–2358.

149. Sheikh S, Nash GB. Continuous activation and deactivation of integrin CD11b/CD18 during de novo expression enables rolling neutrophils to immobilize on platelets. Blood 1996; 87:5040–5050.

150. Cai TQ, Wright SD. Energetics of leukocyte integrin activation. J Biol Chem 1995; 270:14358–14365.

151. Vik DP, Fearon Dt. Neutrophils express a receptor for iC3b, C3dg and C3d that is distinct from CR1, CR2, and CR3. J Immunol 1985; 134:2571–2579.

152. Bilsand CA, Diamond MS, Springer TA. The leukocyte integrin p150,95 (CD11c/CD18) as a receptor for iC3b. Activation by a heterologous beta subunit and localization of a ligand recognition site to the I domain. J Immunol 1994; 152:4582–4589.

153. Freyer DR, Morganroth ML, Rogers CE, Arnaout MA, Todd RF. Modulation of surface CD11/CD18 glycoproteins by human mononuclear phagocytes. Clin Immunol Immunopathol 1988; 46:272–283.

154. Myones BL, Dalzell JG, Hogg N, Ross GD. Neutrophil and monocyte cell surface p150,95 has iC3b-receptor (CR4) activity resembling CR3. J Clin Invest 1988; 82:640–651.

155. Berger M, Norvell TM, Tosi MF, Emancipator SN, Konstan MW, Schreiber JS. Tissue specific Fc and complement receptor expression by alveolar macrophages determines relative importance of IgG and complement in promoting phagocytosis of *P. aeruginosa*. Pediatr Res 1994; 35:68–77.

156. Hirsch CS, Ellner JJ, Russell DG, Rich EA. Complement receptor-mediated uptake and tumor necrosis factor-alpha-mediated growth inhibition of *Mycobacterium tuberculososis* by human alveolar macrophages. J Immunol 1994; 152:743–753.

157. Keizer GD, Borst J, Visser W, Schwarting R, De Vries JE, Figdor CG. Membrane glycoprotein p150,95 of human cytotoxic T cell clones is involved in conjugate formation with target cells. J Immunol 1987; 138:3130–3136.

13

Cellular Responses to the Membrane Attack Complex

CAROLYN MOLD

University of New Mexico Health Science Center,
Albuquerque, New Mexico

I. INTRODUCTION

The discovery and analysis of the complement pathways was based largely on observations of bacterial killing and erythrocyte lysis. These functions are mediated by the membrane attack complex (MAC), a complex of the terminal complement components that inserts into and disrupts membranes. Cytolysis and bacterial killing by the MAC may be its most obvious activities. However, many cells, particularly nucleated cells, are quite resistant to lysis by homologous complement. A number of responses have been described in nucleated cells undergoing sublytic complement attack. Some of these are directly related to resistance to cytolysis. Other responses are proinflammatory and may contribute to the host response to injury or to disease pathogenesis. This chapter will describe briefly the lytic potential of the MAC for different targets. Next the protective responses of nucleated cells to sublytic complement attack will be reviewed. Other responses of nucleated cells and the relationship of these to defense against lysis will be considered. Finally, the systemic inflammatory response to the presence of MAC in cell membranes and specific examples of the contribution of MAC to disease pathogenesis will be discussed.

II. LYSIS BY THE MAC

The membrane attack complex was discovered and named for its ability to cause cell lysis. It does this by disruption of the permeability barrier of cell membranes, with resulting colloid osmotic lysis. The lytic effect of the MAC has been studied most intensively using heterologous erythrocytes and artificial lipid bilayers as targets. As reviewed recently (1–3) and discussed elsewhere in this volume, there is still debate concerning the molecular orientation of the MAC in the membrane, the formation and role of polymerized C9, and the mechanism of membrane lysis. However, it is clear that formation of C5b-8 initiates the insertion of one or more C9 molecules into membranes leading to the loss of membrane integrity and lysis. There is also evidence that different targets have different requirements for MAC lysis. In the simplest cases of heterologous erythrocytes and liposomes, complement-mediated lysis obeys one-hit kinetics and the full lytic potential of the MAC is achieved with complexes composed of $(C5b-8)_1C9_1$ (3). Complexes of this composition have a pore size of 1–3 nm, which can be enlarged to 10 nm by additional C9 (4). The MAC lesions formed on erythrocytes and liposomes are also quite stable. Homologous erythrocytes resist complement-mediated lysis due to the presence of membrane-regulatory proteins, principally CD59 that binds to C8 and C9 and prevents MAC assembly (5, 6, and reviewed in Chapter 7).

III. BACTERIAL KILLING BY THE MAC

In contrast, bacterial killing by the MAC is more complex. Gram-negative bacteria, some of which are susceptible to complement-mediated killing, have an outer membrane containing lipopolysaccharide and an inner cytoplasmic membrane. The lethal hit requires dissipation of the membrane potential at the inner membrane, but is signaled by the insertion of C9 into the outer membrane of the bacterial cell. The full lytic potential of the MAC is achieved with complexes composed of $(C5b-8)_1C9_3$ (7). Although insertion of MAC and disruption of the outer membrane permeability barrier to macromolecules are normally closely coupled to disruption of the cytoplasmic membrane permeability barrier to small molecules (8), the mechanism of this coordinate lysis is not clear. An intriguing observation was made by Tomlinson et al. (9), who found that functional MACs isolated from erythrocyte membranes and passively transferred to the outer membrane of bacterial cells were nonlethal. These studies indicate that MAC-induced permeability changes in the outer membrane are not of themselves sufficient for disruption of the cytoplasmic membrane, which results in lethality. Mechanisms by which the active formation of the initial outer membrane lesion could lead to access of C9 or fragments of C9 to the periplasm and cytoplasmic membrane have been proposed (3). Strategies of microbial resistance to complement killing, and comparisons of bacterial killing by complement to bacterial killing by colicins and cytotoxic neutrophil proteins are areas of active investigation, but are beyond the scope of this chapter.

IV. LYSIS OF NUCLEATED CELLS BY THE MAC

Cytolysis or cell killing by the MAC may be its most dramatic activity. However, many nucleated cells are quite resistant to lysis by complement, particularly lysis by homologous complement. This resistance is due in part to membrane-regulatory proteins that restrict MAC assembly. These are discussed in Chapters 6 and 7. In addition to regulation of MAC assembly, most nucleated cells undergo a protective response triggered by the MAC. A number of responses have been described in nucleated cells undergoing complement attack that may or may not be directly related to resistance to cytolysis. In this section the responses of nucleated cells to complement attack that result in MAC elimination will be reviewed. The next section will consider the signaling pathways for MAC removal and additional cellular responses to terminal complement complexes.

A. Resistance of Nucleated Cells to Lysis Requires an Active Response

Resistance of nucleated cells to lysis by homologous complement is attributable in part to the contribution of membrane regulatory proteins that reduce the stability of the C3 and C5 convertases and regulate MAC formation. However, the resistance of nucleated cells to complement killing is only partly explained by this mechanism. A series of early studies by Goldberg, Green and colleagues (10,11) established that resistance of nucleated cells to complement attack is an active process requiring metabolic activity. These studies further showed that cells attacked by complement could recover from increased permeability to small molecules. Later studies by Ohanian, Schlager, and Borsos (reviewed in 12) examined the effect of a range of metabolic inhibitors on killing of tumor cells by complement. The conclusion from these studies was that lipid turnover probably linked to membrane repair was crucial for resistance to complement lysis.

B. Multiple MAC Lesions Are Required for Lysis of Nucleated Cells

Understanding the mechanisms of nucleated cell resistance to complement killing was advanced by more detailed kinetic analysis comparing permeability changes and cell death. Koski et al. (13) examined the ability of limited concentrations of C6 (or C5b6) added to nucleated cells or erythrocytes sensitized with antibody and C6-deficient serum to increase permeability to small ions (^{86}Rb) and to cause cytolysis. These experiments demonstrated monotonic dose response curves for both erythrocyte lysis and ^{86}Rb release from nucleated cells consistent with the requirement for a single effective channel for these events. However, dose–response curves for killing of nucleated cells were sigmoidal, indicating that multiple effective C6 molecules were required for cytolysis. Similar results were obtained with C5b6 and C9 (14). These data were most consistent with a requirement for multiple MAC lesions to achieve cytolysis of nucleated cells.

C. Nucleated Cells Actively Eliminate MAC

Although the requirement for multiple channels to kill nucleated cells could result from resistance to osmotic lysis through ion pumps or other mechanisms, additional studies soon established that MAC channels on nucleated cells, unlike MAC channels on erythrocytes, are expressed transiently (15). Functional channels formed at sublytic complement concentrations on human tumor cells were eliminated rapidly (with a half-life of approximately 1 min) by incubation of the cells at 37°C. The channels were stable for several hours when cells were incubated at 2°C. At about the same time as these functional studies were reported, Morgan et al. (16) using a neutrophil model and Carney et al. (14) using Ehrlich ascites tumor cells demonstrated by immunofluorescence and electron microscopy the physical removal of MAC from the surface of nucleated cells undergoing sublytic complement attack. This removal of MAC from cell membranes correlated with protection from cytolysis (17).

D. Pathways of MAC Elimination

Although removal of MAC from the membrane appears to be a general protective response of nucleated cells undergoing complement attack, there are some variations in the mechanism used by different cell types. In Ehrlich ascites tumor cells (a mouse cell line), removal of lytic sites generated with human serum was observed for cells bearing C5b-7, C5b-8, or C5b-9, with more rapid removal of the more complete complexes (14). The electron microscopic studies done on C5b-8 complexes indicated accumulation of complexes in clathrin-coated pits followed by endocytosis as the major route of removal of lytic complexes. The endocytic pathway for MAC removal appeared to be similar to other endocytic processes and resulted in the appearance of MAC in multivesicular lysosomal bodies (14) and degradation of protein components of the complex (18).

In most other studies, cells undergoing sublytic complement attack have been found to produce and shed vesicles enriched in MAC components from the cell surface. Vesicle shedding is preceded by the formation of membrane patches enriched in MAC. This pathway of triggered membrane shedding has been called ectocytosis by Stein and Luzio (19) to indicate the right-side-out nature of the shed vesicles. Ectocytosis has been described for human neutrophils, platelets, and myeloid cell lines attacked by human complement as well as for several other homologous and heterologous systems (reviewed in 20). In a quantitative study of the process of removal of MAC from human neutrophils (18), 65% of the bound C9 was released in vesicles and approximately 30% of the bound C9 was internalized indicating that both endocytic and ectocytic pathways were operative.

An interesting variation of the process of MAC removal has been observed *in vivo* by Kerjaschki et al. (21). These authors used immunoelectron microscopy to show that MACs localized in the glomeruli in a model of membranous nephritis were endocytosed at the abluminal surface of glomerular epithelial cells and transported across the cell to be exocytosed and excreted into the urine. Internalized MAC were associated with components of the endocytic pathway. The anti-MAC reactive material recovered in the urine was 30 kDa, suggesting degradation of 120 and 140 kDa proteins present in lysed erythrocyte membranes. Urine MAC was associated with a membrane vesicle-containing $100,000 \times$ g pellet and partitioned into the detergent following Triton X-114 fractionation.

E. Characteristics of Shed Vesicles Containing MAC

The process of vesicle shedding has been studied most extensively on neutrophils. Determination of both the lipid and protein composition of the shed vesicles indicates that sorting of membrane components precedes ectocytosis. Using human neutrophils sensitized with antibody and treated with sublytic concentrations of human serum, Morgan et al. (18) observed the release of vesicles of 0.1–1.0 μm in diameter. By transmission electron microscopy these vesicles were found to be covered with ringlike lesions similar to those found on liposomes or erythrocytes following complement lysis and identified by other studies as polymerized C9. The presence of radioiodinated C8 or C9 in the vesicle fraction confirmed the shedding of MAC by the cells, and showed that approximately 65% of the original cell-associated C8 and C9 was associated with the vesicle fraction. In contrast only 2–3% of cell surface radiolabel appeared in the vesicle fraction after complement attack. Stein and Luzio (19), using the same model, compared the protein and lipid composition of intact neutrophil plasma membranes and shed vesicles. They reported 40% of C9 but less than 2% of surface label associated with vesicles and the two fractions displayed different protein patterns by sodium dodecyl sulfate (SDS)-polyacrylamide gel electrophoresis. When the lipid composition of the two membrane fractions was determined, it was found that compared to plasma membranes the vesicles contained similar amounts of membrane phospholipids but increased amounts of cholesterol and diacylglycerol.

V. NUCLEATED CELL SIGNALS FOR REMOVAL OF MAC

A. Initiation of MAC Removal by Calcium Influx

The studies described above established that the ability of nucleated cells to resist complement lysis is related to the physical removal of MAC from the membrane. The most rapid removal of MAC requires C9 (14,17) and a temperature of 37°C (15). An essential trigger for this process appears to be the increase in intracellular calcium that results from entry of calcium ions through channels following MAC insertion. Initial studies using human neutrophils (16) and platelets (22), and mouse Ehrlich ascites tumor cells (23), demonstrated calcium influx in response to MAC that correlated with elimination of MAC from the cell membrane and resistance of the cell to lysis. For Ehrlich ascites tumor cells, decreasing the extracellular calcium concentration from 0.15 mM to 0.015 mM resulted in nearly single-hit characteristics for C9-dependent lysis of cells bearing C5b-8. Chelation of intracellular calcium increased the sensitivity of the cells to lysis. For neutrophils, a later release of calcium from intracellular stores was observed in the absence of extracellular calcium, and chelation of intracellular as well as extracellular calcium was required to decrease MAC elimination markedly (24). In platelets calcium influx in response to MAC or to other stimuli directly leads to plasma membrane vesiculation (22).

B. Additional Responses Involved in MAC Removal and Cell Survival

A number of secondary signals are directly or indirectly triggered by calcium influx in response to sublytic MAC (see Fig. 1). Of these calcium-stimulated K+ efflux, activation of protein kinases (22), activation of phosphatidylcholine-specific phospholipase C with generation of diacylglycerol (25), and activation of adenylate cyclase resulting in elevation of cAMP (26) have been most clearly implicated in the recovery process.

Although calcium influx through MAC channels appears to be sufficient to trigger the vesiculation response in platelets, evidence has also been presented for MAC signaling through additional pathways. In human B lymphoblastoid cell lines an additional pathway mediated by direct interaction of terminal complement components with pertussis-sensitive GTP-binding proteins has been described (27,28). This pathway was associated with phosphatidylcholine and sphingomyelin hydrolysis by phospholipases, leading to the generation of diacylglycerol and ceramide. This phospholipid turnover did not require calcium influx since it was stimulated by C5b-7 complexes that do not cause an increase in intracellular calcium. Diacylglycerol and ceramide generation were enhanced in cells lacking glycosylphosphatidylinositol(GPI)-anchored proteins including CD59. Treatment of cells with pertussis toxin blocked diacylglycerol generation and prevented removal of C5b-7 and C5b-8 complexes from the cell surface (26,28). Diacylglycerol and calcium are potent activators of protein kinase C, and phosphorylation of the protein kinase C substrate MARCKS was observed in CD59-deficient cells treated with sublytic complement consistent with a synergistic activation by diacylglycerol and calcium (27).

In B cells pertussis-sensitive signaling triggered by C5b-7 and MAC has further been associated with the activation of Ras, Raf, and extracellular signal-regulated kinase 1 (ERK), which are key components of the mitogen-activated protein kinase (MAPK) cascade (29). The ras/ERK pathway links extracellular signals from growth factor receptors to induction of c-*fos* transcription (30). A parallel MAPK cascade termed JNK/SAPK

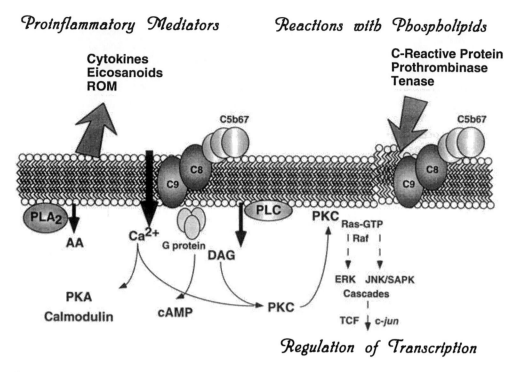

Figure 1 Overview of signaling pathways initiated in response to insertion of the MAC. Intracellular signaling mediators implicated in the cellular response to MAC are indicated in the lower part of the diagram. The upper part of the diagram indicates that cells undergoing sublytic attack by MAC release proinflammatory mediators of various types. In addition there are systemic responses to the presence of MAC in cell membranes. These reactions are initiated in response to altered membrane phospholipids surrounding MAC and in MAC-enriched vesicles shed by the cell.

(for Jun N-terminal/stress-activated protein kinases) is stimulated by ultraviolet (UV)-irradiation and other stress stimuli and results in the phosphorylation of c-Jun and transcriptional activation of the c-*jun* gene (30). Activation of this second pathway in B cells treated with C5b-7 and MAC was demonstrated by increased activity of JNK1 for phosphorylation of its substrate site in c-Jun (29). Although the consequences of activation MAPK pathways by terminal complement components in B cells are not clear, Shin et al. have also studied the effects of sublytic complement attack on myotubes (31) and oligodendrocytes (32). In both cases complement attack resulted in decreased mRNA for cell-specific products due to destabilization of the message. In oligodendrocytes the loss of myelin basic protein and proteolipid protein mRNA was accompanied by induction of c-*jun*, increased uptake of [³H]thymidine, and decreased apoptotic death (33). Cell-cycle induction correlated with activation of c-*jun* and c-*fos* mRNA and JNK activity and was inhibited by antisense c-*jun* oligonucleotides. Both the destabilization of cell-specific mRNA and the induction of DNA synthesis are consistent with a dedifferentiation of oligodendrocytes. However, the two processes are signaled differently, since the regulation of mRNA for myelin basic protein and proteolipid protein was inhibited by the protein kinase A inhibitor H1004 (32), but not by antisense c-*jun* oligonucleotides (33). Halperin et al. (34) reported mitogenic activity of C5b-9 for serum-deprived 3T3 cells both alone and in synergy with other growth factors.

C. Role of CD59

Morgan and colleagues have proposed that MAC may signal by cross-linking CD59 in cell membranes (20). CD59 is a GPI-anchored regulatory protein that binds to homologous C8 and limits C9 incorporation into MAC (5,6). Morgan et al. (35) have demonstrated that cross-linking CD59 with antibody induces tyrosine phosphorylation and release of calcium from internal stores. In addition CD59 is shed from the cell membrane with MAC during vesiculation (20). However, recovery from sublethal complement attack has been described across species and in cells lacking CD59. In addition much of the work on the pertussis-sensitive recovery pathway described above was done in cells lacking CD59 to increase the stability of MAC in the membranes (27,28). Although it is clear that CD59 and other GPI-anchored proteins can signal and that MAC interacts with CD59, direct evidence for MAC signaling through CD59 has not been presented thus far.

D. Protection from Subsequent Attack

The responses discussed above have been related to cell survival and/or MAC removal during sublytic complement attack. Reiter, Fishelson, and co-workers (36–38) have reported that cells surviving sublytic complement attack are protected from subsequent complement-mediated lysis for a period of 3–8 h. Like the initial resistance, induction of this protective response required the complete MAC including C9 and extracellular calcium. Protection was inhibited by actinomycin D and cycloheximide, indicating a requirement for RNA and protein synthesis (36). Cross-protection by MAC, perforin, and streptolysin O (all pore-forming proteins) with the same dependence on extracellular calcium, and RNA and protein synthesis has recently been described (38). This indicates a common resistance mechanism triggered by calcium influx by which cells respond to a loss of membrane integrity. In keeping with the requirement for protein synthesis, synthesis of several high-molecular-weight proteinswas observed in response to MAC in human leukemic cell lines (K562, HL-60, U937) (36). The identity and function of these proteins have not been reported. Sublytic complement attack did not alter expression of CD59 on K562 cells (39).

VI. CELL-SPECIFIC RESPONSES TO MAC

The response of nucleated cells to sublytic complement attack activates a number of pathways which may not be directly related to resistance to lysis. These responses, which are generally proinflammatory, include release of reactive oxygen metabolites, synthesis and release of eicosanoids, and release of cytokines (Fig. 1). The initiation of these responses generally requires calcium influx, stimulation of protein kinases, and activation of phospholipases and may occur through the same mechanisms that protect the cell from lysis. The resulting effects, however, may be cell-type-specific, and can involve secondary autocrine or paracrine responses to the initial release of lipid mediators or cytokines. In addition to the release of mediators, the presence of MAC in the membrane and/or the membrane response to MAC engages other pathways of inflammation and host defense including the coagulation system and acute-phase proteins. This section will consider the specific effects of the MAC on phagocytic cells, platelets, and endothelial cells. The net effect of these responses on the inflammatory state of the host will be considered where it has been studied. Other cell responses closely associated with pathogenic effects will be described in the following section.

A. Responses of Phagocytic Cells to MAC

Superoxide anion and its metabolites (hydrogen peroxide, hydroxyl radical, and hypochlorous acid) are produced by phagocytic cells during the respiratory burst through the action of NADPH oxidase. These reactive oxygen metabolites (ROM) are highly toxic and are used intracellularly to kill microorganisms in the phagolysosome. The release of ROM from phagocytic cells has been implicated in surrounding tissue damage associated with inflammatory responses. Both neutrophils (16,40) and macrophages (41) were found to release ROM in response to complement membrane attack. The responses required extracellular calcium and the complete MAC, suggesting an association with the same signaling pathway needed for MAC removal and cell recovery.

In addition to ROM, phagocytic cells release eicosanoids in response to sublytic MAC. Eicosanoids are diverse activators of pain and inflammation synthesized from arachidonic acid by the cyclooxygenase and lipoxygenase pathways. They are also significant mediators of acute and chronic inflammatory conditions. There are two pathways of eicosanoid production. Prostaglandins, prostacyclins, and thromboxanes are synthesized by the cyclooxygenase pathway, which is initiated by the release of its substrate arachidonic acid from membrane phospholipids by the activation of phospholipase A2. The lipoxygenase pathway, which produces leukotrienes, is activated by increased intracellular calcium. Production of arachidonic acid, prostaglandin E2, and thromboxane in macrophages (41,42) and leukotriene B4 in neutrophils undergoing complement attack (43) has been documented. In rat macrophages and human monocytes, stimulation of eicosanoid release was observed in response to either purified C5b-8 or C5b-9 (41,42). Phospholipid release including lysophosphatidylcholine was associated with this response, indicating phospholipase A2 activation. Phospholipase A2 activation can occur in response to calcium influx induced by ionophore treatment as well (44). In neutrophils C5b-8 was also sufficient to induce rapid release of leukotriene B4 (43), the predominant neutrophil arachidonic acid metabolite. The response was independent of cell lysis, and was rapid, similar to leukotriene B4 synthesis in response to calcium ionophore. A series of uptake and inhibition studies indicated that calcium influx through C5b-8 channels was the primary signal for this response.

B. Platelet Responses to MAC

The responses of platelets to the MAC have been studied extensively by Sims and Wiedmer (reviewed in 45,46). Studies of platelet responses to complement activation were stimulated by reports in the 1970s that C6-deficient rabbits demonstrated prolonged clotting times (47) and that the human platelet response to thrombin was potentiated by the addition of the terminal complement components (48). Generation and accumulation of MAC on platelet membranes can occur in whole blood or plasma independent of the intrinsic complement C3/C5 convertases due to plasmin, elastase, or other platelet-derived protease cleavage of C5. Since platelets lack C3 receptors CR1, CR2, and CR3 as well as receptors for C3a/C4a and C5a, the MAC may be the primary complement-generated signal for platelet responses. Platelets do express CD59 and actively remove MAC by shedding of vesicles from the surface (19,22).

Detailed studies of platelet responses to sublytic MAC ($<10^3$ MAC per platelet) have demonstrated a transient change in membrane potential with an elevation of intracellular calcium due to influx across the plasma membrane (49). These events initiate the recovery process with vesiculation and clearing of MAC from the membrane. In addition the rise in intracellular calcium stimulates phosphorylation of substrates of protein kinase C and other protein kinases (22). The platelet response to this process is secretion of mediators including ATP from platelet storage granules (50), translocation of P-selectin from α-granules to the membrane (51), and a shape change. Platelets stimulated by MAC also produce a small amount of thromboxane A2 (22). These events are dependent on extracellular calcium and can be inhibited by blocking protein kinase C. Despite the activation of granule secretion and shape change, complement attack does not result in platelet aggregation or integrin (GPIIb-IIIa, αIIbβ3) activation for fibrinogen binding (50).

An important feature of the platelet response to MAC is the expression of procoagulant properties due to exposure of membrane binding sites for the tenase (factors VIIIa and IXa) and prothrombinase (factors Va and Xa) enzyme complexes of the coagulation system. These binding sites are generated by transbilayer migration of membrane phospholipids, resulting in transfer of phosphatidylserine (PS) that is normally found in the inner leaflet to the outer leaflet. In platelets treated with MAC, exposure of PS and expression of procoagulant activity required C9 and calcium, the same stimuli that induce the microvesicular shedding of MAC (52). The process could be mimicked by calcium ionophore and differed from the platelet secretory response. The majority of the exposed PS was localized in the shed microparticles rather than the remnant platelet plasma membrane. In an effort to understand the process by which complement attack induces membrane phospholipid rearrangement, transbilayer migration was studied in asymmetrical lipid bilayers containing phosphatidylcholine and PS (53). In this model MAC was found to disorder membrane organization and promote transbilayer migration. The results differed from the observations using platelets, however, in that phospholipid movement in the liposome model was stimulated by C5b-8 without the addition of C9 and was not influenced by calcium. Platelets from patients with paroxysmal nocturnal hemoglobinuria that lack CD59 show enhanced sensitivity to MAC-induced responses (54), which may be related to increased thrombosis in this disorder (55).

C. Endothelial Cell Responses to MAC

The responses of endothelial cells to the MAC will only be mentioned here since they are discussed more fully in Chapter 15. Endothelial cells, like platelets, are induced by sublytic complement attack to secrete granule contents (von Willebrand factor) and translocate P-selectin from granules to the plasma membrane (56). The response requires C9 and extracellular calcium. The MAC also has a procoagulant effect through its action on endothelial cells. In addition to the shedding of MAC-enriched vesicles, exposing on the vesicles a catalytic surface for the prothrombinase complex (57), endothelial cells treated with sublytic concentrations of complement are induced to synthesize tissue factor (58). Tissue factor synthesis is a secondary response to cytokine (IL-1α) release by MAC-treated endothelium. In addition to IL-1, MAC-stimulated endothelial cells have been found to release basic fibroblast growth factor and platelet-derived growth factor (59).

D. Systemic Responses to MAC

The response of individual cells undergoing complement attack is primarily defensive and results in removal of MAC from the membrane. Cells undergoing complement attack also react by the production of reactive oxygen metabolites, and production of eicosanoids and cytokines mainly through signaling pathways set off by the defensive response. These released molecules can then set into play other inflammatory cascades. In addition to inflammatory pathways initiated by the reaction of the cell undergoing attack, the insertion of MAC into cell membranes can bring into play soluble systemic host defense mechanisms. These pathways may be important in several disease states, as discussed below. One example of this type of response is the creation of a procoagulant state by MAC insertion into platelet and endothelial membranes described above. The exposure of anionic phospholipids, particularly PS that are normally sequestered in the inner leaflet of the cell membrane, creates sites for the assembly of the tenase and prothrombinase enzyme complexes that contribute to fibrin clot formation (reviewed in 46). Shed vesicles of recovering platelets and endothelial cells represent the primary sites of these reactions by the coagulation system.

We recently described an additional recognition system for cells undergoing sublytic complement attack (60). In this study the acute-phase serum protein, C-reactive protein (CRP), was shown to bind to human B lymphoblastoid cells as well as mouse myeloma cells and liposomes in association with MAC. CRP (reviewed in 61) is an evolutionarily conserved protein with cyclic pentameric structure, and calcium-dependent ligand binding. In humans the serum levels of CRP are greatly increased (from less than 1 μg/ml to several hundred μg/ml) due to synthesis by hepatocytes in response to cytokines (primarily IL-6 and IL-1) released during inflammation, infection, or tissue injury. Complexes between CRP and polyvalent ligands activate the classical complement pathway and are taken up by receptors on phagocytic cells. In vivo CRP is localized to sites of inflammation. CRP has five binding sites specific for phospholipids and polysaccharides containing phosphocholine that also recognize peptide determinants on protein components of nuclear antigens. In the case of cells undergoing sublytic complement attack, CRP binding required at least C5b-9 and was enhanced following treatment with serum containing C9. It required calcium and was inhibited by phosphocholine. By two-color flow cytometry CRP staining correlated closely with staining for MAC. By two-color immunofluorescence CRP colocalized with MAC and appeared to be shed with MAC in vesiculating cells (Fig. 2). CRP also bound to liposomes treated with MAC, but only if phosphatidylcholine was present in the membrane. These results suggest that CRP recognizes the phosphocholine polar head groups on phosphatidylcholine (and possibly sphingomyelin) in the disordered lipid associated with MAC insertion (1). As there was no evidence for an effect of CRP on the resistance of cells to lysis, the role of CRP may be in the removal of damaged membranes through its opsonic activity.

VII. PATHOGENIC EFFECTS ATTRIBUTABLE TO MAC

The MAC has been identified in lesions in a number of diseases, notably rheumatoid synovium, glomerulonephritis lesions (62,63), demyelinating lesions, atherosclerotic

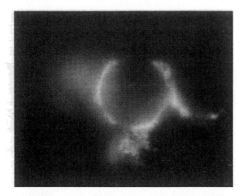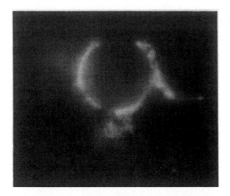

Figure 2 Photomicrographs of two-color analysis demonstrate CRP and MAC colocalization on the surface of Raji cells following complement activation. Cells were incubated with human serum for 2 h at 37°C, then washed and incubated with 200 μg/ml fluorescein-conjugated CRP for 30 min at 37°C, then washed and stained with antihuman C5b-9 monoclonal antibody (Quidel, San Diego, CA) and rhodamine-conjugated goat antimouse IgG. *Left,* FITC-CRP fluorescence; *right,* rhodamine fluorescence for MAC on the same cells.

plaque (64), and ischemic myocardium (65,66). A role for complement activation in several inflammatory diseases is supported by the protective effect of inhibition of complement activation by soluble CR1 and other complement inhibitors in several inflammatory diseases (67; reviewed in 68). However, these inhibitors generally act at the level of C3 or C5 convertases and thus inhibit the potent inflammatory mediator C5a as well as the MAC. This section will review several diseases in which there is experimental evidence for MAC effects on pathogenesis independent of other complement mediators.

A. Rheumatoid Arthritis

Joint inflammation in rheumatoid arthritis is an extremely complex process in which multiple pathways have been implicated. There is long-standing evidence for complement activation within the joint space that correlates with the severity of joint disease (69). Evidence has been presented that MAC attack and recovery is ongoing within the rheumatoid joint (70,71). In addition in vitro studies have documented the ability of isolated MAC to stimulate rheumatoid synovial cells to produce and release several inflammatory mediators. Morgan and colleagues (69,72,73) demonstrated ROM and eicosanoid release from human synoviocytes either in suspension or in culture. Prostaglandin E2 release was directly related to influx of extracellular calcium and stimulated by C5b-8 or C5b-9. MAC stimulation of rheumatoid synoviocytes in culture also induced IL-6, but not IL-1 or tumor necrosis factor, release over a 24 h period. A recent study (74) described the induction of collagenase mRNA synthesis in synovial fibroblasts in response to MAC binding to the membrane. There are, of course, many other stimuli for these mediators in the inflamed joint. Support for an *in vivo* role of the terminal complement components in inflammatory arthritis is provided by the ability of anti-C5 monoclonal antibody to prevent collagen-induced arthritis in mice (75). In addition to blocking the induction of disease in this model, anti-C5 therapy blocked progression and partially reversed joint destruction in established disease. The antibody used blocks complement activation at the level of C5 cleavage so that these experiments do not differentiate pathogenic effects due to C5a from those due to the MAC.

B. Renal Disease

The MAC has been detected by immunofluorescence in renal lesions including glomeruli and basement membranes of kidneys from patients with lupus nephritis (62), and mesangium of kidneys from patients with idiopathic IgA-glomerulonephritis and Henoch-Schönlein purpura nephritis (63). There is experimental evidence that the MAC is important in the development of proteinuria in the passive Heymann nephritis model of membranous nephropathy induced by antibody to glomerular epithelial cells (21) and the antithymocyte serum (ATS) model of mesangioproliferative glomerulonephritis induced by cross-reactivity of ATS with mesangial cells (76). In the most recent of these experimental studies C6-deficient rats demonstrated decreased mesangiolysis, platelet infiltration, mesangial cell proliferation, macrophage infiltration, collagen deposition, and proteinuria in response to ATS (76). These *in vivo* studies are supported by *in vitro* findings of phospholipase A2 activation and eicosanoid production by rat glomerular epithelial cells in response to sublytic MAC (77). Cultured human mesangial cells and glomerular epithelial cells have also been shown to produce type IV collagen and fibronectin in response to sublytic MAC (78). These matrix proteins are believed to contribute to glomerulosclerosis (79).

C. Demyelinating Diseases

There is compelling evidence for the involvement of the MAC in several demyelinating diseases. This area will only be briefly covered here, because it is dealt with more completely in Chapter 23. Several groups of investigators have demonstrated antibody-independent activation of the classical pathway by central nervous system myelin and oligodendrocytes (80–82). Immunofluorescence studies have demonstrated deposition of several complement components in myelin *in vivo* and *in vitro* with MAC antigens most closely associated with altered myelin lamellae (83,84). *In vitro* demyelination of explant cultures induced by antibody from patients with Guillain-Barré syndrome (85) or IgM monoclonal gammopathy and polyneuropathy (83) is dependent on MAC activation, and associated with the insertion of the MAC into myelin lamellae. Formation of C5b-7, C5b-8, or C5b-9 in peripheral myelin activates proteases in oligodendrocytes leading to the cleavage of myelin basic protein (86). Recent studies reported decreased mRNA for myelin basic protein and proteolipid (32) and induction of cell cycle (33) in oligodendrocytes in response to complement treatment that was dependent on activation of the terminal complement components.

VIII. CONCLUSIONS

As our understanding of complement regulation and activation in systems other than the antibody-sensitized sheep erythrocyte has progressed, it has become apparent that the MAC is not just a mechanism for cell lysis. As discussed above, nucleated cells in homologous serum have effective mechanisms to resist lysis by complement. The sequence of intracellular signals and events that contributes to this response seems to be primarily signaled by the influx of extracellular calcium through the lytic pore formed by C5b-8 and more effectively by C5b-9. A number of secondary responses are triggered by the same signals and these mainly result in the production of proinflammatory mediators specific to particular cell types. In addition, several systemic reactions are activated by the changes in membrane phospholipid organization that MAC insertion and removal cause. These include binding of C-reactive protein, and assembly of several enzyme complexes of the blood coagulation system. Lysis of cells by complement also induces responses in the host that result in removal of cells and cell debris. The availability of specific reagents for detection of the MAC has led to the realization that many pathogenic lesions contain MAC. Complement activation has also been implicated as a factor in many of these inflammatory diseases. Although in most cases the effects of MAC have not been fully characterized independent of other inflammatory mediators from the complement system, several examples are given for specific activities of the MAC in contributing to disease pathogenesis.

REFERENCES

1. Esser AF. Big MAC attack: complement proteins cause leaky patches. Immunol Today 1991; 12:316–318.
2. Bhakdi S, Tranum-Jensen J. Complement lysis: a hole is a hole. Immunol Today 1991; 12:318–320.
3. Esser AF. The membrane attack complex of complement. Assembly, structure and cytotoxic activity. Toxicology 1994; 87:229–247.
4. Bhakdi S, Tranum-Jensen J. Membrane damage by complement. Biochim Biophys Acta 1983; 737:343–372.
5. Meri S. Morgan BP, Davies A, Daniels RH, Olavesen MG, Waldmann H, Lachmann PJ. Human protectin (CD59), an 18,000–20,000 MW complement lysis restricting factor, inhibits C5b-8 catalysed insertion of C9 into lipid bilayers. Immunology 1990; 71:1–9.
6. Rollins SA, Sims PJ. The complement-inhibitory activity of CD59 resides in its capacity to block incorporation of C9 into membrane C5b-9. J Immunol 1990; 144:3478–3483.
7. MacKay SLD, Dankert JR. Bacterial killing and inhibition of inner membrane activity by C5b-9 complexes as a function of the sequential addition of C9 to C5b-8 sites. J Immunol 1990; 145:3367–3371.
8. Wright SD, Levine RP. How complement kills *E. coli*. I. Location of the lethal lesion. J Immunol 1981; 127:1146–1150.
9. Tomlinson S, Taylor PW, Luzio JP. Transfer of preformed terminal C5b-9 complement complexes into the outer membrane of viable gram-negative bacteria: effect on viability and integrity. Biochemistry 1990; 29:1852–1869.
10. Green H, Barrow P, Goldberg B. Effect of antibody and complement on permeability control in ascites tumor cells and erythrocytes. J Exp Med 1959; 110:699–713.
11. Green H, Goldberg B. The action of antibody and complement on mammalian cells. Ann NY Acad Sci 1960; 87:352–361.
12. Ohanian SH, Schlager SI. Humoral immune killing of nucleated cells: mechanisms of complement-mediated attack and target cell defense. CRC Crit Rev Immunol 1981; 1:165–209.
13. Koski CL, Ramm LE, Hammer CH, Mayer MM, Shin ML. Cytolysis of nucleated cells by complement: cell death displays multi-hit characteristics. Proc Natl Acad Sci USA 1983; 80:3816–3820.
14. Carney DF, Koski CL, Shin ML. Elimination of terminal complement intermediates from the plasma membrane of nucleated cells: the rate of disappearance differs for cells carrying C5b-7 or C5b-8 or a mixture of C5b-8 with a limited number of C5b-9. J Immunol 1985; 134:1804–1809.

15. Ramm LE, Whitlow MB, Koski CL, Shin ML, Mayer MM. Elimination of complement channels from the plasma membranes of U937, a nucleated mammalian cell line: temperature dependence of the elimination rate. J Immunol 1983; 131:1411–1415.

16. Campbell AK, Morgan BP. Monoclonal antibodies demonstrate protection of polymorphonuclear leukocytes against complement attack. Nature 1985; 317:164–166.

17. Morgan BP, Imagawa DK, Dankert JR, Ramm LE. Complement lysis of U937, a nucleated mammalian cell line in the absence of C9: effect of C9 on C5b-8 mediated cell lysis. J Immunol 1986; 136:3402–3406.

18. Morgan BP, Dankert JR, Esser AF. Recovery of human neutrophils from complement attack: removal of the membrane attack complex by endocytosis and exocytosis. J Immunol 1987; 138:246–253.

19. Stein JM, Luzio JP. Ectocytosis caused by sublytic autologous complement attack on human neutrophils. Biochem J 1991; 274:381–386.

20. Morgan BP. Effects of the membrane attack complex of complement on nucleated cells. Curr Top Microbiol Immunol 1992; 178:115–140.

21. Kerjaschki D, Schulze M, Binder S, Kain R, Ojha PP, Susani M, Horvat R, Baker PJ, Couser WG. Transcellular transport and membrane insertion of the C5b-9 membrane attack complex of complement by glomerular epithelial cells in experimental membranous nephropathy. J Immunol 1989; 143:546–552.

22. Wiedmer T, Sims PJ. Participation of protein kinases in complement C5b-9-induced shedding of platelet plasma membrane vesicles. Blood 1991; 78:2880–2886.

23. Carney DF, Hammer CH, Shin ML. Elimination of terminal complement complexes in the plasma membrane of nucleated cells: influence of extracellular Ca^{2+} and association with cellular Ca^{2+}. J Immunol 1986; 137:263–270.

24. Morgan BP, Campbell AK. The recovery of human polymorphonuclear leucocytes from sublytic complement attack is mediated by changes in intracellular free calcium. Biochem J 1985; 231:205–208.

25. Cybulsky AV, Cyr M-D. Phosphatidylcholine-directed phospholipase C: activation by complement C5b-9. Am J Physiol 1993; 265:F551–F560.

26. Carney DF, Lang TJ, Shin ML. Multiple signal messengers generated by terminal complement complexes and their role in terminal complement complex elimination. J Immunol 1990; 145:623–629.

27. Niculescu F, Rus H, Shin S, Lang T, Shin ML. Generation of diacylglyceride and ceramide during homologous complement activation. J Immunol 1993; 150:214–224.

28. Niculescu F, Rus H, Shin ML. Receptor-independent activation of guanine nucleotide-binding regulatory proteins by terminal complement complexes. J Biol Chem 1994; 269:4417–4423.

29. Niculescu F, Rus HG, Shin ML. Assembly of terminal complement complexes induces activation of both ERK1 and JNK1 in B lymphocytes. Mol Immunol 1996; 33:82 (abstract).

30. Cano E, Mahadevan LC. Parallel signal processing among mammalian MAPKs. Trends Biochem Sci 1995; 20:117–122.

31. Badea T, Lang T, Wade R, Shin ML. Regulation of muscle specific gene expression in myotubes by terminal complement complexes (TCC). Mol Immunol 1996; 33:86 (abstract).

32. Shirazi Y, Rus HG, Macklin WB, Shin ML. Enhanced degradation of messenger RNA encoding myelin proteins by terminal complement complexes in oligodendrocytes. J Immunol 1993; 150:4581–4590.

33. Rus HG, Niculescu F, Shin ML. Sublytic complement attack induces cell cycle in oligodendrocytes. S phase induction is dependent on c-*jun* activation. J Immunol 1996; 156:4892–4900.

34. Halperin JA, Taratuska A, Nicholson-Weller A. Terminal complement complex C5b-9 stimulates mitogenesis in 3T3 cells. J Clin Invest 1993; 91:1974–1978.

35. Morgan BP, van den Berg CW, Davies EV, Hallett MB, Horesji V. Cross-linking of CD59 and of other glycosylphosphatidylinositol-anchored molecules on neutrophils triggers cell activation via tyrosine kinase. Eur J Immunol 1993; 23:2841–2850.

36. Reiter Y, Fishelson Z. Complement membrane attack complexes induce in human leukemic cells rapid expression of large proteins (L-CIP). Mol Immunol 1992; 29:771–781.
37. Reiter Y, Ciobotariu A, Fishelson Z. Sublytic complement attack protects tumor cells from lytic doses of antibody and complement. Eur J Immunol 1992; 22:1207–1213.
38. Reiter Y, Ciobotariu A, Jones J, Morgan BP, Fishelson Z. Complement membrane attack complex, perforin, and bacterial exotoxins induce in K562 cells calcium-dependent cross-protection from lysis. J Immunol 1995; 155:2203–2210.
39. Marchbank KJ, Morgan BP, van den Berg CW. Regulation of CD59 expression of K562 cells: Effects of phorbol myriscate acetate, cross-linking antibody and non-lethal complement attack. Immunology 1995; 85:146–152.
40. Roberts PA, Morgan BP, Campbell AK. 2-chloroadenosine inhibits complement-induced reactive oxygen metabolite production and recovery of human polymorphonuclear leucocytes attacked by complement. Biochim Biophys Res Commun 1985; 126:692–697.
41. Hänsch GM, Seitz M, Betz M. Effect of the late complement components C5b-9 on human monocytes: release of prostanoids, oxygen radicals and of a factor inducing cell proliferation. Int Arch Allergy Appl Immunol 1987; 82:317–320.
42. Hänsch GM, Seitz M, Martinotti G, Betz M, Rauterberg EW, Gemsa D. Macrophages release arachidonic acid, prostaglandin E2, and thromboxane in response to late complement components. J Immunol 1984; 133:2145–2150.
43. Seeger W, Suttorp N, Hellwig A, Bhakdi S. Noncytolytic terminal complement complexes may serve as calcium gates to elicit leukotriene B4 generation in human polymorphonuclear leukocytes. J Immunol 1986; 137:1286–1293.
44. Takenawa T, Homma Y, Nagai Y. Role of calcium in phosphatidylinositol response and arachidonic acid release of formylated tripeptide- or calcium ionophore A23187 stimulated guinea pig neutrophils. J Immunol 1983; 130:2849–2855.
45. Sims PJ, Wiedmer T. The response of human platelets to activated components of the complement system. Immunol Today 1991; 12:338–342.
46. Sims PJ, Wiedmer T. Induction of cellular procoagulant activity by the membrane attack complex of complement. Semin Cell Biol 1995; 6:275–282.
47. Zimmerman TS, Arroyave CM, Müller-Eberhard HJ. A blood coagulation abnormality in rabbits deficient in the sixth component of complement (C6) and its correction by purified C6. J Exp Med 1971; 134:1591–1600.
48. Polley MJ, Nachman RL. The human complement system in thrombin-mediated platelet function. J Exp Med 1978; 147:1713–1726.
49. Sims PJ, Wiedmer T. Repolarization of the membrane potential of blood platelets after complement damage: evidence for a Ca^{++}-dependent exocytotic elimination of C5b-9 pores. Blood 1986; 68:556–561.
50. Ando B, Wiedmer T, Sims PJ. The secretory release reaction initiated by complement proteins C5b-9 occurs without platelet aggregation through glycoprotein IIb-IIIa. Blood 1989; 73:462–467.
51. Wiedmer T, Ando B, Sims PJ. Complement C5b-9-stimulated platelet secretion is associated with a Ca^{2+}-initiated activation of cellular protein kinases. J Biol Chem 1987; 262:13674–13681.
52. Chang C-P, Zhao J, Wiedmer T, Sims PJ. Contribution of platelet microparticle formation and granule secretion to the transmembrane migration of phosphatidylserine. J Biol Chem 1993; 268:7171–7178.
53. van der Meer W, Fugate RD, Sims PJ. Complement proteins C5b-9 induce transbilayer migration of membrane phospholipids. Biophys J 1989; 56:935–946.
54. Wiedmer T, Hall SE, Ortel TL, Kane WH, Rosse WF, Sims PJ. Complement-induced vesiculation and exposure of membrane prothrombinase sites in platelets of paroxysmal nocturnal hemoglobinuria. Blood 1993; 82:1192–1196.

55. Rosse WF. Paroxysmal nocturnal hemoglobinuria. Curr Top Microbiol Immunol 1992; 178:163–173.

56. Hattori R, Hamilton KK, McEver RP, Sims PJ. Complement proteins C5b-9 induce secretion of high molecular weight multimers of endothelial von Willebrand factor and translocation of granule membrane protein GMP-140 to the cell surface. J Biol Chem 1989; 264:9053–9060.

57. Hamilton KK, Hattori R, Esmon CT, Sims PJ. Complement proteins C5b-9 induce vesiculation of the endothelial plasma membrane and expose catalytic surface for assembly of the prothrombinase enzyme complex. J Biol Chem 1990; 265:3809–3814.

58. Saadi S, Holzknecht RA, Patte CP, Stern DM, Platt JL. Complement-mediated regulation of tissue factor activity in endothelium. J Exp Med 1995; 182:1807–1814.

59. Benzaquen LR, Nicholson-Weller A, Halperin JA. Terminal complement proteins C5b-9 release basic fibroblast growth factor and platelet-derived growth factor from endothelial cells. J Exp Med 1994; 179:985–992.

60. Li Y-P, Mold C, Du Clos TW. Sublytic complement attack exposes C-reactive protein binding sites on cell membranes. J Immunol 1994; 152:2995–3005.

61. Kilpatrick JM, Volanakis JE. Molecular genetics, structure, and function of C-reactive protein. Immunol Res 1991; 10:43–53.

62. Biesecker G, Katx S, Koffler D. Renal localization of the membrane attack complex in systemic lupus erythematosus nephritis. J Exp Med 1981; 154:1779–1794.

63. Rauterberg EW, Lieberknecht H-M, Winge A-M, Ritz E. Complement membrane attack (MAC) in idiopathic IgA-glomerulonephritis. Kidney Interntl 1987; 31:820–829.

64. Rus HG, Niculescu F, Constantinescu E, Cristea A, Vlaicu R. Immunoelectron-microscopic localization of the terminal C5b-9 complement complex in human atherosclerotic fibrous plaque. Atherosclerosis 1986; 61:35–42.

65. McManus LM, Kolb WP, Crawford MH, O'Rourke RA, Grover FL, Pinckard RN. Complement localization in ischemic baboon myocardium. Lab Invest 1983; 48:436–437.

66. Mathey D, Schofer J, Schäfer HJ, Hamdock T, Joachim HC, Ritgen A, Hugo F, Bhakdi S. Early accumulation of the terminal complement-complex in the ischaemic myocardium after reperfusion. Eur Heart J 1994; 15:418–423.

67. Mulligan MS, Yeh CG, Rudolph AR, Ward PA. Protective effects of soluble CR1 in complement- and neutrophil-mediated tissue injury. J Immunol 1992; 148:1479–1485.

68. Moore FD Jr. Therapeutic regulation of the complement system in acute injury states. Adv Immunol 1994; 56:267–299.

69. Brodeur JP, Ruddy S, Schwartz LB, Moxley G. Synovial fluid levels of complement SC5b-9 and fragment Bb are elevated in patients with rheumatoid arthritis. Arthritis Rheum 1991; 34:1531–1537.

70. Morgan BP, Daniels RH, Watts MH, Williams BD. In vivo and in vitro evidence of cell recovery from complement attack in rheumatoid synovium. Clin Exp Immunol 1988; 73:467–472.

71. Sanders ME, Kopicky JA, Wigley FM, Shin ML, Frank MM, Joiner KA. Membrane attack complex of complement in rheumatoid synovial tissue demonstrated by immunofluorescent microscopy. J Rheum 1986; 13:1028–1034.

72. Daniels RH, Houston WAJ, Petersen MM, Williams JD, Williams BD, Morgan BP. Stimulation of human rheumatoid synovial cells by non-lethal complement membrane attack. Immunol 1990; 69:237–242.

73. Daniels RH, Williams BD, Morgan BP. Human rheumatoid synovial cell stimulation by the membrane attack complex and other pore-forming toxins in vitro: the role of calcium in cell activation. Immunol 1990; 71:312–316.

74. Jahn B, von Kempis J, Krämer K-L, Filsinger S. Hänsch GM. Interaction of the terminal complement components C5b-9 with synovial fibroblasts: binding to the membrane surface leads to increased levels in collagenase-specific mRNA. Immunology 1993; 78:329–334.

75. Wang Y, Rollins SA, Madri JA, Matis LA. Anti-C5 monoclonal antibody therapy prevents collagen-induced arthritis and ameliorates established disease. Proc Natl Acad Sci USA 1995; 92:8955–8959.

76. Brandt J, Pippin J, Schulze M, Hänsch GM, Alpers CE, Johnson RJ, Gordon K, Couser WG. Role of the complement membrane attack complex (C5b-9) in mediating experimental mesangioproliferative glomerulonephritis. Kidney Int 1996; 49:335–343.

77. Cybulsky AV, Monge JC, Papillon J, McTavish AJ. Complement C5b-9 activates cytosolic phospholipase AZ in glomerular epithelial cells. Am J Physiol 1995; 269:F739–F749.

78. Wagner C, Braunger M, Beer M, Rother K, Hänsch GM. Induction of matrix protein synthesis in human glomerular mesangial cells by the terminal complement complex. Exp Nephrol 1994; 2:51–56.

79. Peten EP, Striker LJ, Carome MA, Elliot SJ, Yang CW, Striker GE. The contribution of increased collagen synthesis to human glomerulosclerosis: a quantitative analysis of aIV collagen mRNA by competitive polymerase chain reaction. J Exp Med 1992; 176:1571–1576.

80. Vanguri P, SIlverman BA, Koski CL, Shin ML. Complement activation by isolated myelin: activation of the classical pathway in the absence of myelin-specific antibodies. Proc Nat Acad Sci USA 1982; 79:3290–3294.

81. Cyong JD, Witkins SS>, Rieger B, Barabrese E, Day NK. Antibody-independent complement activation by myelin via the classical pathway. J Exp Med 1982; 155:587–598.

82. Scolding NJ, Morgan BP, Houston A, Campbell AK, Linington C, Compston DAS. Reversible injury of cultured rat oligodendrocytes by complement. J Neurol Sci 1989; 89:289–300.

83. Monaco S, Bonetti B, Ferrari S, Moretto G, Nardelli E, Tedesco F, Mollnes TE, Nobile-Orazio E, Manfredini E, Bonazzi L, Rizzuto N. Complement-mediated demyelination in patients with IgM monoclonal gammopathy and polyneuropathy. N Engl J Med 1990; 322:649–652.

84. Bruck W, Brück Y, Diederich U, Piddlesden SJ. The membrane attack complex of complement mediates peripheral nervous system demyelination in vitro. Acta Neuropathol 1995; 90:601–607.

85. Sawant-Mane S, Clark MB, Koski CL. In vitro demyelination by serum antibody from patients with Guillain-Barré syndrome requires terminal complement complexes. Ann Neurol 1991; 29:397–404.

86. Vanguri P, Shin ML. Hydrolysis of myelin basic protein in human myelin by terminal complement complexes. J Biol Chem 1988; 263:7228–7234.

14

Regulation by Complement of Acquired Immunity

MICHAEL C. CARROLL
Harvard Medical School, Boston, Massachusetts

DOUGLAS T. FEARON
University of Cambridge, Cambridge, England

I. ENHANCEMENT BY COMPLEMENT OF ACQUIRED IMMUNITY

The proteins of the complement system contain no domains of the immunoglobulin superfamily, and the genes encoding these proteins do not undergo rearrangement, indicating that this innate immune system is distinct from the acquired or adaptive immune system. However, the observation approximately 20 years ago that mice transiently depleted of C3 by treatment with cobra venom factor were impaired in their antibody response to a T-dependent (TD) antigen indicated that complement can influence acquired immunity (1). Subsequent studies of humans (2) and inbred strains of guinea pigs deficient in C2, C3, or C4 (3) provided opportunities not only to confirm these earlier studies but also to demonstrate that the enhancing effect of complement requires an intact classical pathway and promotes the generation of isotypically switched memory B cells, responses that are T-cell-dependent. The role of complement was not obligate, since a 50-fold increase in the dosage of antigen led to near-normal responses in the complement-deficient guinea pigs. These findings indicated that complement, by an unknown cellular mechanism, could facilitate the immune response mediated by the interaction of B and T lymphocytes.

The recent availability of strains of mice bearing targeted disruption of genes encoding the complement components C3 and C4 has allowed for confirmation of the role of the classical pathway in acquired immunity. It has also contributed to the molecular dissection of the mechanism for the enhancing effect in vivo by showing that a gene dosage effect is observed (4,5). Thus, mice heterozygous for C3 or C4 have an intermediate response to soluble antigen when compared to homozygous littermates. Given the relatively high concentration of these proteins in serum, this finding suggests that local synthesis rather than hepatic synthesis is likely to be important. The relevant site may be within the lymphoid compartment because $C3-/-$ mice engrafted with bone marrow from $C3+/+$, major histocompatibility complex (MHC)-matched littermates make an apparently normal immune response to TD antigens, despite the absence of detectable C3 in the serum. Thus, in this model, local synthesis of C3 by bone marrow-derived cells is sufficient for the enhancing effect of complement on the humoral response.

In considering possible mechanisms for the activation of the classical pathway of complement prior to an acquired immune response, preexisiting, cross-reactive, natural antibodies of the IgM isotype may be important (Fig. 1). The capacity of IgM to mediate enhancement of an acquired immune response is dependent both on CR2 (6) and on the ability of IgM to activate C1 (7). Even in individuals who have limited amounts of antigen-specific IgM, it is possible that IgM synthesized within 12 h following immunization, which may not be complement-dependent, can mediate the subsequent, complement-dependent phase of the antibody response. The classical pathway also may be activated by the mannan-binding protein (MBP) system independently of IgM (Fig. 1). Finally, for some antigens, activation of the alternative pathway may be sufficient.

The essential reaction of the complement system that promotes recognition of potential antigen is the covalent attachment of C3b. The bound C3b is capable of continuing the activation of C3, leading to the attachment of additional molecules via the alternative pathway amplification loop. This process will cease when sufficient C3b has been taken up by antigen to mediate binding of the complex by CR1, which can suppress further complement activation through its inhibitory functions. CR1 resides on almost all leukocyte cell types and, in humans, is also present on erythrocytes and glomerular podocytes. CR1 enables erythrocytes to bind C3b-coated antigen–antibody complexes in peripheral blood, and carry them to the liver where the factor I-cofactor function of CR1 causes cleavage of C3b to iC3b and C3dg. This process, which may have evolved to promote the clearance of bacterial toxins, may also limit immune responses to antigen–antibody complexes containing self antigen. The function of CR1 on leukocytes may be to capture C3b-bearing complexes and to promote their transfer, on the same cell, to CR3 and CR2 following cleavage of the C3b to iC3b and C3dg, respectively. CR3 resides mainly on myelomonocytic cells where it mediates adhesive and endocytic functions, whereas CR2 is present on mature B lymphocytes, follicular dendritic cells, and a few T lymphocytes.

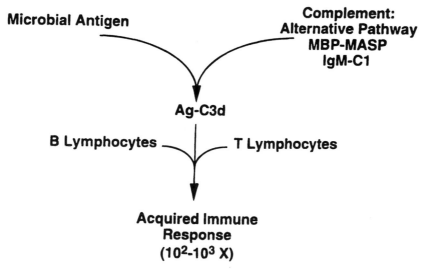

Figure 1   Attachment of C3d to microbial antigens when complement is activated by the classic or alternative pathways in the nonimmune host amplifies the response of B and T cells to that antigen.

Evidence that attachment of C3d to potential antigen is the essential outcome of classical pathway activation comes from experiments using a recombinant antigen, hen egg lysozyme (HEL), coupled to three tandemly repeated copies of C3d (although the physiological fragment generated by cleavage of iC3b by factor I is C3dg, the susceptibility of this fragment to proteolysis to C3d prompted the experimental use of the latter component). Compared to HEL alone, HEL-C3d$_3$ was 10,000-fold more immunogenic in eliciting a T-dependent B-cell response in mice (8). This effect may have been greater than had been observed in earlier studies of complement because every molecule of antigen had been modified, whereas with in vivo activation of complement there is less efficient attachment of C3b to antigen.

The enhancing effect of C3 in this and earlier experiments was shown to be mediated by CR2, or the CR2 site on CR1. The *Cr2* locus is expressed primarily on B cells and follicular dendritic cells (FDCs) in mice (9–11). Pretreatment of mice with a monoclonal antibody that blocks the C3d-binding site on CR1 and CR2 resulted in an impaired immune response to TD antigens similar to that described in mice transiently depleted of C3 (12). Moreover, pretreatment of mice with a soluble form of CR2 receptor, an IgG-CR2 fusion protein, also suppressed the IgG1-4 response to TD antigens (13). Most definitive has been the recent finding that mice bearing a targeted disruption of the *Cr2* locus (*Cr2−/−*) have impaired humoral responses to TD antigens (14,15). Consistent with the requirement for complement in the generation of memory B cells was the observation that germinal center formation was impaired in *CR2−/−* mice. A similar abnormality is observed in C3- and C4-deficient mice (4). Finally, coupling the *Cr2−/−* system with blastocyst complementation of *Rag−/−* mice allowed the demonstration that CR2 on lymphocytes rather than on FDCs was required for this response (16). This finding does not exclude an important role for CR2 on FDCs in the maintenance of memory, as initially suggested by the studies of Klaus and Humphrey (17). Taken together, these experiments indicate that attachment of C3b to antigen and conversion to C3dg (C3d), followed by binding of that C3d to CR2, are critical events in complement enhancement of the acquired immune response.

II. BIOCHEMISTRY OF COMPLEMENT-DEPENDENT ENHANCEMENT OF THE IMMUNE RESPONSE

Most, if not all, mature primary B cells express CR2, whereas only a few T cells have small numbers of this receptor. Therefore, CR2 on B cells is likely to be responsible for mediating the effects of complement on the acquired immune response. During development, CR2 appears at the mature B cell stage, and becomes absent during terminal differentiation to the plasma cell. On human B cells, CR2 resides in the form of two complexes: a CR1–CR2 complex (18) and CR2–CD19–CD81–Leu-13 complex (19) (Fig. 2). On murine B cells, CR2 and CR1 represent alternatively spliced transcripts of the same gene (9–11) so that the homologue of the human CR1-CR2 complex is murine CR1, which contains the binding sites of both types of receptors. A distinct function for the CR1-CR2 complex, or for murine CR1, has not been proven although, as suggested above, it may be that the C3b-binding site of CR1 captures antigens that bear this ligand and promote factor I-mediated processing to C3dg. The close association with CR2 either within the same molecule, as in the mouse, or in the same complex, as in humans, enables retention of the C3dg-coated complex for subsequent signaling purposes.

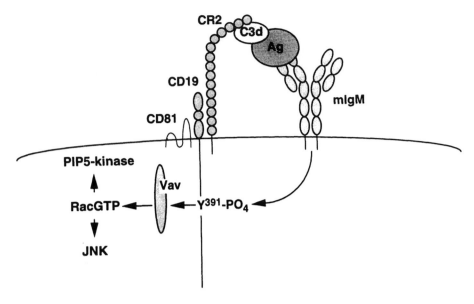

Figure 2 Antigen-bound C3d coligates the CR2–CD19–CD81 and mIgM complexes and amplifies signaling by inducing phosphorylation of CD19. Tyrosine-391 of CD19 binds Vav, a guanine nucleotide exchange factor for the Rac family of small GTPases. RAC-GTP activates PIP5-kinase to induce synthesis of PIP2, and JNK, a MAP kinase that regulates the transcriptional activity of c-jun.

In the complex containing CD19, CD81, and Leu-13, the ratio of CR2 and CD19 is 1:1, and CD81 is always present. Leu-13 is variably present and relatively little is known of this protein. CD81, a member of the tetraspan family, is likely to have important cellular functions related to adhesion and possibly intracellular trafficking, but is expressed by all hematopoietic cell types and forms complexes with other membrane proteins; it will not be considered further in this review. CD19 is expressed only on B cells (20), and is the earliest lineage-specific membrane protein to be expressed during development. It is a member of the Ig superfamily, having two Ig-like domains, and, in contrast to the short, 34 amino acid intracellular domain of CR2, has a cytoplasmic tail of 243 amino acids. Contained within this domain are nine tyrosines, some of which become phosphorylated when mIg is ligated. Phosphorylation of tyrosine-391 causes the binding of Vav (21; unpublished data), and phosphorylation of tyrosines 482 and 513 mediates binding of phosphatidylinositol 3-kinase (PI3-kinase) (22). In a model in vitro system, coligating the CD19-CR2 complex to mIg, as would occur with complexes containing C3d and antigen for which the B cell was specific, lowers the threshold by two orders of magnitude for the number of antigen receptors that must be ligated to induce cellular proliferation. The basis for this effect of CD19 is the enhanced activation of intracellular pathways of signal transduction.

The interaction of CD19 with Vav alters phosphoinositide metabolism and activation of a MAP kinase (Fig. 2). Vav has a dbl homology (DH) domain that may mediate the exchange of GTP for GDP on the members of the Rho GTPases (23). The single SH2 domain of Vav mediates binding to phosphorylated Y391 of CD19, targeting the exchange function of Vav to the plasma membrane where the activated GTPases function. Two enzymes have been shown to be regulated by the interaction of Vav with tyrosine phosphorylated CD19 and recruitment of Rac: phosphatidylinositol 4-phosphate 5-kinase (PIP5-kinase) and JNK. PIP5-kinase synthesizes phosphatidylinositol 4,5-bisphosphate (PIP2), the substrate for phospholipase C. Since PIP2 is rapidly depleted by activated PLC-γ, its resynthesis becomes a rate-limiting step in the generation of IP3 and the maintenance of elevated levels of free intracellular Ca^{2+}. Among the effects of Ca^{2+} is the activation of calcineurin, which mediates the dephosphorylation and translocation to the nucleus of NF-AT, a transcription factor essential in T cells for the expression of IL-2 (24,25). Activated JNK phosphorylates the transcription factor, c-jun (26), which forms part of the AP-1 transcriptional complex that, in the T cell, interacts with NF-AT. Thus, the CD19-Vav interaction may regulate the expression of as yet unidentified genes in the B cell that are important for responses to T-cell-dependent antigens.

A second general mechanism by which C3 attachment to antigen may promote the response to T-dependent antigens is to enhance antigen uptake and processing by B cells and other antigen-presenting cells (6,27,28). Covalent attachment of C3b to antigen alters proteolytic cleavage in a manner that increases the efficiency of processing and interaction with MHC class II. The importance of these effects is likely to relate to the route of immunization, since augmented priming of T cells by complement has not yet been demonstrated in vivo.

III. ROLES OF COMPLEMENT-DEPENDENT IMMUNE RESPONSES IN HEALTH AND DISEASE

The development of molecular cloning has transformed strategies for vaccination because there is now the potential for selecting as targets antigens that are nontoxic and induce protective immunity. A difficulty with this strategy, however, has been that removing these antigens from their usual microbiological context reduces immunogenicity. Presumably this form of antigen does not activate the several innate immune systems that would have been stimulated by intact microorganisms. Therefore, the finding that C3d can serve as a molecular adjuvant when attached to antigen may provide an approach to enhancing the immunogenicity to recombinant antigens.

Individuals who are deficient in C1, C4, or C2 have an increased occurrence of a disease resembling, or identical to, systemic erythematosus (SLE). These persons have an impaired clearance of self antigen–antibody complexes from their blood, which may be associated with increased deposition of complexes within tissues. Such complexes might have a tendency to accumulate and aggregate, culminating in activation of the alternative pathway. This process leads to the attachment of many copies of C3b, and solubilization of the complexes. The solubilized complexes containing self antigen to which C3b, iC3b, and C3dg are attached will go to local lymph nodes. If sufficient C3dg has been bound to self antigen, it is possible that the signaling threshold in tolerized B and T cells may be overcome, causing an autoimmune response. This proposed sequence of events may now be tested for its validity.

Another potential role for complement in autoimmunity is its participation in the regulation of autoreactive B cells. Maintenance of peripheral B cell tolerance relies on multiple checkpoints that naive B cells must pass during activation and expansion (29,30). As with B-cell activation, the threshold of signaling via the B cell receptor is a critical factor in tolerance induction. Thus, it is proposed that CR2 also acts as a coreceptor in recognition of self antigen by autoreactive B cells. This hypothesis is supported by the recent finding that breeding the *Cr2null* allele onto the lupus prone *lpr/lpr* strain of mouse results in a more severe phenotype (S. Goerg and L. Chu, personal communication). Thus, *Cr2null/lpr/lpr* mice are characterized by increased levels of autoantibodies, increased lymphadenopathy and splenomegaly, and reduced survival compared to *CR2+/lpr/lpr* controls. While the mechanism for this increased severity can only be speculated at this point, it is becoming increasingly apparent that complement has a role in the induction phase of autoimmunity.

REFERENCES

1. Pepys MB. Role of complement in induction of the allergic response. Nature 1972; 237:157.
2. Jackson CG, Ochs HD, Wedgewood RJ. Immune response of a patient with deficiency of the fourth component of complement and systemic lupus erythematosus. N Engl J Med 1979; 300:1124–1129.
3. Bitter-Suermann D, Burger R. C3 deficiencies. Curr Top Microbiol Immunol 1990; 153:223–33.
4. Fischer M, Ma M, Goerg S, Zhou X, Xia J, Finco O, Han S, Kelsoe G, Howard R, Rothstein T, Kremmer E, Rosen F, Carroll, M. Regulation of the B cell response to T-dependent antigens by classical pathway complement. J Immunol 1996; 157:549–556.
5. Wessels MR, Butko P, Ma M, Warren HB, Lage A Carroll MC. Studies of group B steptococcal infection in mice deficient in complement C3 or C4 demonstrate an essential role for complement in both innate and acquired immunity. Proc Natl Acad Sci USA 1995; 92:11490–11494.
6. Thornton BP, Vetvicka V and Ross GD. Natural antibody and complement-mediated antigen processing and presentation by B lymphocytes. J Immunol 1994; 152:1727–1737.
7. Heyman B, Pilstrom L, Shulman, MJ. Complement activation is required for IgM-mediated enhancement of the antibody response. J Exp Med 1988; 167:1999–2004.
8. Dempsey PW, Allison ME, Akkaraju S, Goodnow CC, Fearon, DT. C3d of complement as a molecular adjuvant: bridging innate and acquired immunity. Science 1996; 271:348–350.
9. Molina H, Kinoshita T, Inoue K, Carel J-C, Holers VM. A molecular and immunochemical characterization of mouse CR2. J Immunol 1990; 145:2974–2983.
10. Kurtz CB, O'Toole E, Christensen SM, Weis JH. The murine complement receptor gene family. IV. Alternative splicing of Cr2 gene transcripts predicts two distinct gene products that share homologous domains with both human CR2 and CR1. J Immunol 1990; 144:3581–3591.
11. Kinoshita T, Thyphronitis G, Tsokos CG, Finkelman FD, Hong K, Sakai H, Inoue K. Characterization of murine complement receptor type 2 and its immunological cross-reactivity with type 1 receptor. Int Immunol 1990; 2:651–59.
12. Heyman B, Wiersma EJ, Kinoshita T. In vivo inhibition of the antibody response by a complement receptor-specific monoclonal antibody. J Exp Med 1990; 172:665–668.
13. Hebell T, Ahearn JM, Fearon DT. Suppression of the immune response by a soluble complement receptor of B lymphocytes. Science 1991; 254:102–105.
14. Ahearn J, Fischer M, Croix D, Goerg S, Ma M, Xia J, Zhou X, Howard R, Rothstein T, Carroll M. Disruption of the Cr2 locus results in a reduction in B-1a cells and in an impaired B cell response to T dependent antigen. Immunity 1996; 4:251–262.
15. Molina H, Holers V, Li B, Fung Y, Mariathasan S, Goellner J, Strauss-Schoenberger J, Karr R, Chaplin D. Markedly impaired humoral immune response in mice deficient in complement receptors 1 and 2. Proc Natl Acad Sci USA 1996; 93:3357–3361.
16. Croix D, Ahearn J, Rosengard A, Han S, Kelsoe G, Ma M, Carroll M. Antibody response to a T-dependent antigen requires B cell expression of complement receptors. J Exp Med 1996; 183:1857–1864.

17. Klaus GG, Humphrey JH, Kunkl A, Dongworth DW. The follicular dendritic cell: its role in antigen presentation in the generation of immunological memory. Immunol Rev 1980; 53:3–28.

18. Tuveson DA, Ahearn JM, Matsumoto AK, Fearon DT. Molecular interactions of complement receptors on B lymphocytes: a CR1/CR2 complex distinct from the CR2/CD19 complex. J Exp Med 1991; 173:1083–1089.

19. Matsumoto AK, Martin DR, Carter RH, Klickstein LB, Ahearn JM, Fearon DT. Functional dissection of the CD21/CD19/TAPA-1/Leu-13 complex of B lymphocytes. J Exp Med. 1993; 178:1407–1417.

20. Tedder TF, Zhou LJ, Engel P. The CD19/CD21 signal transduction complex of B lymphocytes. Immunol Today 1994; 15:437–442.

21. Weng WK, Jarvis L, LeBien TW. Signaling through CD19 activates Vav/mitogen-activated protein kinase pathway and induces formation of a CD19/Vav/phosphatidylinositol 3-kinase complex in human B cell precursors. J Biol Chem 1994; 269:32514–32521.

22. Tuveson DA, Carter RH, Soltoff SP, Fearon DT. CD19 of B cells as a surrogate kinase insert region to bind phosphatidylinositol 3-kinase. Science 1993; 260:986–989.

23. Adams JM, Houston H, Allen J, Lints T, Harvey R. The hematopoietically expressed vav proto-oncogene shares homology with the dbl GDP-GTP exchange factor, the bcr gene and a yeast gene (CDC24) involved in cytoskeletal organization. Oncogene 1992; 7:611–618.

24. Jain J, Loh C, Rao A. Transcriptional regulation of the IL-2 gene. Curr Opin Immunol 1995; 7:333–342.

25. Crabtree GR, Clipstone NA. Signal transmission between the plasma membrane and nucleus of T lymphocytes. Annu Rev Biochem 1994; 63:1045–1083.

26. Karin M. The regulation of AP-1 activity by mitogen-activated protein kinases. Philos Trans R Soc Lond B Biol Sci 1996; 351:127–134.

27. Arvieux J, Yssel H, Colomb M. Ag-bound C3b and C4b enhance Ag presenting cell function in activation of human T-cell clones. Immunology 1988; 65:229–235.

28. Jacquier M, Gabert F, Villiers M, Colomb M. Modulation of antigen processing and presentation by covalently linked complement C3b fragment. Immunology 1995; 84:164–170.

29. Bretscher P, Cohn M. A theory of self-nonself discrimination: paralysis and induction involve the recognition of one and two determinants on an antigen, respectively. Science 1970; 163:1042–1049.

30. Goodnow C, Cyster J, Hartley S, Bell S, Cooke M, Healy J, Akkaraju S, Rathmell J, Pogue S, Shokat K. Self-tolerance checkpoints in B lymphocyte development. Adv Immunol 1995; 59:279–368.

15

Endothelial Cell Responses to Complement Activation

SOHEYLA SAADI and JEFFREY L. PLATT
Duke University Medical Center, Durham, North Carolina

The physiology of the endothelium and the complement system are intertwined in manifold ways. Both play integral roles in defending the host against infection. Both promote and participate in specific immune responses. Both contribute to repair of tissue damage. Through the function of cell-associated molecules such as decay accelerating factor (DAF), membrane cofactor protein (MCP, CD46), and CD59, endothelium regulates activation of complement (1). At the same time, by altering the metabolism of IL-1α and heparan sulfate proteoglycan, complement regulates the functional state and differentiation of endothelial cells (2,3). In this chapter we first review the physiology and pathophysiology of endothelium and then the mechanisms by which complement influences endothelial physiology in health and disease.

I. PHYSIOLOGY OF ENDOTHELIUM IN HEALTH AND DISEASES

During the past two decades the concept of vascular endothelium has evolved from that of an inert and passive partition between the blood and the blood vessel wall to that of a dynamic structure that plays a pivotal role in maintaining the homeostasis of blood components, blood vessel walls, and surrounding tissues. These dynamic properties reflect in part the ability of endothelium to assume divergent physiologic postures. Thus, "quiescent" endothelium limits the access of blood components to the tissues, inhibits coagulation and inflammation, and regulates vascular tone. "Activated" endothelium allows blood elements to penetrate into blood vessel walls and surrounding tissues, promotes coagulation and inflammation, and mediates profound changes in vascular tone.

A. Quiescent Endothelium

Quiescent endothelial cells maintain blood and tissue homeostasis through four fundamental physiologic functions. First, vascular endothelium forms a barrier regulating the movement of macromolecules, solutes, and blood cells across blood vessel walls into tissues. For example, endothelial cells effectively separate plasma coagulation factors, especially factor VIIa, from tissue factor in underlying matrix and smooth muscle cells, thus preventing spontaneous formation of fibrin thrombi.

While it constitutes an anatomical boundary between blood and tissues, endothelium does not have a uniform "barrier property" along the length of the vascular tree. For example, endothelial cells in the kidney, endocrine glands, and liver have fenestrations that allow ready exchange of solutes while retaining blood cells to a varying extent. On the other hand, endothelial cells in many peripheral tissues, muscle, and brain form an integral boundary where the passage of plasma constituents into tissues is regulated, in part by intercellular junctions such as tight junctions.

Tight junctions vary in number and complexity depending on the location of endothelium (4). For instance, tight junctions are well organized and numerous in brain capillaries, forming the blood–brain barrier where the exchange of macromolecules needs to be tightly regulated (5). On the other hand, tight junctions almost disappear in the high endothelial venules of lymphoid tissue where lymphocyte extravasation and exchange of plasma constituents need to be very efficient (6).

Heparan sulfate proteoglycan also contributes to the barrier function of endothelium. Enzymatic removal of heparan sulfate increases the permeability of endothelium to plasma proteins and allows extravasation of blood cells or metastatic tumor cells (7).

The second function of endothelial cells is regulation of coagulation. In addition to separating plasma coagulation factors from extravascular tissue factor, healthy endothelial cells elaborate cell-associated macromolecules that prevent inadvertent clotting of blood. One such endothelial cell-associated regulator of coagulation is thrombomodulin, a 105 kDa integral membrane protein (for review, see 8). Thrombomodulin complexes with small amounts of thrombin generated at endothelial cell surfaces causing conformational changes in thrombin (Fig. 1A). Complexed with thrombomodulin, thrombin fails to react with its coagulation substrates including fibrinogen while its ability to activate protein C, a potent circulating anticoagulant, is enhanced 1000-fold (9). Activated protein C is a serine protease that, together with its cofactor protein S, inhibits coagulation by inactivating clotting factors Va and/or VIIIa. The physiological relevance of thrombomodulin-protein C/S pathway for the anticoagulant properties of the vascular wall is revealed by the thrombotic disorders frequently found in patients deficient in protein C or in protein S (8). Endothelial cells also inhibit coagulation by elaborating heparan sulfate proteoglycan, a protein polysaccharide component of cell membranes and extracellular matrices. Heparan sulfate proteoglycan binds to and activates antithrombin III (10). Activated antithrombin III is a serpin that inhibits thrombin, factor Xa, and factor IXa (11). Endothelial cells also express tissue factor pathway inhibitor (TFPI), a 45 kDa protein that inhibits tissue factor activity in a two-step stoichiometric reaction (for review, see 12). TFPI first binds to plasma factor Xa and then to tissue factor-factor VIIa complexes that form on endothelial cell surfaces. The interaction of TFPI inactivates factor Xa factor VIIa (Fig. 1B) (13,14). Heparan sulfate proteoglycan enhances the inhibitory effect of TFPI (15). The physiological importance of TFPI is suggested by recent studies in which administration of TFPI was found to prevent venous thrombosis in rabbits (12).

The third function of endothelium is the regulation of leukocyte migration into lymphoid organs and peripheral tissues. Endothelium of most peripheral tissues is nonadherent for leukocytes and these tissues contain few resident white blood cells. Endothelium of lymphatic organs, on the other hand, expresses adhesion molecules such as the "addressins" (MadCAM-1), which interact with adhesion molecules on lymphocytes leading to lymphocyte retention in lymphoid organs (16).

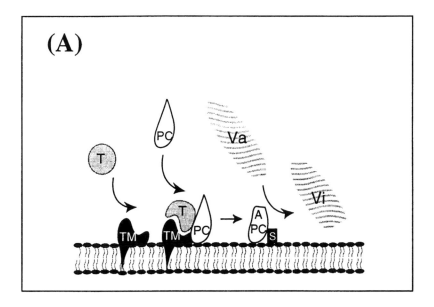

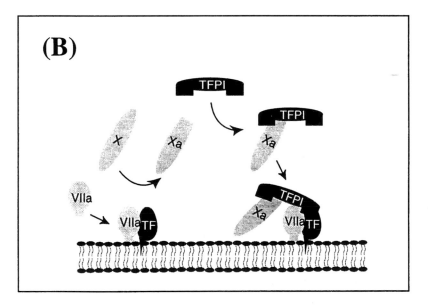

Figure 1 Inhibition of coagulation by normal endothelial cells. (A) Thrombomodulin (TM)/protein C (PC) anticoagulant pathway (8). Thrombin (T) generated as a result of vascular injury binds to thrombomodulin on normal endothelial cell surfaces. Thrombin–thrombomodulin complexes convert protein C to activated protein C (APC). Activated protein C binds to protein S (S) on cell surface. Activated protein C–protein S complexes then convert active factor V (Va) to inactive factor V (Vi) and thus the coagulation cascade stops. (B) Inhibition of coagulation by tissue factor pathway inhibitor (TFPI) (12). TFPI binds to factor Xa (Xa) first and then binds to tissue factor (TF)-factor VIIa(VIIa) complexes on cell surfaces. In this quaternary complex, TFPI inhibits both Xa and TF.

The fourth function of vascular endothelium is to regulate vascular tone. Vascular tone is determined in part by the action of endothelial cell-derived vasodilators and vasoconstrictors on smooth muscle cells (for review, see 17). Under normal conditions, physiological blood flow is maintained by the secretion of small amounts of vasodilatory factors. The best known vasodilator is nitric oxide (NO), the product of nitric oxide synthase (18,19) that is released constitutively from endothelial cells. NO was originally known as "endothelial-derived relaxing factor" (EDRF) (18). EDRF derived its name from the observation that removal of endothelium from a blood vessel causes severe vasoconstriction due to the loss of EDRF. Another vasodilator released from endothelial cells is PGI_2, an unstable prostaglandin constitutively produced in endothelial cells from PGH_2 by the action of PGI_2 synthase (20). The vasodilator activity of PGI_2 was identified shortly after its discovery, based on the observation that PGI_2 and its stable analogue, dehydro-PGI_2 methyl ester, caused relaxation of arterial strips and decreased pulmonary perfusion pressure (21).

B. Activated Endothelium

The normal properties of endothelium change dramatically under conditions of injury and disease. Exposure to agonists such as endotoxin and cytokines, and physical factors such as turbulent blood flow and injury, stimulate endothelial cells to undergo a global change in structure and function over a period of minutes to hours. Endothelial cells that manifest this set of changes are considered to be "activated." Activated endothelial cells contribute to sequestration of infectious agents, the repair of injured tissue, and the return to homeostasis.

Activated endothelium has defective barrier function. One mechanism contributing to the loss of barrier function in activated endothelium is the dissociation of endothelial intercellular junctions, leading to the formation of intercellular "gaps." The formation of gaps allows egress of water and the passage of macromolecules across the endothelial monolayer and exposes coagulation factors in the blood to procoagulant substances in the subendothelium leading to intravascular and extravascular coagulation. Majno and Palade (22) showed that histamine caused formation of gaps in rat vascular endothelium. In their studies, intracellular junctions in endothelium were dissociated within 1 min, allowing leakage of colloidal particles from blood vessels. These gaps were transient and disappeared within 3 h. Histamine, bradykinin, tumor necrosis factor (TNF), and α-thrombin also cause rapid formation of gaps in cultured endothelial cells (23–25).

Activated endothelial cells promote coagulation. One mechanism underlying the procoagulant posture of endothelial cells is the de novo synthesis of tissue factor. Activated endothelial cells upregulate tissue factor, a 47 kDa transmembrane protein normally absent in endothelial cells (for reviews, see 26). Tissue factor initiates coagulation by binding to and serving as a cofactor for coagulation factor VIIa (Fig. 2). Tissue factor–factor VIIa complexes cleave and activate factor X to yield Xa. Factor Xa in turn complexes with factor Va on cell membrane phospholipid. These complexes are referred to as prothrombinase because they catalyze conversion of prothrombin to active thrombin. Mediators of inflammation induce procoagulant activity (27). Bevilaqua et al. showed that IL-1 induces procoagulant activity over a period of 8 h, which depended on the presence of factor VIIa indicative of expression of tissue factor in endothelial cell cultures. Infusion of endotoxin also causes endothelial cells to synthesize tissue factor causing widespread intravascular coagulation (28). Inflammatory mediators such as IL-1, endotoxin, and TNF also decrease

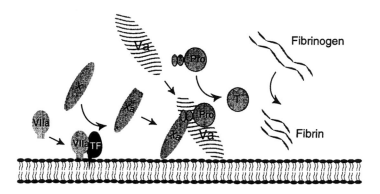

Figure 2 Initiation of coagulation by activated endothelial cells. Activated endothelial cells express tissue factor (TF) that binds to plasma factor VIIa (VIIa) on endothelial cell surfaces (109). Factor X (X) binds to and is cleaved by tissue factor–factor VIIa complexes to yield activated factor X (Xa). Factor Va (Va) associates with factor Xa on cell surfaces to form prothrombinase complexes. Prothrombin (Pro) binds to and is activated by prothrombinase complex to yield thrombin (T), which cleaves fibrinogen to fibrin.

expression of thrombomodulin on surface of endothelial cells, exacerbating a hypercoagulable state (29,30).

Another mechanism underlying the procoagulant posture of activated endothelial cells is impairment of fibrinolysis caused by induction of plasminogen activator inhibitor 1 (PAI-1). Under normal conditions, inadvertent fibrin clots are degraded by a serine protease, plasmin, the activated form of plasminogen. Formation of plasmin from plasminogen is normally catalyzed by plasminogen activators such as the urokinase-like plasminogen activators and the tissue-type plasminogen activators. Activated endothelial cells allow the persistence of fibrin clots by elaborating PAI-1, which binds to plasminogen activators and inhibits generation of plasmin (31,32). Bevilaqua et al. (33) showed that activation of human endothelial cells with IL-1 resulted in concomitant decrease in production of plasminogen activators and increase in production of PAI-1 within 6 h. Emeis and Kooistra (32) showed that endotoxin also induces PAI-1 *in vitro* and that *in vivo* infusion of endotoxin or IL-1 rapidly increases plasma PAI-1 activity.

Activated endothelial cells recruit leukocytes to sites of inflammation (for review, see 34). Recruitment of leukocytes into tissues is mediated in part by the increased expression of cell adhesion molecules and chemokines on endothelial cells. Leukocyte recruitment is thought to occur in three steps: attachment and rolling, arrest, and migration, mediated in part by sequential interactions between cell adhesion molecules on endothelial cell surfaces and infiltrating leukocytes. As a first step in this process, endothelial cells express P-selectin and E-selectin (ELAM-1) that interact with carbohydrate ligands such as sialyl Lewis X on leukocytes. Whereas cell surface expression of pre-existing P-selectin occurs within 5 min following exposure of endothelial cells to oxidants or inflammatory mediators (35,36), expression of E-selectin occurs over 6–8 h following activation of endothelial cells (37). P- and E-selectin cause the initial attachment and rolling of leukocytes on the blood vessel wall. As a second step, endothelial cells increase expression of ICAM-1 and release chemokines that become anchored to endothelial cell-associated heparan sulfate proteoglycan. Chemokines cause expression of β_2 integrins such as LFA-

1 and MAC-1 on the surface of leukocytes. These integrins bind to ICAM-1 on endothelial cells resulting in firm adhesion or "sticking" of leukocytes. In the final step, endothelial cells participate in transmigration of leukocytes. The binding of β_2 integrins on activated leukocytes to PECAM-1 at intercellular junctions of endothelial cells and chemoattractants present in the inflamed tissue direct the migration of leukocytes into injured tissues. IL-1, TNF, and endotoxin can augment leukocyte adhesion to endothelial cells by inducing expression of E-selectin, and increasing expression of ICAM and chemokines (37–40).

Activated endothelial cells also elaborate substances that change vascular tone. Changes in vascular tone are in part due to decreased release of vasodilators and in part due to increased elaboration of vasoconstrictors. For example, endothelial cells exposed to hypoxia synthesize less PGI_2 and exposed to prolonged ischemia release endothelial-derived contracting factors such as thromboxane A2 (TxA_2) and endothelin-1 (ET-1) (41,42). TxA_2 is a product of cyclooxygenase upregulated in response to inflammatory mediators such IL-1α (41). IL-1α also upregulates expression of proendothelin mRNA. The proendothelin protein is proteolytically cleaved to produce ET-1 (43). Vasoconstriction mediated by vasoconstrictors not only leads to ischemia but also, as will be seen below, potentially localizes the effect of inflammatory mediators.

Activation of endothelial cells is orchestrated in part by the transcriptional induction of various genes by nuclear factor-κB (NF-κB) (reviewed in 44,45). In activated endothelial cells, NF-κB binds to κB site(s) on genes such as tissue factor, PAI-1, and adhesion molecules and participates in the initiation of their transcription. NF-κB is a homo- or heterodimer composed of two proteins of the Rel family. The prototype of NF-κB consists of p50/p65 or c-Rel/p65 subunits, which in resting endothelial cells form a complex with a cytoplasmic transcriptional inhibitor, IκB-α. The IκB-α prevents nuclear localization of NF-κB complex and thus NF-κB remains in the cytoplasm and is transcriptionally inactive. Following stimulation, IκB is phosphorylated and subsequently degraded, freeing up NFκB. NFκB then translocates to the nucleus where it binds to κB sites and contributes to activation of endothelial cells.

II. EFFECT OF COMPLEMENT ON ENDOTHELIAL CELLS

Activation of the complement system leads to profound changes in the structure and function of endothelium. Some of these changes resemble the changes seen after endothelial cells are activated by endotoxin, IL-1, and TNF. It will be seen, however, that the pathways through which endothelial cells respond to complement differ in important ways from the pathways through which endothelial cells respond to cytokines and endotoxin. Some of the changes associated with complement activation are caused by locally secreted inflammatory mediators and thus are influenced by regional blood flow. Other changes induced by complement can be attributed to alteration in the metabolism of heparan sulfate proteoglycan. Changes caused by activation of complement on endothelial cells, like those induced by "conventional agonists," may help blood vessels to cope with the harmful effects of infection and blood vessel injury or they might lead to manifestations of vascular diseases. Here we consider some of the changes in endothelial cell functions induced by active complement components. In the section that follows, we describe some prototypic responses of endothelial cells to complement activation in or around blood vessels and how pathological changes might be linked to specific changes in endothelial cell physiology.

A. Effect of Anaphylotoxins on Endothelial Cells

The generation of anaphylotoxins, particularly C5a, in the vicinity of blood vessels can have a profound effect on endothelial cells. One mechanism for these effects involves the activation of neutrophils and macrophages. Another mechanism involves the direct action of anaphylotoxins on endothelial cells.

One way that C5a affects endothelium is by binding to and activating neutrophils, which in turn may damage endothelium. Neutrophils activated by C5a generate reactive oxygen metabolites that may directly mediate the detachment and killing of endothelial cells (46,47). C5a also causes neutrophils to express elastase that may act on endothelial cells to disrupt junctions and impair barrier function (48). Key et al. (49) found that elastase released from activated neutrophils also causes the release of heparan sulfate by cleavage of the proteoglycan core. The effects of heparan sulfate release on endothelial cell function are discussed below. Activated neutrophils release other proteases and membrane phospholipases potentially destructive to endothelium. Activation of neutrophils causes formation of neutrophil aggregates in the vasculature. The intravascular accumulation of neutrophils can physically impair blood flow and thereby exacerbate the ischemic injury (50).

C5a also acts directly on endothelial cells. Recent studies have indicated that endothelial cells have mRNA for C5a receptors and bind C5a in a manner consistent with receptor to ligand interaction (51), leading to generation of signal transduction through G proteins (52).

Interaction of C5a with endothelial cells induces, within minutes, expression of P-selectin on endothelial cell surfaces (36). The expression of P-selectin is transient and is mediated by fusion of Weibel-Palade bodies containing preformed P-selectin with endothelial cell membranes. P-selectin serves as a ligand for adhesion of neutrophils (53) and thus facilitates neutrophil infiltration into tissues (54).

C5a triggers the synthesis of reactive oxidants in endothelial cells. Reactive oxidants are generated by at least two different mechanisms. First, Friedl et al. (55) showed that following exposure of endothelial cells to C5a, xanthine dehydrogenase is converted to xanthine oxidase within 5–10 min. This change promotes the generation of O_2^- and OH^- (56). Second, Murphy et al. (52) showed that stimulation of endothelial cells with C5a generates oxidants independent of xanthine oxidase. This mechanism is insensitive to inhibitors of xanthine oxidase and requires activation of protein kinase C and a pertussis toxin-sensitive G protein. Besides causing direct damage to endothelial cells, oxygen free radicals may activate NFκB (57), leading to induction of tissue factor (58) and perhaps adhesion molecules.

Exposure of endothelial cells to C5a causes activation of endothelial cell-derived serine and/or cysteine proteinases that cleave the core protein of heparan sulfate proteoglycan preferentially from the cell surface (59,60). Endothelial cells activated by C5a release more than 50% endothelial cell-associated heparan sulfate proteoglycan within 30–60 min (61).

Alterations in the metabolism of endothelial cell heparan sulfate proteoglycan by C5a or by elastase may have a major impact on endothelial cell function, since heparan sulfate proteoglycan contributes to a number of important physiological properties. One vital function of heparan sulfate is the maintenance of endothelial cell barrier property (7,62,63). The loss of heparan sulfate leads to edema, exudation of plasma proteins, and transmigration of blood cells as occurs during inflammation. Endothelial cell-associated heparan sulfate also acts as anticoagulant by binding and activating antithrombin III (10). The loss of heparan sulfate proteoglycan can thus favor coagulation by depriving endothelium of activated antithrombin III. Antithrombin III has also been reported to regulate complement activation (64) and thus the loss of this function may augment complement-mediated processes in the vicinity of the affected blood vessel. Heparan sulfate tethers extracellular superoxide dismutase (SOD), a free radical scavenger, to the endothelial cell surfaces; thus, the loss of heparan sulfate probably decreases local antioxidant activity (65). Heparan sulfate released from endothelial cells may modulate local immune reactions through interaction with immune cells (3). For instance, heparan sulfate activates antigen-presenting cells, leading to profound alteration in their ability to stimulate proliferative and cytolytic T-cell responses (66–68).

B. Effects of C3b on Endothelial Cells

Deposition of C3b on endothelial cells provides a ligand for adherence of neutrophils and other phagocytes that express complement receptors. For example, Vercellotti et al. showed that after heterologous complement is activated on the surface of endothelial cells, neutrophils bind to iC3b through CD11b/CD18 (CR3) (69). Binding of iC3b to CR3 signals activation of neutrophils. To this end, CR3 has been shown to play a major role in neutrophil-mediated detachment of endothelial cells and release of H_2O_2 from neutrophils (70).

C. Effects of Terminal Complement Complexes on Endothelial Cells

Formation of membrane attack complex (MAC) has profound effects on the physiology of endothelial cells. At one extreme, formation of MAC may cause endothelial cell lysis leading to leakage of vascular contents and exposure of plasma coagulation factors to procoagulant components in the matrix (71). While MAC might lyse endothelial cells under some circumstances, complement-mediated lysis is probably less common than might be thought. Indeed, endothelial cells appear to resist the cytotoxic effects of complement (61). One mechanism for this resistance involves expression of complement regulatory proteins such as DAF, CD59, and MCP (1). However, even under conditions in which protective effects of these complement regulatory proteins are minimal, such as when cells are exposed to heterologous complement, resistance to lysis is quite apparent (72). For example, exposure of porcine endothelial cells to human complement under conditions mediating heparan sulfate release does not cause endothelial cell death as measured by ^{51}Cr release (60). This intrinsic resistance of endothelial cells to complement-mediated cytotoxicity may reflect rapid elimination of MAC complexes from the plasma membrane (73,74).

One of the most important structural changes in endothelium mediated by terminal complement complexes is disruption of intercellular junctions leading to formation of gaps (72). Formation of gaps is mediated by MAC, C5b678, and C5b67 (72). The gaps, which are approximately 5 μm in diameter, can be detected as early as 5 min after exposure of endothelial cells to complement. The gaps, formed between adjacent cells undergo repair within 60 min. Restoration of monolayer integrity following formation of gaps depends on the assembly of MAC, since C8-deficient serum can induce gap formation but cannot support repair. Restoration of monolayer integrity also depends on secretion of an endothelial cell product(s), since removal of conditioned medium retards this process. Agents that increase the concentration of cAMP in endothelial cells prevent MAC-induced gap formation.

MAC also activates endothelial cells. MAC-treated endothelial cells elaborate procoagulant "activity," promote inflammation, and have an altered physiology similar to endothelial cells stimulated with endotoxin or cytokines. There is a significant difference, however, between the mechanism of endothelial cell activation by endotoxin or cytokines and the mechanisms of endothelial cell activation induced by MAC. Endotoxin or cytokines signal endothelial cells "directly" leading to induction of the functional changes discussed above, such as tissue factor and adhesion molecules. These changes are referred to as a "primary response" because they reflect direct transcriptional activation of the genes for these proteins. MAC, on the other hand, does not directly stimulate expression of the genes associated with endothelial cells activation. Rather, MAC induces de novo synthesis and secretion of IL-1α as a primary response and IL-1α activates endothelial cells in an autocrine fashion (Fig. 3) (75). The pivotal role of IL-1α in MAC-mediated alteration of endothelial cells is demonstrated by the observation that IL-1 receptor antagonist and anti-IL-1α antibodies abolish MAC-induced endothelial cell activation (75,76).

One manifestation of endothelial cell activation induced by MAC is increased procoagulant activity. MAC induces procoagulant functions through at least four mechanisms. First, MAC causes alterations of endothelial cell membrane phospholipid bilayers within 10 min that support prothrombinase activity (77). Second, MAC also induces the formation and shedding of membrane vesicles enriched with binding sites for factor Va and may serve as a nidus for formation of prothrombinase complexes (77). Indeed, approximately 75% of the prothrombinase activity associated with MAC-treated endothelial cells are present on these vesicles. Third, MAC also induces synthesis of tissue factor (75) detected hours after complement activation; as mentioned above induction of tissue factor synthesis depends on production of IL-1α as an intermediate. Upregulation of tissue factor on endothelium can cause widespread coagulation and fibrin deposition. Fourth, MAC also causes the upregulation of PAI-1 through the IL-1α-dependent pathway leading to persistence of fibrin clots.

Formation of MAC on endothelial cells promotes adhesion of leukocytes by two mechanisms. First, MAC, like C5a, within minutes induces expression of P-selectin on the

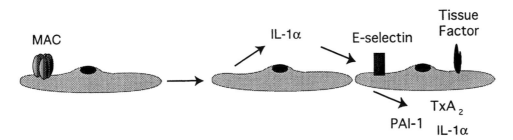

Figure 3 A model for MAC-mediated endothelial cell activation. MAC does not directly activate endothelial cells but causes the elaboration of IL-1α, which acts on endothelial cells as an autocrine to mediate expression of E-selectin, plasminogen activator inhibitor (PAI-1), and tissue factor (TF). Vasoconstriction mediated by thromboxane (TxA₂) retains IL-1α in the vicinity of the stimulated endothelium, allowing propagation of endothelial cell activation.

surfaces of endothelial cells (78). Second, MAC causes *de novo* synthesis and expression of E-selectin that peaks hours later and depends on synthesis of IL-1α by endothelial cells. MAC also seems to enhance the endothelial cell responses to TNF-α by a yet unknown mechanism. Treatment of endothelial cells with TNF-α plus MAC results in augmentation of expression of E-selectin and ICAM-1 in comparison to endothelial cells treated with TNF-α alone (79).

Terminal complement complexes modulate vascular tone. MAC and C5b678 cause the release of PGI$_2$ a, potent vasodilator from endothelial cells within 5 min (80). Endothelial cells release twice as much PGI$_2$ in response to MAC as they do in response to C5b678 (80). MAC also causes *de novo* synthesis of TxA$_2$ in endothelial cells (81) through an IL-1α-dependent mechanism. TxA$_2$ causes vasoconstriction and retardation of the blood flow. The reduction of regional blood flow caused by terminal complement complexes may contribute to activation of endothelial cells by allowing accumulation of IL-1α in the microenvironment and propagation of endothelial cell activation downstream from the initial point of injury. Consistent with this concept are studies demonstrating that removal of conditioned medium from MAC-stimulated endothelial cells abolishes activation of endothelial cells (75).

The mechanism through which assembly of MAC delivers signals to endothelial cells is incompletely understood. MAC causes an increased intracellular concentration of Ca^{2+} (78,80), which may play a role in surface expression of P-selectin (78). Increases in the intracellular concentration of Ca^{2+} are also important in the release of PGI$_2$ from endothelial cells stimulated by MAC (74). Whether the intracellular concentration of Ca^{2+} plays a role in upregulation of IL-1α by MAC is unknown.

The formation of MAC on endothelium may contribute to repair of cellular injury. MAC assembly causes the release of basic fibroblast growth factor and platelet-derived growth factor from endothelial cells (82). These growth factors may induce vascular smooth muscle cells and fibroblasts to undergo proliferation (82). MAC also directly stimulates endothelial cells to undergo proliferation. While under some circumstances, proliferation of smooth muscle is harmful and may cause thickening of blood vessel walls, proliferation of endothelial cells may lead to repair and return to a physiological state. For example, proliferation of endothelial cells mediated by MAC may cause repair of denuded endothelium, reestablishing the integrity of the blood vessel lining.

III. MODELS OF ENDOTHELIAL RESPONSES TO COMPLEMENT ACTIVATION

Activation of complement on endothelium or in its vicinity clearly causes profound changes in the structure and function of blood vessels. We have described above how individual components of complement mediate such changes. At the whole organ level, the changes induced by complement are much more complex due to the presence of active complement components and other effector systems. In some cases, particularly in autoimmune diseases such as systemic lupus erythematosus (83), rheumatoid arthritis (84), and systemic vasculitis (85), the effects of complement may be difficult to differentiate from the effects of other immune mediators. Here we review three models of complement-mediated injury to blood vessels in which the components involved and their localization in blood vessels is established.

A. Hyperacute Rejection

An organ transplanted into a recipient with circulating antidonor antibodies is subject to hyperacute rejection, a severe rejection reaction that destroys an organ graft within minutes to a few hours and is characterized by interstitial hemorrhage, edema, and thrombosis in which platelets are particularly involved (Fig. 4) (86). Hyperacute rejection is initiated by binding of antibodies to endothelium and activation of the recipient's complement. It is seen in allografts in which the recipient is presensitized to donor HLA or in allografts in which recipient and donor are incompatible for ABO blood group antigens. Hyperacute rejection is also seen when an organ transplanted into a phylogenetically disparate recipient, such as when porcine heart is transplanted into a baboon.

Several lines of evidence demonstrate that the pathogenesis of hyperacute rejection depends absolutely on the activation of complement. Complement in the recipient's plasma is consumed early in the course of hyperacute rejection and deposited along endothelium

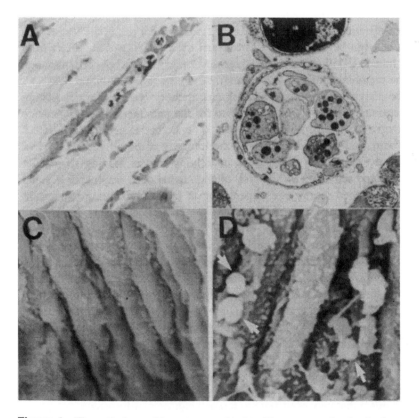

Figure 4 The pathology of hyperacute rejection. Hyperacute rejection is characterized by interstitial hemorrhage and thrombosis, consisting predominantly of platelets occurring within minutes of transplantation. (A) Interstitial hemorrhage from the microvasculature of a newly implanted xenograft. (B) Platelet aggregation within a capillary of a xenograft as an early pathological change observed by transmission electron microscopy. (C) Scanning electron microscopy reveals the intact endothelial lining of a cardiac blood vessel. (D) Scanning electron microscopy reveals attachment of platelets to interstices formed between retracting endothelial cells immediately after reperfusion of a xenograft by the recipient's blood.

of the newly transplanted organ (87). Hyperacute rejection is never observed in recipients treated with complement inhibitors such as cobra venom factor (88), soluble CR1 (89), or intravenous gamma globulin (90), or in recipients with inherited complement deficiencies (91).

Hyperacute rejection of xenogeneic organ grafts illustrates the physiological importance of complement regulation by endothelial cell-associated proteins. Xenografts are especially susceptible to complement-mediated injury because DAF, MCP, and/or CD59 expressed in the graft fail to control effectively the complement system of the heterologous recipient (92). The contribution of complement regulation to the homeostasis of blood vessels was seen in recent experiments in which organs from transgenic pigs expressing human CD59 and DAF did not undergo hyperacute rejection after transplantation into baboons (93). If the pathogenesis of hyperacute rejection can be attributed to complement-induced loss of endothelial cell function, expression of DAF, CD59, and presumably MCP can be seen as integrally linked to the normal function of endothelial cells.

Hyperacute rejection is mediated by terminal complement complexes, as it is not observed in recipients deficient in C6 (91). While the membrane attack complex probably mediates hyperacute rejection in most cases, there is evidence that the tissue lesion seen in hyperacute rejection can be induced by C5b678 and even C5b67. Thus, hearts from pigs transgenic for human CD59 are subject to hyperacute rejection by baboons, although the formation of the membrane attack complex may be substantially inhibited (94).

How does the activation of complement on endothelium lead to the devastating injury seen in hyperacute rejection? One mechanism for the pathogenesis of hyperacute rejection might involve complement-mediated lysis of endothelial cells. The lysis of endothelial cells would lead to the disruption of the integrity of blood vessels, loss of vascular contents, and exposure of platelets to underlying matrix leading to platelet adhesion, aggregation, and activation. While lysis of endothelial cells may occur in some cases, tissue samples obtained shortly after reperfusion of grafts undergoing hyperacute rejection do not generally reveal widespread death of endothelial cells. Thus hyperacute rejection would seem to reflect noncytotoxic effects of complement on blood vessels.

One noncytotoxic mechanism that probably contributes to the development of hyperacute rejection is the alteration in cell shape and formation of intercellular "gaps" induced by terminal complement complexes on endothelial cells (72). The interendothelial cell gaps provide channels through which erythrocytes and plasma components may pass. The importance of this mechanism is suggested by the finding that within 5 min after reperfusion, platelets can be found attached to the intercellular junctions (Fig. 4D). The contribution of interendothelial cell gaps to hyperacute rejection is also suggested by the fact that neither the formation of gaps nor the development of hyperacute rejection requires the formation of MAC. Thus hyperacute rejection is observed in pig-to-primate xenografts expressing human CD59 but not in transgenic organs expressing human DAF (95).

Another mechanism that may contribute to the pathogenesis of hyperacute rejection is the loss of heparan sulfate from endothelial cells (61). Loss of heparan sulfate would deprive endothelial cells of barrier and anticoagulant functions as described above. Stevens et al (96) showed that about 30% of total heparan sulfate is lost from xenografts within 5 min of perfusion by recipient's blood and that therapies that prevent heparan sulfate release also retard hyperacute rejection. The loss of heparan sulfate can not by itself account for hyperacute rejection since it is mediated by C5a and not by terminal complement components. However, loss of heparan sulfate may well confer heightened susceptibility to complement-mediated injury by impairing control of complement and increasing sensitivity to oxidant-mediated injury.

B. Complement-Mediated Acute Lung Injury

The rapid activation of complement within the lining of blood vessels by administration of large doses of cobra venom factor induces severe damage to pulmonary endothelial cells leading to acute pulmonary failure (97). The lesion of acute lung injury mediated by cobra venom factor is characterized histologically by edema, focal hemorrhage, fibrin deposition, and by the formation of neutrophil and platelets aggregates in pulmonary capillaries (98,99), findings indicative of injury to pulmonary blood vessels.

Several lines of evidence demonstrate the importance of C5a in the development of the pulmonary lesions. The role of C5a is suggested by studies in which C5-deficient mice fail to develop acute lung injury upon administration of cobra venom factor and by studies in which infusion of purified C5a peptide causes sequestration of neutrophils in lung capillaries in experimental animals (98,100). Furthermore, venom factor isolated from *Naja n. naja*, which generates C5a, but not venom factor isolated from *Naja h. haje*, which does not, induces acute lung injury (101).

An important process underlying pathology of acute lung injury is thought to be the loss of vascular integrity within 30 min following administration of cobra venom factor (98). The classical concept of the pathogenesis of acute lung injury in this model is that cobra venom factor induces formation of C5a, which activates leukocytes, and the interaction of these activated leukocytes with lung endothelium induces pulmonary damage (99–103). The pivotal role of neutrophils in mediating endothelial damage in this model is suggested by three observations. First, depletion of neutrophils by nitrogen mustard causes 70% reduction in lung injury (99). Second, reconstitution of neutrophil-depleted plasma with isolated neutrophils causes acute lung injury following complement activation in isolated rat lungs (104). Third, administration of anti-CD18 or anti-CD11 antibodies that inhibit adhesion of neutrophils to pulmonary endothelium prevents lung injury in this model (105,106). One way that neutrophils injure endothelial cells in this model is by production of reactive oxidants such as O_2^-, OH^-, and H_2O_2 which are cytotoxic to endothelial cells (99). The role of oxidants in mediating acute lung injury induced by complement activation is supported by the observation that administration of superoxide dismutase and catalase significantly protects against endothelial damage (97,99).

The pathogenesis of acute lung injury may also reflect direct action of C5a on lung endothelium. C5a may act directly on pulmonary endothelial cells to cause loss of heparan sulfate (60) and production of oxidants (55,56) as described above. In addition, C5a may cause vasoconstriction through its action on smooth muscle cells, resulting in ischemia.

C. Goodpasture Syndrome

Binding of complement-activating antibodies to pulmonary and renal basement membranes leads to the development of the Goodpasture syndrome (107,108). The Goodpasture syndrome is characterized by rapidly progressive glomerulonephris and hemorrhagic pneumonitis, both associated with prominent vascular injury. The antibodies that initiate the Goodpasture syndrome recognize an epitope(s) in the noncollagenous domain of type IV collagen in the basement membranes of renal and pulmonary capillaries. Binding of

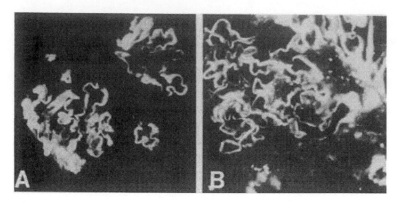

Figure 5 Immunopathology of Goodpasture syndrome. Localization of (A) IgG and (B) C3 by immunofluorescence in the basement membranes of renal glomerular capillaries in a patient with Goodpasture syndrome. Activation of complement in the basement membrane leads to leukocyte chemotaxis, endothelial damage, and loss of vascular integrity. The Goodpasture syndrome thus provides a model for the effect of complement activation in the vicinity of blood vessels. (Courtesy of Drs. Alfred A. Michael and Alfred J. Fish, University of Minnesota Medical School, Minneapolis, Minnesota.)

IgG to this structure activates complement, leading to deposition of C3 and localized inflammation and coagulation (Fig. 5).

Because the antigenic target of the anti-basement-membrane antibodies is definitively apart from the cell membranes of affected capillaries, this syndrome demonstrates how the activation of complement in an extravascular locus can profoundly influence the structure and function of nearby capillaries. However, how exactly complement mediates tissue injury in this syndrome is not certain. There is speculation that generation of C5a promotes chemotaxis of neutrophils and monocytes, which in turn mediate capillary damage by release of oxidants and cytokines. It also seems likely that complement components activated in the basement membranes may interact directly with endothelium, leading to loss of endothelial integrity and development of vascular injury. It is also likely that the sieving properties of capillary endothelial cells may contribute to the pathogenesis. The porous endothelium of the kidney and lung may allow the ready diffusion of C5a but retain carboxypeptidase N. Thus, the regulation of complement in the extravascular space might be less efficient than in the plasma or on endothelial cell surfaces.

ACKNOWLEDGMENT

This work was supported by grants from the National Institutes of Health (HL50985, HL52297, HL46810).

REFERENCES

1.   Morgan BP, Meri S. Membrane proteins that protect against complement lysis. Semin Immunopathol 1994; 15:369–396.

2. Schleef RR, Bevilacqua MP, Sawdey M, Gimbrone Jr. MA, Loskutoff DJ. Cytokine activation of vascular endothelium. J Biol Chem 1988; 263:5797–5803.

3. Ihrcke NS, Wrenshall LE, Lindman BJ, Platt JL. Role of heparan sulfate in immune system–blood vessel interactions. Immunol Today 1993; 14:500–505.

4. Dejana E, Corada M, Grazia Lampugnani M. Endothelial cell-to-cell junctions. FASEB J 1995; 9:910–918.

5. Goldstein GW. Endothelial cell-astrocyte interactions. A cellular model of the blood–brain barrier. Ann NY Acad Sci 1988; 529:31–39.

6. Girard JP, Springer TA. High endothelial venules (HEVs): specialized endothelium for lymphocyte migration. Immunol Today 1995; 16(9):449–457.

7. Kanwar YS, Linker A, Farquhar MG. Increased permeability of the glomerular basement membrane to ferritin after removal of glycosaminoglycans (heparan sulfate) by enzyme digestion. J Cell Biol 1980; 86:688–693.

8. Esmon CT. The roles of protein c and thrombomodulin in the regulation of blood coagulation. J Biol Chem 1989; 264:4743–4746.

9. Esmon NL, Owen WG, Esmon CT. Isolation of a membrane-bound cofactor for thrombin-catalyzed activation of protein C. J Biol Chem 1982; 257:859–864.

10. Rosenberg RD, Rosenberg JS. Natural anticoagulent mechanisms. J Clin Invest 1984; 74:1–6.

11. Lawson JH, Butenas S, Ribarik N, Mann KG. Complex-dependent Inhibition of factor VIIa by antithrombin III and heparin. J Biol Chem 1993; 268:767–770.

12. Broze GS Jr. Tissue factor pathway inhibitor. Thromb Haemostasis 1995; 74:90–93.

13. Rapaport SI. The extrinsic pathway inhibitor: a regulator of tissue factor-dependent blood coagulation. Thromb Haemostasis 1991; 66:6–15.

14. Broze GJ, Jr., Warren LA, Novotny WF, Higuchi DA, Girard JJ, Miletich JP. The lipoprotein-associated coagulation inhibitor that inhibits the factor VII-tissue factor complex also inhibits factor Xa: insight into its possible mechanism of action. Blood 1988; 71:335–343.

15. Kaiser B, Hoppensteadt DA, Jeske W, Wun TC, Fareed J. Inhibitory effects of TFPI on thrombin and factor Xa generation in vitro—modulatory action of glycosaminoglycans. Thromb Res 1994; 75:609–616.

16. Michie SA, Streeter PR, Bolt PA, Butcher EC, Picker LJ. The human peripheral lymph node vascular addressin. An inducible endothelial antigen involved in lymphocyte homing. Am J Pathol 1993; 143(6):1688–1698.

17. Luscher TF, Boulanger CM, Dohi Y, Yang Z. Endothelium-derived contracting factors. Hypertension 1992; 19:117–130.

18. Palmer RMJ, Ferridge AG, Moneada S. Nitric oxide release accounts for the biological activity of endothelium-derived relaxing factor. Nature 1987; 327:524–526.

19. Radomski MW, Palmer RMJ, Moncada S. Glucocorticoids inhibit the expression of an inducible, but not the constitutive, nitric oxide synthase in vascular endothelial cells. Proc Natl Acad Sci USA 1990; 87:10043–10047.

20. Ristimaki A, Viinikka L. Modulation of prostacyclin production by cytokines in vascular endothelial cells. Prostaglandins Leukot Essent Fatty Acids 1992; 47:93–99.

21. Hyman AL, Chapnick BM, Kadowitz PJ, et al. Unusual pulmonary vasodilator activity of 13, 14-dehydroprostacyclin methyl ester: comparison with endoperoxides and other prostanoids. Proc Natl Acad Sci USA 1977; 74:5711–5715.

22. Majno G, Palade GE. The effect of histamine and serotonin on vascular permeability: an electron microscopic study. J Biophys Biochem Cytol 1961; 11:571–603.

23. Arfors CE, Rutili G, Svensjo E. Microvascular transport of macromolecules in normal and inflammatory conditions. Acta Physiol Scand Suppl 1979; 463:93–103.

24. Campbell WN, Ding X, Goldblum SE. Interleukin-1 α and -β augment pulmonary artery transendothelial albumin flux in vitro. Am J Physiol 1992; 263:L128–L136.

25. Gerlach H, Lieberman H, Bach R, Godman G, Brett J, Stern D. Enhanced responsiveness of endothelium in the growing/motile state to tumor necrosis factor/cachectin. J Exp Med 1989; 170:913–931.

26. Nemerson Y. Tissue factor: then and now. Thromb Haemostasis 1995; 74:180–184.
27. Belivacqua MP, Pober JS, Majeau GR, Cotran RS, Gimbrone Jr MA. Interleukin 1 (IL-1) induces biosynthesis and cell surface expression of procoagulant activity in human vascular endothelial cells. J Exp Med 1984; 160:618–623.
28. Drake TA, Cheng J, Chang A, Taylor FB. Expression of tissue factor, thrombomodulin, and E-selection in baboons with lethal *Escherichia* sepsis. Am J Pathol 1993; 142:1458–1470.
29. Nawroth PP, Stern DM. Modulation of endothelial cell hemostatic properties by tumor necrosis factor. J Exp Med 1986; 163:740–745.
30. Hirokawa K, Aoki N. Regulatory mechanisms for thrombomodulin expression in human umbilical vein endothelial cells in vitro. J Cell Physiol 1991; 147:157–165.
31. Nachman RL, Hajjar KA, Silverstein RL, Dinarello CA. Interleukin 1 induces endothelial cell synthesis of plasminogen activator inhibitor. J Exp Med 1986; 163:1595–1600.
32. Emeis JJ, Kooistra T. Interleukin 1 and lipopolysaccharide induce an inhibitor of tissue-type plasminogen activator in vivo and in cultured endothelial cells. J Exp Med 1986; 163:1260–1266.
33. Bevilacqua MP, Schleef RR, Gimbrone Jr. MA, Loskutoff DJ. Regulation of the fibrinolytic system of cultured human vascular endothelium by interleukin 1. J Clin Invest 1986; 78:587–591.
34. Springer TA. Traffic signals for lymphocyte recirculation and leukocyte emigration: the multistep paradigm. Cell 1994; 76:301–314.
35. Patel KD, Zimmerman GA, Prescott SM, McEver RP, McIntyre TM. Oxygen radicals induce human endothelial cells to express GMP-140 and bind neutrophils. J Cell Biol 1991; 112:749–759.
36. Foreman KE, Vaporciyan AA, Bonish BK, et al. C5a-induced expression of P-selectin in endothelial cells. J Clin Invest 1994; 94:1147–1155.
37. Bevilacqua MP, Pober JS, Mendrick DL, Cotran RS, Gimbrone Jr. MA. Identification of an inducible endothelial-leukocyte adhesion molecule. Proc Natl Acad Sci USA 1987; 84:9238–9242.
38. Bevilacqua MP, Stengelin S, Gimbrone Jr. MA, Seed B. Endothelial leukocyte adhesion molecule I: an inducible receptor for neutrophils related to complement regulatory proteins and lectins. Science 1989; 243:1160–1164.
39. Bevilacqua MP, Pober JS, Wheeler ME, Cotran RS, Gimbrone MA. Interleukin 1 acts on cultured human vascular endothelium to increase the adhesion of polymorphonuclear leukocytes, monocytes, and related leukocyte cell lines. J Clin Invest 1985; 76:2003–2011.
40. Pober JS, Gimbrone MA, Jr., LaPierre LA, et al. Overlapping patterns of activation of human endothelial cells by interleukin 1, tumor necrosis factor, and immune interferon. J Immunol 1986; 137:1893–1896.
41. Maier JAM, Hla T, Maciag T. Cyclooxygenase is an immediate-early gene induced by interleukin-1 in human endothelial cells. J Biol Chem 1990; 265(19):10805–10808.
42. Yanagisawa M, Kurihara H, Kimura S, et al. A novel potent vasoconstrictor peptide produced by vascular endothelial cells. Nature 1988; 332:411–415.
43. Yoshizumi M, Kurihara H, Morita T, et al. Interleukin 1 increases the production of endothelin-1 by cultured endothelial cells. Biochem Biophys Res Commun 1990; 166:324–329.
44. Collins T, Read MA, Neish AS, Whitley MZ, Thanos D, Maniatis T. Transcriptional regulation of endothelial cell adhesion molecules: NF-κB and cytokine-inducible enhancers. FASEB J 1995; 9:899–909.
45. Mackman N. Regulation of the tissue factor gene. FASEB J 1995; 9:883–889.
46. Hardy MM, Flickinger AG, Riley DP, Weiss RH, Ryan US. Superoxide dismutase mimetics inhibit neutrophil-mediated human aortic endothelial cell injury in vitro. J Biol Chem 1994; 269:18535–18540.
47. Varani J, Ginsburg I, Schuger L, et al. Endothelial cell killing by neutrophils: synergistic interaction of oxygen products and proteases. Am J Pathol 1989; 135:435–438.

48. Owen CA, Campbell MA, Sannes PL, Boukedes SS, Campbell EJ. Cell surface-bound elastase and cathepsin G on human neutrophils: a novel, non-oxidative mechanism by which neutrophils focus and preserve catalytic activity of serine proteinases. J Cell Biol 1995; 131(3):775–789.

49. Key NS, Platt JL, Vercellotti GM. Vascular endothelial cell proteoglycans are susceptible to cleavage by neutrophils. Arterio Thromb 1992; 12:836–842.

50. Kloner RA, Ganote CE, Jennings RB. The no-reflow phenomenon after temporary coronary occlusion in the dog. J Clin Invest 1974; 54:1496–1508.

51. Haviland DL, Mccoy RL, Whitehead WT, et al. Cellular expression of the C5a anaphylatoxin receptor (C5aR): demonstration of C5aR on nonmyeloid cells of the liver and lung. J Immunol 1995; 154:1861–1869.

52. Murphy HS, Shayman JA, Till GO, et al. Superoxide responses of endothelial cells to C5a and TNF-α: divergent signal transduction pathways. Am J Physiol 1992; 263:L51–L59.

53. Geng JG, Bevilacqua MP, Moore KL, et al. Rapid neutrophil adhesion to activated endothelium mediated by GMP-140. Nature 1990; 343:757–760.

54. Hausman MS, Snyderman R, Mergenhagen SE. Humoral mediators of chemotaxis of mononuclear leukocytes. J Infect Dis 1972; 125:595–602.

55. Friedl HP, Till GO, Ryan US, Ward PA. Mediator-induced activation of xanthine oxidase in endothelial cells. FASEB J 1989; 3:2512–2518.

56. Zimmerman BJ, Granger DN. Reperfusion injury. Surg Clin North Am 1992; 72:65–83.

57. Barchowsky A, Munro SR, Morana SJ, Vincenti MP, Treadwell M. Oxidant-sensitive and phosphorylation-dependent activation of NF-κB and AP-1 in endothelial cells. Am Physiol Soc 1995; L829–L836.

58. Golino P, Ragni M, Cirillo P, et al. Effects of tissue factor induced by oxygen free radicals on coronary flow during reperfusion. Nature Med 1996; 2:35–40.

59. Ihrcke NS, Platt JL. Shedding of heparan sulfate proteoglycan by stimulated endothelial cells: evidence for proteolysis of cell surface molecules. J Cell Physiol 1996; 168:625–637.

60. Platt JL, Dalmasso AP, Lindman BJ, Ihrcke NS, Bach FH. The role of C5a and antibody in the release of heparan sulfate from endothelial cells. Eur J Immunol 1991; 21:2887–2890.

61. Platt JL, Vercellotti GM, Lindman BJ, Oegema TR, Jr., Bach FH, Dalmasso AP. Release of heparan sulfate from endothelial cells: implications for pathogenesis of hyperacute rejection. J Exp Med 1990; 171:1363–1368.

62. Savion N, Vlodavsky I, Fuks Z. Interaction of T lymphocytes and macrophages with cultured vascular endothelial cells: attachment, invasion, and subsequent degradation of the subendothelial extracellular matrix. J Cell Physiol 1984; 118:169–178.

63. Nakajima M, DeChavigny A, Johnson CE, Hamada J, Stein CA, Nicolson GL. Suramin: a potent inhibitor of melanoma heparanase and invasion. J Biol Chem 1991; 266:9661–9666.

64. Weiler JM, Linhardt RJ. Antithrombin III regulates complement activity in vitro. J Immunol 1991; 146:3889–3894.

65. Abrahamsson T, Brandt U, Marklund SL, Sjoquist P. Vascular bound recombinant extracellular superoxide dismutase type C protects against the detrimental effects of superoxide radicals on endothelium-dependent arterial relaxation. Circ Res 1992; 70:264–271.

66. Wrenshall LE, Cerra FB, Carlson A, Bach FH, Platt JL. Regulation of T lymphocyte responses by heparan sulfate. J Immunol 1991; 147:455–459.

67. Wrenshall LE, Carlson A, Cerra FB, PLatt JL. Modulation of cytolytic T-cell responses by heparan sulfate. Transplantation 1994; 57:1087–1094.

68. Wrenshall LE, Cerra FB, Singh RK, Platt JL. Heparan sulfate initiates signals in murine macrophages leading to divergent biological outcomes. J Immunol 1995; 154:871–880.

69. Vercellotti GM, Platt JL, Bach FH, Dalmasso AP. Enhanced neutrophil adhesion to xenogeneic endothelium via C3bi. J Immunol 1991; 146:730–734.

70. Von Asmuth E, Van Der Linden C, Leeuwenberg J, Buurman WA. Involvement of the CD11b/CD18 integrin, but not of the endothelial cell adhesion molecules ELAM-1 and ICAM-1 in tumor necrosis factor-α-induced neutrophil toxicity. J Immunol 1991; 147:3869–3875.

71. Gerlach H, Esposito C, Stern D. Modulation of endothelial hemostatic properties: an active role in the host response. Annu Rev Med 1990; 41:15–24.

72. Saadi S, Platt JL. Transient perturbation of endothelial integrity induced by antibodies and complement. J Exp Med 1995; 181:21–31.

73. Carney DF, Hammer CH, Shin ML. Elimination of terminal complement complexes in the plasma membrane of nucleated cells: influence of extracellular Ca^{2+} and association with cellular Ca^{2+}. J Immunol 1986; 137:263–270.

74. Carney DF, Koski CL, Shin ML. Elimination of terminal complement intermediates from the plasma membrane of nucleated cells: the rate of disappearance differs for cells carrying C5b-7 or C5b-8 or a mixture of C5b-8 with a limited number of C5b-9. J Immunol 1985; 134:1804–1809.

75. Saadi S, Holzkhecht RA, Patte CP, Stern DM, Platt JL. Complement-mediated regulation of tissue factor activity in endothelium. J Exp Med 1995; 182:1807–1814.

76. Parker W, Saadi S, Lin SS, Holzknecht ZE, Bustos M, Platt JL. Transplantation of discordant xenografts: a challenge revisited. Immunol Today 1996; 17:373–378.

77. Hamilton KK, Hattori R, Esmon CT, Sims PJ. Complement proteins C5b-9 induce vesiculation of the endothelial plasma membrane and expose catalytic surface for assembly of the prothrombinase enzyme complex. J Biol Chem 1990; 265:3809–3814.

78. Hattori R, Hamilton KK, McEver RP, Sims PJ. Complement proteins C5b-9 induce secretion of high molecular weight multimers of endothelial von Willebrand factor and translocation of granule membrane protein GMP-140 to the cell surface. J Biol Chem 1989; 264:9053–9060.

79. Kilgore KS, Shen JP, Miller BF, Ward PA, Warren JS. Enhancement by the complement membrane attack complex of tumor necrosis factor-α-induced endothelial cell expression of E-selectin and ICAM-1. J Immunol 1995; 155:1434–1441.

80. Suttorp N, Seeger W, Zinsky S, Bhakdi S. Complement complex C5b-8 induces PGI_2 formation in cultured endothelial cells. Am J Physiol 1987; 253:C13–C21.

81. Bustos M, Coffman TM, Saadi S, Platt JL. Modulation of eicosanoid metabolism in endothelial cells in a xenograft model: role of cyclooxygenase-z. J Clin Invest 1997; 100:1150–1158.

82. Benzaquen LR, Nicholson-Weller A, Halperin JA. Terminal complement proteins C5b-9 release basic fibroblast growth factor and platelet-derived growth factor from endothelial cells. J Exp Med 1994; 179:985–992.

83. Biesecker G, Katz S, Koffler D. Renal localization of the membrane attack complex in systemic lupus erythematosus nephritis. J Exp Med 1981; 154:1779–1794.

84. Corvetta A, Pomponio G, Rinaldi N, Luchetti MM, Di Loreto C, Stramazzotti D. Terminal complement complex in synovial tissue from patients affected by rheumatoid arthritis, osteoarthritis and acute joint trauma. Clin Exp Rheumatol 1992; 10:433–438.

85. Kissell JT, Mendell JR, Rammohan KW. Microvascular deposition of complement membrance attack complex in dermatomyositis. N Eng J Med 1986; 314(6):329–334.

86. Platt JL. Hyperacute Xenograft Rejection. Austin: R.G. Landes Company, 1995:

87. Platt JL, Fischel RJ, Matas AJ, Reif SA, Bolman RM, Bach FH. Immunopathology of hyperacute xenograft rejection in a swine-to-primate model. Transplantation 1991; 52:214–220.

88. Leventhal JR, Dalmasso AP, Cromwell JW, et al. Prolongation of cardiac xenograft survival by depletion of complement. Transplantation 1993; 55:857–866.

89. Pruitt SK, Kirk AD, Bollinger RR, et al. The effect of soluble complement receptor type 1 on hyperacute rejection of porcine xenografts. Transplantation 1994; 57:363–370.

90. Magee JC, Collins BH, Harland RC, et al. Immunoglobulin prevents complement mediated hyperacute rejection in swine-to-primate xenotransplantation. J Clin Invest 1995; 96:2404–2412.

91. Brauer RB, Baldwin III WM, Daha MR, Pruitt SK, Sanfilippo F. Use of C6-deficient rats to evaluate the mechanism of hyperacute rejection of discordant cardiac xenografts. J Immunol 1993; 151:7240–7248.

92. Platt JL, Vercellotti GM, Dalmasso AP, et al. Transplantation of discordant xenografts: a review of progress. Immunol Today 1990; 11:450–456.

93. Platt JL, Logan JS. Use of transgenic animals in xenotransplantation. Transplant Rev 1996; 10:69–77.

94. Diamond LE, McCurry KR, Oldham ER, et al. Characterization of transgenic pigs expressing functionally active human CD59 on cardiac endothelium. Transplantation 1996; 61:1241–1249.

95. Cozzi E, White DJG. The generation of transgenic pigs as potential organ donors for humans. Nature Med 1995; 1:964–966.

96. Stevens RB, Wang YL, Kaji H, et al. Administration of nonanticoagulant heparin inhibits the loss of glycosaminoglycans from xenogeneic cardiac grafts and prolongs graft survival. Transplant Proc 1993; 25:382.

97. Till GO, Ward PA. Systemic complement activation and acute lung injury. Fed Proc 1986; 45(1):13–18.

98. Tvedten HW, Till GO, Ward PA. Mediators of lung injury in mice following systemic activation of complement. Am J Pathol 1985; 119:92–100.

99. Till GO, Johnson KJ, Kunkel R, Ward PA. Intravascular activation of complement and acute lung injury. J Clin Invest 1982; 69:1126–1135.

100. O'Flaherty JT, Showell HJ, Ward PA. Neutropenia induced by systemic infusion of chemotactic factors. J Immunol 1977; 118(5):1586–1589.

101. Till GO, Morganroth ML, Kunkel R, Ward PA. Activation of C5 by cobra venom factor is required in neutrophil-mediated lung injury in the rat. Am J Pathol 1987; 129:44–53.

102. Stimler NP, Hugli TE, Bloor CM. Pulmonary injury induced by C3a and C5a anaphylatoxins. J Pathol 1980; 100(2):327–338.

103. Henson PM, Larsen GL, Webster RO, Mitchell BC, Goins AJ, Henson JE. Pulmonary microvascular alterations and injury induced by complement fragments: synergistic effect of complement activation, neutrophil sequestration, and prostaglandins. Ann NY Acad Sci 1982; 384:287–300.

104. Morganroth ML, Till GO, Kunkel RG, Ward PA. Complement and neutrophil-mediated injury of perfused rat lungs. Lab Invest 1986; 54(5):507–513.

105. Mulligan MS, Varani J, Warren JS, et al. Roles of β_2 integrins of rat neutrophils in complement- and oxygen radical-mediated acute inflammatory injury. J Immunol 1992; 148:1847–1857.

106. Mulligan MS, Smith CW, Anderson DC, et al. Role of leukocyte adhesion molecules in complement-induced lung injury. J Immunol 1993; 150:2401–2406.

107. Hellmark T, Segelmark M, Bygren P, Wieslander J. Glomerular basement membrane autoantibodies. In: Peter JB, Shoenfeld Y, eds. Autoantibodies. Amsterdam: Elsevier Science, 1996:291–298.

108. Glassock RJ. Renal involvement in multisystem diseases. In: Massry SG, Glassock RJ, eds. Textbook of Nephrology. Baltimore: Williams & Wilkins, 1995:818–822.

109. Rapaport SI, Rao LVM. The tissue factor pathway: how it has become a "prima ballerina." Thromb Haemostasis 1995; 74:7–17.

16

The Complement System in Reproduction

TERESA J. OGLESBY
Washington University School of Medicine, St. Louis, Missouri

Complement (C) and its regulatory proteins have recently attracted attention in the study of reproduction, in part, because of the following observations. Fluids of the female reproductive tract contain a functional C system and C3 is synthesized in large amounts by the uterus. Reproductive tissues and gametes have an unexpectedly diverse distribution of C regulators. Certain trophoblast–lymphocyte cross-reactive (TLX) antibodies recognize the C regulatory protein, membrane cofactor protein (MCP, CD46) and block fertilization in vitro. Finally, careful characterization of the C inhibitory properties of seminal plasma suggests new roles for prostasomes, which are vesicular organelles necessary for sperm maturation.

This chapter reviews expression and, in certain instances, function of C and its regulators and receptors pertinent to the human (unless noted otherwise) female and male reproductive tracts, fertilization, and placental development. Since relating C to reproduction is a relatively new undertaking, observations are often descriptive. Basic reproductive tract and placental anatomy, histology, and physiology, helpful in interpreting the C studies, have been reviewed and pertinent chapters in several texts are used as general references.

I. FEMALE REPRODUCTIVE TRACT

From menarche until menopause, the female reproductive tract undergoes functional changes related to cyclic hormonal secretion (Fig. 1) in preparation for pregnancy. Examples of distinct C regulator expression on reproductive epithelia and oocytes are summarized in Table 1.

A. Ovary and Oocytic Development

The ovaries store all eggs an individual will possess and secrete hormones necessary to drive the menstrual cycle and maintain secondary sexual characteristics (reviewed in 1,2). The monthly ovulatory process (Fig. 1B) begins with growth of multiple follicles, only one of which will ovulate in response to a surge of luteinizing hormone (LH) and the peak of follicle-stimulating hormone (FSH) secretion (Fig. 1A). Because only one oocyte

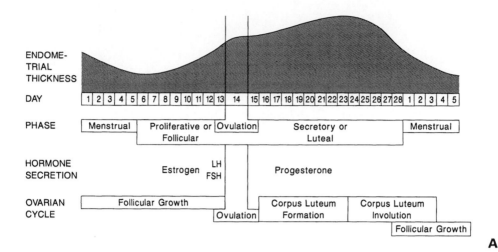

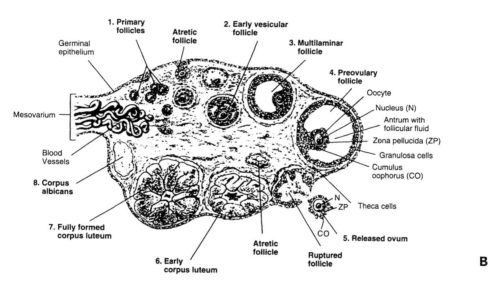

Figure 1   The menstrual cycle. (A) Endometrial height and follicular development (ovarian cycle) in relation to menstrual phase, predominant hormonal influence, and day of cycle. (B) Schematic representation of the ovary with stages of follicular development (1–4), ovulation (5), corpus luteum (6,7) and corpus albicans (8) formation. (Modified from Blaustein, A (ed). In Pathology of the Female Genital Tract, 2nd ed. New York: (Springer-Verlag, 1982; as adapted from Gray's Anatomy of the Human body, 35th ed, Philadelphia: Lea & Febiger.)

per cycle ovulates, atresia or degeneration of other developing follicles occurs throughout the cycle.

Initially, the oocyte is surrounded by a single layer of follicular cells, termed granulosa cells, that proliferate under the cooperative influence of FSH, LH, and estradiol. Concomitantly, the zona pellucida, a complex, acellular matrix of glycoproteins, forms between the oocyte and granulosa cells, some of which are destined to form the cumulus oophorus. The outermost theca layer of the developing follicle is derived from stromal cells that differentiate into the internal and external thecal layers: at follicular maturation

Table 1 Characteristics of C Regulatory Protein Expression on the Female Reproductive Tract

Cells/tissue		MCP[a]	DAF[a]	CD59[a]
Epithelia				
Cervix	Basal	+++	0	+++
	Surface	++	++	+++
Endometrial glands[b]	Proliferative	+++	+	++
	Secretory	+++	++	++
Ovarian surface		+++	0/+	+++
Fallopian tube[b]		+++	+	+/++
Oocytes	Developing follicles	+++	0	+/0
	At ovulation	0–+++	++	+++
Postfertilization	Preimplanted blastocyst	+–+++	++	+++

Source: From refs. 6,10,11,18–20.
[a] Immunohistochemical anlyses: 0, absent; +, weak; ++, moderate; +++, strong.
[b] DAF and CD59 exhibit apical staining.

the theca interna, a precursor of the corpus luteum, is responsible for hormonal secretion and is highly vascularized.

The antrum of a multilaminar follicle forms by coalescence of follicular fluid collections. This viscous, hyaluronic-acid-rich fluid contains C components (3–5) and remains at the site of extrusion of the ovum from the ovarian surface. The concentration of follicular fluid C varies substantially but the finding of C3, C4, and C5 degradation products suggests that some degree of C activation accompanies ovulation, potentially via activation of the fibrinolytic system.

Having developed in a C-containing milieu, it is not surprising that the oocyte expresses C-regulatory proteins and receptors, although there is not complete consensus on this in the literature. MCP is found (6–8), but not universally (9–10), on the plasma membrane of zona-free and zona-intact oocytes. MCP is also strongly expressed on the oocyte in developing follicles in fresh, frozen ovaries, where staining appears to coincide with the nuclear material of the oocyte (11).

In contrast, DAF and CD59 are weakly expressed or absent on the developing oocyte (11), but are expressed in variable quantity on the plasma membrane of mature oocytes and within the zona pellucida (8,10). Cumulus cells, freshly obtained or cultured following removal from oocytes, express CD59 strongly and MCP moderately, without relation to degree of differentiation (8). DAF expression is weak or undetectable on fresh cumulus cells and variable on cultured cells (8).

Anderson et al. (9) have shown CR1 and CR3, but not CR2, on the surface of zona-free fresh eggs, as well as impressive dimeric C3b binding. Taylor and Johnson (8) found most oocytes to lack C receptors, although up to 20% of aged, fixed oocytes stained for CR1, CR2, and CR3. Fenichel et al. (10) also did not detect CR1, and it was not present on the oocyte within developing follicles (11). The presence of C regulators, and to a lesser extent receptors, suggests a mechanism to protect the developing and mature oocyte from C damage and possibly a direct role in fertilization, as discussed later.

B. Corpus Luteum and Corpus Albicans

A corpus luteum forms after ovulation by transformation of the follicular remnant into a vascular, glandular structure capable of hormonal secretion. It persists as the corpus luteum of pregnancy if fertilization ensues, or involutes to a corpus albicans if not. Cytoprotection of this structure may be particularly important before the placenta is fully functional. Corpora lutea express MCP, DAF, and CD59, and corpora albicantia primarily DAF and CD59 (11). Unexpectedly, heavy DAF staining was seen on the theca lutein, or progesterone-secreting cell population, in contrast to scant DAF on the thecal population in the developing follicle, suggesting that expression may be under hormonal control.

C. Uterus: Endometrium, Cervix, and Cervical Secretion

Striking uterine changes parallel oocytic development (1). The uterine endometrium responds to estrogen by glandular proliferation; thereafter, the glands become actively secretory in response to progesterone (Fig. 1). An elaborate vasculature simultaneously develops, with prominent spiral arterioles extending from the myometrium into the endometrium. The endometrium then either forms the bed for implantation of the fertilized ovum or is sloughed during menstruation.

C3 is the predominant protein secreted by rat endometrial epithelium in response to estrogen (12,13); its secretion is blocked in the presence of antiestrogens (14) and progesterone (13,15,16). Human endometrium also secretes C3 and factor B, coincident with the secretory or luteal phase of the menstrual cycle (17,18). Concomitant C regulatory proteins expression by endometria is well documented: MCP (11,18,19) and CD59 (11,18,20) are present at all phases of the menstrual cycle. Although DAF expression may be enhanced on secretory endometria (18), it is also found on proliferative samples (11). Infiltrating mononuclear cells, but not endometrial epithelia, express CR1 and CR3. CR2 has not been observed.

The local presence of C, along with its regulators and receptors, implies a role, albeit undetermined, in mammalian reproduction. Physiologically, the diverse biological effects of C3 cleavage may influence local host defense, especially in rodent models, or mediate immune regulation during pregnancy when there is exposure to foreign antigens and substantial cellular remodeling occurs.

In contrast, pathological C activation may contribute to the inflammation and infertility associated with endometriosis. Increased C3 synthesis in endometrial explants is most pronounced in early disease when the samples are highly cellular and is variable at later stages (21). A clear relationship to upregulation of C regulatory proteins as a means of controlling this process has not been established.

The endocervix, contiguous with the uterine body, is the site of cervical mucus secretion. The physical state of this complex material, with high- and low-viscosity components, varies with the menstrual cycle. The mucus column functions as a barrier until midcycle when sperm penetrate readily. Like follicular fluid, cervical mucus contains functional C, as a result of synthesis or transudation (22,23), as well as DAF and CD59 (19).

DAF is preferentially expressed on the mature surface of exocervical stratified epithelia, while MCP expression is most prominent on the basal (immature) layer and CD59 expression is comparable throughout (11). Since MCP and DAF are now recognized as receptors for pathogens (reviewed in Chapters 7 and 18), this distribution may influence acquisition or chronicity of infections. The relationship of expression to abnormal cellular maturation, such as cervical neoplasia, is unknown.

II. MALE REPRODUCTIVE TRACT

The male reproductive system produces spermatozoa and the fluids necessary to support final sperm maturation in the female tract. C regulatory protein expression on the male reproductive tract and its fluids is summarized in Table 2.

A. Testes and Development of Spermatozoa

The testes are the site of testosterone production by Leydig cells, and of spermatogenesis, the constant process by which spermatogonia differentiate to spermatozoa (reviewed in 24). Spermatogenesis takes place in the specialized germinal epithelia lining the seminiferous tubules. The main cell populations are the supporting Sertoli cells and the germ cells, arranged in a gradient of increasing maturity from periphery to tubular lumen. Haploid spermatids terminally differentiate by spermiogenesis. This striking morphological change includes formation of an enzyme-containing acrosome that will form the anterior of the

Table 2 Characteristics of C Regulatory Protein Expression on the Male Reproductive Tract[a]

Cells/tissue	MCP[a]	Mol. mass kDa[b]	DAF[a]	Mol. mass kDa[b]	CD59[a]
Sperm					
Immature[c](testes)	+++		0/+		++
Testicular lysate		60,50–55,45 (3 bands)		70	
Capacitated	0		+, diffuse		++,diffuse
Acrosome reacted (AR)	++,iam		+,iam		++,diffuse
AR sperm lysate		38–44		44–54	
Prostatic epithelia	+++		0		++
Prostatic lysate		60		−	
Seminal plasma					
Normal[d]	682	60	1064	70	26.8
Postvasectomy[d]	562		511		14.7
Prostasomes	++		+++		+++
Non-prostasome fraction	0		+, gpi intact		+, gpi intact

Source: From refs 25−29,36−38,46,51,52.
[a] Immunohistochemical staining: 0, absent; +, weak; ++, moderate; +++, strong.
[b] Immunoblotting analyses of indicated cell/tissue lysates; Mol. mass of CD59 18—20 kDa in all samples; −, none detected
[c] Staining patterns in text.
[d] Concentration of seminal plasma MCP and DAF=ng/ml; CD59-μg/ml. Seminal plasma MCP and DAF exist as single, broad electrophoretic bands at indicated. Mol. mass. AR, acrosome reacted; iam, inner acrosomal membrane; gpi, glycolipid anchor.

sperm (Fig. 2A), acquisition of a flagellum, elongation and condensation of nuclear material, and extensive cytoplasmic phagocytosis by Sertoli cells. The end result is a mature fertilizing gamete.

Developing spermatozoa express C regulatory proteins, as documented by immuno-histochemical analyses of testes. MCP staining shows weak reactivity with immature germ cells and intense reactivity in the head (acrosomal) region of condensing spermatids (25–29). Western blotting of testicular lysates reveals three MCP bands, of 60–62 kDa, 54–56 kDa, and 45–47 kDa (28,29) and, in one case, a single band of about 45 kDa (27). These studies have proven useful in determining the source of MCP on mature sperm and in seminal plasma, as discussed later.

Simpson and Holmes (29) documented that testicular CD59 expression is weak on the germinal epithelial layer containing spermatogonia and Leydig cells and intense on differentiating germinal epithelium, whereas DAF staining is weak on germinal epithelia and on the acrosomal region of condensing sperm heads. DAF from testicular membranes has a distinctly lower mol. mass of 55 kDa compared to the about 70 kDa form detected on most other cells.

From the testes, mature, but virtually immotile, spermatids are released to the tubular lumen and pass to the head of the epididymis. During transit and epididymal storage further maturation changes occur, particularly glycosylation and deglycosylation of membrane proteins and the onset of strong, directional motility.

The final stages of sperm maturation, capacitation, and the acrosome reaction take place in the female tract following ejaculation. These are discussed in the section on fertilization, along with the unique biochemical properties and cellular localization of sperm MCP, DAF, and CD59.

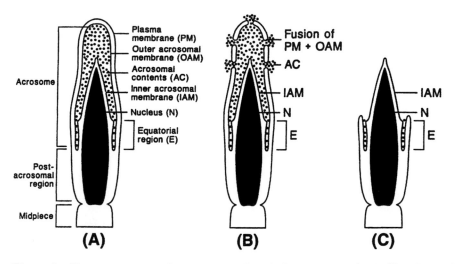

Figure 2 The acrosome reaction (AR). (A) Pre-AR human sperm in profile. (B) During AR. Acrosomal contents, primarily enzymes, released as plasma and outer acrosomal membranes fuse and acrosomal cap becomes fenestrated. (C) Post-AR sperm. IAM and equatorial region are exposed on the mature sperm. (Modified from Yanagimachi R. In Fertilization and Embryonic Development In Vitro. Mastroianni and Biggers, eds. New York: Plenum Press, 1981.)

B. Accessory Sex Glands, Seminal Plasma, and Prostasomes

Semen is composed of seminal plasma and a small volume of spermatozoa ($2–3 \times 10^8$ total cells) in fluid derived from the epididymis and vas deferens (reviewed in 24,30). Seminal plasma is derived mainly from seminal vesicle and prostatic secretions. It provides a carbohydrate energy source for sperm, immobilizes ejaculated sperm near the cervical os, and has immunomodulatory properties, including C inhibition. The source of seminal plasma proteins is determined by comparison of fluids from normal and vasectomized men. Sperm and material of testicular and epididymal origin appear only in normal samples while postvasectomy samples contain secretions from the seminal vesicles and prostate, structures distal to the transection site of the vas deferens. This distinction is important in evaluating the origin and potential function of C regulatory proteins on spermatozoa and in seminal plasma.

Seminal vesicle epithelia secrete fluid rich in prostaglandins and fructose and the proteins that facilitate semen coagulation following ejaculation. High concentrations of E series prostaglandins in seminal plasma may supress the female immune response potentially triggered by alloantigenic sperm proteins.

In contrast, prostatic fluid contains high concentrations of mono- and divalent cations, citric acid, acid phosphatase, and proteolytic enzymes that liquefy coagulated semen. MCP (28,29) and CD59 (29) are strongly expressed on prostatic epithelia, whereas DAF is undetectable. MCP on prostatic membranes exists as a single 60 kDa band and CD59 as a 18–20 kDa band. Variable expression of CD59 and DAF on glandular epithelia, as at other sites, is common and suggests that hormonal activity or cellular maturity may affect their expression.

Low-speed centrifugation of liquified semen removes most intact spermatozoa, leaving an essentially cell-free supernatant (31). Preparative ultracentrifugation of cell-free seminal plasma results in a pellet containing complex vesicular organelles derived from prostatic epithelia called prostasomes. Prostasomes are bi- or trilaminar structures, $\approx$150 nm in diameter, surrounded by a plasma membrane. They arise by either exocytosis or by direct release from the intracellular compartment as intact vesicles (31) and are capable of direct binding to spermatozoa through hydrophobic interactions (32).

The physiological role of prostasomes has not been fully explored. They contribute to the immunosuppressive activity of seminal plasma, as evidenced by diminished mitogen-stimulated lymphoproliferation and decreased macrophage phagocytosis in their presence (33). Sperm motility is also enhanced by interaction with prostasomes (34,35).

Seminal plasma also has potent C inhibitory activity and characterization of C has focused on regulatory proteins and the significance of their association with prostasomes. MCP in seminal plasma exists predominantly as a single broad band of 60 kDa, indistinguishable from that of prostate membrane preparations (28,36). A 60 kDa MCP form is also present in testicular lysates, but detection of comparable quantities of MCP in the seminal plasma of fertile and vasectomized men suggests the source to be the prostate (37). O- and N-linked sugars are present on seminal plasma MCP and C3 cofactor activity has been clearly demonstrated (28). Seminal plasma MCP has been termed "soluble" (28,38). However, Simpson and Holmes (36) demonstrated convincingly by detergent extractions that MCP was membrane associated, putatively with prostasomes, as confirmed by Kitamura et al. (39) and Rooney et al. (37).

DAF and CD59 concentrations in postvasectomy seminal plasma are approximately half that of normal donors (37). Seminal plasma CD59 has many potential sites of origin within the male tract. Seminal plasma DAF (70 kDa) may originate from the epididymis or seminal vesicles (37) since it is not found on the prostate (36) and testicular DAF is expressed in small quantity and has a distinctly different molecular mass (55 kDa).

SP40, 40 or clusterin (40–43), a fluid phase inhibitor of the membrane attack complex, is present in human seminal plasma at up to 15 mg/ml. Main sources of clusterin are the testes, epididymes, and seminal vesicles. Only a small number of abnormal or immature sperm express clusterin.

Human clusterin (42) shares 77% homology with sulfated glycoprotein-2 or SGP-2, a major secretory protein of rat Sertoli cells (44). In contrast to human clusterin (43), rat clusterin is associated with the plasma membrane of normal developing and mature spermatozoa (45). Rodent and human studies suggest that this protein is important in male fertility, whether in a role similar to a conventional C regulatory protein or via its adhesive, non-C-related, properties (42,43).

Several interesting observations resulted from characterization of seminal plasma CD59 and DAF. Initially it was shown that CD59 was present at >20 μg/ml in unfractionated seminal plasma and that cells exposed to seminal plasma incorporated functional CD59 (46). The majority of the CD59 was prostasome-associated, suggesting a physiological mechanism for protein replacement and a pathological mechanism for microbial persistence in the reproductive tracts. Subsequently, DAF and CD59 were also found in the nonprostasome fractions, as high-molecular-mass aggregates, with their lipid anchors intact (37). Prostasomes bound to nucleated and nonnucleated cell surfaces but did not transfer their contents to the cytoplasm or fuse with the cell membranes. Cells also acquired CD59, putatively through the lipid anchor, during incubation with the nonprostasome fraction. This suggests two basic mechanisms for spermatozoa to acquire seminal plasma proteins that may affect their survival, maturation, or fertilization capacity. The expression of C regulatory proteins on prostasomes per se also provides a mechanism for their own preservation from C attack, and for that of mature sperm when there is no active protein synthesis.

III. SELECTED ASPECTS OF FERTILIZATION

Mammalian fertilization and the final maturational events of spermatozoa, capacitation and the acrosome reaction (Fig. 2) take place in the female tract, where an intact C system is present.

A. Sperm Maturation: Capacitation and the Acrosome Reaction

Capacitation (reviewed in 47–49) results in numerous changes to the topology and net charge of the sperm surface but not to its morphology. The process proceeds over 3–15 h, physiologically, as ejaculated sperm contact cervical mucus, or in vitro, by exposure to follicular fluid or hypertonic media. Capacitated sperm are capable of binding to the oocyte zona pellucida and undergoing the acrosome reaction (reviewed in 49) as follows (Fig. 2). The outer acrosomal membrane fuses with the sperm plasma membrane, allowing release of enzymes and exposure of the antigenically distinct inner acrosomal membrane covering the anterior sperm surface and equatorial region. Acrosome-reacted spermatozoa represent the fully mature gamete, capable of further penetration through the zona pellucida in a process facilitated by acrosin, a trypsinlike inner acrosomal protease that also cleaves C3.

Characterization of C regulatory proteins on human spermatozoa provided several unexpected observations. First, capacitated, non-acrosome-reacted sperm express CD59 strongly, and DAF weakly, from head to tail (8,29,50) whereas no MCP is present (8,51). After the acrosome reaction, MCP is revealed on the inner acrosomal membrane and equatorial region (8,9,25,29,51). The equatorial region is often the site of contact with the oolemma: proteins expressed there are strategically located for interaction during fertilization. DAF expression is predominantly on the inner acrosomal membrane (8,29,52) following the acrosome reaction, while CD59 staining remains diffuse, with occasional postequatorial staining (29,53).

Next, sperm MCP (51) and DAF (52), in contrast to all other cells, were shown to have substantially lower than expected size-MCP at 38–44 kDa and DAF at 44–54 kDa. O-linked glycosylation of the serine and threonine rich (ST) domains of MCP and DAF contributes significantly to their mass and alternative splicing of the ST of MCP accounts in part for its isoforms (see Chapter 7). Sperm MCP mol. mass also bears no relation to the donor's peripheral blood mononuclear cell MCP phenotype. The C-regulatory activities of MCP and DAF are intact despite glycosylation differences (51,52). The origin of the lower mol. mass forms has not been elucidated. The most likely explanation is differential glycosylation of the ST domains during sperm maturation (51), since removal of the ST region adversely affects DAF (54) and MCP function and the size of MCP and DAF does not change after the acrosome reaction (52).

Expression of functional C regulatory proteins on spermatozoa provides a mechanism for their safe transit through the female tract where C activation is possible through the classical or alternative pathways, as suggested by in vitro models (50,55,56), or via physiological turnover of C3. The causative relationship of antisperm antibodies and C activation to infertility is still debated but it appears that normal protective mechanisms can be overridden in certain cases (56).

B. Zona Binding and Gamete Fusion

Two major processes in fertilization, zona pellucida binding and sperm–oolemmal fusion, are the subject of continuing study (49,57–60). Sperm binding to the zona pellucida occurs prior to or concomitant with initiation of the acrosome reaction and is species-specific. Zona binding in mice is mediated primarily through the glycoprotein zona-binding protein 3 or ZP3 (57). ZP3 interacts with one or more putative egg binding proteins on sperm including β-galactosyl-transferase (61,62); p95, a protein possibly autophosphorylated by tyrosine kinase activity (63,64); and sp56 (65). The latter, a 56 kDa murine sperm-specific protein, has homology to C proteins via its seven CCP modules (66). β-Galactosyl-transferase (62) and sp56 (67) each interact with an O-linked carbohydrate moiety of ZP3, suggesting that carbohydrate-mediated cellular adhesion may be important in zona binding.

Oolemmal fusion with a spermatozoon is immediately followed by reactions in the oolemma and the zona to prevent polyspermy and to activate the oocyte (reviewed in 68,69). Sperm contact with the oolemma occurs at the equatorial or postacrosomal region. Fusion of male and female pronuclei produces a diploid zygote, and cell division leads to formation of a preimplantation blastocyst that travels through the C-containing fallopian tube to reach the uterus. At the preimplantation stage MCP, DAF, and CD59 are consistently expressed (6,8,10); however, there is not consensus about when expression begins.

The mechanism of gamete recognition and subsequent membrane fusion has been likened to that of viral infection of eukaryotic cells (reviewed in 68). Identification of several putative fusion and binding proteins suggests that multiple interactions may be necessary for fertilization. Several lines of investigation support a role for C, although a precise mechanism is not determined, nor are the anticipated alternative functions of these proteins, clearly proven.

In independent findings, MCP monoclonal antibodies H316 (25) and MH61 (70) were reported to inhibit human sperm penetration of zona-free hamster eggs. Later, the ability of MCP monoclonal antibodies TRA-2-10 and MH61 to inhibit human sperm penetration of human zona-free eggs was directly compared (7). A significant decrease in sperm binding and pronuclei formation was found when both sperm and eggs (but not one or the other) were preincubated with TRA-2-10 only. The epitope recognized by TRA-2-10 (and H316) is within the first CCP module of MCP (71), while MH61 blocks C3-regulatory activities that are associated primarily with CCP 3 and 4 (71). CCP 1 is critical for measles virus binding (72) and is thus a potential site of interaction for a novel non-C ligand(s).

Anderson and colleagues (9) have proposed that C3b and its degradation products, as generated by proteolytic cleavage or alternative pathway activation, may interact with C3 receptors and regulators expressed differentially on the sperm inner acrosomal membrane and the oolemma to effect gamete binding. Evidence supporting this entailed immunohistochemical demonstration of MCP on acrosome-reacted sperm and the receptors CR1 and CR3 on zona-free oocytes; intense C3b dimer binding to zona-free oocytes; demonstration of C3 α chain cleavage by the acrosomal protease acrosin; and the concentration-dependent ability of C3b dimers to enhance or inhibit egg penetration. Along with a mechanism for fertilization based upon C3 cleavage, they also suggest that oocyte CR3 may interact with the sperm PH-30, a disintegrin.

Other C-related interactions in vitro include C1q binding to receptors on sperm, and alteration of sperm–egg binding and penetration in the presence of C1q (73) and significant, dose-dependent decreases in both human sperm binding to zona-free hamster eggs and in sperm penetration in the presence of an anti-CD59 monoclonal antibody (53).

IV. IMPLANTATION AND PLACENTAL DEVELOPMENT

Once the rapidly dividing zygote reaches the uterine cavity, 4–5 days after fertilization, two cell populations separate: an inner cell mass becomes the embryo, and the outer cell mass, or trophoblast, becomes the placenta. After superficial attachment to the endometrial epithelium, the trophoblast rapidly proliferates and differentiates into cytotrophoblast cells that encircle the blastocyst and migrate into the endometrial epithelium. Within the maternal endometrial surface and the underlying stroma (decidua) the cytotrophoblast cells fuse and become the multinucleate syncytiotrophoblast. By week two, chorionic villi form (Fig. 3). They acquire an extraembryonic mesodermal core and surrounded by villous cytotrophoblast and syncytiotrophoblast layers. Capillaries derived from the mesoderm eventually become part of the fetal circulation. By the 8th week, chorionic villi are restricted to a circular area that forms the placenta. The peripheral surface of the chorion (smooth) is covered by the remnant of the trophoblast, the chorionic laeve, which fuses

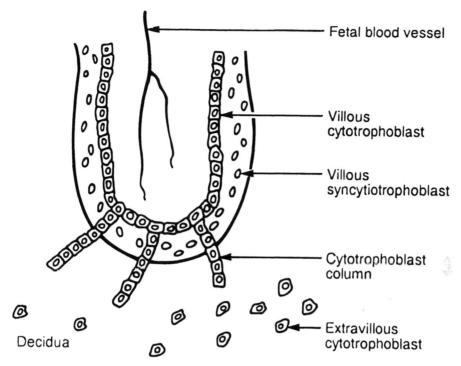

Figure 3 Early chorionic villus with trophoblast populations. Villous syncytiotrophoblast (multinucleate) and cytotrophoblast columns arise from villous cytotrophoblast. Extravillous cytotrophoblast includes cells free in decidua (interstitial), in maternal vessels (endovascular), and isolated giant cells. Trophoblast populations are characterized in Table 3 and in the text. (From Ref. 82.)

with the amnion to form the amniochorionic membrane (Fig. 4). The fully developed placenta actively synthesizes proteins, has a vast surface area for nutrient transport and waste removal, serves as an endocrine organ, and is essential to sustaining pregnancy (reviewed in 74,75).

A. Trophoblast Populations, the Fetomaternal Interface, and Trophoblast–Lymphocyte Cross-Reactive Antibodies

The fetomaternal interface is anatomically and immunologically difficult to conceptualize (76–79). The focus will thus be on characterization of the trophoblast, documented sites of C deposition, and the differential expression of C regulatory proteins (Table 3).

The collective term "trophoblast" (Fig. 3) describes several fetal cell populations (77,80–82) as follows. Villous cytotrophoblast is located between the mesenchymal core and the villous syncytiotrophoblast and is the source of cells that differentiate to become the amorphous villous syncytiotrophoblast. Villous cytotrophoblast does not have direct maternal contact and progressivley decreases with placental development.

Villous syncytiotrophoblast is exposed to maternal blood and represents the major fetomaternal interface. In this strategic location, syncytiotrophoblast neither expresses HLA molecules nor contains mRNA for them at any stage of pregnancy.

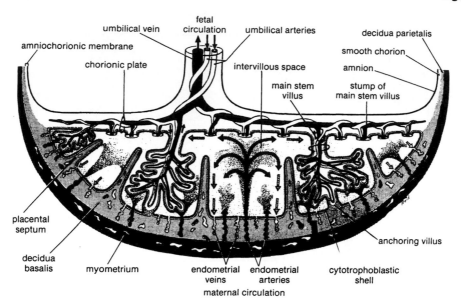

Figure 4 Schematic representation of the term placenta. Fetally derived structures: amniochorionic membrane, chorionic plate, main stem villi containing cytotrophoblastic shell and anchoring villus, amnion, smooth chorion. Maternal tissues: decidua basalis, decidua parietalis, placental septae, and myometrium. Contact sites include maternal blood bathing projections from fetal mainstem villi (villous chorion), anchoring villi abutting decidua basalis, amniochorionic membrane, and decidua parietalis. The respective fetal (umbilical vein and two arteries) and maternal circulation (endometrial, spiral or uteroplacental arteries and veins) are as shown. (From Ref. 75.)

Extravillous cytotrophoblast includes the trophoblast columns that anchor the villi, the interstitial cytotrophoblast cells that exist free in the decidua, the endovascular trophoblast that invade maternal vessels, the chorionic trophoblast, abutting the uterine wall and associated with the chorionic laeve and isolated trophoblast giant cells. To varying degrees, extravillous cytotrophoblast have contact with maternal decidua and vasculature. Extravillous cytotrophoblast express the nonclassical, nonpolymorphic, putatively nonantigenic HLA-G molecule whose function is unknown.

Maternal exposure to fetal antigens may also result from pulmonary embolization of placental fragments, from trophoblast found in the maternal peripheral circulation, and from fetal leukocytes and erythrocytes that enter the maternal circulation at delivery. Despite this, and the fact that as many as 60% of multiparous women develop anti-HLA antibodies, severe immunological sequelae usually do not result (reviewed in 78).

TLX antibodies, which occur in the sera of a subset of women who have experienced recurrent abortions, may represent an exception (reviewed in 5,83,84). They are thought to arise in response to an alloantigen(s) common to trophoblast and lymphocytes. TLX also describes a set of monoclonal antibodies produced against placental membranes and hematopoietic cell lines (85–89). Unexpectedly, monoclonals such as H316, GB24, E4.3, and TRA-2-10 recognize MCP (all isoforms, including sperm MCP) (71,90,91). It is unlikely that MCP represents the sole TLX alloantigen; certain maternal sera do react with C3b-bound MCP but not all sera with TLX antibodies immunoprecipitate MCP.

Table 3 Characteristics of the Fetoplacental Unit

Trophoblast population	Maternal exposure	HLA[a] surface	HLA[a] mRNA	MCP[b,c]	DAF[b,c]	CD59[b,c]
First trimester						
Syncytiotrophoblast	Blood	0	0	++	++	++++
Villous cytotrophoblast	None	0	+	++++	0/+	++++
Cytotrophoblast columns	+/− Decidua			++	++++	++++
Interstitial extravillous cytotrophoblast	Decidua	++	++	++	+	++++
Term						
Syncytiotrophoblast	Blood	0	+/0	+++	+++	++++
Basal plate (BP) and chorionic (C) extravillous cytotrophoblast	Decidua	+	+	++	++++, BP ++,C	++++

Source: From refs 77,79,93,94.

[a] HLA=class I HLAG, described in text.

[b] Immunohistochemical staining: 0, absent; +, absent; +, weak; ++, moderate; +++, strong; ++++, extremely intense.

[c] Immonoblotting analyses of cell or tissue lysates. MCP phenotype varied among individual samples, 2 bands at 55−65 kDa. In all samples DAF, 70 kDa; CD59, 18−20 kDa.

B. C Regulatory Proteins on the Placenta

MCP, DAF, and CD59 are differentially expressed on trophoblast populations (Table 3), from as early as several weeks of gestation, and vary with placental age (77,79,85,92–94).

Villous cytotrophoblast, most isolated in terms of maternal exposure and actively dividing during the first trimester, has intense MCP and considerably less DAF expression. Increased MCP on neoplastic cells suggests that cellular proliferation or immaturity may be a factor in expression, as may be the case with trophoblast. DAF expression, in contrast, appears to intensify with advancing placental age and with distance from the villi and thus enhanced maternal contact, for example on apical syncytiotrophoblast. Here, some degree of C activation and cellular maturation may influence DAF expression while its apical expression may enhance efficiency of C inactivation. CD59, as the primary MAC regulator, is intensely expressed on all populations, throughout pregnancy.

C. C Deposition on Normal and Pathological Placentae

Immunohistological analyses of normal preterm and term placentae have shown differential C deposition with C1q staining in chorionic villi, in contrast to C3c, C3d, and C9 detected on the trophoblast basement membrane (95). Sinha et al. (96) confirmed the anatomical localization of C deposition on normal tissue and found significantly more C deposition on preeclamptic placentae. Presence of the potentially cytolytic MAC, detected by anti-C9 neoantigen, was confirmed in a direct comparison of normal and preeclamptic term placentae (97). The most intense C9 staining in normal placentae was located in the fibrinoid area of the basal plate decidua where it was not colocalized with S-protein, indicating some degree of continuing C activation. Less C9 was found in the mature villi, in association with S protein. Preeclamptic placentae showed more intense deposition in the same locations.

Tedesco et al. (98) also established that a syncytiotrophoblast population could be lysed in vitro by C via classical pathway activation or reactive lysis, and that the susceptibility was enhanced when MCP and CD59 function was blocked.

Vascular deposition of C1, C4, C3d, and C9, in addition to fibrinogen, has been described in the uteroplacental spiral arteries and interstitial trophoblast, but not veins or endometrial glands, of normal placentae (99).

Uteroplacental arteries are a prime site for local C activation. They contain endovascular trophoblast and undergo histological change, following fibrinoid deposition, to facilitate high blood flow and low resistance. Differential C deposition is seen on endometrial vessels in subinvolution of the uteroplacental arteries, a cause of postpartum hemorrhage (100). The normally involuted vessels contain substantial immunoglobulin, fibrinogen, and C in contrast to virtually no deposition on the abnormal subinvoluted vessels. A physiological role of C is presumably related to normal reendothelialization of the vessels and vascular remodeling.

The role C plays in normal and pathological pregnancies remains unknown. As noted, C deposition and villitis (101) in normal placentae suggests a physiological mechanism for removal of immune complexes in the chorionic villi (95) and a mechanism for dealing with local cellular turnover, or continuous low-grade C activation, particularly since significant systemic C activation in normal pregnancy is not typical (reviewed in 102). Similar deposition, in some cases quantitatively more impressive, has been seen in diabetes, systemic lupus erythematosus, preeclampsia, and intrauterine growth retardation in which integrity of the placental bed is suspect (reviewed in 103). In such cases, C activation, with its myriad proinflammatory sequelae, may follow immunological attack of placental trophoblast or endothelia and overcome cytoprotective mechanisms.

REFERENCES

1. Blandau RJ. The female reproductive system. In: Weiss L, ed. Histology: Cell and Tissue Biology, 5th ed. New York: Elsevier Biomedical, 1983:914–943.
2. Greenwald GS, Roy SK. Follicular development and its control. In: Knobil E, Neill JD, Greenwald GS, Markert CL, Pfaff DW, eds. The Physiology of Reproduction, 2nd ed. New York: Raven Press, 1994:629–724.
3. Perricone R, De Carolis C, Moretti C, Santuari E, De Sanctis G, Fontana L. Complement, complement activation and anaphylatoxins in human ovarian follicular fluid. Clin Exp Immunol 1990; 82:359–362.
4. Perricone R, Pasetto N, De Carolis C, et al. Functionally active complement is present in human ovarian follicular fluid and can be activated by seminal plasma. Clin Exp Immunol 1992; 89:154–157.
5. Vanderpuye OA, Labarrere CA, McIntyre JA. The complement system in human reproduction. Am J Reprod Immunol 1992; 27:145–155.
6. Roberts JM, Taylor CT, Melling GC, Kingsland CR, Johnson PM. Expression of the CD46 antigen, and absence of class I MHC antigen, on the human oocyte and preimplantation blastocyst. Immunology 1992; 75:202–205.
7. Taylor CT, Biljan MM, Kingsland CR, Johnson PM. Inhibition of human spermatozoon-oocyte interaction in vitro by monoclonal antibodies to CD46 (membrane cofactor protein). Hum Reprod 1994; 9:907–911.

8. Taylor CT, Johnson PM. Complement-binding proteins are strongly expressed by human preimplantation blastocysts and cumulus cells as well as gametes. Mol Hum Reprod 1996; 2:52–59.

9. Anderson DJ, Abbott AF, Jack RM. The role of complement component C3b and its receptors in sperm-oocyte interaction. Proc Natl Acad Sci USA 1993; 90:10051–10055.

10. Fenichel P, Donzeau M, Cervoni F, Menezo Y, Hsi BL. Expression of complement regulatory proteins on human eggs and preimplantation embryos. Am J Reprod Immunol 1995; 33:155–164.

11. Oglesby TJ, Longwith JE, Huettner PC. Human complement regulator expression by the normal human female reproductive tract. Anat Rec 1996; 46:78–86.

12. Sundstrom SA, Komm BS, Ponce-de-Leon H, Yi Z, Teuscher C, Lyttle CR. Estrogen regulation of tissue-specific expression of complement C3. J Biol Chem 1989; 264:16941–16947.

13. Kuivanen PC, Capulong RB, Harkins RN, DeSombre ER. The estrogen-responsive 110K and 74K rat uterine secretory proteins are structurally related to complement component C3. Biochem Biophys Res Commun 1989; 158:898–905.

14. Galman MS, Sundstrom SA, Lyttle CR. Antagonism of estrogen- and antiestrogen-induced uterine complement component C3 expression by ICI 164, 384. J Steroid Biochem 1990; 36:281–286.

15. Brown EO, Sundstrom SA, Komm BS, Yi Z, Teuscher C, Lyttle CR. Estrogen regulation of tissue-specific expression of complement C3. Biol Reprod 1990; 42:713–719.

16. Hasty LA, Lyttle CR. Progesterone and RU486 regulation of uterine complement C3 after prior induction with estradiol. Biol Reprod 1992; 47:285–290.

17. Hasty LA, Brockman WO, Lambris JD, Lyttle CR. Hormonal regulation of complement factor B in human endometrium. Am J Reprod Immunol 1993; 30:63–67.

18. Hasty LA, Lambris JD, Lessey BA, Pruksananonda K, Lyttle CR. Hormonal regulation of complement components and receptors throughout the menstrual cycle. Am J Obstet Gynecol 1994; 170:168–175.

19. Jensen TS, Bjorge L, Wollen AL, Ulstein M. Identification of the complement regulatory proteins CD46, CD55, and CD59 in human fallopian tube, endometrium, and cervical mucosa and secretion. Am J Reprod Immunol 1995; 34:1–9.

20. Ratnoff WD, Brockman WW, Hasty LA. Immunohistochemical localization of C9 neoantigen and the terminal complement inhibitory protein CD59 in human endometrium. Am J Reprod Immunol 1995; 34:72–79.

21. Isaacson KB, Galman M, Coutifaris C, Lyttle CR. Endometrial synthesis and secretion of complement component-3 by patients with and without endometriosis. Fertil Steril 1990; 53:836–841.

22. Price RJ, Boettcher B. The presence of complement in human cervical mucus and its possible relevance to infertility in women with complement dependent sperm immobilising antibodies. Fertil Steril 1979; 32:61–66.

23. Schumacher GFB. Immunology and spermatozoa and cervical mucus. Hum Reprod 1988; 3:289–300.

24. Dym M. The male reproductive system. In: Weiss L, ed. Histology: Cell and Tissue Biology, 5th ed. New York: Elsevier Biomedical, 1983:1000–1053.

25. Anderson DJ, Michaelson JS, Johnson PM. Trophoblast/leukocyte-common antigen is expressed by human testicular germ cells and appears on the surface of acrosome-reacted sperm. Biol Reprod 1989; 41:285–293.

26. Fenichel P, Dohr G, Grivaux C, Cervoni F, Donzeau M, Hsi BL. Localization and characterization of the acromosal antigen recognized by GB24 on human spermatozoa. Mol Reprod Dev 1990; 27:173 178.

27. Cervoni F, Fenichel P, Akhoundi C, Hsi BL, Rossi B. Characterization of a cDNA clone coding the human testis membrane cofactor protein (MCP, CD46). Mol Reprod Dev 1993; 34:107–113.

28. Seya T, Hara T, Matsumoto M. Membrane cofactor protein (MCP, CD46) in seminal plasma and on spermatozoa in normal and "sterile" subjects. Eur J Immunol 1993; 23:1322–1327.

29. Simpson KL, Holmes CH. Differential expression of complement regulatory proteins decay-accelerating factor (CD55), membrane cofactor protein (CD46) and CD59 during human spermatogenesis. Immunology 1994; 81:452–461.

30. Luke MC, Coffey DS. The male sex accessory tissues: structure, androgen action, and physiology. In: Knobil E, Neill JD, Greenwald GS, Markert CL, Pfaff DW, eds. The Physiology of Reproduction, 2nd ed. New York: Raven Press, 1994:1435–1487.

31. Ronquist G, Brody I. The prostasome: its secretion and function in man. Biochim Biophys Acta 1985; 822:203–218.

32. Ronquist G, Nilsson BO, Hjerten S. Interaction between prostasomes and spermatozoa from human semen. Arch Androl 1990; 24:147–157.

33. Kelly RW, Holland P, Sibinski G, et al. Extracellular organelles (prostasomes) are immunosuppressive components of human semen. Clin Exp Immunol 1991; 86:550–556.

34. Stegmayr B, Ronquist G. Stimulation of sperm progressive motility by organelles in human seminal plasma. Scand J Urol Nephrol 1982; 16:85–90.

35. Stegmayr B, Ronquist G. Promotive effect on human sperm motility by prostasomes. Urol Res 1982; 10:253–257.

36. Simpson KL, Holmes CH. Presence of the complement-regulatory protein membrane cofactor protein (MCP, CD46) as a membrane-associated product in seminal plasma. J Reprod Fertil 1994; 102:419–424.

37. Rooney IA, Heuser JE, Atkinson JP. GPI-anchored complement regulatory proteins in seminal plasma. J Clin Invest 1996; 97:1675–1686.

38. Hara T, Kuriyama S, Kiyohara H, Nagase Y, Matsumoto M, Seya T. Soluble forms of membrane cofactor protein (CD46, MCP) are present in plasma, tears, and seminal fluid in normal subjects. Clin Exp Immunol 1992; 89:490–494.

39. Kitamura M, Namiki M, Matsumiya K, et al. Membrane cofactor protein (CD46) in seminal plasma is a protasome-bound form with complement regulatory activity and measles virus neutralizing activity. Immunology 1995; 84:626–632.

40. Jenne DE, Tschopp J. Molecular structure and functional characterization of a human complement cytolysis inhibitor found in blood and seminal plasma: identity to sulfated glycoprotein 2, a constituent of rat testis fluid. Proc Natl Acad Sci USA 1989; 86:7123–7127.

41. Choi NH, Mazda T, Tomita M. A serum protein SP-40, 40 modulates the formation of membrane attack complex of complement on erythrocytes. Mol Immunol 1989; 26:835–840.

42. Kirszbaum L, Sharpe JA, Murphy B, et al. Molecular cloning and characterization of the novel, human complement-associated protein, SP-40, 40: a link between the complement and reproductive systems. EMBO J 1989; 8:711–718.

43. O'Bryan MK, Baker HWG, Saunders JR, et al. Human seminal clusterin (SP-40, 40): isolation and characterization. J Clin Invest 1990; 85:1477–1486.

44. Collard MW, Griswold MD. Biosynthesis and molecular cloning of sulfated glycoprotein 2 secreted by rat Sertoli cells. Biochemistry 1987; 26:3297–3303.

45. Sylvester S, Morales C, Oko R, Griswold M. Localization of sulfated glycoprotein-2 (Clusterin) on spermatozoa and in the reproductive tract of the male rat. Biol Reprod 1991; 45:195–207.

46. Rooney IA, Atkinson JP, Krul ES, et al. Physiologic relevance of the membrane attack complex inhibitory protein CD59 in human seminal plasma: CD59 is present on extracellular organelles (prostasomes), binds cell membranes and inhibits complement-mediated lysis. J Exp Med 1993; 177:1409–1420.

47. Langlais J, Roberts KD. A molecular membrane model of sperm capacitation and the acrosome reaction of mammalian spermatozoa. Gamete Res 1985; 12:183–224.

48. Wassarman PM. Early events in mammalian fertilization. Annu Rev Cell Biol 1987; 3:109–142.

49. Yanagimachi R. Mammalian fertilization. In: Knobil E, Neill JD, Greenwald GS, Markert CL, Pfaff DW, eds. The Physiology of Reproduction, 2nd ed. New York: Raven Press, 1994:189–317.

50. Rooney IA, Davies A, Morgan BP. Membrane attack complex (MAC)-mediated damage to spermatozoa: protection of the cells by the presence on their membranes of MAC inhibitory proteins. Immunology 1992; 75:499–506.

51. Cervoni F, Oglesby TJ, Adams EM, et al. Identification and characterization of membrane cofactor protein (MCP) on human spermatozoa. J Immunol 1992; 148:1431–1437.

52. Cervoni F, Oglesby TJ, Fenichel P, et al. Expression of decay accelerating factor (CD55) of the complement system on human spermatozoa. J Immunol 1993; 151:939–948.

53. Fenichel P, Cervoni F, Hofmann P, et al. Expression of the complement regulatory protein CD59 on human spermatozoa: characterization and role in gametic interaction. Mol Reprod Dev 1994; 38:338–346.

54. Coyne KE, Hall SE, Thompson ES, et al. Mapping of epitopes, glycosylation sites, and complement regulatory domains in human decay accelerating factor. J Immunol 1992; 149:2906–2913.

55. D'Cruz OJ, Haas Jr. GG, Wang B, DeBault LE. Activation of human complement by IgG antisperm antibody and the demonstration of C3 and C5b-9-mediated immune injury to human sperm. J Immunol 1991; 146:611–620.

56. D'Cruz OJ, Haas Jr. GG. The expression of the complement regulators CD46, CD55, and CD59 by human sperm does not protect them from antisperm antibody- and complement-mediated immune injury. Fertil Steril 1993; 59:876–884.

57. Wassarman PM. The biology and chemistry of fertilization. Science 1987; 235:553–560.

58. Ward CR, Kopf GS. Molecular events mediating sperm activation. Dev Biol 1993; 158:9–34.

59. Dunbar BS, Avery S, Lee V, et al. The mammalian zona pellucida: its biochemistry, immuno-chemistry, molecular biology, and developmental expression. Reprod Fertil Dev 1994; 6:331–347.

60. Schultz RM, Kopf GS. Molecular basis of mammalian egg activation. Curr Top Dev Biol 1995; 30:21–62.

61. Benau DA, McGuire EJ, Storey BT. Further characterization of the mouse sperm surface zona-binding site with galactosyltransferase activity. Mol Reprod Dev 1990; 25:393–399.

62. Miller DJ, Macek MB, Shur BD. Complementarity between sperm surface B-1, 4-galactosyl-transferase and egg-coat ZP3 mediates sperm egg binding. Nature 1992; 357:589–592.

63. Burks DJ, Carballada R, Moore HD, Saling PM. Interaction of a tyrosine kinase from human sperm with the zona pellucida at fertilization. Science 1995; 269:83–86.

64. Leyton L, Tomes C, Saling PM. LL95 monoclonal antibody mimics functional effects of ZP3 on mouse sperm: evidence that the antigen recognized is not hexokinase. Mol Reprod Dev 1995; 42:347–358.

65. Bleil JD, Wassarman PM. Identification of a ZP3-binding protein on acrosome-intact mouse sperm by photoaffinity crosslinking. Proc Natl Acad Sci USA 1990; 87:5563–5567.

66. Bookbinder LH, Cheng A, Bleil JD. Tissue- and species-specific expression of sp56, a mouse sperm fertilization protein. Science 1995; 269:86–89.

67. Cheng A, Le T, Palacios M, et al. Sperm–egg recognition in the mouse: characterization of sp56, a sperm protein having specific affinity for ZP3. J Cell Biol 1994; 125:867–878.

68. Myles DG. Molecular mechanisms of sperm–egg membrane binding and fusion in mammals. Dev Biol 1993; 158:35–45.

69. Green DPL. Mammalian fertilization as a biological machine: a working model for adhesion and fusion of sperm and oocyte. Hum Reprod 1993; 8:91–96.

70. Okabe M, Nagira M, Kawai Y, Matsno S, Mimura T, Mayumi T. A human sperm antigen possibly involved in binding and/or fusion with zona-free hamster eggs. Fertil Steril 1990; 54:1121–1126.

71. Adams EM, Brown MC, Nunge M, Krych M, Atkinson JP. Contribution of the repeating domains of membrane cofactor protein (CD46) of the complement system to ligand binding and cofactor activity. J Immunol 1991; 147:3005–3011.

72. Manchester M, Valsamakis A, Kaufman R, et al. Measles virus and C3 binding sites are distinct on membrane cofactor protein (MCP; CD46). Proc Natl Acad Sci USA 1995; 92:2303–2307.

73. Fusi F, Bronson RA, Hong Y, Ghebrehiwet B. Complement component C1q and its receptor are involved in the interaction of human sperm with zona-free hamster eggs. Mol Reprod Dev 1991; 29:180–188.

74. Padykula HA. The Human Placenta. In: Weiss L, ed. Histology: Cell and Tissue Biology, 5th ed. New York: Elsevier Biomedical, 1983:966–999.

75. Moore KL. The placenta and fetal membranes. In: Moore KL, ed. The Developing Human, 4th ed. Philadelphia: W. B. Saunders, 1988:104–130.

76. Young M. The nature of the feto-maternal physiological relationship. In: Stern CMM, ed. Immunology of Pregnancy and its Disorders. Boston: Kluwer Academic Publishers, 1989:1–32.

77. Hunt JS, Hsi BL. Evasive strategies of trophoblast cells: selective expression of membrane antigens. Am J Reprod Immunol 1990; 23:57–63.

78. Billington WD. The normal fetomaternal immune relationship. Clin Obstet Gynaecol 1992; 6:417–438.

79. Holmes CH, Simpson KL. Complement and pregnancy: new insights into the immunobiology of the fetomaternal relationship. Clin Obstet Gynaecol 1992; 6:439–460.

80. Bulmer JN, Johnson PM. Antigen expression by trophoblast populations in the placenta and their possible immunological relevance. Placenta 1985; 6:127–140.

81. Loke YW. Human trophoblast antigens. In: Stern CMM, ed. Immunology of Pregnancy and its Disorders. Boston: Kluwer Academic Publishers, 1989:61–90.

82. Rooney IA, Oglesby TJ, Atkinson JP. Complement in human reproduction: activation and control. Immunol Res 1993; 12:276–294.

83. McIntyre JA. In search of trophoblast-lymphocyte crossreactive (TLX) antigens. Am J Reprod Immunol 1988; 17:100–110.

84. McIntyre JA. Immune recognition at the maternal-fetal interface: overview. Am J Reprod Immunol 1992; 28:127–131.

85. Johnson PM, Cheng HM, Molloy CM, Stern CMM, Slade MB. Human trophoblast-specific surface antigens identified using monoclonal antibodies. Am J Reprod Immunol 1981; 1:246–254.

86. Sparrow RL, McKenzie IFC. HuLy-m5: a unique antigen physically associated with HLA molecules. Hum Immunol 1983; 7:1–15.

87. Andrews PW, Knowles BB, Parkar M, Pym B, Stanley K, Goodfellow PN. A human cell-surface antigen defined by a monoclonal antibody and controlled by a gene on human chromosome 1. Ann Hum Genet 1985; 49:31–39.

88. Stern PL, Beresford N, Thomspon S, Johnson PM, Webb PD, Hole N. Characterization of the human trophoblast-leukocyte antigenic molecules defined by a monoclonal antibody. J Immunol 1986; 137:1604–1609.

89. Hsi BL, Yeh C-JG, Fenichel P, Samson M, Grivaux C. Monoclonal antibody GB24 recognizes a trophoblast-lymphocyte cross-reactive antigen. Am J Reprod Immunol Microbiol 1988; 18:21–27.

90. Purcell DFJ, McKenzie IFC, Lublin DM, et al. The human cell surface glycoproteins HuLy-m5, membrane cofactor protein (MCP) of the complement system, and trophoblast-leukocyte common (TLX) antigen, are CD46. Immunology 1990; 70:155–161.

91. Cho SW, Oglesby TJ, Hsi BL, Adams EM, Atkinson JP. Characterization of three monoclonal antibodies to membrane cofactor protein (MCP) of the complement system and quantification of MCP by radioassay. Clin Exp Immunol 1991; 83:257–261.

92. Holmes CH, Simpson KL, Wainwright SD, et al. Preferential expression of the complement regulatory protein decay accelerating factor at the fetomaternal interface during human pregnancy. J Immunol 1990; 144:3099–3105.

93. Hsi BL, Hunt JS, Atkinson JP. Differential expression of complement regulatory proteins on subpopulations of human trophoblast cells. J Reprod Immunol 1991; 19:209–223.

94. Holmes CH, Simpson KL, Okada H, et al. Complement regulatory proteins at the feto-maternal interface during human placental development: distribution of CD59 by comparison with membrane cofactor protein (CD46) and decay accelerating factor (CD55). Eur J Immunol 1992; 22:1579–1585.

95. Faulk WP, Jarret R, Keane M, Johnson PM, Boackle RJ. Immunological studies of human placentae: complement components in immature and mature chorionic villi. Clin Exp Immunol 1980; 40:299–305.

96. Sinha D, Wells M, Faulk WP. Immunological studies of human placentae: complement components in pre-eclamptic chorionic villi. Clin Exp Immunol 1984; 56:175–184.

97. Tedesco F, Radillo O, Candussi G, Nazzaro A, Mollnes TE, Pecorari D. Immunohistochemical detection of terminal complement complex and S protein in normal and pre-eclamptic placentae. Clin Exp Immunol 1990; 80:236–240.

98. Tedesco F, Narchi G, Radillo O, Meri S, Ferrone S, Betterle C. Susceptibility of human trophoblast to killing by human complement and the role of the complement regulatory proteins. J Immunol 1993; 151:1562–1570.

99. Wells M, Bennett J, Bulmer JN, Jackson P, Holgate CS. Complement component deposition in utero-placental (spiral) arteries in normal human pregnancy. J Reprod Immunol 1987; 12:125–135.

100. Andrew A, Bulmer JN, Morrison L, Wells M, Buckley CH. Subinvolution of the uteroplacental arteries: an immunohistochemical study. Int J Gynecol Pathol 1993; 12:28–33.

101. Labarrere CA, McIntyre JA, Faulk WP. Immunohistologic evidence that villitis in human normal term placentas is an immunologic lesion. Am J Obstet Gynecol 1990; 162:515–522.

102. Abramson SB, Buyon JP. Activation of the complement pathway: comparison of normal pregnancy, preeclampsia, and systemic lupus erythematosus during pregnancy. Am J Reprod Immunol 1992; 28:183–187.

103. Bulmer JN. Immune aspects of pathology of the placental bed contributing to pregnancy pathology. Clin Obstet Gynaecol 1992; 6:461–488.

17

Bacteria and Complement

FRANZ PETRY and MICHAEL LOOS
Johannes Gutenberg-University, Mainz, Germany

I. HISTORICAL REVIEW

In the second half of the 19th century, shortly after it became clear from the work of Louis Pasteur (1822–1895) and Robert Koch (1843–1910) that microorganisms cause infectious diseases, extensive studies were undertaken to elucidate the mechanisms of protection from and resistance to infections. This early history of the investigation of immunity is characterized by the dispute between two opposing schools, the protagonists of the "cellular" and the "humoral" theories. Eli Metchnikoff (1845–1919) was the first to recognize the general significance of the phenomenon of phagocytosis in animal tissues (1–3). In 1883, he published his first papers on the theory of phagocytosis. Despite initial struggle, the phagocytes were soon accepted as the principal, if not the only, defenses of the body against bacterial invasion.

Only a few years later, in 1888, Nutall found that blood of different species had bactericidal activity against *Bacillus anthracis, B. megaterium, B. subtilis*, and *Staphylococcus aureus* (4). He observed that destruction took place independently of leukocytes and that bactericidal activity was destroyed by heating at 55°C for 30–60 min. Investigating the effect of certain molds on the clotting of plasma, von Grohmann, in 1884, observed that the development of these organisms was arrested when treated with plasma (5). Furthermore, he showed that after exposure to plasma anthrax bacilli had a greatly reduced virulence in guinea pigs. Although he was not directly investigating the bactericidal activity of serum, Buchner gave him credit for making the first observations in this field (6,7). In 1889, Buchner confirmed the observations by Nutall and found that cell-free serum has a bactericidal activity against a variety of gram-positive and gram-negative bacteria. Dialysis of fresh serum against water at 0°C for 18–36 h eliminated bactericidal activity, but there was no loss of activity following dialysis against 0.75–0.80% sodium chloride solution buffered with sodium bicarbonate. He concluded that the ability of fresh serum to kill bacteria was due to serum proteins with enzymatic activity. Buchner named the heat-labile, bactericidal activity "alexine."

Another humoral defense was described by von Behring and Kitasato in 1890, who found that the serum of animals that had received a series of injections of nonlethal doses of tetanus toxin had the power to neutralize tetanus toxin specifically and to protect normal animals from otherwise lethal doses of toxin (8). In addition, Pfeiffer and Issaeff (1894) made the observation that when living cholera vibrios were introduced into the peritoneal cavity of guinea pigs previously inoculated with killed cultures of vibrios, they were dissolved (i.e., they underwent bacteriolysis). They found that the bacteriolytic power of serum from animals that had been immunized with microorganism was far greater than that from nonimmunized animals (9).

In 1896, Bordet showed that the lysis of vibrios was independent of cells (10,11). He found that the addition of a small volume of normal serum restored the bactericidal activity of heat-inactivated serum from an immunized animal. Therefore, Bordet suggested that the bactericidal action of serum was due to two factors. One was relatively heat stable and specific for cholera vibrio. This "preventive substance" was not always present in normal serum, but appeared in large amounts in the "immune serum" in response to immunization; this factor was later called "sensitizer," "amboceptor," or as it is commonly known today, "antibody." It caused "clumping" of the organisms but was incapable of killing these bacteria in the absence of a second factor. This second factor turned out to be identical to Buchner's alexine, since it was responsible for the lysis of the bacteria and could be destroyed by heat. The "alexine" was detected in all normal sera. This agent did not increase during immunization; later it was called "addiment" or "complement" by Paul Ehrlich.

Until 1955, antibody was thought to hold a dominant role, if not the monopoly, in host defense mechanism. Therefore, it was surprising when Pillemer and his colleagues described an antibody-independent pathway of complement activation. They found that incubation of serum with zymosan (a suspension of boiled yeast cell walls) depleted serum of C3 activity with little apparent loss of C1, C4, and C2 (12). This new pathway for complement activation involved a hitherto unknown serum protein termed "properdin," bypassing the early C components C1, C4, and C2 (12–17).

In addition to zymosan, many other high-molecular-weight polysaccharides and bacterial cell walls were found to fix C3 and activate C by the "alternative," properdin-mediated, pathway. Therefore, it was thought that this new antibody-independent pathway might play a role in host defense. This idea was further supported by studies of the interaction between bacteria-derived lipopolysaccharides and the C-system. Bladen (18), Gewurz (19), and their co-workers found that lipopolysaccharides (LPS) isolated from gram-negative bacterial cell wall and zymosan preferentially induce consumption of C3-C9 (the late-acting C components) from serum.

In the middle of the 1970s, Loos and his co-workers demonstrated an antibody-independent interaction of surfaces of Gram-negative bacteria with the early C components, C1, C4, and C2 (20,21). These studies showed that activation of the classical pathway, especially by serum-sensitive bacteria, is based on the direct interaction of lipopolysaccharides with C1q. The interaction of the first component of complement with the bacterial surface leads to the activation of the whole C cascade and finally to bacteriolysis. This antibody-independent binding of C1 to bacterial surfaces has an important function in host defense during the preimmune phase.

Since it was mentioned at the beginning that the early history of the investigation of immunity was characterized by the dispute between the protagonists of the cellular and the humoral theories, it should be noted that today, almost a century later, it is well established that Metchnikoff's macrophages are one of the prominent cell types for serum complement production. However, the individual C components are not merely liberated into the fluid phase as an artifact of in vitro manipulation, as was assumed by Metchnikoff. The living macrophages synthesize and secrete most of the C components (22,23). Furthermore, phagocytosis, especially of microorganisms, requires an intact humoral defense system (i.e., complement alone or antibodies partially cooperating with complement).

II. COMPLEMENT AND BACTERIA

A. Envelope of the Gram-Negative Bacterial Cell

The cell envelope of gram-negative bacteria consists of three essential layers, namely the cytoplasmic (or inner) membrane, the peptidoglycan (or murein) layer, and the outer membrane. Both membranes are made of phospholipids and proteins. In addition, the outer layer of the outer membrane contains lipopolysaccharides (LPS) as well as many proteins serving passive and active transport functions for ions and nutrients. LPS contains three covalently linked domains: lipid A, core polysaccharide (PS), and O-polysaccharide (O-PS). Lipid A consists of a diglucosamine subunit and attached fatty acids. The core PS contains residues unique to prokaryotes (2-keto 3-deoxyoctonate and heptoses) and is relatively invariable among a wide variety of gram-negative bacteria. The O-PS, composed of repeating subunits of oligosaccharides, imparts serological specificity to gram-negative organisms. The length of the O-PS side chain can vary from a single O-antigen repeating unit to more than 55–60 units (24). Not all gram-negative organisms contain O-PS-bearing repeating O-antigen subunits. In particular, many pathogens that reside on the respiratory mucosa, such as *Haemophilus influenzae* (25) and *Neisseria meningitidis* (26), or the genitourinary mucosa, such as *Neisseria gonorrhoea* (27), apparently contain relatively short oligosaccharide moieties attached to the lipid A moiety.

Several soluble proteins are located between the two membranes in a compartment known as the periplasmic space. The two membranes are interconnected by zones of adhesion. The outer membrane is not always the outermost layer of the cell envelope as it is often covered with a rather amorphous capsular layer. Finally, appendices such as flagella, fimbriae, or pili are anchored in the cell envelope.

Although many high-grade gram-negative bacterial pathogens, such as certain strains of *Salmonella typhi*, lack a polysaccharide capsule, the presence of a capsule is generally considered to be an important virulence determinant.

B. Cell Wall of the Gram-Positive Bacterial Cell

Gram-positive bacteria present a remarkable contrast in many ways to the gram-negative organisms. The complex outer membrane is lacking and a hypertrophied peptidoglycan layer that can reach a thickness of 160 nm (compared to 3 nm of the enteric bacteria) is the outermost structure. In addition to the gram-positive cell wall, the capsular polysaccharides, which are found on essentially pathogenic gram-positive organisms, are of major importance in the interactions of the organism with the host defense mechanisms. The basic scaffolding of the peptidoglycan layer is provided by a repeating disaccharide (-*N*-acetyl-glucosamine-*N*-acetyl muramic acid-). The muramic acid is derivatized with a short amino acid side chain, and these amino acid side chains are often cross-linked with another four to five amino acid peptide bridge (28). Unusual amino acids, such as D-forms, are found. The exact composition of the side chain and of the peptide bridge varies among the genera and species of the gram-positive bacteria. Within this carbohydrate and amino acid framework is a second major constituent of the gram-positive cell wall, the teichoic acid. Teichoic acids in general are glycolipids, which also vary in precise structure from genus to genus. The exact details of the manner in which these teichoic acids interact with the peptidoglycan is not known. However, they clearly play an essential role in normal bacterial physiology. Their importance has been most clearly and dramatically demonstrated by work with *S. pneumoniae* by Tomasz' laboratory (29–31). These workers showed that pneumococcal autolysin, an enzyme that is essential for normal cell division, is regulated by the pneumococcal teichoic acid-containing structure, termed Forssman antigen. Simply substituting ethanolamine for choline in pneumococcal growth medium, a change that alters cell wall teichoic acid, renders autolysin incapable of bringing about normal cell division (32). Interesting is that the pneumococcal teichoic acid is antigenically cross-reactive with the glycolipid Forssman antigen present on many mammalian cells (33,34). In addition, there are protein components of the gram-positive cell walls. Many of these components must represent specific transport proteins for nutrients essential to bacterial growth. Some cell wall proteins may also play a role in interactions of the bacteria with host defense mechanisms. For example, protein A of *S. aureus* binds IgG by its Fc piece and this may activate complement (35). M protein of the group A streptococcal cell wall is quite clearly antiphagocytic. The structural connections between these important intrinsic cell wall proteins and the previously described carbohydrate and lipid components of gram-positive cell walls are not understood at present.

C. Mechanisms of Complement Activation by Gram-Negative Bacteria

1. Classical Pathway

The classical pathway of complement is primarily triggered by binding of macromolecular C1, consisting of the components C1q, C1r, and C1s, to immune complexes. C1q binds to the Fc-portion of immunoglobulins (IgM and IgG) and this binding leads to internal activation of the serine esterases C1r and C1s.

Gram-negative bacteria can activate complement by both the alternative and the classical pathway in the presence or absence of antibodies. The mode of interaction of complement with gram-negative organisms is ascribable to specific constituents within the cell wall.

A direct interaction of some bacterial LPS preparations with the first component of complement, C1, and its subcomponent C1q in the absence of antibodies was first demonstrated by Loos et al. (20). From these findings it was assumed that the lipid A region of the LPS molecule is the C1-binding site of LPS. Later results by Morrison and Kline confirmed this interpretation (36). This C1q-LPS interaction appears to be influenced by core region sugars and the O-specific chains of the LPS; whereas the lipid A portion, which is almost identical in all LPS, has a strong C1q-binding capacity. In addition to the binding of C1 to isolated LPS, C1 was also shown to bind to some serum-sensitive gram-negative bacteria such as *Klebsiella* spp., *Escherichia* spp., *Shigella* spp., *Salmonella* spp. (21,37–40), *Mycoplasma* spp. (41), and retroviruses (42).

The binding of C1q to strains of *Salmonella minnesota* (smooth and rough form) has been demonstrated direct by electron microscopic studies. The bacteria were treated with purified C1q, anti-C1q (IgG) and anti-IgG labeled with ferritin (43) (Fig. 1, upper part). The S form did not bind C1q since no ferritin grains were detectable on the outer membrane of the S form. A conspicious ferritin layer surrounds the Re form, indicating that a large amount of cell-bound C1q could be detected by the antibodies on the bacterial surface.

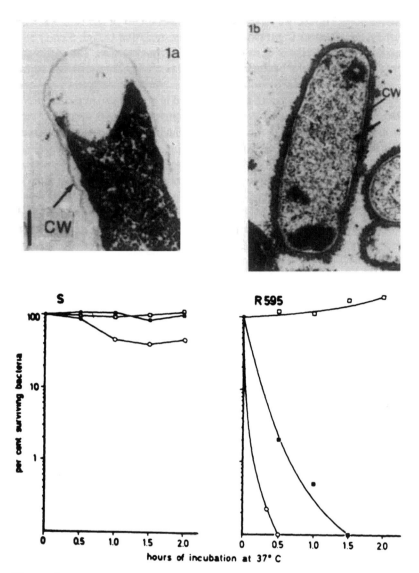

Figure 1 Upper part: Ultrathin sections of the S and Re forms of *Salmonella minnesota*. The bacteria were treated with purified C1q, anti-C1q IgG, and anti-IgG labeled with ferritin. No ferritin is detected on the outside the cell wall (CW) of the S form (1a), whereas the cell wall of the Re form (1b) is surrounded by an intense layer of ferritin (*arrow*), indicating the presence of C1q antigen. The bar represents 200 nm (43). Lower part: Bactericidal activity of a selective complete C1q deficient human serum (10%) before (□) and after (■) the addition of highly purified C1q (6.5 × 10¹⁰ effective molecules per ml [i.e., 1/200 of the amount of 1 ml NHS]) on the S form (left) and the Re form (right) of *S. minnesota*. Buffer-treated bacteria were used as 100% controls. The open circles represent the data obtained with 10% NHS on the same number of bacteria (10^3/ml).

Because of these observations, we have studied the interaction of the first reacting C component initiating the classical C pathway, with serum-sensitive (rough forms) and serum-resistant (smooth forms) strains of *S. minnesota* and *S. typhimurium*. The participation of the classical C pathway in the bacterial reaction was clearly demonstrated using human (HS) and guinea pig sera (GPS) with a selective complete deficiency in one individual C component (44–46). The smooth strain survived in normal and in the deficient sera. In contrast, the rough strains, which were serum-sensitive in normal sera, were not killed in either normal HS depleted of C1 via IgG-CNBr-Sepharose 4B or patient serum completely deficient in C1q (Fig. 1, lower part). The killing capacity could be restored by addition of purified C1q. The first complement component has, under physiological conditions, no affinity for the serum-resistant smooth forms of *S. minnesota* and *S. typhimurium*. The lack of the O-antigenic sugar chains causes the high C1-binding affinity to the rough forms. C1q is only bound in high amounts by the deep rough mutants (Rd and Re). The inhibition of LPS-synthesis by diazaborine (47) completely abrogates C1q binding to such pretreated bacteria. Therefore, LPS appears to be essential for any interaction with C1.

However, LPS is not the only C1 acceptor on the bacterial cell surface. The high-affinity binding of C1 contrasts with the low affinity of C1q for the bacteria. Stemmer and Loos (48) showed that C1 binds to outer membrane proteins (OMP) isolated from *S. minnesota*. OMP (Mr 39 000) binds to C1q and C1 to the same extent. These data are in agreement with observations by Galdiero and co-workers (49).

It is likely that membrane proteins are more available for C1 on core-deficient R mutants than on S forms. Therefore, a different binding mechanism for C1 to the R forms may be the reason for the irreversible attachment of C1 to the serum-sensitive gram-negative bacteria. This C1 attachment, resulting in the activation of the classical pathway, may be the cause of the serum sensitivity of gram-negative bacteria.

As described by Grossman and Leive (50), not only the chain length but also the structure of the LPS network is of importance for biological interactions. Earlier reports by Betz and co-workers (37,38) suggested that *E. coli* J5 activated complement in HS via the classical pathway. In their studies with native precursor C1, it was demonstrated that binding and activation of C1 occurs in the absence of antibodies. They used [^{125}I]C1 to demonstrate binding and activation of precursor C1 at physiological ionic strength. In agreement with our own experiments with serum-sensitive *Salmonella* strains, they found that approximately 2000 molecules of C1 were bound and activated by *E. coli* J5. If we assume that a single lytic event is sufficient to kill a bacterium, as already proposed by Inoue and co-workers (51), the number of the bound C1 molecules should be sufficient to account for the bactericidal activity of nonimmune HS. Further calculations by Inoue et al. (52) revealed that a single killing hit in their system corresponded to 1450 lesions on the bacterial surface. They hypothesized that many lesions formed on the bacterial surface might not directly induce killing unless they were formed at precise targets (e.g., where the inner membrane is bound tightly with the outer membrane). Consequently, the significance of the observations described above depends on the subsequent effect of activated complement components on the bacterium.

Betz and co-workers (38) investigated the role of specific antibodies on the binding and activation of purified C1. They showed an increase of radio-labeled C1 binding by *E. coli* J5 in the presence of specific IgG or IgM. However, the rate of C1 activation was decreased if bacteria were preincubated with immune Ig. Furthermore, preincubation of bacteria with NHS (60 min, 4°C) to absorb so-called "natural antibodies" did not accelerate the killing rate of such pretreated, "serum-sensitive" R forms, providing further evidence that antibodies are not necessary for the classical pathway-mediated killing (44).

More recently, *Legionella pneumophila* have been shown to bind C1q and activate the classical pathway in the absence of antibody. The binding of C1q could be attributed to a major OMP but not to *L. pneumophilia* LPS (53).

In serum-sensitive strains of *Klebsiella pneumoniae*, direct binding of C1q to two major outer membrane proteins, presumably the porins of these bacteria, was demonstrated and classical pathway activation was measured as C4 consumption and loss of total hemolytic activity. Again, no C1q binding to other components of the bacterial membrane, especially rough LPS was seen (54).

2. Lectin Pathway

In addition to the classical and alternative pathway of complement activation, a third "lectin pathway," has recently been established. Mannan-binding protein, MBP, is a member of the collectin family, a group of proteins with a collagenlike domain and a globular domain that has C-type (Ca^{2+} dependent) lectin characteristics. In order to differentiate the abbreviation MBP from myelin basic protein and major basic protein, the term mannan binding lectin (MBL) has been suggested. Two MBL-associated serine proteases (MASP) were characterized showing similarities to C1r and C1s (55). MBL was shown to bind to a number of bacterial, fungal, and viral pathogens and can lead to complement activation via C4 cleavage and subsequent C3-convertase formation.

A first report on the binding of MBL to *Salmonella montevideo* was published in 1989 (56). Recent studies have demonstrated significant binding of MBL to noncapsulated *Listeria monocytogenes*, *Haemophilus influenzae*, *N. cinera*, and *N. subflava* (57). Lipo-oligosaccharide (LOS) of *N. meningitidis* plays an important role for MBL binding (58).

3. Alternative Pathway

In vivo, small amounts of C3b are constantly formed as a result of nonenzymatic hydrolysis of the internal thiol ester bond within native C3. C3b can bind covalently to activator surfaces and will trigger the binding of factor B in the presence of Mg^{2+}.

Upon enzymatic hydrolysis by factor D the C3 convertase of the alternative pathway, C3bBb, is generated. An important activator surface of the alternative pathway is provided by gram-negative bacteria and it has been shown by Pillemer in initial studies of the alternative pathway that LPS is a potent activator molecule. In experiments with purified complement components, Schreiber and co-workers (59) could clearly demonstrate that *E. coli* K12 could be killed in the absence of immunoglobulins or other serum components.

Current understanding of alternative pathway activation suggests that LPS provides a "protected site" for C3b deposition and C3 convertase formation, a state at which inactivation of bound C3b by factors H and I is relatively inefficient. This idea was confirmed for LPS from *E. coli* 04 by the demonstration that the affinity of factor H for C3b bound to the LPS molecules was far lower than that of factor B (60). It appears that the polysaccharide portion of the LPS molecule can activate the alternative pathway. Studies by Grossman and Leive (50) using LPS-coated erythrocytes demonstrated that LPS-molecules bearing as few as five O-antigen repeats are as efficient as LPS molecules bearing 18–40 O-antigen repeats in activating the alternative pathway.

Substantial differences exist between different LPS O-polysaccharides in their capacity to activate complement. Galanos et al. (61) demonstrated major differences among the LPS from various strains of *Salmonella* and *E. coli* in their ability to deplete complement activity from serum. It seems likely that differences in the degree of LPS aggregation played a role in these findings (62). Likewise, Morrison (63) demonstrated a substantial difference in the capacity of LPS from different organisms and of different serotypes to elicit a serum-dependent respiratory burst from neutrophils. The fine specificity of the differential AP-activating capacity of LPS was demonstrated in studies comparing LPS from *Salmonella* strains varying only in the substitution of abequose for tyvulose (epimers of one another) in the O-antigen repeat unit of the O-polysaccharide (50).

Further experiments by Joiner and co-workers (64) demonstrated the antibody requirement for the alternative pathway mediated killing of *E. coli* 0111. They had shown that bacterial IgG (not Fab') changes the nature of association of C5b-9 with the outer membrane, leading to insertion of bactericidal C5b-9 into the outer membrane. They, therefore, sought to determine the mechanism by which IgG mediates this process. Equivalent or greater amounts of C3 and C9 were deposited when IgG was added at intermediate steps in the complement cascade as when IgG was added at the initiation of complement activation. The results provide further evidence that killing is not a direct function of the number of C5b-9 complexes bound. More importantly, these results show that to mediate killing IgG must be present at the time of, or preceding, C3 deposition and C5 convertase formation. C3b bound to IgG molecules on the bacterial surface obviously serves an additional role, since killing does not occur in the absence of IgG despite equivalent C5b-9 deposition.

Rough mutants which are characterized by truncated O-specific chains of LPS are much more susceptible to C5b-C9-mediated killing (65). This fact emphasizes the protective role of long polysaccharide side chains of smooth forms of bacteria that may activate complement but prevent the membrane attack complex C5b-9 to form on and insert in the bacterial outer membrane.

In addition to the activation of the alternative pathway by LPS, C3 binding to the major OMP of *Legionella pneumophila* has been demonstrated (66). In Western blot analysis the authors showed exclusive binding of C3 to *L. pneumophila* MOMP, whereas binding to LPS could not be seen. It was further shown that MOMP-bearing liposomes mediated phagocytosis by human monocytes after opsonization with C3.

4. Terminal Sequence

A wide variety of gram-negative bacteria are killed after exposure to serum by a process that requires the participation of either the classical or alternative pathway of complement and the generation of macromolecular C5b-9 protein complexes. These form stable lesions embedded in the envelope of susceptible bacteria (serum-sensitive bacteria), resembling those visualized on membranes of complement-exposed erythrocytes (18, 67–72).

Complexes are formed from the fluid phase proteins (C5b, C6, C7, C8, and C9) of the terminal complement membrane attack pathway by spontaneous association following enzymatic cleavage of C5. Polymerization is accompanied by the appearance of terminal apolar regions on the cylindrical C5b-9 complex that facilitate insertion into hydrophobic domains of target membranes, leading to the death of serum-sensitive bacteria (69, 73–76). Complement acts on target membranes by forming ion-permeable channels that allow the flux of small molecules across the membrane resulting in osmotic imbalance and bursting.

As the gram-negative cell envelope consists of three layers, it is clear that these bacteria present a more complex target that requires a more complex mechanism for disruption than that described for red-cell lysis. Complement has been shown to damage the outer membrane of gram-negative bacteria (77–80). Complement treatment releases periplasmic enzymes and admits extracellular lysozyme into the periplasmic space. The destruction of the outer membrane, however, is unlikely to be lethal for gram-negative bacteria, as the bacteria are capable of rapid cell division and may be able to undertake a repair of damaged sites on the cell envelope. In addition, they may display an altered phenotype in response to environmental pressure. Killing may also be dependent upon an energy-dependent process requiring an input of bacterially generated ATP (81). These factors must be taken into account when considering the mechanisms of complement-mediated bactericidal action.

D. Complement Activation by Gram-Positive Bacteria

1. Classical Pathway

Intact gram-positive bacteria do not activate the classical complement pathway directly like gram-negative bacteria. The most prominent constituent of the cell wall, isolated muramyl-dipeptide, did not interact with C1 or C1q (82). Additional studies of the interaction of the classical pathway components with isolated lipoteichoic acids (LTA), however, revealed that C1 activation depended on the density of the negative charges of the phosphate groups of LTA (83). The biological significance of this observation is not yet clarified.

Pneumococci are able to activate the classical pathway when sensitized with antibody of the appropriate class. However, there appear to be significant differences in the ability of pneumococcal anticapsular antibodies isolated from different species to activate the classical pathway. For example, a number of studies have shown that either rabbit anticapsular antibody or rabbit anti-cell-wall antibody is capable of activating the classical pathway (84, 85). In contrast, experiments performed using antipneumococcal antibodies isolated from convalescent human sera have failed to demonstrate significant activation of the classical pathway (86–88).

The reason(s) for the relative inability of human antibodies to activate the classical pathway is (are) unknown, but may relate to the sensitivity of the assays used for detecting activation and/or to the class or subclass of antibodies to the pneumococcus which is present in immune human sera. Pneumococci may also activate the classical pathway when C-reactive protein (CRP) complexes with pneumococcal C polysaccharide (89,90). In experiments performed using highly purified C polysaccharide and human CRP, activation of the classical pathway was independent of antibody to the C polysaccharide. However, like the activation of complement by immune complexes, there was consumption of the early components of the classical pathway (C1, C4, C2) and of C3–C9.

Two different approaches revealed the regions on C1q and CRP that are important for the interaction of the proteins. Inhibition experiments using synthetic peptides (91) could localize the binding sites of CRP on the C1q A-chain at positions 14–26 and 76–92; both regions are within the collagenous part of the C1q A-chain. The C1q binding site on human CRP has been mapped by site-directed mutagenesis (92). The data indicate that the negative charge of residue Asp-112 plays a major role in the formation of the C1q-binding site of CRP.

In group A streptococci (*S. pyogenes*) two cell surface proteins, Arp and Ser, have binding capacities for immunoglobulins and C4 binding protein (C4bp). Bound C4bp retained its ability to act as a cofactor of factor I in cleaving C4. The presence of either or both of these proteins in strains of group A streptococci may therefore interfere with the activation of the classical pathway (93).

2. Alternative Pathway

In the absence of antibody, gram-positive cell walls activate complement by the alternative pathway. This activation, which has been demonstrated in an number of organisms, has been studied most carefully in *S. aureus* and *S. pneumoniae*. Alternative pathway activation in serum by gram-positive organisms leads to the generation of both C3b and iC3b bound covalently to the bacterial surface (94). Studies quantitating the two forms of C3 have generally shown that C3b is the predominant form bound to intact bacteria. Studies on whether the peptidoglycan, the teichoic acid, or some unspecified component of cell walls is responsible for alternative pathway activation have been less conclusive. Winkelstein and Tomasz (95) examined this question using purified components of the pneumococcal cell wall, and demonstrated that pneumococcal teichoic acid can activate the alternative pathway, but that pneumococcal peptidoglycan cannot. On the other hand, results from similar experiments performed with isolated components of *S. aureus* cell wall led to the opposite conclusion (96,97). These studies showed that while peptidoglycan activated the alternative pathway, *S. aureus* teichoic acid was without effect. Structural or chemical differences between the cell wall components of pneumococci and staphylococci may explain these differences. However, it is important to realize that purification of these components requires quite harsh conditions that may alter the native properties of these molecules as found in the bacterial cell wall.

A second way through which *S. pyogenes* can interfere with complement activation emanates from the binding affinity of the C-domain of the M protein for factor H, the alternative pathway analogue to C4bp, and for membrane cofactor protein (MCP), the cofactor of factor I on host cells. Besides the inhibition of the alternative pathway C3 convertase and C5 convertase (98), the binding of M protein to MCP may play an important role in attachment to keratinocytes, the most abundant cell type in the skin, where many *S. pyogenes* infections occur (99).

E. Opsonization

Complement-mediated phagocytosis undoubtedly plays an important role when the nonimmune host is first challenged with a microorganism. Liang-Takasaki and colleagues (100) have related the virulence of various strains of *Salmonella typhimurium* to differences in their O-antigenic structure, with the less virulent being more likely to fix C3 by the alternative complement pathway and more likely to be taken up by phagocytic cells. Clas and Loos (46) reported that *S. minnesota* can bind C1 independently of antibody and activate the classical pathway. Horwitz and Silverstein (101) have shown that nonencapsulated *E. coli* can be phagocytized by neutrophils upon addition of normal serum, while the encapsulated form requires bacteria-specific antibody.

In studying the interaction of bacterial LPS with the macrophage membrane, Euteneuer and Loos (102) found that LPS and porins (omp) from bacterial cell walls are involved in the binding of gram-negative bacteria to macrophages. This antibody independent attachment and ingestion of gram-negative bacteria is mediated by endogenous macrophage-membrane associated C1q (23,103).

Because gram-positive organisms are not killed directly by complement, complement has a very different role to play in host defense against these bacteria. The object of complement activation in host defense against these bacteria is to lead to their opsonization. A number of complement components may play a role in the recognition and ingestion of bacteria by phagocytic cells, but the most important complement protein in achieving this effect is the component C3. Activation of either the classical or alternative pathway results in the fixation of opsonically active C3b to the pneumococcal surface. *S. pneumoniae* that are incubated in sera in which both the classical and the alternative pathways are intact (e.g., normal sera) are opsonized at a more rapid rate than *S. pneumoniae* incubated in sera in which just the alternative pathway is functional (e.g. C4- or C2-deficient sera). The requirements for complement-dependent opsonization of the *Pneumococcus* appear to vary considerably from serotype to serotype. While some serotypes can be efficiently opsonized by C3b in the absence of detectable anticapsular antibody, others require opsonization by both C3b and anticapsular antibody for optimal ingestion by phagocytic cells. A number of studies have focused on the interaction of the *Pneumococcus* and C3b at the molecular level in order to explore the relationship between the fixation of C3b to the *Pneumococcus* and opsonization (104).

The opsonic potential of C3b depends on the number of C3-molecules activated by the microorganisms, the number of C3b-molecules fixed to the bacterial surface and its location on the cell wall in regard to its accessibility to phagocytic cells. Studies by Law et al. (105) have examined the site of C3b binding on the pneumococcal surfaces in an attempt to clarify this point. Native C3 contains an intramolecular thioester in its α-chain, which after activation of C3 to C3b can undergo transesterification with hydroxyl groups on suitable receptor surfaces. Nascent C3b must bind to an acceptor surface soon after it is cleaved from the parent molecule or its labile binding site disappears. Therefore, nascent C3b would be expected to bind on, or in close proximity to, the subcellular organelle responsible for initiating its activation. Thus, activation of the alternative pathway by intact pneumococci results in fixation of C3b to the cell wall deep into the capsule, a location where the capsule may act as a mechanical barrier to the recognition of C3b by the phagocytic cell. In contrast, activation of the classical pathway by anticapsular antibody results in fixation of C3b to the capsular polysaccharide, a location where the C3b might potentially be more accessible to act as an opsonic ligand for phagocytic cells. In fact, studies by Brown et al. (84) have shown that when C3b is fixed to the pneumococcal capsule, it is relatively more accessible than when it is fixed to the cell wall. Thus, the mechanism by which the C3b is activated (alternative pathway vs. classical pathway) may influence where on the encapsulated organism it becomes attached (cell wall vs. capsule), which in turn may influence its opsonic potential (104).

F. Conclusions

Complement was first described by investigators studying the bactericidal activity of blood and serum. Many isolated components of gram-negative bacteria, mainly lipopolysaccharides (LPS), have been shown to activate either the classical or the alternative or both pathways of complement. However, whether these components as they occur in an intact bacterium are able to activate the complement system is very much dependent on the cell wall composition and the environment within the cell wall. Most gram-negative bacteria can activate complement by both pathways; some of them are susceptible to the membrane attack complex (MAC), some of them appear to be resistant to the MAC, especially those bearing longer than normal O-polysaccharide side chains. However, the deposition of complement activation products like C1q, C4b, C3b, iC3b, C3dg, and C3d on the surface of complement-activating microbes may result in opsonization and subsequent phagocytosis. In this regard most of the gram-positive bacteria are resistant to the MAC but susceptible to phagocytosis.

Interesting and at the moment still poorly understood, is that some pathogens use antibody-independent activation of complement and opsonization for entrance into phagocytic cells as a mechanism to escape the attack of the immune system and to survive within cells by preventing the fusion of phagosomes with lysosomes. This is one possible way of how pathogens may escape the overall complement activity, which, besides macrophages, plays the most important role in natural resistance to microorganisms.

REFERENCES

1. Metchnikoff E. Arb Zool Inst Univ Wien 1883; 5:141.
2. Metchnikoff E. Sur la proprieté bactéricide des humeurs. Revue critique. Ann Immunol (Paris) 1889; 3:664–671.
3. Metchnikoff E. Immunity in Infective Diseases. London: Cambridge University Press 1905: 195.
4. Nutall G. Experimente über die bakterienfeindlichen Einflüsse des tierischen Körpers. Z Hyg Infektionskr 1888; 4:353–394.
5. Grohmann W von. Über die Einwirkung des zellfreien Blutplasmas auf einige pflanzliche Mikroorganismen (Schimmel-Spross—Pathogene und nicht pathogene Spaltpilze). Ph.D. dissertation, Dorpat, 1884.
6. Buchner H. Über die nähere Natur der bakterientödtenden Wirkung des zellfreien Blutserums. I. und II. Zentralbl Bakteriol 1889; 5:817–823.
7. Buchner H. Über die nähere Natur der bakterientödtenden Substanzen im Blutserum. Zentralbl Bakteriol 1889; 6:561–565.
8. Behring E von, Kitasato S. Über das Zustandekommen der Diphtherie-Immunität und der Tetanus-Immunität bei Tieren. Dtsch Med Wochenschr 1890; 16:1113–1145.
9. Pfeiffer R, Isaeff R. Über die spezifische Bedeutung der Cholera-Immunität. Z Hyg Infektionskr 1894; 17:335–440.
10. Bordet J. Sur l'agglutination et la dissolution des globules rouges par le serum d'animaux injectiés de sang defibrine. Ann Inst Pasteur (Paris) 1898; 12:688–695.
11. Bordet J. Sur le mode d'action des serums préventifs. Ann Inst Pasteur (Paris) 1896; 10:193–219.
12. Pillemer L, Schoenberg MD, Blum L, Wurz L. Properdin system and immunity. II. Interaction of the properdin system with polysaccharides. Science 1955; 122:545–549.
13. Pillemer L. Recent advances in the chemistry of complement. Chem Rev 1943; 33:1–26.
14. Pillemer L, Blum L, Lepow IH, Ross OA, Todd EW, Wardlaw AC. The properdin system and immunity. I. Demonstration and isolation of a new serum protein, properdin, and its role in immune phenomena. Science 1954; 120:279–285.
15. Pillemer L, Blum L, Pensky J, Lepow IH. The requirement for magnesium ions in the inactivation of the third component of human complement (C3) by insoluble residues of yeast cells (zymosan). J Immunol 1953; 71:331–338.
16. Pillemer L, Lepow IH, Blum L. The requirement for hydrazine-sensitive serum factor and heat-labile serum factors in the inactivation of human C3 by zymosan. J Immunol 1953; 71:339–345.
17. Pillemer L, Blum L, Lepow IH, Wurz L, Todd EW. The properdin system and immunity. III. The zymosan assay of properdin. J Exp Med 1956; 103:1–43.
18. Bladen HA, Evans RT, Mergenhagen SE. Lesions in *Escherichia coli* membranes after action of antibody and complement. J Bacteriol 1966; 91:2377–2381.
19. Gewurz H, Shin HS, Mergenhagen SE. Interactions of the complement system with endotoxic lipopolysaccharide: consumption of each of six terminal complement components. J Exp Med 1968; 128:1049–1057.

20. Loos M, Bitter-Suermann D, Dierich M. Interaction of the first (C1), the second (C2) and the fourth (C4) component of complement with different preparations of bacterial lipopolysaccharides and with lipid A. J Immunol 1974; 112:935–940.

21. Loos M, Wellek B, Thesen R, Opferkuch W. Antibody-independent interaction of the first component of complement with gram-negative bacteria. Infect Immun 1978; 22:5–9

22. Bentley C, Zimmer B, Hadding U. The macrophage as a source of complement components. In: Pick E, ed. Lymphokines 4. New York: Academic Press, 1981:197–230.

23. Loos M. Biosynthesis of the collagen-like C1q molecule and its receptor functions for Fc and polyanionic molecules on macrophages. Curr Top Microbiol Immunol 1983; 102:1–56.

24. Goldmann RC, Leive L. Heterogeneity of antigenic sidechain length in lipopolysaccharide from *Escherichia coli* 0111 and *Salmonella typhimurium* LT2. Eur J Biochem 1980; 107:145–149.

25. Flesher AR, Insel RA. Characterization of lipopolysaccharide of *Haemophilus influenzae*. Infect Dis 1978; 138:719–730.

26. Tsai CM, Boykins R, Frasch CE. Heterogeneity and variation among *Neisseria meningitidis* lipopolysaccharides. J Bacteriol 1983; 155:498–504.

27. Guymon LF, Esser M, Shafer WM. Pyocin-resistant lipopolysaccharide mutants of *Neisseria gonorrhoeae*: alterations in sensitivity to normal human serum and polymyxin B. Infect Immun 1982; 36:541–547.

28. Tomasz A. Surface components of *Streptococcus pneumoniae*. Rev Infect Dis 1981; 3:190–211.

29. Tomasz A. Choline in the cell wall of a bacterium: novel type of polymer-linked choline in pneumococcus. Science 1967; 157:694–697.

30. Tomasz A, McDonnel A, Westphal M, Zanati E. Coordinated incorporation of nascent peptidoglycan and teichoic acid into pneumococcal cell walls and conservation of peptidoglycan during growth. J Biol Chem 1974; 250:337–341.

31. Holtje JV, Tomasz A. Purification of the pneumococcal N-acetylmuramyl-L-alanine amidase to biochemical homogeneity. J Biol Chem 1976; 251:4199–4207.

32. Mosser JL, Tomasz A. Choline-containing teichoid acid as a structural component of pneumococcal cell wall and its role in sensitivity of lysis by an autolytic enzyme. J Biol Chem 1970; 245:287–298.

33. Fujiwara M. The Forssman antigen of pneumococcus. Jpn J Exp Med 1967; 37:581–592.

34. Fujiwara M. Immunological properties of antipneumococcus rabbit serum as heterophile antibodies. Jpn J Exp Med 1968; 38:1–10.

35. Forsgren A, Sjoquist J. Protein A from S. aureus I. Pseudo-immune reaction with human γ-globulin. J Immunol 1966; 97:822–827.

36. Morrison DC, Kline FL. Activation of the classical and properdin pathway of complement by bacterial lipopolysaccharides (LPS). J Immunol 1976; 118:362–368.

37. Betz SJ, Isliker H. Antibody-independent interactions between *E. coli* J5 and human complement components. J Immunol 1981; 127:1748–1754.

38. Betz SJ, Page N, Estrade C, Isliker H. The effect of specific antibody on antibody-independent interactions between *E. coli* J5 and human complement. J Immunol 1982; 128:707–711.

39. Clas F, Loos M. Killing of the S- and Re-Forms of *Salmonella minnesota* via the classical pathway of complement activation in guinea-pig and human sera. Immunology 1980; 40:547–556.

40. Skarnes RC. Humoral bactericidal systems: nonspecific and specific mechanisms. Infect Immun 1978; 19:512–522.

41. Bredt W, Wellek B, Brunner H, Loos M. Studies on the interaction between *Mycoplasma pneumoniae* and the first component of complement. Infect Immun 1977;15:7–12.

42. Bartholomew RM, Esser AF. Differences in activation of human and guinea-pig complement by retroviruses. J Immunol 1978; 121:1748–1751.

43. Clas F, Golecki JR, Loos M. Electron microscopic study showing the antibody-independent binding of C1q, a subcomponent of the first component of complement, to serum-sensitive salmonellae. Infect Immun 1984; 45:795–797.

44. Clas F, Loos M. Antibody-independent killing of gram-negative bacteria via the classical pathway. Behring Inst Res Commun 1984; 76:59–74.

45. Clas F, Schmidt G, Loos M. The role of the classical pathway for the bactericidal effect of normal sera against Gram-negative bacteria. Curr Top Microbiol Immunol 1985; 121:19–72.

46. Clas F, Loos M. Antibody independent binding of the first component of complement (C1) and its subcomponent C1q to the S- and R-forms of *Salmonella minnesota*. Infect Immun 1981; 31:1138–1144.

47. Hogenauer G, Woisetschlager M. A diazaborine derivative inhibits lipopolysaccharide biosynthesis. Nature 1981; 239:662–664.

48. Stemmer F, Loos M. Evidence for direct binding of the first component of complement, C1, to outer membrane proteins of *S. minnesota*. Curr Top Microbiol Immunol 1985; 121:73–83.

49. Galdiero F, Tufano MA, Sommese L, Folgore A, Tedesco F. Activation of complement systems by porins extracted from *S. typhimurium*. Infect Immun 1984; 46:559–563.

50. Grossmann N, Leive L. Complement activation via the alternative pathway by purified *Salmonella* lipopolysaccharide is affected by its structure but not its O-antigen length. J Immunol 1984; 132:376–385.

51. Inoue K, Akiyama Y, Kinoshita T, Higashi Y, Amano T. Evidence for a one-hit theory in the immune bactericidal reaction and demonstration of a multi-hit response for hemolysis by streptolysin O and *Clostridium perfringens* theta toxin. Infect Immun 1976; 13:337–344.

52. Inoue K, Kinoshita T, Okada M, Akiyama Y. Release of phospholipids from complement-mediated lesions on the surface structure of *Escherichia coli*. J Immunol 1977; 119:65–72.

53. Mintz CS, Arnold PI, Johnson W, Schutz DR. Antibody-independent binding of complement component C1q by *Legionella pneumophila*. Infect Immun 1995; 63:4939–4943.

54. Alberti S, Marques G, Camprubi S, Merino S, Tomas JM, Vivanco F, Benedi VJ. C1q binding and activation of the complement classical pathway by *Klebsiella pneumoniae* outer membrane proteins. Infect Immun 1993; 61:852–860.

55. Vorup-Jensen T, Stover C, Paulsen K, Laursen SB, Eggleton P, Reid KBM, Willis AC, Schwaeble W, Lu J, Holmskov U, Jensenius JC, Thiel S. Cloning of cDNA encoding a human MASP-like protein (MASP-2). Mol Immunol 1996; 33:81 (abstract).

56. Kuhlmann M, Joiner K, Ezekowitz RA. The human mannose-binding protein functions as an opsonin. J Exp Med 1989; 169:1733–1745.

57. Van Emmerik LC, Kuijper EJ, Fijen CA, Dankert J, Thiel S. Binding of mannan-binding protein to various bacterial pathogens of meningitis. Clin Exp Immunol 1994; 97:411–416.

58. Turner MW. Mannose-binding lectin: the pluripotent molecule of the innate immune system. Immunol Today 1996; 17:532–540.

59. Schreiber RD, Morrison DC, Podack ER, Müller-Eberhard HJ. Bactericidal activity of the alternative complement pathway generated from 11 isolated plasma proteins. J Exp Med 1979; 149:870–882.

60. Pangburn MK, Morrison DC, Schreiber RD, Müller-Eberhard HJ. Activation of the alternative complement pathways: recognition of surface structures on activators of bound C3b. J Immunol 1980; 124:977–987.

61. Galanos C, Luderitz O. The role of the physical state of lipopolysaccharides in the interaction with complement. High molecular weight as prerequisite for the expression of anti-complementary activity. Eur J Biochem 1976; 65:403–408.

62. Wilson ME, Morrison DC. Evidence for the different requirements in physical state for the interaction of lipopolysaccharides with the classical and the alternative pathway of complement. Eur J Biochem 1982; 128:137–141.

63. Morrison DC. Bacterial endotoxins and pathogenesis. Rev Infect Dis 1983; 5:5733–5747.

64. Joiner KA. Studies on the mechanism of bacterial resistance to complement-mediated killing and on the mechanism of action of bactericidal antibody. Curr Top Microbiol Immunol 1985; 121:99–133.

65. Taylor PW. Bactericidal and bacteriolytic activity of serum against gram-negative bacteria. Microbiol Rev 1983; 47:46–83.

66. Bellinger-Kawahara C, Horwitz MA. Complement component C3 fixes selectively to the major outer membrane protein (MOMP) of *Legionella pneumophila* and mediates phagocytosis of liposome-MOMP complexes by human monocytes. J Exp Med 1990; 172:1201–1210.

67. Bladen HA, Gewurz H, Mergenhagen SE. Interaction of the complement system with the surface and endotoxic lipopolysaccharide of *Veillonella alcalescens*. J Exp Med 1967; 125:767–786.

68. Harriman GR, Podack ER, Braude AI, Corbeil LC, Esser AF, Curd JG. Activation of complement by serum-resistant *Neisseria gonorrhoeae*. Assembly of the membrane attack complex without subsequent cell death. J Exp Med 1982; 156:1235–1249.

69. Kroll HP, Bhakdi S, Taylor PW. Membrane changes induced by exposure of *Escherichia coli* to human serum. Infect Immun 1983; 42:1055–1066.

70. Kroll HP, Voigt WH, Taylor PW. Stabile insertion of C5b-9 complement complexes into the outer membrane of serum treated susceptible *Escherichia coli* cells as a prerequisite for killing. Zentralbl Bakteriol Mikrobiol Hyg (A) 1984; 258:316–326.

71. Swanson J, Goldschneider I. The serum bacericial system: ultrastructural changes in *Neisseria meningitidis* exposed to normal rat serum. J Exp Med 1969; 129:51–79.

72. Taylor PW, Kroll HP. Effect of lethal doses of complement on the functional integrity of target enterobacteria. Curr Top Microbiol Immunol 1985; 121:135–156.

73. Joiner KA, Brown EJ, Hammer CH, Frank MM. Mechanism of bacterial resistance to serum killing. Clin Res 1982; 30:518–522.

74. Joiner KA, Hammer CH, Brown EJ, Frank MM. Studies on the mechanism of bacterial resistance to complement-mediated killing. I. Terminal complement components are deposited and released from *Salmonella minnesota* S218 without causing bacterial death. J Exp Med 1982; 155:797–808.

75. Joiner KA, Hammer CH, Brown EJ, Frank MM. Studies on the mechanism of bacterial resistance to complement-mediated killing. II. C8 and C9 release C5b67 from the surface of *Salmonella minnesota* S218 because the terminal complex does not insert into the bacterial outer membrane. J Exp Med 1982; 155:809–819.

76. Taylor PW, Kroll HP. Interaction of human complement proteins with serum-sensitive and serum-resistant strains of *Escherichia coli*. Mol Immunol 1984; 21:609–620.

77. Davis SD, Boatman ES, Gemsa D, Ianneta A, Wedgwood RJ. Biochemical and fine structural changes induced in *Escherichia coli* by human serum. Microbios 1969; 1B:69–86.

78. Feingold DS, Goldmann JN, Kuritz HM. Locus of the action of serum and the role of lysozyme in the serum bactericidal reaction. J Bacteriol 1968; 96:2118–2126.

79. Feingold DS, Goldmann JN, Kuritz HM. Locus of the lethal event in the serum bactericidal reaction. J Bacteriol 1968; 96:2127–2131.

80. Inoue K, Yonemasu K, Takamizawa A, Amano T. Studies on the immune bacteriolysis. XIV. Requirement of all nine components of complement for immune bacteriolysis. Biken J 1986; 11:203–206.

81. Taylor PW, Kroll HP. Killing of an encapsulated strain of *E. coli* by human serum. Infect Immun 1983; 39:122–131.

82. Loos M, Seidl PH, Schleifer KH. Teichoic acid-free peptidoglycan of *S. aureus* RM59 does not activate complement (Abstract). Second International Workshop on the Biological Properties of Peptidoglycan, München, May 20, 1985, p. 45.

83. Loos M, Clas F, Fischer W. Interaction of purified lipoteichoic acid with the classical complement pathway. Infect Immun 1986; 53:595–599.

84. Brown EJ, Hosea SW, Hammer CH, Burch CG, Frank M. A quantitative analysis of the interaction of anti-pneumococcal antibody and complement in experimental pneumococcal bacteria. J Clin Invest 1982; 69:85–98.

85. Johnston RB, Klemperer MR, Alper CA, Rosen F. The enhancement of bacterial phagocytosis by serum. The role of complement components and two co-factors. J Exp Med 1969; 129:1275–1290.

86. Coonrod JD, Rylkp-Bauer B. Complement-fixing antibody response in pneumococcal pneumonia. Infect Immun 1977; 18:617–623.

87. Horsfall FL Jr, Goodner K. Lipids and immunological reactions. II. Further experiments on the relation of lipids to the type-specific reactions in anti-pneumococcus sera. J Immunol 1936; 31:135–142.

88. Stats D, Bullowa JGM. Failure of the human convalescent type-specific anti-pneumococcal antibody to fix complement. J Immunol 1942; 44:41–48.

89. Kaplan MH, Volanakis JE. Interaction of C-reactive protein complexes with the complement system. J Immunol 1974; 112:2135–2147.

90. Osmond AP, Mortensen RF, Siegel J, Gewurz H. Interactions of C-reactive protein with the complement system. III. Complement dependent passive hemolysis initiated by CRP. J Exp Med 1975; 142:1065–1072.

91. Jiang H, Robey FA, Gewurz H. Localization of sites through which C-reactive protein binds and activates complement to residues 14–26 and 76–92 of the human C1q A chain. J Exp Med 1992; 175:1373–1379.

92. Agrawal A, Volanakis JE. Probing the C1q-binding site on human C-reactive protein by site-directed mutagenesis. J Immunol. 1994; 152:5404–5410.

93. Thern A, Stenberg L, Dahlback B, Lindahl G. Ig-binding surface proteins of *Streptococcus pyogenes* also bind human C4b-binding protein (C4BP), a regulatory component of the complement system. J Immunol 1995; 154:375–386.

94. Brown EJ, Joiner KA, Gaither TA, Hammer CH, Frank MM. The interaction of C3b bound to pneumococci with factor H (B1H globulin), factor I (C3b/C4b inactivator), and properdin factor B of the human complement system. J Immunol 1983; 131:409–414.

95. Winkelstein JA, Tomasz A. Activation of the alternative complement pathway by pneumococcal cell wall teichoic acid. J Immunol 1978; 120:174–178.

96. Verbrugh HA, Van Dijk WC, Peters R, van Erne ME, Peterson PK, Verhoef J. Opsonic recognition of staphylococci mediated by cell wall peptidoglycan: antibody-independent activation of human complement and opsonic activity of peptidoglycan antibodies. J Immunol 1980; 124:1167–1172.

97. Wilkinson BJ, Kim Y, Petersen PK. Factors affecting complement activation by *Staphylococcus aureus* cell walls, their components, and mutants altered in teichoic acid. Infect Immun 1981; 32:216–224.

98. Hong K, Kinoshita T, Takeda J, Kozono H, Pramoonjago P, Kim YU, Inoue K. Inhibition of the alternative C3 convertase and classical C5 convertase of complement by group A streptococcal M protein. Infect Immun 1990; 58:2535–2541.

99. Okada N, Liszewski MK, Atkinson JP, Caparon M. Membrane cofactor protein (CD46) is a keratinocyte receptor for the M protein of the group A streptococcus. Proc Natl Acad Sci USA 1995; 92:2489–2493.

100. Liang-Takasaki CJ, Grossman N, Leive L. Salmonellae activate complement differentially via the alternative pathway depending on the structure of their lipopolysaccharide O-antigen. J Immunol 1983; 130:1867–1870.

101. Horwitz MA, Silverstein SC. Influence of *Escherichia coli* capsule on the complement fixation and on phagocytosis and killing by human phagocytes. J Clin Invest 1980; 65:82–94.

102. Euteneuer B, Störkel S, Loos M. Differences in attachment and phagocytosis of *S. minnesota* by mouse peritoneal macrophages. Curr Top Microbiol Immunol 1985; 121:85–97.

103. Clas F, Euteneuer B, Stemmer F, Loos M. Interaction of fluid-phase C1/C1q and macrophage-membrane associated C1q with Gram-negative bacteria. Behring Inst Mitt 1989; 84:236–254.

104. Winkelstein JA. Complement and host's defence against pneumococcus. CRC Rev 1984; D11:187.

105. Law SK, Lichtenberg NA, Levine RP. Evidence for an ester linkage between the labile binding site of C3b and receptive surfaces. J Immunol 1979; 123:1388–1394.

18

Complement and Viruses

NEIL R. COOPER

The Scripps Research Institute, La Jolla, California

I. INTRODUCTION

Virus particles are differentiated from other infectious agents by their relatively simple structure and small size, and by their absolute dependence on cellular proteins for infection and replication. They are thus obligate intracellular parasites. Although members of the 71 recognized virus families differ enormously in structure, all virions contain a DNA or RNA genome closely associated with a variable number of viral proteins that subserve various functions related to infection or replication. Viral particles are either nonenveloped or enveloped. Nonenveloped virions are surrounded by a coat or shell composed of multiple copies of virus-encoded protein subunits, termed the capsid, which often possesses icosahedral symmetry. In the case of enveloped viruses, the capsid is surrounded by a lipid bilayer membrane acquired from the cell of origin (Fig. 1). Cellular proteins are generally excluded from assembled virions, although certain cell membrane proteins are found on some enveloped viruses, as considered later. Fully assembled viral particles are only found extracellularly.

Host defense against viral infection is complex and includes multiple intrinsic, or nonspecific, as well as elicited, specific mechanisms. Despite these formidable host defense mechanisms, viral infections are common. Viruses are perhaps the most successful human pathogens for a number of reasons. As replicating agents, they have the ability to provide a continuing or increasing antigenic challenge to the host, and through mutation, to elude specific defenses. Except for the late stages of viral replication or during viral transit between cells, viral antigens are intracellular, and thus inaccessible to the actions of antibody (Ab) and complement. Certain persistent viruses target cells of the immune system for infection. Finally, members of a number of viral families have evolved mechanisms to subvert host defenses.

This chapter focuses, first, on complement dependent host defense mechanisms. Complement activation by viral particles, both alone, and together with Ab, will be reviewed, and the various processes by which the complement system inactivates virus particles and virus-infected cells will be summarized. In the second portion of this review, the processes which various viruses have evolved to use complement molecules to facilitate infection, or to avoid complement mediated destruction will be considered. Strikingly,

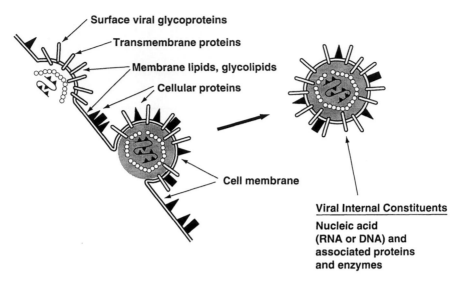

Figure 1 Schematic representation of a moderately complex enveloped virus and the stages of maturation by budding from the membrane of infected cells.

many of these mimic the processes which protect normal mammalian cells from damage by the activated complement system.

II. COMPLEMENT-MEDIATED HOST DEFENSE MECHANISMS

Ab molecules bound to surface viral Ags efficiently activate the complement system. In addition, however, free viral particles activate either the classical or the alternative complement pathway in the complete absence of Ab. Virus-infected cells likewise directly activate the complement system in the absence of Ab; when present, Ab augments such activation. These findings indicate that complement possesses the ability to discriminate self from nonself. In this context, complement functions as the humoral equivalent of the NK cell. The characteristics of Ab-dependent and Ab-independent complement activation by members of various virus families, and by virus-infected cells, and the functional consequences to the virus, and to the infected cell, are summarized in this section.

A. Complement Activation by Viruses

1. *Antibody-Dependent Complement Activation*

Viral components are antigenic and elicit the formation of specific Abs (1,2). On subsequent infection with the same virus, or with an antigenically related virus, such Abs form immune complexes with viral antigens (Ags) expressed on the viral surface, or on the membrane of infected cells. In the case of IgG Ab, the repeating array of viral envelope proteins probably facilitates the formation of clusters of IgG molecules, a requirement for efficient C1 binding and activation. Ab dependent activation of the classical pathway may lead to viral neutralization by one of the mechanisms considered below. In addition,

Ab-dependent alternative pathway activation may occur. In fact alternative pathway activation by some viruses, such as influenza, only occurs in the presence of specific Ab (3).

2. Antibody-Independent Classical Pathway Activation

Members of a number of virus families have been found to bind C1 and activate the classical complement pathway in human serum, or in mixtures of the purified components in the absence of Ab (4,5). These include all type C retroviruses of avian, rodent, and feline origin thus far examined (more than 20), which avidly bind C1q and activate C1 and the classical pathway (6,7); this is mediated by the p15E envelope protein of these viruses (8). The human lentiviruses, human immunodeficiency virus type I (HIV-1), and human T-cell leukemia virus type I (HTLV-1) also possess this property (9,10); for HIV-1, such activation has been reported to be mediated by the gp41 and gp120 viral glycoproteins (9,11,12). In the case of human complement, such activation leads to lysis of the animal retroviruses, but the human lentiviruses, as considered subsequently, are resistant to lytic destruction by human complement because of the presence of host cell membrane cofactor protein (MCP) (CD46), decay-accelerating factor (DAF) (CD55), and CD59 on the viral envelope. Less complete evidence also exists for classical pathway activation by sindbis virus (13), a togavirus, and Newcastle Disease and measles viruses (14,15), which are both paramyxoviruses.

Binding of mannose binding protein (MBP) to high-mannose-containing oligosaccharides on gp120 of HIV-1 and HIV-2 (16), and to influenza virus (17), an orthomyxovirus, has been found to trigger activation of this parallel classical pathway. Since high-mannose-containing carbohydrates are present on many enveloped viruses, it is anticipated that additional examples of MBP-dependent classical pathway activation will be described.

3. Antibody Independent Alternative Pathway Activation

C3b molecules formed in human serum bind covalently, via ester bonds, to hydroxyl groups on carbohydrates and proteins in the fluid phase, and on cell surfaces; amide bonds can also form with amino groups. On normal mammalian cells, amplification of such bound C3b molecules is prevented by the actions of a number of plasma and cell membrane complement regulatory molecules including factors H and I, and CR1, DAF, and MCP; cytolytic damage by assembling C5b-9 that escapes such control is prevented by membrane-associated CD59 (Fig. 2). Viruses, with the exceptions noted later, generally lack complement regulatory molecules. For this reason, nonenveloped and enveloped viruses efficiently activate the alternative complement pathway, often leading to the deposition of enormous numbers of C3 molecules on the virion surface (4,5,18). Alternative pathway activation in human serum lacking specific Ab has been demonstrated for a number of viruses. These include: sindbis virus (13,19); vesicular stomatitis virus (19), a rhabdovirus; simian virus 5 (19), a paramyxovirus; and Epstein-Barr virus (EBV) (20), a herpesvirus. In the case of EBV, alternative pathway activation is mediated by the viral glycoprotein, gp350/220 (21). The resistance of virus-triggered alternative pathway activation to control by factors H and I in plasma suggests the presence of proteins or structures that interfere with factor H binding, but this has not been investigated.

B. Consequences of Complement Activation by Viruses

1. Complement-Dependent Viral Lysis

Most, and probably all enveloped viruses are susceptible to complement-mediated lysis. Complement-mediated lysis of numerous viruses has been demonstrated, including mem-

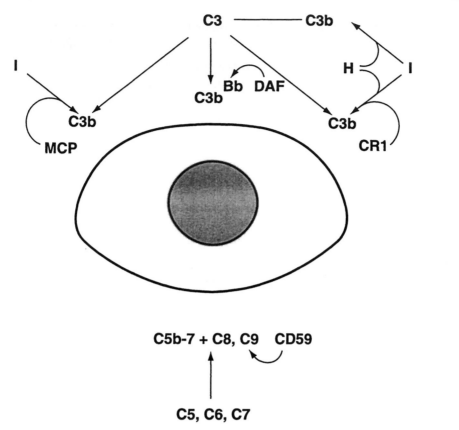

Figure 2 Complement regulatory proteins that protect normal mammalian cells from complement-mediated destruction. CR1, complement receptor type I; DAF, decay accelerating factor; H, factor H; I, factor I; MCP, membrane cofactor (Modified, Cooper N. R. Immunol Today 12:327, 1991.)

bers of the alphavirus, coronavirus, herpesvirus, orthomyxovirus, paramyxovirus, and retrovirus families (1,4,5,18). Complement-mediated lysis of enveloped viruses has the same morphological, physical, and functional consequences as observed for lysis of cells (i.e., the appearance of typical circular lesions produced by the C5b-9 complex, disruption of viral integrity and release of intraviral constituents, and loss of viability) (22,23).

2. *Viral Neutralization by Envelopment with Complement Proteins*

Studies have revealed that enveloped viruses, although susceptible to lysis, are neutralized with completion of the C4 or C3 reaction steps. Among the viruses considered earlier, this has been observed with influenza, vesicular stomatitis, and Newcastle disease viruses, and with EBV; C4- or C3-dependent neutralization has also been observed for herpes simplex virus, a herpesvirus; equine arteritis virus, a togavirus; and vaccinia virus, a poxvirus (3,18,20,23–26). Nonenveloped viruses, such as polyomavirus, a papovavirus, are also neutralized upon completion of the C3 reaction step (27). A thick coat of complement protein on the viral surface is readily visualized in electron microscopic studies

(22,23,27,28). It is likely that this layer of complement protein interferes with the ability of the various viruses to bind to their normal cell surface receptors. Envelopment with complement proteins is likely to be the most common mechanism by which complement mediates viral neutralization.

3. Virus Destruction by Complement-Mediated Opsonization

C3 fragments bound to virus particles as a consequence of complement activation can mediate viral attachment to complement receptors on various cell types. For example, EBV, which only binds to B lymphocytes, acquires the ability to bind to monocytes and neutrophils via CR1 and CR3 after complement activation (18) (Nemerow and Cooper, unpublished studies). Ingestion of complement-coated EBV is followed by viral degradation in phagolysosomes. Although not yet investigated, such reactions are likely to be important in localized viral infections characterized by a surrounding inflammatory reaction. With certain viruses, as considered subsequently, bound C3 may divert complement-coated virus particles from the cell type they normally infect, and even increase viral pathogenicity by permitting the virus to infect other cell types via complement receptors.

C. Complement Activation by Virus-Infected Cells

Virus-encoded proteins are expressed on the membrane of cells infected with a number of enveloped viruses (Fig. 1). Changes in normal cell membrane properties also occur as a consequence of virus infection. As a consequence, cells infected with many viruses efficiently activate the human complement system in the absence of Ab; Ab, when present, augments such activation. Examples include cells infected with measles, mumps, and parainfluenza viruses, which are paramyxoviruses; HIV-1, HTLV-1, herpes simplex virus types I and II, EBV, and influenza virus (2,11,18,29–37). In extensive studies using entirely homologous systems consisting of specific human antiviral Ab or F(ab')$_2$ fragments, human complement, and many types of human cells (epithelial, fibroblastic, lymphoid and neural) infected with many viruses (herpesviruses, orthomyxoviruses, and paramyxoviruses), complement activation has been found to be exclusively mediated by the alternative complement pathway, and to lead to lysis of the cells (32,34,36). However, subsequent studies have shown that human cells infected with HIV-1 and HTLV-1 are resistant to lysis, although they efficiently activate the alternative pathway (11). Since cells infected with the multiple viruses listed above are of human origin, viral infection must alter the expression or distribution of the complement regulatory proteins that normally prevent such unrestricted alternative pathway activation. In this regard, studies with many strains of measles virus show that infection leads to downregulation of MCP (38,39). Classical pathway activation by virus-infected human cells is uncommon; there is only a single report of this property (with HIV) (40) and this finding has been disputed (11).

III. MANIPULATION OF THE COMPLEMENT SYSTEM BY VIRUSES TO FACILITATE INFECTION

Efficient complement activation by free viruses and by virus-infected cells can lead to viral neutralization and destruction of the infected cell, as considered above. However, viruses have evolved numerous mechanisms to evade recognition by specific immune mechanisms and to avoid destruction by the complement system, properties which account for their success as human pathogens, despite the existence of numerous nonspecific and specific antiviral host defense mechanisms. Among these, some viruses have developed the ability to bind to and infect cells via membrane complement receptors and regulatory factors. Some viruses have evolved the ability to use complement-regulatory molecules, such as CR1, DAF, MCP, and CD59 acquired from the cell of origin of the virus, to avoid complement-mediated destruction. Most remarkably, however, some viruses encode proteins that possess CR1, DAF, MCP, or CD59-like properties; these proteins enable such viruses to avoid destruction by the complement system. The use of complement-like molecules by various viruses to facilitate infection and/or to avoid destruction is a developing theme that suggests that complement plays a more central role in antiviral host defense than is commonly appreciated. The various incestuous relationships between viruses and the complement system that facilitate infection are summarized in this section.

A. Use of Cellular Complement Receptors and Regulatory Molecules as Viral Receptors

1. Infection Mediated by Binding of C3-Coated Viral Particles to Cellular C3 Receptors

C3 fragments bound to the surface of viral particles as a result of complement activation could mediate viral binding to C3 receptors on various cell types. As considered before, this type of reaction could lead to phagocytosis and destruction of the virus. In the case of West Nile virus, a flavivirus, viral infection via this mechanism has been reported (41) (Table 1). Several groups have reported that C3 fragments on HIV-1 acquired as a result of complement activation either enable the virus to bind to and infect cells through complement receptors or augment infection. Thus, complement-coated HIV-1 acquires the ability to infect T cell lines via CR1 or CR2 (10,42–44), thymocytes via CR1 or CR2 (43), B cells via CR1 and CR2 (45), B cell lines via CR2 (46), and monocytes/macrophages via CR3 (47). The importance and biological significance of these reactions are not yet clear.

Table 1 Complement Molecules Serving as Viral Receptors

Virus family	Virus	Complement dependence	Cellular receptor
Paramyxovirus	Measles virus	0	MCP (CD46)
Picornaviruses	Coxsackie group B viruses	0	DAF (CD55)
	Echo viruses	0	DAF (CD55)
	Enterovirus 70	0	DAF (CD55)
Herpesvirus	Epstein-Barr virus	0	CR2 (CD21)
Flavivirus	West Nile virus	+	CR3 (CD11b, CD18)
Retrovirus	HIV	+	CR1 (CD35)
			CR2 (CD21)
			CR3 (CD11b, CD18)

2. Infection Mediated by Complement-Independent Interactions of Viral Particles with Cellular Complement Receptors and Regulatory Molecules

Viruses representing several families initiate infection by binding to C3 receptors or other membrane-associated complement regulatory molecules (Table 1). The first example to be reported is the use, by EBV, of CR2 to bind to and infect human B cells (48–53). The major EBV glycoprotein, gp350/220, is the viral ligand for CD21 (54,55); binding is mediated by a nine amino acid primary sequence homologous to the CR2-binding region in C3dg, the natural CR2 ligand (50). This appears to be an example of convergent evolution. The evidence for the conclusion that CR2 is the EBV receptor comes from a variety of approaches including inhibition experiments with monoclonal and polyclonal Abs to CR2; binding studies with purified and recombinant CR2, EBV gp350/220 glycoprotein, and portions of these molecules; and transfection studies. The use of CR2 by EBV as its receptor explains the selective tropism of this virus for B lymphocytes.

Several other viruses have been recently shown to also use normal cell membrane complement proteins as receptors (Table 1). These include measles virus, which initiates infection of epithelial, fibroblastic, and lymphoid cells by binding to MCP (56–58). The evidence includes inhibition of infection by mAbs to CD46, and acquisition of ability of rodent cells transfected with MCP to be productively infected by measles virus. Measles virus binds to the N-glycan of SCR2 on the MCP molecule (59). The viral hemagglutinin mediates viral binding to MCP (60).

A number of serotypes of echovirus (6,7,11,12,20, and 21), which are nonenveloped viruses of the picornavirus family, bind to and infect susceptible human epithelial cells via DAF (61,62) (Table 1). The evidence for this conclusion derives from the findings that mAbs to DAF block infection, and hamster cells transfected with DAF acquire the ability to bind echoviruses. The specificity of the blocking mAb suggests that SCR2 or SCR3, or a combined epitope mediates binding (61,62). Of note, infection of the transfected rodent cells does not occur, indicating that other, likely species-specific cellular factors are necessary for infection. Other echovirus serotypes use different cellular receptors, one of which, the VLA-2 integrin, has been identified (61).

A number of coxsackievirus group B strains (B1, B3, and B5), which are also picornaviruses, also use DAF as their cellular receptor (62,63) (Table 1). The approaches used to show that these coxsackie strains use DAF as their cellular receptor are similar to those noted above (i.e., inhibition of binding and infection by mAbs to DAF, and acquisition of ability of rodent cells transfected with human DAF to bind certain coxsackievirus strains). As with echovirus binding, the specificity of the mAbs suggests involvement of SCR2, SCR3, or both (62,63). However, studies with hamster cells transfected with DAF cDNAs with various deleted SCRs showed that only SCR2 was required for coxsackievirus binding (63). Also as observed with the echovirus strains, binding of coxsackievirus strains to DAF-transfected hamster cells does not lead to infection, indicating that postreceptor species, or cell-specific events are also important for infection. Other group B coxsackievirus strains, use different, as yet, unidentified cellular receptors. Another picornavirus family member, enterovirus 70, has also been shown to use DAF as the cellular receptor mediating infection (64). Additional examples of the use of membrane complement molecules as receptors for viruses are likely to be found. The viral proteins mediating attachment of these picornaviruses to the complement molecules are not known.

B. Use of Complement Regulatory Epitopes to Evade Complement Mediated Viral Destruction

1. Viral Capture of Cellular Complement Regulatory Molecules

The envelopes of viruses that mature by budding from cell membranes express viral glycoproteins, as well as cell membrane-derived lipids and carbohydrates (Fig. 1). Most cell membrane proteins are excluded from the areas of the cell membrane where maturation of enveloped viruses occur. However, it has recently become evident that some viruses acquire normal membrane complement regulatory molecules from their cells of origin during viral maturation, and use these proteins to evade complement-mediated attack (Fig. 1).

Examples of this process include human cytomegalovirus (HCMV), a herpesvirus family member, and three retrovirus family members, human T-cell leukemia virus type 1 (HTLV-1), HIV-1, and simian immunodeficiency virus (SIV) (Table 2). Western blot analyses revealed the presence of MCP, DAF and CD59 in purified HCMV preparations [5,65; (Bradt BM, Cooper NR, *unpublished data*]). Furthermore, purified HCMV was found to possess factor-I-dependent C3b cleaving activity, which was inhibitable by a blocking mAb to human MCP, and decay-accelerating activity for the alternative pathway C3 convertase, which was inhibitable by a blocking mAb to human DAF (5); Bradt BM, Cooper NR, unpublished data), findings indicating that the proteins are not only host cell derived, but also are functionally active. DAF and CD59 were also detectable in purified HTLV-1 preparations by mAb to these proteins in Western blotting studies, virus capture experiments, and induction of complement-dependent viral lysis (65) (Table 2). Functional integrity of the host-cell derived proteins present on HTLV-1 was demonstrated by showing that removal of these proteins from the viral envelope (by treatment with phosphatidylinositol-specific phospholipase C) rendered HTLV-1 susceptible to complement-dependent destruction in the presence of HTLV-1-specific Abs, while reconstitution of the treated virus with purified DAF and CD59 restored resistance to complement-mediated inactivation (65). Similar approaches to those described for HTLV-1 were used to show that HIV-1 and SIV acquire functionally active DAF and CD59 from host cells during viral maturation

Table 2 Viral Capture of Functional Cellular Complement Regulatory Proteins

Virus family	Virus	Captured proteins
Herpesvirus	HCMV	MCP (CD46)
		DAF (CD55)
		CD59
Retroviruses	HTLV-1	DAF (CD55)
		CD59
	HIV	MCP (CD46)
		DAF (CD55)
		CD59
	SIV	MCP (CD46)
		DAF (CD55)
		CD59

(66–69) (Table 2). DAF and CD59 have also been demonstrated on the HIV envelope by electron microscopy (70). HIV-1 and SIV have also been found to possess host-cell derived MCP by virus capture with mAb to human MCP (68).

2. Viral Gene Products Possessing Complement Regulatory Functions

Viruses from two different families express viral genome-encoded proteins with complement regulatory functions (Table 3). Three of these are herpesvirus family members. This is of considerable interest since herpesviruses persist in latent form in host cells for the life of the individual after initial infection; continuing evasion of host defense mechanisms is obviously therefore a requirement for such persistence. The first of these to be characterized is the gC envelope glycoprotein of herpes simplex viruses types 1 and 2 (HSV-1, HSV-2), gC (Table 3). Glycoprotein C from HSV-1 and HSV-2 (gC-1, gC-2) binds C3b (71–74). This viral glycoprotein does not contain partial or complete SCRs, and no other structural similarities of the widely separated C3b binding regions with CR1, or other C3b-binding proteins, have been identified (73,75). Viral gC-1 accelerates decay of the alternative pathway C3 convertase, but unlike CR1, gC-1 lacks MCP activity (76).

gC-1 also possesses no classical pathway-related functions, which findings further differentiate its actions from those of known complement regulatory proteins. Expression of gC-1 protects HSV-1 from complement-mediated damage (72). HSV-1 strains expressing mutant gC-1 molecules lacking C3b binding activity replicate to considerably lower levels (10–1000 fold) *in vivo*, and they are less pathogenic (77). In C3-deficient guinea pigs, the gC mutant strains and wild type HSV-1 strains exhibit comparable viral titers and severity of disease (77), which suggest that gC contributes to pathogenesis in vivo by protecting the virus from complement-mediated destruction.

Purified EBV serves as a factor-I-dependent cofactor for cleavage of C3b, iC3b, C4b, and iC4b, and it accelerates decay of the alternative pathway C3 convertase (78) (Table 3). However, unlike CR1 and MCP, EBV does not bind C3b, and these activities do not appear to result from the actions of host cell proteins acquired from the cell of origin, because the viral functional properties differ significantly from those of cellular CR1, MCP, and DAF. For example, EBV, unlike CR1 and MCP, does not bind C3b; unlike MCP, EBV serves as a cofactor for factor-I-mediated cleavage of iC3b and iC4b; and

Table 3 Viral Gene Products Possessing Complement Regulatory Functions

Virus family	Virus	Viral protein	Complementlike structural features	Complement function
Herpesvirus	HSV	gC-1, gC-2	None	Binds C3b, posseses DAF-like activity
	EBV	Unknown	None	Posseses MCP and DAF-like activities
	HVS	65–75 kDA	Contains 4 SCRs	Blocks complement activation at the C3 step
	HVS	20 kDA	Homologous to CD59	Blocks C5b-9 action
Poxvirus	VV	gp35 (VCP)	Contains 4 SCRs	Binds C3b and C4b, possesses CR1, MCP and DAF-like activities

unlike DAF, EBV does not accelerate decay of the classical pathway C3 convertase (78). Furthermore, the viral genome does not contain full or partial SCRs. The viral protein(s) responsible for these actions have not been identified.

Herpesvirus saimiri (HVS) expresses an envelope protein composed of four SCRs, which is 29–46% identical to human MCP or DAF, depending on the SCR compared (79) (Table 3). Cells transfected with and expressing this HVS gene exhibit resistance to complement-mediated damage; the site of action is at the C3 step (80). In addition, HVS contains a second protein that is 48% identical in sequence to human CD59, and cells expressing the HVS CD59 homologue are resistant to C5b-9 action (81,82). The CD59 homologue is, like mammalian CD59, linked to the membrane via a glycosyl-phosphatidyl-inositol tail (82).

Finally, vaccinia virus (VV), a member of the poxvirus family, expresses a 35 kDa protein that contains four SCRs, and is 38% identical to the four amino terminal SCRs of the eight SCR human C4bp complement-regulatory protein (83) (Table 3). This protein binds C4b, and prevents formation and accelerates the decay of the alternative and classical pathway C3 convertases; it also serves as a cofactor for factor-I-mediated cleavage of C3b and C4b (84). Unlike CR1, it is a cofactor only for the first cleavage of C3b (85). Studies with chimeras have shown that all four SCRs are required for the expression of functional activity (86). A VV deletion mutant lacking this protein was found to be attenuated in vivo and in vitro (87), which suggests that this protein plays a role in viral pathogenesis.

IV. SUMMARY

Viral particles and virus-infected cells activate the complement system in the absence of Ab. In this context, the complement system represents the humoral equivalent of the NK cell. It also subserves the recognition functions normally associated with antibody and specific T-cell immunity. Such activation occurs because of the presence of specific viral proteins that bind C1q or MBP, and/or because they lack mammalian complement regulatory proteins that prevent complement activation by normal cells. In addition, viral proteins expressed on the surface of viral particles and virus-infected cells form immune complexes with specific Abs and efficiently activate the complement system. As a result of Ab-independent or dependent complement activation, viral particles and infected cells become coated with complement components, including C3. Viral particles may be inactivated by envelopment in complement protein, by lysis, or by interacting with phagocytic cells. Virus-infected cells may also be lysed by the activated complement system.

However, viruses have evolved multiple mechanisms that enable them to manipulate the complement system, either to facilitate infection, or to avoid complement-mediated destruction despite efficient complement activation. Thus, some viruses bearing C3 fragments acquired as a result of complement activation bind to and infect cells through complement receptors. Other viruses have evolved proteins that enable them to directly bind to and infect cells through complement receptors and other complement regulatory molecules, including CR2, MCP, and DAF. Such viruses clearly use the complement system to facilitate infection. Another principal mechanism is the acquisition, by some viruses, of complement regulatory molecules including MCP, DAF, and CD59, from the cells in which they mature. More interesting is that several other viruses encode proteins that possess MCP, DAF, or CD59-like functional properties. Both types of mechanisms enable such viruses to avoid complement-mediated destruction by mimicking the complement regulatory processes that protect normal mammalian cells from destruction by the activated complement system. The existence of complement regulatory molecules in many different viruses suggests a common requirement to circumvent C3 and C3 receptor and C5b-9 mediated events for these diverse pathogens to produce disease.

ACKNOWLEDGMENTS

I wish to thank Catalina Hope and Joan Gausepohl for assistance with preparation of the manuscript. Studies from my laboratory were supported by NIH grants (CA14692, AI25016, CA52241 and GCRC grant 2 MO1 RR00833). This is publication No. 10271-IMM.

REFERENCES

1. Cooper NR. Humoral immunity to viruses. In: Fraenkel-Conrat H, ed. Comprehensive Virology. New York: Plenum Press, 1979:123–170.
2. Cooper NR, Nemerow GR. Complement, viruses and virus infected cells. Semin Immunopathol 1983; 6:327–347.
3. Beebe DP, Schreiber RD, Cooper NR. Neutralization of influenza virus by normal human sera: mechanisms involving antibody and complement. J Immunol 1983; 130:1317–1322.
4. Cooper NR. Complement dependent neutralization of viruses. In: Rother K, Till G, eds. The Complement System. Berlin: Springer-Verlag, 1988: 342–348.
5. Cooper NR. Interactions of the complement system with microorganisms. In: Erdei A, ed. New Aspects of Complement Structure and Function. Austin: R.G. Landes Co. 1994:133–149.
6. Cooper NR, Jensen FC, Welsh RM Jr, et al. Lysis of RNA tumor viruses by human serum: direct antibody independent triggering of the classical complement pathway. J Exp Med 1976; 144:970–984.
7. Welsh RM, Cooper NR, Jensen FC, et al. Human serum lyses RNA tumour viruses. Nature 1975; 257:612–614.
8. Bartholomew RM. Lysis of oncornaviruses by human serum: lysis of oncornaviruses by human serum: isolation of the viral complement (C1) receptor and identification as p15E. J Exp Med 1978; 147:844.
9. Ebenbichler CF, Thielens NM, Vornhagen R, et al. Human immunodeficiency virus type 1 activates the classical pathway of complement by direct C1 binding through specific sites in the transmembrane glycoprotein gp41. J Exp Med 1991; 174:1417–1424.
10. Dierich MP, Ebenbichler CF, Marschang P, et al. HIV and human complement: mechanisms of interaction and biological implication. Immunol Today 1993; 14(9):435–439.
11. Sölder BM, Schultz TF, Hengster P, et al. HIV and HIV-infected cells differentially activate the human complement system independent of antibody. Immunol Lett 1989; 22:135–146.
12. Süsal C, Kirschfink M, Kröpelin M, et al. Complement activation by recombinant HIV-1 glycoprotein gp120. J Immunol 1994; 152:6028–6034.
13. Hirsch RL, Winkelstein JA, Griffin DE. The role of complement in viral infections III. Activation of the classical and alternative complement pathways by Sindbis virus. J Immunol 1980; 124:2507–2510.
14. Welsh RM. Host cell modification of lymphocytic choriomeningitis virus and Newcastle disease virus altering viral inactivation by human complement. J Immunol 1977; 118:348–354.
15. Schluederberg A, Ajello C, Evans B. Fate of rubella genome ribonucleic acid after immune and nonimmune virolysis in the presence of ribonuclease. Infect Immun 1976; 14:1097–1102.

16. Haurum JS, Thiel S, Jones IM, et al. Complement activation upon binding of mannan-binding protein to HIV envelope glycoproteins. AIDS 1993; 7:1307–1313.

17. Reading PC, Hartley CA, Ezekowitz RAB, et al. A serum mannose-binding lectin mediates complement-dependent lysis of influenza virus-infected cells. Biochem Biophys Res Commun 1995; 217:1128–1136.

18. Cooper NR, Nemerow GR. Complement dependent mechanisms of virus neutralization. In: Ross G, ed. Immunobiology of the Complement System. New York: Academic Press, 1986:139–162.

19. McSharry JJ, Pickering J, Caliguiri A. Activation of the alternative complement pathway by enveloped viruses containing limited amounts of sialic acid. Virology 1981; 114:507–515.

20. Mayes JT, Schreiber RD, Cooper NR. Development and application of an enzyme linked immunosorbent assay for the quantitation of alternative complement pathway activation in human serum. J Clin Invest 1984; 73:160–170.

21. Mold C, Bradt BM, Nemerow GR, et al. Activation of the alternative complement pathway by Epstein-Barr virus and the viral envelope glycoprotein, gp350. J Immunol 1988; 140:3867–3874.

22. Nemerow GR, Cooper NR. Isolation of Epstein-Barr virus and studies of its neutralization by human IgG and complement. J Immunol 1981; 127:272–278.

23. Welsh RM, Lampert PW, Burner PA, et al. Antibody and complement interactions with purified lymphocytic choriomeningitis virus. Virology 1976; 73:59.

24. Leddy JP, Simons RL, Douglas RG. Effect of selective complement deficiency on the rate of neutralization of enveloped viruses by human sera. J Immunol 1977; 118:28.

25. Linscott WD, Levinson WE. Complement components required for virus neutralization by early immunoglobulin antibody. Proc Natl Acad Sci USA 1969; 64:520.

26. Nemerow GR, Jensen FC, Cooper NR. Neutralization of Epstein-Barr virus (EBV) by nonimmune human serum: role of cross reacting antibody to herpes simplex virus (HSV-1) and complement (C). J Clin Invest 1982; 70:1081–1091.

27. Oldstone MBA, Cooper NR, Larson DL. Formation and biologic role of polyoma virus–antibody complexes. J Exp Med 1974; 140:549.

28. Berry DM, Almeida JD. The morphological and biological effects of various antisera on avian infectious bronchitis virus. J Gen Virol 1968; 3:97.

29. Okada H, Tanaka H, Okada N. Cytolysis of Sendai virus-infected guinea-pig cells by homologous complement. Immunol 1983; 49:29–35.

30. Okada H, Okada N. Sendai virus infected cells are readily cytolysed by guinea-pig complement without antibody. Immunology 1981; 43:337–344.

31. Sissons JGP, Oldstone MBA, Schreiber RD. Antibody-independent activation of the alternative complement pathway by measles virus-infected cells. Proc Natl Acad Sci USA 1980; 77 No. 1:559–562.

32. Sissons JGP, Schreiber RD, Perrin LH, et al. Lysis of measles virus infected cells by the purified cytolytic alternative complement pathway and antibody. J Exp Med 1979; 150:445–454.

33. McConnell I, Lachmann PJ. Complement and cell membranes. Transplant Rev 1976; 32:72.

34. Perrin LH, Joseph BS, Cooper NR, et al. Mechanism of injury of virus infected cells by antiviral antibody and complement: participation of IgG, Fab'$_2$ and the alternative complement pathway. J Exp Med 1976; 143:1027–1041.

35. Mold C, Nemerow GR, Bradt BM, et al. CR2 is a complement activator and the covalent binding site for C3 during alternative pathway activation by Raji cells. J Immunol 1988; 140:1923–1929.

36. Sissons JGP, Cooper NR, Oldstone MBA. Alternative complement pathway mediated lysis of measles virus infected cells-induction by IgG antibody bound to individual viral glycoproteins and comparative efficacy of F(ab')$_2$ and Fab' fragments. J Immunol 1979; 123:2144–2149.

37. Joseph B, Cooper NR, Oldstone MBA. Immunologic injury of cultured cells infected with measles virus I: role of IgG antibody and the alternative complement pathway. J Exp Med 1975; 141:761–774.

38. Naniche D, Wild F, Rabourdin-Combe C, et al. Measles virus haemagglutinin induces down-regulation of gp57/67, a molecule involved in virus binding. J Gen Virol 1993; 74:1073–1079.

39. Schneider-Schaulies J, Dunster LM, Kobune F, et al. Differential downregulation of CD46 by measles virus strains. J Virol 1995; 69:7257–7259.

40. Spear GT, Landay AL, Sullivan BL, et al. Activation of complement on the surface of cells infected by human immunodeficiency virus. J Immunol 1990; 144:1490–1496.

41. Cardosa MJ, Peterfield JS, Gordon S. Complement receptors mediate enhanced flavivirus replication in macrophages. J Exp Med 1983; 158:258–263.

42. Boyer V, Desgranges C, Trabaud M-A, et al. Complement mediates human immunodeficiency virus type 1 infection of a human T cell line in a CD4- and antibody-independent fashion. J Exp Med 1991; 173:1151–1158.

43. Delibrias C-C, Mouhoub A, Fischer E, et al. CR1(CD35) and CR2(CD21) complement C3 receptors are expressed on normal human thymocytes and mediate infection of thymocytes with opsonized human immunodeficiency virus. Eur J Immunol 1994; 24:2784–2788.

44. Gras GS, Dormont D. Antibody-dependent and antibody-independent complement-mediated enhancement of human immunodeficiency virus type 1 infection in a human, Epstein-Barr virus-transformed B-lymphocytic cell line. J Virol 1991; 65(1):541–545.

45. Legendre C, Gras G, Krzysiek R, et al. Mechanisms of opsonized HIV entry in normal B lymphocytes. FEBS Lett 1996; 381:227–232.

46. Boyer V, Delibrias C, Noraz N, et al. Complement receptor type 2 mediates infection of the human CD4-negative Raji B-cell line with opsonized HIV. Scand J Immunol 1992; 36:879–883.

47. Soelder BM, Reisinger EC, Koeffler D. Complement receptors and HIV entry into cells. Lancet 1989; 2:271–272.

48. Fingeroth JD, Weis JJ, Tedder TF, et al. Epstein-Barr virus receptor of human B lymphocytes is the C3d receptor CR2. Proc Natl Acad Sci 1984; 81:4510–4514.

49. Frade R, Barel M, Ehlin-Henriksson B, et al. gp140, the C3d receptor of human B lymphocytes, is also the Epstein-Barr virus receptor. Proc Natl Acad Sci USA 1985; 82:1490–1493.

50. Nemerow GR, Houghten RA, Moore MD, et al. Identification of the epitope in the major envelope protein of Epstein-Barr virus that mediates viral binding to the B lymphocyte EBV receptor (CR2). Cell 1989; 56:369–377.

51. Nemerow GR, Wolfert R, McNaughton ME, et al. Identification and characterization of the Epstein-Barr virus receptor on human B lymphocytes and its relationship to the C3d complement receptor. J Virol 1985; 55:347–351.

52. Cooper NR, Moore MD, Nemerow GR. Immunobiology of CR2, the B lymphocyte receptor for Epstein-Barr virus and the C3d complement fragment. Annu Rev Immunol 1988; 6:85–113.

53. Nemerow GR, Luxembourg AT, Cooper NR. CD21/CR2: its role in EBV infection and immune function. Epstein Barr Rep 1994; 1:59–64.

54. Nemerow GR, Mold C, Keivens-Schwend V, et al. Identification of gp350 as the viral glycoprotein mediating attachment of Epstein-Barr virus (EBV) to the EBV/C3d receptor of B cells: sequence homology of gp350 and C3 complement fragment C3d. J Virol 1987; 61:1416–1420.

55. Tanner J, Weis J, Fearon D, et al. Epstein-Barr virus gp350/220 binding to the B lymphocyte C3d receptor mediates adsorption, capping and endocytosis. Cell 1987; 50:203–213.

56. Naniche D, Varior-Krishnan G, Cervoni F, et al. Human membrane cofactor protein (CD46) acts as a cellular receptor for measles virus. J Virol 1993; 67:6025–6032.

57. Dörig RE, Marcil A, Chopra A, et al. The human CD46 molecule is a receptor for measles virus (Edmonston strain). Cell 1993; 75:295–305.

58. Manchester M, Liszewski MK, Atkinson J-P, et al. Multiple isoforms of CD46 (membrane cofactor protein) serve as receptors for measles virus. Proc Natl Acad Sci 1994; 91(6):2161–2165.

59. Maisncr A, Alvarez J, Liszewski MK, et al. The N-glycan of the SCR 2 region is essential for membrane cofactor protein (CD46) to function as a measles virus receptor. J Virol 1996; 70:4973–4977.

60. Nussbaum O, Broder CC, Moss B, et al. Functional and structural interactions between measles virus hemagglutinin and CD46. J Virol 1995; 69:3341–3349.

61. Bergelson JM, Chan M, Solomon KR, et al. Decay-accelerating factor (CD55), a glycosylphosphatidylinositol-anchored complement regulatory protein, is a receptor for several echoviruses. Proc Natl Acad Sci USA 1994; 91:6245–6248.

62. Shafren DR, Bates RC, Agrez MV, et al. Coxsackieviruses B1, B3, and B5 use decay accelerating factor as a receptor for cell attachment. J Virol 1995; 69:3873–3877.

63. Bergelson JM, Mohanty JG, Growell RL, et al. Coxsackievirus B3 adapted to growth in RD cells binds to decay-accelerating factor (CD55). J Virol 1995; 69:1903–1906.

64. Karnauchow TM, Tolson DL, Harrison BA, et al. The HeLa cell receptor for enterovirus 70 is decay-accelerating factor (CD55). J Virol 1996; 70:5143–5152.

65. Spear GT, Lurain NS, Parker CJ, et al. Host cell-derived complement control proteins CD55 and CD59 are incorporated into the virions of two unrelated enveloped viruses. J Immunol 1995; 155:4376–4381.

66. Schmitz J, Zimmer JP, Kluxen B, et al. Antibody-dependent complement-mediated cytotoxicity in sera from patients with HIV-1 infection is controlled by CD55 and CD59. J Clin Invest 1995; 96:1520–1526.

67. Stoiber H, Pinter C, Siccardi AG, et al. Efficient destruction of human immunodeficiiency virus in human serum by inhibiting the protective action of complement factor H and decay accelerating factor (DAF, CD55). J Exp Med 1996; 183:307–310.

68. Montefiori DC, Cornell RJ, Zhou Y, et al. Complement control proteins, CD46, CD55, and CD59, as common surface constituents of human and simian immunodeficiency viruses and possible targets for vaccine protection. Virology 1994; 205:82–92.

69. Marschang P, Sodroski J, Wurzner R, Dierich P. Decay-accelerating factor (CD55) protects human immunodeficiency virus type 1 from inactivation by human complement. Eur J Immunol 1995; 25:285–290(abstract).

70. Dourmashkin RR, Davies A, Davis D, Lachmann PJ. Enumeration of complement regulatory proteins on the surface of HIV particles by electron microscopy. Mol Immunol 1996; 33:14(abstract).

71. Friedman HM, Cohen GH, Eisenberg RJ, et al. Glycoprotein C of herpes simplex virus 1 acts as a receptor for the C3b complement component on infected cells. Nature 1984; 309:633–635.

72. McNearney TA, ODell C, Holers VM, et al. Herpes simplex virus glycoproteins gC-1 and gC-2 bind to the third component of complement and provide protection against complement mediated neutralization of viral infectivity. J Exp Med 1987; 166:1525–1535.

73. Seidel-Dugan C, Ponce de Leon M, Friedman HM, et al. Identification of C3b-binding regions on Herpes simplex virus type 2 glycoprotein C. J Virol 1990; 64:1897–1906.

74. Eisenberg RJ, Ponce de Leon M, Friedman M, et al. Complement component C3b binds directly to purified glycoprotein C of herpes simplex virus types 1 and 2. Microb Pathog 1987; 3:423–435.

75. Hung S-L, Peng C, Kostavasili I, et al. The interaction of glycoprotein C of herpes simplex virus types 1 and 2 with the alternative complement pathway. Virology 1994; 203:299–312.

76. Fries LF, Friedman HM, Cohen GH, et al. Glycoprotein C of herpes simplex virus 1 is an inhibitor of the complement cascade. J Immunol 1986; 137:1636–1641.

77. Friedman HM, Wang L, Burger R, Lambris J, Eisenberg RJ, Cohen GH, et al. The role of herpes simplex virus type 1 glycoprotein C, A C3b binding protein, in pathogenesis. Mol Immunol 1996: 33:63(abstract).

78. Mold C, Bradt BM, Nemerow GR, et al. Epstein-Barr virus regulates activation and processing of the third component of complement. J Exp Med 1988; 168:949–969.

79. Albrecht J-C, Fleckenstein B. New member of the multigene family of complement control proteins in herpesvirus saimiri. J Virol 1992; 66:3937–3940.

80. Fodor WL, Rollins SA, Bianco-Caron S, et al. The complement control protein homolog of herpesvirus saimiri regulates serum complement by inhibiting C3 convertase activity. J Virol 1995; 69:3889–3896.

81. Albrecht J-C, Nicholas J, Cameron KR, et al. Herpesvirus saimiri has a gene specifying a homologue of the cellular membrane glycoprotein CD59. Virology 1992; 190:527–530.
82. Rother RP, Rollins SA, Fodor WL, et al. Inhibition of complement-mediated cytolysis by the terminal complement inhibitor of herpesvirus saimiri. J Virol 1994; 68:730–737.
83. Kotwal GJ, Moss B. Vaccinia virus encodes a secretory polypeptide structurally related to complement control proteins. Nature 1988; 335:176–178.
84. McKenzie R, Kotwal GJ. Regulation of complement activity by vaccinia virus complement-control protein. J Infect Dis 1992; 166:1245–1250.
85. Sahu A, Isaacs SN, Lambris JD. Modulation of complement by recombinant vaccinia virus complement control protein. Mol Immunol 1996; 33:61 Abstract.
86. Rosengard AM, Turka LA, Korb LC, Baldwin WM, III, Sanfilippo F, Ahearn JM. Functional comparison of vaccinia virus complement-control protein and human CR1. Mol Immunol 1996; 33:67(abstract).
87. Isaacs SN, Kotwal GJ, Moss B. Vaccinia virus complement-control protein prevents antibody-dependent complement-enhanced neutralization of infectivity and contributes to virulence. Proc Natl Acad Sci USA 1992; 89:628–632.

19

Complement Deficiencies and Infection

PETER DENSEN

University of Iowa College of Medicine, Iowa City, Iowa

I. INTRODUCTION

For patients with inherited disorders, these afflictions are most often seen as a curse. To the biologist, these "experiments of nature" provide a window onto the elucidation of the full range of activities in which a given protein participates. Indeed, the insights provided by both the detailed clinical investigation of patients with these disorders and the study of animals with these defects have been so revealing that this principle has become a fundamental pillar of modern molecular biology in the form of "knock out" mice bred precisely for this purpose.

The utility of inherited disorders in providing unanticipated insights into the normal actions and interactions of individual proteins as well as protein systems is well illustrated by the complement cascade. Indeed, these natural and assisted experiments of nature have dispelled the notion espoused by Macfarlane Burnet that "the classical phenomenon of complement lysis of red cells is a laboratory artifact of no real significance for immunity" (1). This rather dim view of the complement system has been progressively replaced by the growing delineation of the complement system as an essential mechanism contributing broadly to all aspects of inflammation. These aspects include not just those reactions that promote inflammation (the classical characteristics of rubor, calor, tumor, and dolor, mediated in part by the complement anaphylatoxins) and innate host defense but also those that promote immune complex processing as well as the immune response. This growing understanding has been accompanied by the realization that, like the clotting cascade, the complement system is comprised of plasma proteins designed to function normally in a highly localized manner at the interface between plasma (or other body fluids) and cell surfaces. There exist on the surface of host cells a number of proteins whose function it is to protect these cells from the injurious potential of complement activation and in doing so to help differentiate self from nonself. This chapter will illustrate what the infectious consequences of complement deficiency states tell us about the function of the complement cascade and, conversely, what these associations tell us about host defense against specific microbial pathogens. Other chapters address this theme with respect to the processing of immune complexes and the immune response.

II. CLINICAL PATTERNS OF INFECTION IN
COMPLEMENT-DEFICIENT PATIENTS

Several reviews of complement deficiency states have documented the increased susceptibility to infection experienced by complement-deficient patients (2–4). Nevertheless,
reviews such as these are subject to an inherent ascertainment bias as well as the potential
for underreporting of conditions that typify the disorder and an overreporting of unusual
conditions that may or may not be truly associated with the deficiency state. A number
of studies comparing the prevalence of complement deficiency states in the general
population and populations bearing the putative clinical hallmarks of the deficiency (e.g,
infection, systemic lupus erythematosus [SLE]) have confirmed the major associations
noted in individual case reports and emphasize that the *relative* frequency of these reported
associations among the different deficiency states probably is reflective of the true state
of affairs (3, 5, 6).

About half or more of complement-deficient persons experience at least one infection. *Meningococcus* is the single most common documented cause (67%) of infection in
these patient as a whole. However, a more instructive pattern emerges upon scrutiny of
the frequency of these infections with respect to deficiencies affecting the different functional units within the complement system, which arise as a consequence of the structural
organization of the cascade itself. The clinical syndrome produced by complement deficiencies within a given functional unit is similar despite the involvement of distinct proteins.
These functional units include the early classical pathway components (C1, C4, and C2);
alternative pathway components (factors D, B, and P); C3 and factors H and I: regulatory
components whose absence is associated with low concentrations of C3; and the terminal
or late-acting complement components (C5, C6, C7, C8, and C9) (Table 1). Viewed in
this manner, relatively distinctive clinical patterns of disease emerge that are helpful to
clinicians likely to encounter patients with infectious diseases and reflective of the unique
functional aspects of the proteins comprising each unit as well as the bacteriological
properties of the organisms responsible for the infections.

III. FUNCTIONAL CONSEQUENCES IN THE
DIFFERENT TYPES OF COMPLEMENT
DEFICIENCY

A. Deficiencies of Classical Pathway Proteins

Although individual components within the early portion of the classical pathway, especially C1q, are very important with respect to the processing of immune complexes (see
chapter 20), they do not appear to have a direct affect on host defense. Instead, the
infectious consequences of a deficiency of one of these components stem largely from
decreased complement activation via the classical pathway and consequent impairment
in C3-mediated functions. Thus, patients with classical pathway deficiencies are similar
to those with C3 deficiency with respect to the age of initial infection and the sites at
which these infections commonly occur, but they differ in the frequency of infection and
its recurrence. This difference reflects the ability of patients with classical pathway defects
to utilize the alternative pathway to deposit C3 on bacteria, an ability that improves as
the patient ages and acquires specific antibodies that facilitate alternative pathway activation and efficiency (7).

Table 1 Clinical Patterns of Infection in Complement Deficiency

	Deficiency state			
Clinical variable	CP (C1, C2, C4)	AP (P, D, B)	C3 (C3, H, I)	LCCD (C5–C9)
Functional defect	↓C' act. ↓IC metab. ↓Immun. resp.	↓C' act.	↓ops./phag. ↓SBA ↓Immun. resp. ↓IC metab. ↓CTX	↓SBA (↓CTX)[a]
% with Infection	40%	57%	78%	64%
Median age at first infection (yr)	2	14	2	17
Site of infection (%)				
Sinopulmonary	56	25	57	4
CNS	23	39	28	72
Blood	20	36	14	24
Organisms				
S. pneumonia	33	4	21	5
H. influenzae	6	3	3	1
N. meningitidis	9	36	26	262
N. gonorrhoeae	1	2	0	29
Other[b]	32	7	11	8
Recurrent Infection with Same Org. (%)	6.3	3.5	56	50[c]

CP, classic pathway; AP, alternative pathway; IC metab., immune complex metabolism; C' act., complement activation; Immun. resp., immune response; ops./phag., opsonophagocytosis; CTX, chemotaxis; SBA, serum bactericidal activity.
[a] C5 deficiency only.
[b] Other. CP: gm. neg. rods (8), *S. aureus* (6), beta *Streptococcus* (4), M. Tb (4), misc. (10); AP: gm. neg. rods (5), misc. (2); C3: gm. neg. rods (4), beta *Streptococcus* (3), *S. aureus* (1), misc. (3); LCCD: toxoplasma (4), M. Tb. (2), misc. (2).
[c] Recurrent disease not reported in C9 deficiency.

A secondary effect of these deficiencies is a decrease in the immune responsiveness of these patients to infection, which is reflected in lower than expected serum IgG concentrations, especially IgG2 and IgG4 (8). These antibody subclasses are particularly important in the host defense against encapsulated bacteria; which are precisely the organisms to which these patients are most susceptible. These clinical observations are supported in general by experiments in complement-deficient animals documenting a suboptimal immune response to T-dependent antigens and a failure to undergo isotype switching from IgM to IgG. Decreased antibody concentrations in these complement deficiencies is postulated to arise as a consequence of decreased C3 deposition on specific organism constituents, for example, capsular polysaccharide, and impaired signaling through the CR2 receptor for C3dg on B lymphocytes (9–11) (see chapter 14). Indeed, the age of the patient at the time of first infection, the organisms causing infection, and the anatomical sites at which infection occurs in these complement-deficient individuals closely mimic those observed in patients with the primary immunoglobulin deficiencies.

In addition to these well-documented effects, the chemical preference of the C4B allotype to form covalent ester linkages with available hydroxyl groups that predominate on sugars, such as those making up bacterial capsular polysaccharides, has been postulated to be another risk factor for infection in patients with homozygous C4B deficiency. However, initial reports to this effect have not been borne out by subsequent studies (12–16). Thus, the infectious consequences in patients with these deficiencies results from the defect itself as well as the secondary effects of the defect on antibody production.

B. Deficiencies of Alternative Pathway Proteins

Inherited deficiencies of alternative pathway proteins are less prevalent than those of the classical pathway and conclusions drawn about the effects of these deficiencies largely reflect consequences of properdin deficiency, which is the most common of these disorders. Although factors H and I are properly considered as components of the alternative pathway, the functional consequence of the deficiencies is a markedly reduced C3 concentration. These proteins are more appropriately considered in that functional context.

Even though a number of immune modulating effects of factor B have been described in vitro, the only recognized clinical consequence of alternative pathway deficiencies is defective complement activation. Indeed, detailed studies of factor-B-deficient knock-out mice have not documented an immune modulating effect of factor B in vivo (17). This conclusion has been supported by the limited observations made in the sole homozygous factor-B-deficient patient described to date (18). In addition, defective complement activation may be clinically apparent only in the absence of specific antibody, which otherwise serves as an effective activator of the classical pathway. Interesting is that the predominant infectious consequence of these deficiencies is meningococcal infection. The clinical picture in these patients is similar to that in patients with late complement component deficiencies with respect to causative organism, age of first infection, and site of infection. This observation suggests that the clinical consequences of these deficiencies may most often reflect impaired serum bactericidal activity through the alternative pathway rather than any direct effect on associated C3-dependent opsonophagocytosis. This paradox is most likely attributable to the failure to deposit C3 on the bacterial capsule in the absence of specific antibody, or a requirement for both capsular antibody and C3 for the effective opsonophagocytic elimination of meningococci. In addition, there may be a unique requirement for complement activation via the alternative pathway in the normal host defense against meningococci.

Recurrent infection is uncommon in individuals with a deficiency of one of the alternative pathway proteins, probably because of their ability to utilize the classical pathway once a specific antibody response has been initiated (19). A second reason may be as a consequence of the relatively high mortality rate observed in properdin deficiency, although this is not as great as originally believed (3,20). Recurrent infection has been observed in the few factor-D-deficient individuals discovered to date, suggesting that additional functional consequences may yet be described in deficiency states affecting the alternative pathway proteins.

C. C3 Deficiency States

As might be anticipated from its concentration in serum and its location at the juncture of the classical and alternative pathways with the late-acting complement components, patients with C3 deficiency exhibit a profound defect in multiple complement-mediated functions that contributes to their increased susceptibility to infection. Foremost among these defects are impaired opsonophagocytosis, serum bactericidal activity, and immune responsiveness (21). The contribution of these defects to the enhanced susceptibility of these patients to infection has been amply confirmed in C3-deficient animals, which also demonstrate impaired immune responses to both T-cell-independent and -dependent antigens. In addition, some C3-deficient patients fail to develop granulocytosis in response to bacterial infection both because of the absence of the C3e cleavage product that promotes this response and because of a secondary defect in the generation of C5a, a complement-derived chemotaxin. Like patients with classical pathway defects, patients with C3 deficiency also exhibit abnormalities in the processing of immune complexes. As a consequence of this multitude of defects, very few patients with C3 deficiency remain healthy; 78% suffer from repeated infections and 79% experience autoimmune disorders, with considerable overlap between these two groups. Infection typically begins early in life; involves the sinopulmonary track, meninges, and bloodstream; is caused by encapsulated bacteria, particularly *S. pneumoniae* and *N. meningitidis*; and recurs frequently.

D. Late Complement Component Deficiencies

With the exception of individuals with C5 deficiency, the sole defect in persons with late complement component deficiencies (LCCD) is the inability to assemble the membrane attack complex (MAC) and their consequent inability to generate complement-dependent bactericidal activity. Up to two-thirds of these individuals will experience at least one episode of meningococcal infection and about half of these persons will experience recurrent disease. The striking propensity of these individuals to develop exclusively meningococcal or systemic gonococcal infection underscores the critical importance of serum bactericidal activity in the host defense against *Neisseria*. That this defect in serum bactericidal activity is directly responsible for the increased susceptibility of these patients to infection is indicated by two fundamental observations. First, serum from C9-deficient individuals is able to kill meningococci, albeit at a slower rate than complement-sufficient serum (22). Second, the risk of developing meningococcal disease among C7- and C9-deficient Japanese is approximately 5,000- and 700-fold greater than that in complement-sufficient Japanese, respectively (23,24). Thus, although C9-deficient individuals clearly are at increased risk of developing meningococcal disease, this risk is 7 fold less than that in other patients with LCCD whose serum does not support any direct bactericidal activity against this organism. The combination of these in vitro and in vivo data indicate a dose–response relationship between the rate of meningococcal killing and the risk of infection and directly implicates the absence of bactericidal activity as the mechanism underlying the increased risk of patients with LCCD for neisserial disease.

Among the LCCDs, C5 and C9 deficiency deserve additional comment. First, although the migration of neutrophils to skin windows in C5-deficient individuals is unequivocally impaired, this defect does not appear to contribute to the susceptibility of these persons to meningococcal infection or to the severity of the disease that they experience since the clinical aspects of meningococcal disease in these patients is indistinguishable from that in patients with other LCCDs (24). Second, although there has been some question as to whether C9-deficient individuals display an increased susceptibility to meningococcal disease, the carefully collected data by several Japanese investigators cited above convincingly address this issue. Interesting is that accompanying observations indicate that recurrent meningococcal disease has yet to be reported in C9-deficient individuals and that disease in these individuals has manifest itself as the meningitis syndrome, not meningococcemia (24). If these observations are borne out in future reports, they would suggest that specific antibody enhances the efficiency of the limited bactericidal activity generated by C5–C8 and that token amounts of bactericidal activity are sufficient to protect the bloodstream although not the meninges. This is probably because the level of complement and antibody in the cerebrospinal fluid bathing these structures is quite low, even in normal individuals. These deductions are supported in part by the absence of an enhanced susceptibility to infection in individuals who have either subtotal C6 deficiency or who are heterozygous for the null allele for any of the terminal complement components.

IV. SITE OF INFECTION IN COMPLEMENT-DEFICIENT INDIVIDUALS

Understanding the functional activities that are defective in complement-deficient individuals and then observing the sites at which they commonly experience infection implies that certain functions may be particularly relevant to host defense at these sites. Thus the common occurrence of recurrent infections involving the sinopulmonary tree in patients with a deficiency of one of the early components of the classical pathway or of C3 itself suggests that opsonophagocytosis may be a particularly important means of preventing microbial invasion from mucosal membranes. The striking association between meningococcal meningitis and defects that impair complement-dependent killing likewise suggests a particular role of the membrane attack complex either in preventing this organism from spreading via the bloodstream to the meninges or in host defense in this location. Both opsonophagocytic and complement-dependent bactericidal activity appear to play an important role in eliminating organism from the bloodstream and in maintaining its sterility. Clearance of encapsulated bacteria, such as *S. pneumoniae*, from the bloodstream is critically dependent on C3 and a functional spleen, especially in the nonimmune host (25–27).

V. ORGANISMS CAUSING INFECTION IN COMPLEMENT-DEFICIENT HOSTS

Although infection is a frequent manifestation of complement deficiency, the precise cause of many of these infections is unknown, especially for those deficiencies in which infection of the sinopulmonary tree is common. Clinicians frequently make little attempt to identify the causative agents in patients presenting with sinusitis, otitis, and bronchitis even when these infections recur on a frequent basis and especially if the patient is not known to have an immune deficiency. As the perceived severity of the infection increases, from pneumonia to bacteremia and meningitis, it becomes more likely that cultures will be obtained. This fact coupled with the sterile nature of the bloodstream and cerebrospinal fluid make data obtained in these infections and from these sources increasingly meaningful predictors of microbiological associations with complement deficiency states.

   With these caveats in mind, *Neisseria sp.*, especially *Neisseria meningitidis, Streptococcus Streptococcus pneumoniae*, and *Haemophilus influenzae* account for 88% of the infectious episodes in which a specific microbial infection is identified [Table 1 (3)]. These findings should not be interpreted to mean that the role of complement in host defense is limited to these organisms, especially given the extensive in vitro and in vivo experimental data that exist in this regard for other bacteria, viruses, and parasites. Rather, they point to complement as a major host defense mechanism against these pathogens and to the redundancy that exists with respect to the protective mechanisms brought into play against most microorganisms.

Opsonophagocytosis is particularly relevant for the elimination of encapsulated organisms and the role of C3 as an opsonin deserves special attention because its deposition on the bacterial surface is a critical determinant of the outcome of the encounter between the host and the organism. First, covalent C3 deposition serves to localize complement activation to specific topographical locations on the organism surface. In the case of C3 deposited on the outer membrane of gram-negative bacteria, localization brings assembly of the MAC into close apposition with the membrane into which it must be inserted if it is to express its bactericidal potential. However in the case of encapsulated bacteria, deposition of C3 in this location, mediated either by activation of the alternative pathway or by antibody specific for subcapsular antigens, hinders effective interaction between the C3 and its receptors on phagocytic cells. In contrast, antibody to capsular antigens promotes C3 deposition on the capsular surface (28). Deposited C3 is clustered about the antibody in a topographical configuration that promotes the synergistic interaction of these two ligands with their respective receptors on phagocytic cells that then effectively engulf and kill the organism. These considerations probably account for the prevalence of infection caused by encapsulated bacteria in individuals with a deficiency of one of the early components of the classical pathway or with C3 deficiency itself.

Although opsonophagocytosis is an important component of host defense against meningococci, direct complement-mediated bactericidal activity is uniquely relevant to host defense against systemic neisserial infection. As a consequence, meningococci and gonococci predominate as causes of infection in any complement deficiency that selectively impairs this activity. The absence of a similar association with infections caused by *H. influenzae* remains enigmatic.

VI. MENINGOCOCCAL DISEASE AND COMPLEMENT DEFICIENCY

The fact that meningococci are the most common cause of infection in complement deficiency states suggests a unique relationship between this organism and the complement system. In the case of LCCD this suggestion has led to the identification of a number of variables that provide additional insight into the role of the complement system in the pathophysiology of this infection and, by extension, other diseases as well (2,24). Unique features that differentiate meningococcal disease in LCCD patients from that in normal individuals include frequency of infection; age at first infection; serogroup of the infecting meningococcus recurrent disease; disease relapse; and mortality.

LCCD individuals experience a 5–10,000-fold increase in the risk of infection compared to complement sufficient individuals. As discussed above, the absence of serum bactericidal activity appears directly responsible for this increased susceptibility, although it is possible that the inoculum needed to cause infection in deficient persons might also be lower than that in normal persons.

The difference in age at the time of the first meningococcal infection in complement-sufficient persons and persons with LCCD is both striking and puzzling (24). The median age of infection in the normal population is 3 years, whereas it is between 14 and 17 years in the complement-deficient patients. The major risk factor for meningococcal disease in the normal population is the absence of protective antibody, which inversely correlates with the peak incidence of meningococcal disease observed in the first 2 years of life. Acquisition of protective antibody begins early in life, hence 56% of all meningococcal infections in the general population occur before the age 5. In contrast, only 10% of the meningococcal infections in LCCD individuals occur within the same time period. The absence of a similar early peak in the age specific incidence of meningococcal infection in complement-deficient persons indicates that simple stochastic considerations, such as a lifetime of risk, do not explain the older age at which these persons acquire their first infection. This observation leads to a paradox in which deficient individuals pass through the period of life when the deficiency might be expected to increase maximally their susceptibility to meningococcal disease without evincing evidence of that susceptibility, only to emerge later in life with an increased risk of infection. The shift in the age at which individuals experience meningococcal infection is also observed in persons with properdin deficiency, as well as in the normal population during epidemics, and raises the possibility that yet to be identified factors may enhance the susceptibility of deficient persons to infection later in life (24).

Meningococcal disease in complement-deficient individuals is caused by uncommon serogroups, particularly groups Y and W-135, more often than in normal individuals (2,29). In converse fashion, the prevalence of these deficiencies is increased among individuals with meningococcal disease caused by these serogroups (29). The basis for this observation is not known with certainty, but group B isolates appear to be more readily ingested and killed by phagocytic cells in the absence of capsular antibody than isolates belonging to other serogroups (30).

Recurrent meningococcal infection is common in complement-deficient hosts and distinctly uncommon in the normal population, an observation that has been attributed to cross-protective antibodies reactive with subcapsular meningococcal antigens, particularly lipopolysaccharide. Such antibodies are believed to function more effectively to focus the bactericidal potential of the complement cascade on the cell wall. In the absence of bactericidal activity, these antibodies could confer protection only if they functioned in an opsonic capacity, which, as discussed above, they do poorly (28). Hence, protection against meningococcal infection in complement-deficient hosts is strictly dependent on the presence and persistence of antibody specific for each of the capsular serogroups.

In addition to these considerations, attention has recently been drawn to functional differences among the various polymorphic forms of the FcγRIIa receptors on phagocytic cells and the possible linkage of the poor IgG2 binding allotype to meningococcal disease in the general population (31). Extension of this line of inquiry to a small number of LCCD patients who had or had not experienced meningococcal disease revealed a statistically significant association of the FcγRIIa allotype with infection, whereas neutrophils from persons with LCCD without infection were more likely to bear FcγRIIIb and to phagocytose and kill meningococci effectively (32, 33). This observation suggests a possible explanation for the fact that not all individuals with LCCD become infected with meningococci.

Relapse of meningococcal disease, defined as infection with the same serogroup occurring less than 1 month following the initial infection, is relatively common in complement-deficient persons and distinctly uncommon in normal persons. This observation suggests that complement deficiency may contribute to the intracellular survival of meningococci, a suggestion for which there is some experimental support.

The most striking aspect of meningococcal disease in LCCD individuals is that despite a several-thousand-fold increase in the risk of infection, mortality resulting from infection is actually reduced by as much as 10-fold compared with complement-sufficient hosts. Thus, the identical defect that predisposes to infection appears to provide protection from the lethal consequences of the disease. This remarkable observation suggests that the host's exuberant response to meningococci is as much responsible for the clinical manifestations and outcome as the organism itself. This deduction is supported by the close correlation that exists between the extent of complement activation and mortality in patients with meningococcal disease and suggests that the latter is in part dependent upon the assembly of the membrane attack complex (34, 35).

Some clinical observations suggest that meningococcal disease may be milder in complement-deficient persons (36), although this is not universally accepted. Experimental evidence suggests that LCCD individuals may be able to tolerate a given load of organisms and endotoxin better than complement-sufficient individuals (37). The most striking of these pieces of evidence is the report of a C6-deficient individual who developed detectable circulating endotoxin and went into shock shortly after receiving fresh frozen plasma to replace C6 as part of her treatment for severe meningococcal disease (38). The increased release of endotoxin from gram-negative bacteria following insertion of the membrane attack complex in vitro is well documented and there is a direct correlation between the concentration of circulating endotoxin and outcome in meningococcal disease (34, 35). Patients with LCCD are unable to assemble the MAC and thus might be exposed to lower levels of circulating endotoxin for a given organism load. Insertion of the MAC into host cell membranes during fluid-phase complement activation would also be minimized. Thus, the net result of the inability to form the MAC would be an increased susceptibility to infection, decreased endotoxin release during infection, an increased ability to tolerate released endotoxin, and less complement-mediated damage to host cells.

VII. SCREENING FOR COMPLEMENT DEFICIENCY STATES

Complement deficiency should be suspected in patients who bear the clinical correlates of the absence of complement's functional effects, most notably SLE or recurrent infection. The clinical patterns illustrated in Table 1 are particularly useful for this purpose. A somewhat more complex issue is whether all individuals with meningococcal infection should be routinely screened for these deficiencies. Studies addressing this issue report strikingly different figures for the prevalence of associated complement deficiency in persons with meningococcal disease detected in different countries. For example, the prevalence of these deficiencies among individuals with meningococcal infection in Denmark was <1%, in the United States about 10%, and in Japan 50%. This apparent discrepancy can be resolved by plotting the different prevalence figures as a function of the logarithm of the incidence of meningococcal disease in the various countries, which reveals a straight line inverse relationship between these two variables (3, 39). Thus, the higher the incidence of meningococcal disease, the lower the prevalence of associated complement deficiency states.

This relationship can be explained by considering the major determinant of risk for developing meningococcal disease: the concentration of protective antibody. The level of protective immunity in the population in countries in which the incidence of meningococcal disease is high must be low. Hence the number of persons at risk for disease as a consequence of insufficient antibody greatly exceeds the number at risk as a consequence of complement deficiency. As the level of immunity in the population increases the incidence of meningococcal disease declines. In contrast, the prevalence of complement deficiencies in the general population remains constant regardless of the incidence of meningococcal disease and thus assumes proportionately greater significance as a risk factor for disease acquisition as this incidence falls. Based on these considerations it seems reasonable to routinely screen individuals with meningococcal disease for complement deficiency states when the incidence of disease is about 10 cases or less per million in the general population (3, 39).

The likelihood that a complement deficiency will be detected can also be increased by considering the unique features of meningococcal disease in complement-deficient hosts discussed above. The yield of screening will be increased the most if the individual being screened has a prior history or a family history of meningococcal disease. Consideration of the serogroup of the infecting organism and limiting the population to be screened to those individuals 10 years of age and older will have a lesser but significant impact on the probability that screening individuals with meningococcal disease will uncover an associated complement deficiency (32).

VIII. MANAGEMENT OF COMPLEMENT-DEFICIENT INDIVIDUALS

In addition to the treatment of associated infectious and autoimmune complications, two major issues that should be addressed in the management of complement-deficient individuals and their families are genetic and disease counseling, and vaccination. All complement-deficient individuals, regardless of the location of the defect within the cascade, should receive the tetravalent meningococcal vaccine. Individuals who are missing one of the early components of the classical pathway or C3 should also receive the pneumococcal and conjugate *H. influenzae* vaccines. Indeed, given the low cost and high potential benefit of these vaccines, all three vaccines should probably be administered to any individual with complement deficiency.

For C1-, C4-, and C2-deficient individuals these recommendations are based not only on the observed frequency with which these three organisms cause infection but also on *in vitro* observations that antibody can facilitate activation of the alternative pathway, which remains intact in these patients. Although not well studied, conjugate vaccines, like that for *H. influenzae*, which initiate a T-cell-dependent response, appear to stimulate the production of higher antibody concentrations and a longer persistence of the antibody in C2-deficient individuals than the do pure polysaccharide vaccines. The T-cell dependence of this vaccine may help to circumvent the qualitative defect in antibody production observed in these patients (8). However, clinical studies confirming the value of vaccination in these patients have not been published.

Several studies have documented the ability of properdin deficient persons to respond appropriately to the meningococcal vaccine. The resulting antibody response initiates complement-dependent killing of appropriate meningococci in properdin-deficient serum indistinguishable with respect to the kinetics and extent of killing from that in the serum from normal individuals (19, 40).

Neither clinical nor in vitro studies have explored the potential ability of vaccination to help protect C3-deficient individuals from infection with these three organisms. The theoretic basis for such an approach lies in the ability of antibody alone to facilitate phagocytic elimination of organisms, albeit it at a reduced rate of killing. This property would be most relevant to the clearance of organisms from the bloodstream via the spleen and liver, organs in which the structural architecture and lining of the sinusoids with tissue macrophages contribute greatly to surface phagocytosis (25–27).

The best theoretic and clinical data supporting the utility of vaccination of complement-deficient individuals comes from studies of patients with LCCD. The theoretical basis for vaccinating these patients lies in the demonstrated ability of antibody to capsular polysaccharides to facilitate C3 deposition on the organism surface. In vitro studies employing pre- and postvaccination serum have documented the ability of these patients to respond to the tetravalent meningococcal vaccine and for that response to facilitate phagocytic killing of the appropriate meningococci. More important is that recent clinical investigations have documented that vaccination substantially reduces the likelihood of subsequent infection by organisms covered by the vaccine (41, 42). Survival analysis indicated that vaccination reduced the frequency of infection from 0.15 to 0.04 episodes per individual per year and the interval between infections was prolonged from 3.6 years to more than 6 years (42). Thus, these studies, like those in other groups of complement-deficient individuals, attest to the utility of vaccination as an immunological means to circumvent the major clinical manifestation of inherited defects of the complement system.

REFERENCES

1. Burnet SM. Cellular Immunology. Melbourne: Cambridge University Press, 1970.
2. Ross SC, Densen P. Complement deficiency states and infection: epidemiology, pathogenesis and consequences of neisserial and other infections in an immune deficiency. Medicine 1984; 63:243–273.
3. Figueroa JE, Densen P. Infectious diseases associated with complement deficiencies. Clin Microbiol Rev 1991; 4:359–395.
4. Platonov A, Beloborodov VB, Vershinina IV. Meningococcal disease in patients with late complement component deficiencies: studies in the U.S.S.R. Medicine 1993; 72:374–392.
5. Johnston RB. The complement system in host defense and inflammation: the cutting edges of a double edged sword. Pediatr Infect Dis J 1993; 12:933–941.
6. Ratnoff WD, Fearon DT, Austen KF. The role of antibody in the activation of the alternative complement pathway. Semin Immunopathol 1983; 6:361–371.
7. Densen P, Sanford M, Burke T, Densen E, Wintermeyer L. Prospective study of the prevalence of complement deficiency in meningitis. 30th Interscience Conference on Antimicrobial Agents and Chemotherapy 1990 (Abst. #320), p. 140.
8. Bird P, Lachmann PJ. The regulation of IgG subclass production in man: low serum IgG4 in inherited deficiencies of the classical pathway of C3 activation. Eur J Immunol 1988; 18:1217–1222.
9. Matsumoto AK, Kopicky-Burd J, Carter RH, et al. Intersection of the complement and immune systems: a signal transduction complex of the B lymphoctye-containing complement receptor type 2 and CD19. J Exp Med 1991; 173:55–64.
10. Erdei A, Fust G, Gergely J. The role of C3 in the immune response. Immunol Today 1991; 12:332–337.

11. Ochs HD, Wedgwood RJ, Frank MM, et al. The role of complement in the induction of antibody responses. Clin Exp Immunol 1983; 53:208–216.

12. Rowe PC, McLean RH, Wood RA, Leggiadro RJ, Winkelstein JA. Association of homozygous C4B deficiency with bacterial meningitis. J Infect Dis 1989; 160:448–451.

13. Bishof NA, Welch TR, Beischel LS. C4B deficiency: a risk factor for bacteremia with encapsulated organisms. J Infect Dis 1990; 162:248–250

14. Fasano MB, Densen P, McLean RH, Winkelstein JA. Prevalence of homozygous C4B deficiency in patients with deficiencies of terminal complement components and meningococcemia. J Infect Dis 1990; 162:1220–1221.

15. Cates KL, Densen P, Lockman JC, Levine RP. C4B deficiency is not associated with meningitis or bacteremia with encapsulated bacteria. J Infect Dis 1992; 165:942–944.

16. Ekdahl K, Truedsson L, Sjöholm AG, Braconier JH. Complement analysis in adult patients with a history of bacteremic pneumococcal infections or recurrent pneumonia. Scand J Infect Dis 1995; 27:111–117.

17. Matsumoto M, Fukuda W, Goellner J, Strauss-Schoenberger J, Huang G, Karr RW, Colten HR, Chaplin DD. Generation and characterization of mice deficient for factor B. Mol Immunol 1996; 33 Suppl 1:63 (Abstract 249).

18. Densen P, Weiler J, Ackermann L, Barson B, Zhu Z-B, Volanakis J. Functional and antigenic analysis of human factor B deficiency. Mol Immunol 1996; 33 Suppl 1:68 (Abstract 270).

19. Densen P, Weiler JM, Griffiss JM, Hoffman, LG. Familial properdin deficiency and fatal meningococcemia: correlation of the bactericidal defect by vaccination. N Engl J Med 1987; 316:922–926.

20. Sjöholm AG. Absence and dysfunction of properdin as a basis for susceptibility to meningococcal disease. Immunopathol Immunother Forum 1989; 4:3–12.

21. Singer L, Colten HR, Wetsel RA. Complement C3 deficiency: human, animal, and experimental models. Pathobiology 1994; 62:14–28.

22. Harriman GR, Esser AF, Podack ER, Wunderlich AC, Braude AI, Lint TF, Curd JG. The role of C9 in complement-mediated killing of Neisseria. J Immunol 1981; 127:2386–2390.

23. Nagata M, Hara T, Aoki T, Mizuno Y, Akeda H, Inaba S, Tsumoto K, Ueda K. Inherited deficiency of ninth component of complement: an increased risk of meningococcal meningitis. J Pediatr 1989; 114:260–264.

24. Densen P. Human complement deficiency states and infection. In: Whaley K, Loos M, Weiler JM, eds. Complement in Health and Disease. 2nd ed. Immunology and Medicine. Vol. 20. Dordrecht, The Netherlands: Kluwer Academic Publishers, 1993.

25. Hosea SW, Brown EJ, Frank MM. The critical role of complement in experimental pneumococcal sepsis. J Infect Dis 1980; 142:903–909.

26. Brown EJ, Hosea SW, Frank MM. The role of the spleen in experimental pneumococcal bacteremia. J Clin Invest 1981; 67:975–982.

27. Van Wyck DB, Witte MH, Witte CL. Synergism between the spleen and serum complement in experimental pneumococcemia. J Infect Dis 1982; 145:514–519.

28. Brown EJ, Joiner KA, Cole RM, Berger M. Localization of complement component 3 on Streptococcus pneumoniae: anti-capsular antibody causes complement deposition on the pneumococcal capsule. Infect Immun 1983; 39:403–409.

29. Fijen CA, Kuijper EJ, Hannema AJ, Sjöholm AG, van Putten JP. Complement deficiencies in patients over ten years old with meningococcal disease due to uncommon serogroups. Lancet 1989; 2:585–588.

30. Ross SC, Rosenthal J, Berberich HM, Densen P. Killing of Neisseria meningitidis by human neutrophils: implications for normal and complement-deficient individuals. J Infect Dis 1987; 155:1266–1275.

31. Bredius RGM, Derkx BHF, Fijen CAP, de Wit TPM, de Haas M, Weening RS, van de Winkel JGJ, Out TA. Fcγ receptor IIa (CD32) polymorphism in fulminant meningococcal septic shock in children. J Infect Dis 1994; 170:848–853.

32. Fijen CAP, Bredius RGM, Kuijper EJ. Polymorphism of IgG Fc receptors in meningococcal disease (letter). Ann Intern Med 1993; 119:636.

33. Fijen CAP, Bredius RGM, Kuijper EJ, Out TA, de Haas M, de Wit TWJ, Daha MR, Dankert J, van de Winkel JGJ. Complement deficiency and the role of Fcγ receptors, properdin and C3 in phagocytosis of meningococci. In: Fijen CAP, ed. Meningococcal Disease and Complement Deficiencies in the Netherlands. Amsterdam: University of Amsterdam, 1995; 157–175.

34. Brandtzaeg P, Mollnes TE, Kierulf P. Complement activities and endotoxin levels in systemic meningococcal disease. J Infect Dis 1989; 160:58–65.

35. Brandtzaeg P, Kierulf P, Gaustad P, Skulberg A, Bruun JN, Halvorsen S, Sorensen E. Plasma endotoxin as a predictor of multiple organ failure and death in systemic meningococcal disease. J Infect Dis 1989; 159:195–204.

36. Platonov AE, Beloborodov VB. Late complement component deficiency (LCCD) in the USSR: the situation in 1991. Compl Inflamm 1991; 8:211 (abstract).

37. Brown DL, Lachmann PJ. The behaviour of complement and platelets in lethal endotoxin shock in rabbits. Int Arch Allergy 1973; 45:193–205.

38. Lehner PJ, Davies KA, Walport MJ, Cope AP, Wurzner R, Orren A, Morgan BP, Cohen J. Meningococcal septicaemia in a C6-deficient patient and effects of plasma transfusion on lipopolysaccharide release. Lancet 1992; 340(2):1379–1381.

39. Densen P. Complement. In: Mandell GL, Bennett JE, Dolin R, eds. Principles and Practice of Infectious Diseases. 4th ed. New York: Churchill Livingstone, 1995:58–78.

40. Söderstrom C, Braconier JH, Danielsson D, Sjöholm AG. Bactericidal activity for Neisseria meningitidis in properdin-deficient sera. J Infect Dis 1987; 156:107–12.

41. Fijen CAP, Kuijper EJ, van Leeuwen Y, Daha MR, Dankert J. Antibody response of complement deficient patients to tetravalent meningococcal polysaccharide vaccine. Proceedings of the Ninth International Pathogenic Neisseria Conference, Winchester, England, September 26–30, 1994:440 (abstract).

42. Platonov AE, Vershinina IV, Dankert J, Kuijper EJ, Gustafson L, Käyhty H. Long-term follow-up of late complement component deficient patients vaccinated with meningococcal polysaccharide vaccine: antibody persistence and efficacy of vaccination. Abstracts of the Tenth International Pathogenic Neisseria Conference, Baltimore, Maryland, September 8–13, 1996:235 (abstract).

20

Processing and Clearance of Immune Complexes by Complement and the Role of Complement in Immune Complex Diseases

KEVIN A. DAVIES and MARK J. WALPORT
Royal Postgraduate Medical School, Hammersmith Hospital, London, England

I. WHAT ARE IMMUNE COMPLEXES AND WHEN DO THEY FORM IN VIVO?

A. Physiology of Immune Complexes

Immune complexes consist of any combination of antibody with antigen. There is enormous variability in the composition of immune complexes. In addition to antigen and antibody there may be complement proteins associated with immune complexes, covalently bound in the case of C3 and C4, or noncovalently in the case of C1q. The properties of the immune complex vary according to the antibody isotype and according to the antigen, which may be soluble or particulate, for example, bacteria or cells.

The formation of an immune complex is the physiological consequence of an adaptive humoral immune response. The binding of antibody to antigen promotes removal of foreign antigens, stimulation of an adaptive immune response, and the development of specific immunological memory.

B. Pathophysiology of Immune Complexes

Immune complexes may also be an important cause of pathological tissue injury. This occurs in two situations. The first of these is when antigen persists because it is not cleared effectively by formation of immune complexes. Important examples of this are when the antigen is an autoantigen that cannot be removed from the body and, in the case of persistent infection, where the immune response is ineffective in controlling the infection and there is persistent production of antigens from the infectious agent. The second circumstance in which immune complexes cause tissue injury is when the physiological clearance mechanisms are overwhelmed by formation of a large amount of immune complexes. A good example of this is serum sickness, which is discussed in Section IV.C.

II. PROCESSING AND CLEARANCE OF IMMUNE COMPLEXES BY COMPLEMENT

Complement plays a critical role in several stages of the processing of immune complexes. Incorporation of complement proteins into immune complexes modifies the lattice structure. Covalently incorporated cleavage products of C3 and C4 then influence the fate of immune complexes by acting as ligands, first, for receptors on cells that transport immune complexes through the body and, second, for receptors on cells that take up and process immune complexes. The consequences of cellular uptake of immune complexes are the catabolism of foreign antigen and presentation of antigen to T and B lymphocytes, leading to a specific adaptive immune response to the antigen. These processes will be discussed in detail in the next section. For the purposes of this discussion, it is convenient to classify immune complexes into those containing soluble antigens, such as proteins, and those containing particulate antigens, such as cells and bacteria, because the clearance mechanisms are somewhat different for soluble and particulate immune complexes.

A. Clearance of Soluble Immune Complexes

1. Role of Complement in Modifying Immune Complex Lattice Structure

The importance of the incorporation of proteins of the complement system into immune complexes was first recognized during the 1940s with the finding that immune precipitates contained more nitrogen when they formed in normal serum compared with heat-treated serum (1). Heidelberger found that the presence of complement reduced the rate of immune precipitation, a phenomenon rediscovered 20 years later by investigators developing radio-immunoassays, who observed that complement interfered with the precipitation reaction (2,3). It was later discovered that complement not only inhibits the formation of immune precipitates but can also solubilize preformed immune precipitates (4). Inhibition of immune precipitation is primarily mediated through activation of the classical pathway of complement (5,6), in contrast with solubilisation of immune precipitates, which is mediated by the alternative pathway (4). The ability of complement to inhibit immune precipitation has been studied in several in vitro model systems. For example, it was demonstrated that complexes formed between bovine serum albumin (BSA) and rabbit anti-BSA at 37°C were kept soluble more easily when formed in antibody excess. During the first minutes of the reaction, immune complexes were kept soluble by classical pathway components alone, but at later stages the alternative pathway was essential (6). The binding of C3 fragments is necessary for maintaining immune complex solubility. The binding of C3 and C4 is covalent and, in the case of ovalbumin/rabbit anti-ovalbumin immune complexes studied in vitro, involved amide bonds between C3b and the IgG heavy chain (7).

There are two probable explanations for the modification of immune complex solubility by complement (C3b). The first is that the incorporation of complement proteins into the lattice reduces the valency of antibody for antigen by occupying sites of interaction between antibody and antigen (reviewed in 8) The second is that complement incorporation interferes with noncovalent Fc–Fc interactions, which promote the rapid aggregation of immune complexes (9).

The isotype of the antibody in the immune complex determines the efficiency of inhibition of immune precipitation, since only isotypes that activate the classical pathway will induce complement-mediated inhibition of immune precipitation. Inhibition of immune precipitation occurs with IgG and IgM complexes but not with IgA complexes (10). The ability of an immune complex to activate the classical pathway of complement does not correspond necessarily to its ability to incorporate C3b into the lattice. For example, complexes of monoclonal IgM rheumatoid factor and IgG, found in patients with mixed essential cryoglobulinaemia, deplete complement rapidly but do not incorporate C3 into the complex (11).

When immune precipitates form they may activate the alternative pathway of complement. The solubilization of immune precipitates is associated with covalent binding of C3b to antigen and antibody molecules. A fraction of antibody may be released from the complex during solubilization, although the mechanism by which bound C3b interferes with primary antigen–antibody bonds is unclear. The solubilization reaction is relatively inefficient, and requires a large amount of complement activation. Calculations suggest a requirement for approximately 1 molecule of C3b to bind per antibody molecule in order to produce solubilization (12). Since less than 10% of activated C3 binds to an immune aggregate, it follows that large quantities of complement are consumed during solubilization. This may result in deposition of the membrane attack complex and release of complement split products and anaphylatoxins in the surrounding tissues.

The degree of complement activation required for solubilization can be generated only by alternative pathway amplification; insoluble immune aggregates appear to form "protected" surfaces to which factor H has little access, thereby providing sites where amplification of complement activation is favored (13). All the proteins of the alternative pathway, including properdin, are required. Activation of the classical pathway alone does not suffice to solubilize immune precipitates, although partial solubilization by classical pathway activation has been demonstrated in vitro using immune precipitates (14). However, the classical pathway does not appear to be necessary for complex solubilization since serum deficient in C1, C4, or C2 shows no impairment in solubilization, apart from a slight delay in its initiation (15).

In summary, there are two important differences between the processes of inhibition of immune complex precipitation and solubilization of precipitates. First, the capacity of the complement system to inhibit immune precipitation is 10 times greater than its capacity for solubilization. This probably reflect the ease of prevention of Fc–Fc interactions and lattice enlargement, compared with disruption of a lattice that is already formed. Second, the reactions differ in their inflammatory potential since inhibition of immune precipitation generates smaller amounts of the anaphylatoxins C3a and C5a than does solubilization (16).

2. Immune Adherence, Complement Receptor Type I, and Immune Complex Transport

Immune complexes that form within or enter the circulation may have to travel some distance around the body before arrival in one of the organs of the fixed mononuclear phagocytic system. There is evidence that the majority of immune complexes travel through the circulation bound to receptors on the surface of circulating cells rather than free in plasma. On arrival in the fixed mononuclear phagocytic system, they are transferred from the carrier cell to fixed macrophages.

This binding of immune complexes to receptors on carrier cells was first described for complement-coated microorganisms many years ago. Bull injected pneumococci intravenously into immune rabbits and observed the clustering of bacteria around platelets in blood taken by cardiac puncture (17). Rieckenberg (18) found that the serum of rats that had recovered from infection with *T. brucei* would cause blood platelets to adhere to *T.*

brucei in vitro. It was subsequently found in humans and other primates that erythrocytes rather than platelets were the main cell in blood to which opsonized trypanosomes would bind (19).

The role of complement in mediating these binding reactions was initially suggested by Kritschewsky and Tscherikower, working in Moscow, who observed that sera inactivated at 55°C would not mediate binding (20). It was then shown that erythrocyte adherence reactions could be abolished by heat treatment of sera and by dilute ammonia (which inactivates C4 [21–23]). The observation that treatment of serum with cobra venom factor (CVF) prevented adherence reactions showed an essential role for C3 [23]. Adherence could be reconstituted by the addition of CVF-treated serum to ammonia-treated serum.

These early observations were mainly published in French and German journals, and then in British journals of tropical medicine, and were overlooked between the late 1930s and early 1950s. Indeed, in the excellent short monograph entitled Complement or Alexin by Osborn, published in 1937 (24), and in the review of complement by Ecker and Pillemer, published in 1942 (25), no mention is made of any of the work on complement-dependent adherence reactions described above.

The next phase of research was initiated in 1953 by Nelson who rediscovered adherence reactions between human erythrocytes and specifically opsonized treponemes and pneumococci (26). He observed that there was a heat-labile component in the adherence reaction and also that absorption of guinea pig sera with heterologous antibody–antigen complexes would abolish their ability to mediate adherence, confirming that the activity was due to complement. He coined the term "immune adherence" to describe these reactions.

The modern era of studies on immune adherence followed the isolation by Fearon (27) of the molecule responsible for the adherence reactions of human erythrocytes, the C3b/iC3b receptor (complement receptor type 1, CR1, CD 35). This receptor bound large immune complexes and was shown to play a role in the transport of soluble immune complexes in vivo in primates (reviewed in 28). CR1 is a receptor for C3b and iC3b with diverse activities, discussed in Chapters 8, 12, and 20. These include the uptake by phagocytic cells of C3b and iC3b-coated immune complexes and particles; the activation of B cells by antigen in the form of complement-coated immune complexes; acting as a cofactor for Factor-I-mediated cleavage of C3b to iC3b and then C3dg; and as a transport molecule for immune complexes, both soluble and particulate. Here we will focus on the role of CR1 as a transport molecule.

The sites of expression of CR1 vary substantially between different species. In humans and other primates the majority of CR1 in the circulation is located in a clustered form on erythrocytes. The actual number of CR1 molecules per erythrocyte is extremely low, varying between 50 and approximately 1000 receptors per cell in humans (29,30). This compares with 5,000–50,000 receptors per neutrophil depending on the state of cellular activation (31). However, in spite of this unfavorable comparison, red cells play an important role in the binding and transport of C3b and iC3b-coated immune complexes and particles through the circulation. There are two reasons for this. The first is the vast numerical majority of red cells over other cell types: approximately 1000 erythrocytes for every neutrophil. The second is the spatial organisation of the receptor on the cell surface, which on red cells is clustered (32). This promotes very high avidity interactions with ligand, in comparison to neutrophils and lymphocytes on which the receptor is expressed as cell surface monomers. This is discussed in more detail in section II.A.3. In other species a hybrid molecule sharing the activities expressed by human CR1 and

CR2 is expressed on leukocytes and platelets, reviewed in (33), and no complement receptor is expressed on erythrocytes.

There are two types of genetic polymorphism of CR1, each of which may show functional variation in respect of the transport of immune complexes. The first is a structural polymorphism. Four alleles of CR1 have been characterized with molecular weights of ~210-kDa (F' (or C) allotype), ~250-kDa (F (or A) allotype), ~290-kDa (S (or B) allotype), and ~330-kDa. This variation of ~40-kD between allelic variants is due to variable internal repetition of the long homologous repeats forming the structural core of CR1. The ~210-kDa (F' [or C]) allotype has reduced binding affinity for C3b dimers, corresponding to absence of one long homologous repeat containing a C3b binding site (34). This uncommon variant appears to have an increased prevalence among patients with SLE (35), although it is very uncommon even in this population. The possible contributory role of CR1 defects in the pathophysiology of autoimmune disease is discussed further in section III.B.1.

The second type of inherited polymorphism of CR1 is a numerical polymorphism of receptor expression in the normal population, numbers varying between 50 and 500 CR1/erythrocyte. This numerical variation of CR1 expression on erythrocytes was first identified following the discovery of normal subjects whose erythrocytes failed to show immune adherence and was shown to be an inherited trait (36). Subsequent studies have confirmed the numerical polymorphism by direct enumeration of the receptor using radioligand binding assays (37).

3. Interaction of Immune Complexes with Other Circulating Cells

How important is the interaction between immune complexes and other cells in the circulation such as polymorphonuclear leucocytes (PMN)? Neutrophils have both complement and Fc receptors and, on resting PMN, the number of CR1/cell is approximately 10-fold higher than on erythrocytes (33), raising the possibility that PMN might have a role to play in immune complex binding and transport. However, the kinetics of the interaction between neutrophil CR1 and immune complexes are quite different to the kinetics of erythrocyte CR1-immune complex binding (38). Nonopsonized immune complexes react only very slowly with PMN and precoating the complexes with C3b accelerates the reaction by 1–2 orders of magnitude. Only CR1 appears to be involved in this efficient binding, since it is inhibited by a monoclonal antiCR1 antibody. In spite of the greater numbers per cell, PMN do not bind C3b-coated immune complexes better than erythrocytes. This discrepancy was explained by electron microscopic studies showing that, in contrast to the distribution on erythrocytes, CR1 are not clustered on PMN. The activation of PMN with various agents, including C5a, IL-8, and FMLP, does not modify this distribution, in spite of stimulating a 5–10-fold increase in the total number of CR1 expressed on the PMN surface (39). These observations suggest that in primates, at least, CR1-dependent binding of immune complexes to circulating leukocytes is not of major importance in immune complex processing, and indeed, one of the primary roles of erythrocyte CR1 may be in preventing potentially harmful interactions between immune complexes, leukocytes, and endothelium, by maintaining the complexes within the central stream of the vessel. In support of this hypothesis are in vitro observations that erythrocyte CR1 can protect cultured human umbilical vascular endothelial cells from immune complex/PMN-mediated injury (40).

4.   In Vivo Studies of Soluble Immune Complex Processing

The major site of clearance of immune complexes is the fixed mononuclear phagocytic system. In most species, including primates, lagomorphs, and rodents, the liver and spleen are the primary sites in the circulation in which tissue macrophages are located (41). However, pulmonary intravascular macrophages are also found in pigs, cows, sheep, goats, and cats, and these have been shown to be important in both the clearance of particles (42) and soluble immune complexes (43). Important findings that have emerged from the study of the mechanisms of immune complex processing include identification of the sites of processing of immune complexes; the finding that the nature of the antigen in the complex may influence clearance kinetics; observations that immune complex uptake by the mononuclear phagocytic system is saturable; and characterization of receptors on circulating cells that act as transport receptors for immune complexes in the circulation. Each of these is discussed in the following section.

In rodents and lagomorphs soluble immune complexes, injected intravenously were predominantly removed in the liver and spleen (44–47), as in humans, but the complexes were not transported in the circulation bound to erythrocytes, which in these species do not bear CR1. Platelets in these species carry C3b receptors and rapid in vivo binding of immune complexes to platelets has been observed following intravenous injection. For example, model dsDNA/anti-dsDNA complexes bound to guinea pig and rabbit platelets, both in vitro and in vivo (44).

Evidence for the importance of antigen as well as antibody in determining the clearance kinetics of immune complexes came from studies of the clearance in mice of immune complexes containing as antigen either orosomucoid or ceruloplasmin or their desialylated derivatives (48). The asialo-orosomucoid-containing complexes were cleared 20-fold more rapidly than those containing the sialylated molecule. Blocking studies showed that the rapid clearance phase was mediated by a hepatocyte carbohydrate receptor.

Saturation of immune complex clearance mechanisms was seen in rabbits injected with increasing doses of soluble immune complexes in which, following saturation of hepatic uptake, there was spillover of immune complexes into other organs (46). The extent to which this mechanism operates in human disease is unclear.

The physiological importance of erythrocyte complement receptor type 1 in immune complex clearance was first shown in a series of experiments in baboons (49–51). Large radiolabeled immune complexes comprising BSA/anti-BSA were initially employed (reviewed in 52). Following intraaortic infusion, these complexes bound rapidly to erythrocytes, and were subsequently cleared during transit through the hepatic, but not renal circulation (49). The effect of complement-depletion was evaluated by CVF treatment (50). In decomplemented animals, the immune complexes did not bind to red cells, and were cleared more rapidly, depositing in other organs including the kidney. It was subsequently shown that IgA-containing complexes, which fixed complement poorly, also failed to bind to baboon erythrocyte CR1, were cleared rapidly, and localized in other organs (51).

The liver and spleen are not the main sites of IC clearance in all species. In pigs, ruminants, and cats, the anatomy of the fixed mononuclear phagocytic system is different and intravascular pulmonary macrophages play an important role in the clearance of immune complexes (43) (Fig. 1A) and also in the clearance of bacteria (42). Immune complex processing in pigs was associated with a fall in peripheral blood mononuclear cell numbers (43), not seen in studies of immune complex clearance in humans (see

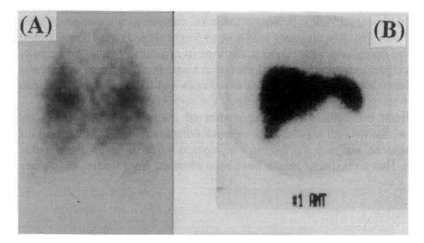

Figure 1 (A) Soluble immune complexes injected intravenously into a pig localize in the lung, as a consequence of uptake by pulmonary macrophages. (Adapted from Ref. 43.) (B) Immune complex uptake in the liver and spleen in a normal human subject, demonstrated by gamma-scintigraphy following the injection of model ^{125}I-labeled HBSAg:anti-HBSAg complexes. (Adapted from Ref 55.)

below) in whom binding of immune complexes to erythrocyte CR1 may act as a buffer protecting leukocytes and endothelium from complex-mediated injury.

5. In Vivo Studies of Soluble Immune Complex Processing in Humans

Three main model immune complexes have been employed to explore the in vivo processing of exogenously administered soluble immune complexes in humans. These are heat-aggregated IgG, tetanus toxoid (TT)/anti-TT, and hepatitis B surface Ag (HBsAg)/anti-HBsAg immune complexes. ^{125}I-Labeled heat-aggregated IgG injected intravenously into normal subjects was shown by gamma-scintigraphy to be cleared in the liver and spleen (53). The complement and CR1-dependent nature of soluble immune complex clearance mechanisms were first studied in vivo using ^{125}I-labeled tetanus-toxoid/antitetanus-toxoid complexes (54). Either native complexes or complexes preopsonized in vitro with autologous serum were injected into normal volunteers, and into patients with immune complex disease or hypocomplementemia. Immune complexes bound to erythrocyte CR1 receptors in a complement-dependent manner, and CR1 number correlated with the level of uptake. Two phases of clearance were seen. In subjects with low CR1 numbers and hypocomplementaemia there was a very rapid initial disappearance of immune complexes. The second phase of clearance was approximately monoexponential, and the observed elimination rate correlated inversely with CR1 numbers and the binding of immune complexes to red cells. The findings in patients with systemic lupus erythematosus (SLE) and complement deficiency are discussed further in section III.B.3.

Similar in vivo studies of soluble immune complex clearance have been performed using ^{123}I-labeled HBsAg anti-HBsAg immune complexes. The fate of these immune complexes was followed by blood sampling and gamma-scintigraphy to define the site and kinetics of processing in normal subjects, patients with SLE, and a single patient with homozygous C2-deficiency (55,56). In normal subjects, complexes were cleared in the liver and spleen, with a median clearance half-time of 5 min (Fig. 2). At 10 min around 40% of the injected complexes were bound in the liver in normal subjects. The majority of the injected complexes bound to red cell CR1 at 2 mins. In all subjects there was a very close correlation between in vivo binding to red cells and CR1 number. The results of similar studies using this model in SLE patients are reviewed in section III.B.3.

One significant criticism of all of the studies of immune complex processing described above is that they all involve large immune complex prepared in vitro, in the absence of complement, and may not therefore be representative of immune complexes that form in vivo. However, similar results have been obtained from studies of immune

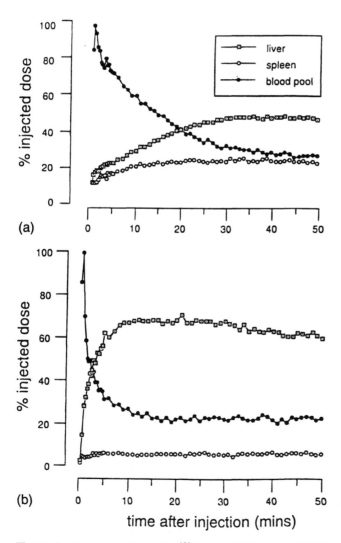

Figure 2 Clearance of soluble ^{123}I-labeled HBSAg:anti-HBSAg complexes in a normal control (a) and a patient with active SLE (b). IC are taken up more rapidly into the liver in the patient, but splenic uptake is greatly reduced. (Adapted from Ref. 55.)

complexes that form in vivo. The successive infusion of human anti-dsDNA antibodies and dsDNA into monkeys and rabbits led to rapid formation of immune complexes that bound to red cell CR1 (57). The formation and fate of immune complex formed in vivo in patients receiving radioimmunotherapy has also been studied (58). The successive administration of a radiolabeled mouse antitumor antibody and a human antimouse antibody resulted in the formation of immune complexes comprising the two antibody species. Rapid clearance of complexes was observed with binding of approximately 10% of the complexed material to CR1. Systemic complement activation and a 30% fall in erythrocyte CR1 numbers were observed. External gamma-counter monitoring indicated that clearance took place primarily in the liver.

B. Clearance of Particulate Complexes

1. Clearance of an Autoantigen: Erythrocytes

The site of clearance of particulate immune complexes depends on the class of antibody bound to the antigen. This is well illustrated by studies of autoimmune hemolytic anemia, which is an important clinical example of a persistent immune complex disease involving a particulate auto-antigen, erythrocytes. Cold agglutinin disease is mediated by IgM anti-I antibodies, which stimulate efficient classical pathway activation and fixation of C4 and C3 to erythrocytes. The role of anti-I and complement in mediating cell lysis was first studied in a rabbit model (59). IgM cold agglutinin was injected into C3-depleted and C6-deficient rabbits. The latter developed thrombocytopenia, neutropenia, and a fall in hemoglobin and packed cell volume (PCV), with only minimal hemoglobinemia, and sharp fall in plasma C3. Circulating red cells could be readily agglutinated with anti-C3 antibodies, and in vivo immune adherence of platelets to red cells occurred. In the C3-depleted animals injection of the anti-I IgM produced no significant hematological changes.

The fate of erythrocytes in cold agglutinin disease has been modeled in primates using radiolabeled cells coated with an IgM cold agglutinin (60). The liver was the main site of red cell uptake. Transient retention of cells in this organ occurred, thought to be mediated by reversible binding to complement receptors. In patients with cold agglutinin disease, circulating red cells are characterized by shape change to a microspherocytic form, accompanied by the presence of many thousands of C3dg molecules bound per erythrocyte. Three conclusions may be drawn from these observations. The first is that phagocytic uptake of erythrocytes that have bound IgM and fixed C3 and C4 is very inefficient. The second is that during the transient retention of red cells in the liver, it is probable that the C3 is catabolized to C3dg and that erythrocyte shape changes occur. The third is that there is no clearance receptor in the circulation for C3dg-coated particles.

In contrast, in IgG-mediated warm hemolytic anemia, uptake of erythrocytes occurs predominantly in the spleen by Fc-dependent pathways. ^{51}Cr-labeled incompatible red cells, transfused into recipients with non-complement-fixing antibodies, were removed from the circulation monoexponentially with a half-time of 18–20/min (61). Splenic uptake was also monoexponential, with a similar half-time. No uptake was detectable elsewhere, notably in the liver. As the spleen exclusively removed cells, and this organ receives only small fraction of the cardiac output, it was reasoned that the splenic extraction efficiency was very high. It was subsequently demonstrated that the site of sensitized red cell destruction was dependent on the degree of antibody coating, with more heavily coated cells being destroyed predominantly by the liver (62).

Radiolabeled erythrocytes, coated with IgG, have been extensively studied as a probe of mononuclear phagocytic function in various disease (reviewed in 63). In humans and other species, these cells are cleared largely in the spleen. The mechanisms by which this probe exhibits primarily splenic clearance, while cells coated with IgM and C3, and soluble immune complexes, discussed above, localize predominantly in the liver, are poorly understood. Tissue macrophages in the liver and spleen bear both Fc- and complement receptors (CR1, CR3, and CR4) (64), while follicular dendritic cells within the spleen and lymph nodes also bear CR2. The Fc-receptors primarily involved in interaction with complexes or aggregated immunoglobulin are the relatively low affinity receptors, Fcγ-RII and Fcγ-RIII (65,66). The binding and retention of an immune complex within the liver and spleen will partly reflect the specific receptor(s) with which it interacts.

There is evidence from in vitro experiments performed using magnetic anti-IgG probes that the potential availability of IgG on red cells to interact with fixed cellular receptors may be different, depending on whether the immunoglogulin is distributed at multiple sites on the red cell surface, adjacent to the cell-membrane, or presented in immune complexes bound to clustered CR1, away from the erythrocyte cell membrane (67). In the latter case, IgG may be safely stripped from the cells as a consequence of interaction with fixed macrophages in the liver and spleen, with little resultant damage to the erythrocyte, as demonstrated in the in vivo clearance models discussed in Section II.A.4. In the case of the antibody-coated erythrocytes used to study reticuloendothelial function in vivo, multiple more intimate contacts with receptors on fixed macrophages may result in cellular destruction, especially in the spleen (reviewed in 68).

The anatomy of the splenic circulation may favor the uptake of particulate rather than soluble immune complexes. The hematocrit in the spleen is high in comparison with that in major arteries and veins (reviewed in 69). The opposite is the case in the sinusoids of the liver, which have a low hematocrit in comparison with major blood vessels. This reflects observations that hepatic sinusoidal macrophages are very efficient at clearing soluble immune complexes from plasma and the splenic macrophages play an important role in handling IgG-coated erythrocytes. In patients who have had splenectomies the peripheral blood is characterized by the presence of abnormal red cells bearing denatured hemoglobin, known as Heinz bodies, and nuclear remnants, known as Howell-Jolly bodies, illustrating the role of the spleen in processing abnormal erythrocytes (70).

2. Bacterial and Endotoxin Clearance

In vivo bacterial clearance has not been studied experimentally in humans, but has been evaluated in a variety of animal models. There is a number of important interspecies differences. In most species clearance of bacterial immune complexes takes place in the liver and spleen, but in dogs, ruminants, and pigs, there is also appreciable lung uptake. Variations in the site of clearance may have a major influence on the pathophysiological consequences of bacteraemia. For example, pigs are extremely susceptible to adult respiratory distress syndrome (ARDS) (71). Equivalent doses (on a weight basis) of *Pseudomonas aeruginosa* administered in parallel to pigs and dogs were well tolerated by the latter, but were associated with acute pulmonary failure in pigs, in which there was selective lung uptake of the organisms. It is interesting to note that in pigs complement- but not neutrophil-depletion abrogated the development of ARDS. These findings suggest that the susceptibility of pigs to ARDS may be specifically related to the pulmonary vascular location of the mononuclear phagocytic system. The local release of inflammatory mediators within the lung, as a consequence of the uptake and processing of bacteria by fixed macrophages within this organ, may predispose the animal to ARDS.

The role of natural antibody and complement in the clearance of endotoxin from the circulation remains unclear. Recently reported experiments in mice rendered C3 or C4 deficient by gene targeting, have demonstrated defective lipopolysaccharide (LPS) clearance in the complement-deficient animals, and enhanced mortality (72). RAG-/- mice, which are unable to produce immunoglobulin, also exhibit defective LPS processing (73).

However, attempts in humans to enhance LPS clearance, and reduce mortality in septic shock, by the administration of exogenous IgM anti-lipid A antibodies, have proved largely unsuccessful (reviewed in 74), even though the reagents used have been shown in vitro to complex with LPS, fix complement, and mediate binding to erythrocyte CR1 (75,76).

III. ROLE OF COMPLEMENT IN IMMUNE COMPLEX DISEASE

The activities of complement in immune complex disease are paradoxical. Abundant data show that complement causes inflammatory injury to tissues in patients and experimental animals in which immune complexes form in the circulation or in situ in tissues. However, it is also clear that either inherited or acquired deficiency of classical pathway complement proteins, and to a lesser extent of C3, are associated with greatly increased susceptibility to immune complex disease in the form of an illness closely resembling SLE. The following sections review these associations.

A. Complement Deficiency and SLE

1. Clinical Data

Data showing a link between complement deficiency and the development of SLE may be classified into three categories. The first is the association of homozygous inherited deficiency of certain complement proteins with disease. The second is evidence showing a link between partial inherited deficiency of C4 and disease susceptibility to SLE. The third set of data shows an association between acquired complement deficiency and the development of SLE.

Homozygous deficiency of C1q, C1r, C1s, C4, or C2 have each been strongly associated with the development of SLE. There is a hierarchy of severity and susceptibility to SLE according to the position of the missing protein in the pathway of activation of the classical pathway. Greater than 90% of patients with homozygous C1q deficiency develop SLE, typically at an early age (77). A wide range of autoantibodies to extractable nuclear antigens incuding anti-Ro, anti-Sm, and anti-RNP are found in these patients, although anti-dsDNA antibodies are uncommon. The typical clinical expression of disease includes severe rashes with a significant proportion of patients developing glomerulonephritis and/or cerebral lupus. In contrast, only about a third of patients with C2 deficiency develop SLE (78). The autoantibody profile tends to be mainly restricted to the presence of anti-Ro antibodies and the severity of disease shares a similar spectrum to that seen in lupus patients without homozygous complement deficiency.

By total contrast, C3 deficiency is usually not associated with the development of full-blown SLE, and typically presents with recurrent pyogenic infections (79). Up to a third of C3-deficient patients develop a prominent rash in association with pyogenic infections, which in one case was associated with a dense neutrophilic cutaneous infiltrate (reviewed in 80). Autoantibodies are only exceptionally identified in patients with C3 deficiency although about a quarter of C3 deficient patients develop a mesangiocapillary glomerulonephritis. Factor I and Factor H deficiency are each associated with severe secondary C3 deficiency, due to failure of regulation of the alternative pathway and amplification loop of C3 cleavage (81). These patients show a similar phenotype to C3 deficiency and typically experience recurrent pyogenic infections with only occasional development of glomerulonephritis without significant autoantibody formation.

Many studies show associations between specific gene products of the major histo-compatibility complex and the development of the majority of autoimmune diseases including SLE. Because of the phenomenon of linkage disequilibrium it is always extremely difficult to dissect which associations between MHC gene products and diseases are primary and which are due to other linked genes in the MHC. Four complement genes are located in the class III region of the MHC: C4A, C4B, C2, and Factor B. All show extensive genetic polymorphism, which in the case of C4A and C4B includes frequent null (nonexpressed) alleles. The finding that homozygous complement deficiency was associated with SLE prompted testing of the hypothesis that single null alleles of C4 may show an association with the disease. This found to be the case (82,83), and the original findings have been confirmed in several different ethnic populations (84). Because the specific allelic associations between different genes of the MHC vary in different races, the discovery that null alleles, particularly of C4A, are associated with SLE in a number of races strengthens the likelihood that the C4 null allele is the relevant gene. However, this is an extremely difficult question to resolve with certainty and not all studies have found the association between C4A null alleles and SLE (85).

A further recent association of a partial deficiency of a complement protein with SLE is the finding of an increased prevalence of alleles of mannose binding protein associated with reduced serum levels of the protein among two populations of patients with SLE (86). The significance of these results is not certain.

The third association of complement deficiency with SLE is that of acquired complement deficiency. Patients with hereditary angioedema due to heterozygous C1 inhibitor deficiency show prolonged depression of C4 and C2 levels due to partially unregulated activity of C1r and C1s. There is an increased prevalence of both antinuclear antibodies and the development of both SLE and a range of other autoimmune disorders, including glomerulonephritis, Sjögren's syndrome, inflammatory bowel disease, and thyroiditis in patients with hereditary angioneurotic edema (HAE) (87,88) and disordered regulation of both cell-mediated and humoral immunity has been described in these patients (89). Patients with prolonged acquired C3 deficiency due to the presence of the autoantibody, C3 nephritic factor may likewise develop SLE many years after presentation with partial lipodystrophy or mesangiocapillary glomerulonephritis with dense deposits (90).

The evidence is extremely strong that these associations of complement deficiency with SLE are physiological and not due to the ascertainment artefact that complement is predominantly measured in patients with diseases associated with complement activation. This would mean that any examples of complement deficiency uncovered would inevitably be associated with those diseases. Large surveys of healthy populations have shown the extreme rarity of inherited homozygous complement deficiency in healthy individuals (91,92). The finding that both inherited and acquired deficiencies of several different complement proteins show similar associations rules out the explanation that the association is due to effects of linked genes.

A number of animal models of complement deficiency have been described. Guinea pigs with C2, C3, and C4 deficiency do not develop spontaneous SLE. Dogs from a colony with C3 deficiency develop a very similar glomerulonephritis to that seen in C3 deficient humans (93). Recently pigs have been discovered in Norway that develop a severe, early onset mesangiocapillary glomerulonephritis. They have been shown to have hereditary Factor H deficiency (94). Mice with targeted deletions of C4 (95), C3 (72), Clq, Factor B (96), and the *Cr2* locus (97) have recently been bred. Our own preliminary data show that Clq-deficient mice develop antinuclear antibodies and some of the mice have died of crescentic glomerulonephritis (unpublished data).

2. Hypotheses About Mechanisms

The clinical data reviewed above show that a physiological activity of the early part of the classical pathway of complement protects against the development of SLE. Three activities of complement may be relevant to this association. The first is the role of complement in the processing of immune complexes. Failure of normal mechanisms of immune complex processing and clearance may result in the inefficient clearance of immune complexes by the fixed mononuclear phagocytic system with deposition of immune complexes in many tissues, causing inflammation, the release of autoantigens and stimulation of an autoimmune response. Evidence for the abnormal processing of immune complexes in hypocomplementaemic patients is discussed in detail in section III.B.

The second role of complement that may be relevant to the association between complement deficiency and SLE relates to the role of complement in antigen processing and presentation in germinal centers. This is discussed in detail in Chapter 14 by Fearon. Complement appears to play an important role in two aspects of the generation of a humoral adaptive antibody response. Follicular dendritic cells, an important depot for antigen in primary and secondary lymphoid follicles, bear CR1, CR2, and CR3. In complement deficiency, antigen does not localize to follicular dendritic cells and this is accompanied by a failure to generate a normal secondary immune response. Second, B lymphocytes bear complement receptors, CR1 and CR2, and ligation of complement by B cells lowers the threshold for B cell activation. At first sight the effects of complement deficiency on these physiological activities should diminish, rather than enhance, the development of an autoantibody response. There is evidence that B cells compete with each other for entry into lymphoid follicles and that autoreactive B cells in the presence of autoantigens do not compete successfully with naive B cells with antibodies reactive with foreign antigens (reviewed in 98). In the absence of complement, follicular dendritic cells may be less able to retain B cells with specificity for foreign antigens and this may shift the competitive balance between B cells such that autoreactive B cells may successfully compete for entry to lymphoid follicles where autoantigen presentation may occur driving the development of SLE.

The third role is that of complement in host defense against infection. It could be that the classical pathway of complement normally provides defense against an infectious agent that induces SLE. Complement is known to play an important role in host defense against pyogenic infections (see Chapters 12, 17, and 19). However, these are unlikely to play an important role in the induction of SLE, since other failures of host defense associated with recurrent pyogenic disease are not associated with development of the disease. There is evidence for a role of complement in host defense against C-type retroviruses (99,100) and it remains a possibility that SLE is an autoimmune response following infection by an unidentified retrovirus.

B. Are There Primary or Secondary Defects in Immune Complex Clearance or Processing Mechanisms?

1. CR1 Defects

The role of CR1 in the clearance of soluble and particulate immune complexes has been discussed above. The average number of receptors per red cell of CR1 varies widely between individuals. The level of expression on erythrocytes is under genetic control at the CR1 locus (30,36). The molecular mechanism of this has not been established, but a restriction fragment length polymorphism within the CR1 gene is correlated with high or low expression of CR1 on red cells (101,102). It was found that patients with SLE expressed reduced numbers of receptors per cell compared with healthy individuals, reviewed in (37). This raised the possibility that low expression of CR1 might constitute a disease susceptibility gene for the development of SLE. However, a number of studies showed that low expression of CR1 in patients with SLE and in a number of other diseases associated with complement activation on erythrocyte surfaces or in plasma was due to acquired mechanisms (37).

CR1 on erythrocytes in patients with immune complex diseases, notably SLE, has been extensively studied, and evidence to date suggests that in SLE at least, there is an acquired reduction in CR1 numbers on these cells (29), discussed further in section III.B.3.

2. Abnormal Fc Receptor Function

A long-standing hypothesis is that defects in mononuclear phagocytic function predispose to the development of SLE by impairment of immune complex clearance. This hypothesis stems from experimental studies of the clearance of colloidal carbon particles in animals (41), which showed that uptake by the mononuclear phagocytic system was saturable. It was subsequently shown that immune complex clearance was also saturable. Immune complexes injected into rabbits showed saturable uptake in the liver, followed by spillover into other organs (46). However, in spite of the attractive experimental data there is no evidence that shows that saturation of soluble immune complex clearance mechanisms occurs in human disease.

Several approaches have been taken to studying whether there is impaired processing of immune complexes in patients with SLE by the mononuclear phagocytic system. Studies of the clearance of IgG-coated erythrocytes by the spleen showed delayed uptake in SLE. Correlations were found between clearance rate, disease activity, and levels of circulating immune complexes in patients with lupus (103,104). However, as discussed in section II.B., IgG-coated erythrocytes may not be an appropriate surrogate measure for Fc- and complement-dependent clearance mechanisms of soluble immune complexes. As discussed above, the clearance of soluble immune complexes in a C2-deficient patient with SLE was totally corrected by complement repletion, excluding a primary defect in mononuclear phagocytic function as the explanation for defective immune complex clearance in that patient (56).

An alternative approach to the study of mononuclear phagocytic cell function in SLE is the study of genetic variation in Fc and complement receptors. Some support for the hypothesis that Fc-receptor fuction is abnormal in SLE has come from recent studies of a functionally important polymorphism of the Fc-receptor, FCγRIIa. An allotypic variant of FcγRIIa, FcγRIIa-HR (FcγRIIa-R131), has been shown in vitro to reduce the capacity of phagocytic cells to bind and internalize IgG-containing immune complexes and IgG-opsonized erythrocytes (105). This receptor primarily binds IgG2. Several groups have studied whether there is an overrepresentation of this allotypic variant in patients with SLE, either by genotype analysis, or by determination of receptor phenotype on peripheral blood leukocytes by FACS analysis using variant-specific monoclonal antibodies. An excess of FcγRIIa-R131 homozygotes was found in African-American patients with lupus nephritis (106) and in Dutch patients with SLE (107). However, we were unable to confirm this finding in groups of white, Afro-Caribbean, or Chinese patients with lupus (108). Further studies are needed to test whether this polymorphic variant of FcγRIIa is a disease susceptibility gene for SLE or, more specifically, for lupus nephritis.

3. Immune Complex Processing in Patients with Abnormal Complement and CR1 Function

In humans, the in vivo clearance of soluble immune complexes in disease has been studied using all of the three models described in section II.A.5: ie IgG aggregates, tetanus toxoid complexes, and anti-HBsAgHBsAg complexes. Significant differences in the clearance of radiolabeled aggregated gamma-globulin were seen between normal subjects and patients with SLE (109). Mean half-time for initial clearance of AIgG was shorter in patients than in controls, and binding of AIgG to erythrocytes was significantly lower in patients compared with normal subjects. In patients, the liver/spleen uptake ratios were significantly higher than in normals, attributable to reduced splenic uptake of AIgG. Accelerated clearance of AIgG was also observed in two C3-deficient patients studied using the same model complexes (110).

These findings are similar to observations in patients with SLE and hypocomplementemia using ^{125}I-labeled tetanus-toxoid / anti-tetanus toxoid complexes as probes of the pathways of immune complex processing (54). Immune complexes bound to erythrocyte CR1 in a complement-dependent manner, and CR1 number correlated with the level of uptake. The most striking finding was the enhanced rapid initial clearance of complexes in patients with lupus and low complement levels, most marked in a patient with Clq deficiency.

The explanation for these results, particularly for the rapid initial clearance of immune complexes in hypocomplementaemic patients, came from studies using ^{123}I-labeled hepatitis B surface antigen (HBsAg) / anti-HBsAg immune complexes. As in normal individuals, the liver and spleen were the main sites of complex uptake (Fig. 1B); however, the initial clearance of immune complexes from blood was more rapid in patients with SLE than in normal controls, as a consequence of more rapid uptake in the liver. In the SLE group, however, there was release of up to 12% of the immune complex from the liver after 30–40 min, which was not seen in normal subjects. Typical clearance curves for a normal subject and an SLE patient are shown in Figure 2. The binding of immune complexes to erythrocytes was greatly reduced in the patients, as a consequence of hypocomplementemia and reduced CR1 numbers. In a C2-deficient patient studied before and after therapy with FFP, there was no uptake of immune complexes in the spleen prior to therapy, but both the kinetics and sites of complex clearance reverted to normal after normalization of classical pathway complement activity (56).

The most striking findings from these studies of in vivo immune complex processing in SLE patients are that more rapid initial clearance of complexes from the circulation takes place in patients than normals, followed by release of immune complexes back into the circulation; and that splenic uptake of immune complexes is reduced in patients. The impaired uptake of complexes in the spleen in SLE may be related to the mode of delivery of immune complexes to the fixed mononuclear phagocytic system. Reduced binding to red cell CR1 was observed in all three models in SLE patients, with a resultant increase in the numbers of complexes delivered to the fixed macrophage system in the fluid phase. The anatomical organization of the spleen favours specifically the uptake of particles (reviewed in 68). The intrasplenic hematocrit is relatively high compared with major blood vessels, and splenic macrophages play a key role in the processing of IgG-coated erythrocytes (discussed in section II.B.). By analogy, it might be expected therefore that immune complexes bound to erythrocyte CR1 would be selectively processed in the spleen, while complexes presented in the fluid phase would localize in the liver.

What is the explanation for the observed release of immune complexes back into the circulation from the liver? One possibility is that only immune complexes are able to interact efficiently with both complement- and Fc-receptors on fixed macrophages, with subsequent internalization and processing retained efficiently within the liver and spleen. Immune complexes bearing low amounts of C3, which are delivered in the fluid phase may bind rapidly to the relatively low-affinity Fcγ-receptors (II and III), but ligation of these receptors alone may be insufficient to trigger internalization of the complexes.

C. Role of Complement in Causing Inflammation

1. General Mechanisms

The activation of complement by immune complexes may induce tissue injury by three major mechanisms. First, complement proteins attached covalently (C3 and C4) or noncovalently (Clq) to immune complexes may ligate receptors on leukocytes and lymphocytes, triggering these cells to express effector activities. Second, formation of the membrane attack complex has been characterized as a powerful proinflammatory stimulus. The third proinflammatory consequence of complement activation by immune complexes is anaphylatoxin generation.

Tissue architecture is an important factor in determining the precise nature of inflammatory tissue injury. A good example of this is glomerulonephritis, in which the glomerular basement membrane is a barrier to the exit of leukocytes from glomerular capillaries. Tissue injury in membranous glomerulonephritis, in which immune complexes form in the subepithelium, is induced by the complement membrane attack complex in the absence of inflammatory leukocytes (111). In contrast, when immune complexes form, or are deposited, in the subendothelium, as in SLE or Goodpasture's disease, tissue injury is induced by a combination of leukocytes and complement (112).

The availability of animals with gene-targeted deletions of complement- and Fc-receptors has allowed a further examination of the proximal triggering mechanisms of inflammation by immune complexes. A popular model system for exploring the mechanisms of inflammation induced by immune complexes is the reverse passive Arthus reaction, in which antibody is injected into the skin or introduced into the lungs of an animal injected intravenously with antigen. In skin, the reverse passive Arthus reaction is dependent on both Fc- and complement-mediated pathways (113–115). Depletion of complement alone did not significantly reduce the inflammatory response. Deficiency of FcγRIII diminished the response to a variable degree, which was correlated inversely with the level of haemolytic complement expressed in individual animals (114). Complete abolition of the response was only seen in FcγRIII animals following depletion of complement with cobra venom factor. These findings may be seen as confirmation of much earlier experiments performed using C5-deficient mice and mice in which complement had been depleted using cobra venom factor, which showed that, at low concentrations of antibody, complement-dependent inflammatory pathways dominated, whereas, at high concentrations, complement-independent pathways were more apparent (115).

The results from studies of the reverse passive Arthus reaction in the lung are broadly consistent with those in the skin, although in this model complement depletion or deficiency of C5 seem to block the inflammatory response more effectively than in the skin (116). The observation that C5 deficiency has some protective effect against the Arthus reaction in the lung (116), as in the skin, implies a role for the anaphylatoxin, C5a and/or the membrane attack complex.

What is the cell type responsible for triggering tissue injury in response to immune complexes in the Arthus reaction? Several lines of evidence support an important role for mast cells. Experiments in a strain of mice lacking mast cells because of deficiency of stem cell factor, c-kit, showed a markedly reduced, although not abolished, reverse passive Arthus reaction (117). These mice were reconstituted with mast cells derived from animals deficient or sufficient in the Fc-receptor γ-chain (118). The Arthus response was only restored to normal in mice reconstituted with mast cells bearing FcγRIII, showing that immune complexes in this model trigger mast cells to release their mediators and cause inflammation by ligation of FcγRIII.

The role of C5a in mediating the inflammatory response to immune complexes in the reverse passive Arthus reaction has been shown by experiments in two further knock-out strains of mice which reveal an additional layer of complexity of the mechanisms of inflammation. Intrapulmonary immune complex formation was explored (119) in mice with gene-targeted deletions of either the NK-1R substance P receptor or the C5a receptor. The inflammatory response following intrapulmonary immune complex formation was abolished in NK-1R -/- mice and was also absent in C5aR -/- mice. These results show an important additional facet of the inflammatory response to immune complexes: the involvement of the tachykinin substance P. This neurotransmitter, found in C type nerve fibers, is also found in macrophages and mast cells, as is the NK-1 receptor.

2. Factors Influencing In Situ Immune Complex Formation or Their Deposition from the Circulation

When antigen meets antibody in solution at equivalence or in antibody excess, rapid precipitation occurs. This reaction requires intact IgG molecules, as distinct from $F(ab')_2$ fragments, suggesting that Fc–Fc interactions are important in promoting precipitation (120). Nucleation phenomena are also important (i.e., large complexes promote the aggregation of small complexes on their surface) (9). These interactions bring the reacting molecules into close proximity and this is followed by formation of an "infinite lattice" of alternating antigen-antibody bonds. The formation of an "infinite lattice" results in the precipitation of an insoluble immune complex.

Such a lattice can also build up on an antigen or antibody located within tissues, either an intrinsic component of tissue, or "planted" from the circulation. Such in situ formation of immune complexes has been demonstrated in experimental glomerulonephritis, in which planted antigen (or antibody), when exposed successively to further antibody and antigen, leads to the development of large, microscopically visible, deposits (121). The mechanisms of subepithelial immune deposit formation in the Heymann model of experimental nephritis are discussed further in Section IV.A.1.

Diseases such as SLE and bacterial endocarditis, in which immune complexes are thought to be important in pathogenesis, are associated with continuous antibody overproduction driven by persistent antigen. In these diseases, immune complexes are formed in large antibody excess and are likely to be large, complement-activating aggregates. The immobilization of these immune complexes in tissues, either from in situ formation or deposition from the bloodstream, causes inflammation and organ injury. An intact complement system may play an important role in limiting such injury by inhibiting the formation of large immune complexes (see above, Section B) and promoting their disposal by the mononuclear phagocytic system. Complement may also contribute to the tissue injury caused by immune complexes in tissues.

3. Effects of Autoantibodies to Complement in Amplifying Immune Complex Injury to Tissues

Several autoantibodies to complement components may have a role in amplifying the proinflammatory effects of immune complexes. The two best characterized examples are C3 nephritic factor (C3 NeF), and antibodies to the collagenous part of the C1q molecule (anti-C1q[CLR]).

C3 NeF is an IgG autoantibody directed against neoantigenic determinants on the alternative pathway C3 convertase, C3bBb. C3 NeF stabilizes the enzyme, causing dysregulated complement activation, leading to a severe secondary deficiency of C3 (reviewed in 122). The clinical associations of C3 NeF are partial lipodystrophy and type II membranoproliferative glomerulonephritis, defined by electrondense deposits in the glomerulus. These deposits do not generally contain immunoglobulin, although C3 is usually demonstrable locally.

The mechanism of the association of C3 NeF with glomerulonephritis is not understood. One hypothesis is that C3 NeF causes secondary C3 deficiency, which in turn is responsible for the development of nephritis. In support of this hypothesis are observations that homozygous C3 deficiency is associated in some humans and in dogs with development of mesangiocapillary glomerulonephritis, although not with the typical electrondense deposits that define type II mesangiocapillary glomerulonephritis. In C3-deficient dogs the histological appearances resemble those of type I human MPGN, with an increase in mesangial matrix, thickening of the capilliary wall, and electrondense deposits in the mesangium and subendothelial space. These deposits typically contain IgG and IgM. In humans, homozygous deficiency of factor H or Factor I is also associated with inability to regulate the alternative pathway C3 convertase enzyme and severe secondary deficiency of C3. A few patients with Factor H or Factor I deficiency have been reported to develop mesangiocapillary glomerulonephritis (81). Recently, pigs with hereditary Factor H deficiency have been identified and a colony has been developed. These animals have a runting disease associated with severe mesangiocapillary glomerulonephritis (94).

The mechanism of the association of C3 deficiency with glomerulonephritis remains uncertain. Attempts to induce renal injury in experimental animals rendered hypocomplementemic by nonimmune mechanisms have been generally unsuccessful (123,124), and nephritis in the context of NeF may coexist with normal complement levels (122).

A second possible explanation for the association of C3 Nef with glomerulonephritis is that C3 NeF acts as a local activator of complement in the kidney. This explanation could also account for the association of Factor H and I deficiencies with glomerulonephritis, in which C3, locally synthesized in the kidney may undergo unregulated activation and cause local tissue injury. In support of this hypothesis are in vitro experiments showing that heat-killed kidney cells may activate complement and bind a NeF-stabilized C3 convertase (125). There is also a report of a patient with mesangiocapillary glomerulonephritis, hypocomplementemia, and systemic candidiasis. The glomerular deposits in this patient contained both C3 and *Candida albicans* a known alternative pathway activator (126). However, if this hypothesis is correct, a different explanation would be necessary to explain the association of primary C3 deficiency with glomerulonephritis.

The pathogenic role of anti-C1q(CLR), IgG autoantibodies to neoepitopes on the collagenous part of the C1q molecule remains similarly poorly understood. These antibodies show a number of specific clinical associations, notably with SLE and hypocomplementemic urticarial vasculitis syndrome (127,128), and are strongly associated with classical pathway complement activation, often with very low levels of C3, C4, and C1q. It is possible that they may augment activation of the complement system by immune complexes in tissues. This idea is supported by the observation that anti-C1q antibodies, purified from two patients with SLE, deposited in mouse glomeruli in the presence of human C1q (129).

A number of other autoantibodies to complement neoantigens have been described. For example, IgG autoantibodies that stabilize the classical pathway convertase, C4b2a, have been described in a patient with poststreptococcal glomerulonephritis and in some patients with SLE (130,131).

IV. COMPLEMENT AND IMMUNE COMPLEXES IN SPECIFIC DISEASES

A. Complement and Immune Complexes in Glomerulonephritis

Within the glomerulus, immune deposits are typically found in one of three extracellular locations: the mesangium, the subendothelium or the subepithelium. The first two sites are associated with proliferative glomerular lesions, while subepithelial deposits are characteristic of membranous glomerulonephritis. Glomerular pathology, particularly that associated with SLE, is often complex, and mixed lesions are common (132). Subepithelial immune deposits are generally thought to develop as a result of in situ immune complex formation (133). It is less certain whether mesangial and subendothelial deposits form in situ, from deposited circulating immune complexes, or from a mixture of both.

1. Subepithelial Immune Complexes

A widely studied model of subepithelial immune complex formation is Heymann nephritis, a model of membranous nephropathy in the rat, in which subepithelial granular IC deposits result from the binding of free antibody to an antigen expressed on the surface of glomerular epithelial cells (134). Complement-dependent (C5-9) tissue injury results (135). This pattern of glomerular injury can result from immune complex formation with either "fixed" or "planted" glomerular antigens. The original Heymann nephritis involves a fixed glomerular antigen, a glycoprotein (GP330) localized along the epithelial cell membrane and coated pits (136). The binding of divalent antibody is thought to cause antigenic modulation and redistribution of the IC on the surface of the cell, with resultant capping and shedding of the aggregates into the nearby slit pore areas and lamina rara externa (137). A very similar mechanism is likely to operate in idiopathic membranous nephritis in humans, although the relevant autoantigen has not been characterized.

The precise role of known autoantibodies in the context of lupus nephritis remains, however, unresolved. In animal models, polyspecific anti-DNA antibodies have been shown to bind directly to cell membrane antigens (138), and to localize under certain conditions in glomeruli (139). It remains, however, very difficult to induce experimentally the formation of subepithelial deposits containing exogenous antigens by the infusion of immune complexes (140). Highly cationic, preformed IC can produce this picture, possibly due to the attraction of cationic antigens or antibodies to anionic glomerular structures. The subepithelial localization of immune deposits may result from filtration forces, while granularity may result from condensation of IC containing polyvalent antigens into larger deposits detectable by electron microscopy (141). In lupus one of the main candidate antigens for involvement in IC formation is dsDNA, an anionic antigen, and Izui and co-workers have demonstrated localization of injected DNA to glomeruli (142). It is also possible that the cationic nature of anti-DNA antibodies may also be important, and cationic anti-DNA antibodies have been successfully eluted from mice with lupus nephritis (143,144).

2. Subendothelial and Mesangial Complex Formation

Each of these sites is potentially accessible to circulating macromolecules, and trapping of circulating IC may have an important role to play in immune deposit formation at these sites. In support of this idea are experiments showing the localization of injected immune compexes to mesangium, although it has proved difficult to induce glomerular injury following the injection of preformed immune complexes (reviewed in 145). However, it has been shown that if antigen localization to the mesangium is succeeded by further accretion of antibody, immune deposit formation occurs, with induction of focal proliferative nephritis (146). Direct antibody-induced mesangial cell damage has also been demonstrated experimentally (147).

Experimental nephritis associated with subendothelial deposits is similarly difficult to induce by the injection of preformed immune complexes. It is possible to produce subendothelial deposit formation experimentally by induction of antigen expression on the endothelial cell surface, followed by infusion of an appropriate antibody (148), but such deposits are rapidly shed into the circulation. By contrast, in the classical animal models of serum sickness, it has always been difficult to discern deposition of circulating IC from local immune deposit formation

B. Infectious Disease

There are a number of well-documented associations between infection and immune complex disease. Two examples on which we will focus here are cryoglobulinemia associated with viral hepatitis, and subacute bacterial endocarditis. Both conditions are characterized by classical pathway complement consumption.

1. Cryoglobulinemia and Hepatitis Infection

A cryoglobulin comprises an antibody or an immune complex, the physicochemical properties of which cause it to precipitate from serum at temperatures below 37°C. Cryoglobulinemia may occur in patients with SLE, rheumatoid arthritis, and Sjögren's syndrome, and is also associated with infections and lymphoproliferative disorders.

Cryoglobulins have been classified into three types (149). Type 1, monoclonal paraproteins of IgG or IgM isotype, typically occurs in patients with myeloma, CLL, or

Waldenström's macroglobulinaemia. Type 2, comprising a monoclonal rheumatoid factor, is typically seen in mixed essential cryoglobulinaemia, but also in association with autoimmune or lymphoproliferative disorders. Type 3, "mixed cryoglobulinaemia," comprises polyclonal IgG and/or IgM, and complement.

Mixed cryoglobulinemia may occur in association with infections such as cytomegalovirus (CMV), Epstein Barr virus (EBV), kala-azar, and infective endocarditis. Hepatitis B and C (HCV) infections are commonly associated with type 2 cryoglobulinemia, particularly in southern Europe (150–153). In a series of 63 French patients with mixed cryoglobulinemia, anti-HCV antibodies were detected in the serum of 33, while 30 showed negative findings (152). Cryoglobulin levels were higher in the anti-HCV positive group, hemolytic complement activity was lower, and cutaneous symptoms more severe. HCV RNA sequences were detected in the majority of sera and cryoprecipitates derived from the anti-HCV-positive group. HBV DNA was not detectable in any of the cryoprecipitates studied. In an analysis of 113 consecutive anti-HCV-positive patients studied in Cambridge, UK, 21 had detectable cryoglobulins, of which 19 of 21 were type 3 and 2 of 21 type 2 (154). HCV RNA was also detected in the majority of cryoprecipitates. Cryoglobulins were detected in 24 of 65 Japanese patients with hepatitis C (155).

2. Infective Endocarditis

Chronic bacterial infection may also be associated with immune complex formation and complement activation. Perhaps the best example of this association is infective endocarditis resulting from chronic bacterial colonization of cardiac valvular structures, most commonly by streptococci (156–158). Circulating immune complexes have also been detected in the serum of 40% patients with bacteremia due to infection of an intravascular catheter or access device, and in 70% patients with *Staphylococcus aureus* bacteremia related to chronic deep tissue infection (159), in whom chronic hypocomplementemia may be a feature. The hypocomplementaemia observed in infective endocarditis is caused partly by classical pathway activation by immune complexes, and probably also by activation of complement by the bacteria. Vegetations on mitral and aortic valves removed at emergency surgery from patients with *S. viridans* endocarditis have been shown to contain IgG, C3, IgM, and bacterial antigens, and both endocardial and subendocardial deposition of C5b-9 has also been demonstrated (160). Antisarcolemmal antibodies that cross-react with bacterial antigens have been demonstrated in infective endocarditis, and there is evidence that these cross-reactive antibodies have complement-dependent cytolytic potential in vitro (161). However, attempts to demonstrate bacterial antigens or antimicrobial antibodies in circulating immune complexes have proved generally unsuccessful (162).

Persistence of circulating immune complexes in infective endocarditis may be associated with tissue injury, typically vasculitis affecting the skin, arthritis, or glomerulonephritis (163). It has been demonstrated in vitro that sera from patients with endocarditis and high levels of immune complexes exhibit defective complement-mediated inhibition of immune precipitation (164). Rheumatoid factors are frequently detected in endocarditis, and a number of groups have demonstrated a fall in both rheumatoid factor and immune complex levels, and a rise in the ability of serum to inhibit immune precipitation, following successful treatment of infective endocarditis (158,164).

C. Serum Sickness

Type III hypersensitivity reactions in response to injected proteins and drugs constitute a clear example of disease in humans caused by immune complexes. The three most common antigens are horse and rabbit serum, usually given as antithymocyte globulin, penicillin, and streptokinase. An excellent animal model of serum sickness was developed by Dixon and Cochrane (165).

1. Antithymocyte Globulin

In recent years, antithymocyte globulin (ATG) has been used mainly in the treatment of marrow and renal allograft rejection, and rarely in patients with systemic autoimmune disorders, including SLE, systemic sclerosis, Wegener's granulomatosis, rheumatoid arthritis (166,167), and in hematological diseases, including bone marrow failure (168), and aplastic anemia (169). The most commonly used preparations are horse and rabbit serum, and severe serum sickness is uncommon in transplant recipients. This may reflect the fact that these patients are also given large doses of corticosteroids, which may limit the inflammatory effects of immune complexes. In contrast, serum sickness was reported in all of a cohort of 10 patients treated for severe aplastic anemia with antithymocyte globulin (ATG) (169), and in 30 of 35 subjects receiving equine ATG for bone marrow failure (168). Biopsies of lesional skin showed immune deposits (comprising IgM, IgE, IgA, and C3) in dermal vessels. Elevated levels of immune complexes were detectable using a C1q-binding assay; C3, C4, and CH50 (measured on day 10) fell 50–80% from baseline, and all affected patients exhibited evidence of an acute-phase response.

2. Streptokinase

Thrombolytic therapy is now widely used in the treatment of myocardial infarction. Streptokinase (SK) is the most frequently used thrombolytic agent (170,171), although recombinant tissue plasminogen activating factor is now increasingly used for this purpose. Streptokinase is a nonenzymatic protein (Mr 47 kDa) produced by group C streptococci. The normal therapeutic regimen for the treatment of myocardial infarction is intravenous administration of approximately 3 g protein over 1 h. The reported frequency of hypersensitivity reactions to the drug varies between 1.7 and 18% (172), of which most are mild and self-limiting, taking the form of type 1 hypersensitivity reactions. However, there is also a number of well-documented cases of serum sickness (173–175) following SK treatment, manifested by transient rash, febrile illness, or mild renal impairment. Reactions are typically described 8–10 days after therapy, and are usually self-limiting, although acute renal failure has been reported (173).

3. Penicillin

Penicillin sensitivity is a common clinical problem, and beta-lactam antibiotics are the drugs most frequently implicated in immunologically mediated adverse reactions. The most common clinical pattern of hypersensitivity reaction (a urticarial rash, angioedema, and anaphylaxis) is mediated by a type I, IgE-mediated reaction (176). However, type II reactions, which may result in a hemolytic anemia (177), and immune complex-mediated hypersensitivity are also well-recognized, although uncommon, side effects of penicillin and related antibiotics. In a large retrospective study performed in Massachussets in a population of 230,000 patients, the records of 3487 children treated with the antibiotics amoxycillin, cefaclor, septrin, or penicillin V were evaluated (178). Twelve cases only of serum sickness were identified, of which five were cefaclor-associated, and only two were amoxycillin- or penicillin-related. Symptoms developed after 7–11 days in all cases, and in all but one case occurred in children with a heavy life-time exposure to antibiotics. As with streptokinase allergy, there is a poor relationship between the results of radioallergoabsorbent tests for penicillin antibodies (IgE) and the development of serum sickness

(179). Although rare, serum sickness in the context of penicillin therapy may have serious consequences, resulting in classical pathway complement consumption, hemolysis with the formation of hemoglobin–haptoglobin complexes, disseminated intravascular coagulation (180), and death (181). It has been possible in rare cases to demonstrate intrarenal deposition of immune complexes containing antipenicillin IgG antibody and C3 (181).

REFERENCES

1. Heidelberger M. Quantitative chemical studies on complement or alexin. I. A method. J Exp Med 1941; 73:691–694.
2. Morgan CR, Sorenson RL, Lazarow A. Further studies of an inhibitor of the two antibody immunoassay system. Diabetes 1964; 13:579–584.
3. Utiger RD, Daughaday WH. Studies on human growth hormone. I. A radioimmunoassay for human growth hormone. J Clin Invest 1962; 41:254–261.
4. Miller GW, Nussensweig V. A new complement function: solubilization of antigen–antibody aggregates. Proc Natl Acad Sci USA 1975; 72:418–422.
5. Schifferli JA, Morris SM, Dash A, Peters DK. Complement-mediated solubilization in patients with systemic lupus erythematosus, nephritis or vasculitis. Clin Exp Immunol 1981; 46:557–564.
6. Schifferli JA, Bartolotti SR, Peters DK. Inhibition of immune precipitation by complement. Clin Exp Immunol 1980; 42:387–394.
7. Hong K, Takata Y, Sayama K, et al. Inhibition of immune precipitation by complement. J Immunol 1984; 133:1464–1470.
8. Lachmann PJ, Walport MJ. Deficiency of the effector mechanisms of the immune response and autoimmunity. In: Whelan J, ed. Autoimmunity and Autoimmune Disease, Ciba Foundation Symposium #129. Chichester: Wiley Ltd., 1987:149–171.
9. Moller NP, Steengaard J. Fc mediated immune precipitation. I. A new role of the Fc portion of IgG. Immunology 1983; 38:631–640.
10. Johnson A, Harkin S, Steward MW, Whaley K. The effects of immunoglobulin isotype and antibody affinity on complement-mediated inhibition of immune precipitation and solubilization. Mol Immunol 1987; 24:1211–1217.
11. Ng YC, Peters DK, Walport MJ. Monoclonal rheumatoid factor-IgG immune complexes. Poor fixation of opsonic C4 and C3 despite efficient complement activation. Arthritis Rheum 1987; 31:99–107.
12. Takahashi M, Tack BF, Nussenzweig V. Requirements for the solubilization of immune aggregates by complement: assembly of a factor B-dependent C3-convertase on the immune complexes. J Exp Med 1977; 145:86–100.
13. Fries LF, Gaither TA, Hammer CH, Frank MM. C3b covalently bound to IgG demonstrates a reduced rate of inactivation by factors H and I. J Exp Med 1984; 160:1640–1655.
14. Spath PJ, Pascual M, Meyer Hanni L, Schaad UB, Schifferli JA. Solubilization of immune precipitates by complement in the absence of properdin or factor D. FEBS Lett 1988; 234:131–134.
15. Volanakis JE. Complement-induced solubilization of C-reactive protein–pneumococcal C-polysaccharide precipitates: evidence for covalent binding of complement proteins to C-reactive protein and to pneumococcal C-polysaccharide. J Immunol 1982; 128:2745–2750.
16. Schifferli JA, Steiger G, Paccaud JP. Complement mediated inhibition of immune precipitation and solubilization generate different concentrations of complement anaphylatoxins (C4a, C3a, C5a). Clin Exp Immunol 1986; 64:407–414.
17. Bull CG. The agglutination of bacteria in vivo. J Exp Med 1915; 22:484–491.

18. Rieckenberg H. Eine neue immuninitasreaktion bei experimentaller trypanosomen-infection: die blutpattchen-probe. Immunitatsforsch 1917; 26:53–64.

19. Duke HL, Wallace JM. "Red-cell adhesion" in trypanosomiasis of man and animals. Parasitology 1930; 22:414–456.

20. Kritschewsky IL, Tscherikower RS. Uber anti-korper, die micro-organismen mit blutpattchen beladen (thrombozytobarinen). Z Immunitatsforsch 1925; 42:131–149.

21. Gordon J, Whitehead HR, Wormall A. The action of ammonia on complement. The fourth component. Biochem J 1926; 20:1028–1035.

22. Wallace JM, Wormall A. Red cell adhesion in trypanosomiasis of man and other animals. II Some experiments on the mechanism of the reaction. Parasitology 1931; 23:346–359.

23. Brown HC, Broom JC. Studies in trypanosomiasis. II. Observations on the red cell adhesion test. Trans R Soc Trop Med Hyg 1938; 32:209–222.

24. Osborne TWB. Complement or Alexin. London: Oxford University Press, 1937.

25. Ecker EE, Pillemer L. Complement. Ann NY Acad Sci 1942; 43:63–83.

26. Nelson RA, Jr. The immune adherence phenomenon: an immunologically specific reaction between micro-organisms and erythrocytes leading to enhanced phagocytosis. Science 1953; 118:733–737.

27. Fearon DT. Identification of the membrane glycoprotein that is the C3b receptor of the human erythrocyte, polymorphonuclear leukocyte, B lymphocyte, and monocyte. J Exp Med 1980; 152:20–30.

28. Hebert LA, Cosio FG. The erythrocyte–immune complex–glomerulonephritis connection in man. Kidney Int 1987; 31:877–885.

29. Walport MJ, Ross GD, Mackworth-Young C, Watson JV, Hogg N, Lachmann PJ. Family studies of erythrocyte complement receptor type 1 levels: reduced levels in patients with SLE are acquired, not inherited. Clin Exp Immunol 1985; 59:547–554.

30. Wilson JG, Wong WW, Schur PH, Fearon DT. Mode of inheritance of decreased C3b receptors on erythrocytes of patients with systemic lupus erythematosus. N Engl J Med 1982; 307:981–986.

31. Fearon DT, Collins LA. Increased expression of C3b receptors on polymorphonuclear leukocytes induced by chemotactic factors and by purification procedures. J Immunol 1983; 130:370–375.

32. Paccaud J-P, Carpentier J-L, Schifferli JA. Direct evidence for the clustered nature of complement receptors type 1 on the erythrocyte membrane. J Immunol 1988; 141:3889–3894.

33. Fearon DT. Cellular receptors for fragments of the third component of complement. Immunol Today 1984; 5:105–110.

34. Wong WW. Structural and functional correlation of the human complement receptor type 1. J Invest Dermatol 1990; 94:64S–67S.

35. Van Dyne S, Holers VM, Lublin DM, Atkinson JP. The polymorphism of the C3b/C4b receptor in the normal population and in patients with systemic lupus erythematosus. Clin Exp Immunol 1987; 68:570–579.

36. Klopstock A, Schartz J, Bleiberg Y, Adam A, Szeinberg A, Schlomo J. Hereditary nature of the behaviour of erythrocytes in immune adherence–haemagglutination phenomenon. Vox Sang 1965; 10:177–187.

37. Walport MJ, Lachmann PJ. Erythrocyte complement receptor type 1, immune complexes and the rheumatic diseases. Arthritis Rheum 1987; 31:153–158.

38. Paccaud JP, Carpentier JL, Schifferli JA. Difference in the clustering of complement receptor type 1 (CR1) on polymorphonuclear leukocytes and erythrocytes: effect on immune adherence. Eur J Immunol 1990; 20:283–289.

39. Paccaud JP, Schifferli JA, Baggiolini M. NAP-1/IL-8 induces up-regulation of CR1 receptors in human neutrophil leukocytes. Biochem Biophys Res Commun 1990; 166:187–192.

40. Beynon HLC, Davies KA, Haskard DO, Walport MJ. Erythrocyte complement receptor type 1 and interactions between immune complexes, neutrophils and endothelium. J Immunol 1994; 153:3160–3167.

41. Biozzi G, Benacerraf B, Halpern BN. Quantitative study of the granulopectic activity of the reticuloendothelial system II. B J Exp Path 1953; 34:441–457.

42. Niehaus GD, Shumacker PR, Saba TM. Reticuloendothelial clearance of blood-borne particulates relevance to experimental lung microembolization and vascular injury. Ann Surg 1980; 191:479–487.

43. Davies KA, Chapman PT, Norsworthy PJ, et al. Clearance pathways of immune complexes in the pig. Insight into the adaptive nature of antigen clearance in humans. J Immunol 1995; 155:5760–5768.

44. Taylor RP, Kujala G, Wilson K, Wright E, Harbin A. In vivo and in vitro studies of the binding of antibody/dsDNA immune complexes to rabbit and guinea pig platelets. J Immunol 1985; 134:2550–2558.

45. Edberg JC, Kujala GA, Taylor RP. Rapid immune adherence reactivity of nascent, soluble antibody/DNA immune complexes in the circulation. J Immunol 1987; 139:1240–1244.

46. Haakenstad AO, Mannik M. Saturation of the reticuloendothelial system with soluble immune complexes. J Immunol 1974; 112:1939–1948.

47. Finbloom DS, Plotz PH. Studies of reticuloendothelial function in the mouse with model immune complexes: II. Serum clearance, tissue uptake and reticuloendothelial saturation in NZB/W mice. J Immunol 1979; 123:1600–1603.

48. Finbloom DS, Magilavy DB, Harford JB, Rifai A, Plotz PH. Influence of antigen on immune complex behavior in mice. J Clin Invest 1981; 68:214–224.

49. Cornacoff JB, Hebert LA, Smead WL, VanAman ME, Birmingham DJ, Waxman FJ. Primate erythrocyte-immune complex-clearing mechanism. J Clin Invest 1983; 71:236–247.

50. Waxman FJ, Hebert LA, Cornacoff JB, et al. Complement depletion accelerates the clearance of immune complexes from the circulation of primates. J Clin Invest 1984; 74:1329–1340.

51. Waxman FJ, Hebert LA, Cosio FG, et al. Differential binding of immunoglobulin A and immunoglobulin G1 immune complexes to primate erythrocytes in vivo: immunoglobulin A immune complexes bind less well to erythrocytes and are preferentially deposited in glomeruli. J Clin Invest 1986; 77:82–89.

52. Cornacoff JB, Hebert LA, Birmingham DJ, Waxman FJ. Factors influencing the binding of large immune complexes primate erythrocyte CR1 receptor. Clin Immunol Immunopathol 1984; 30:255–264.

53. Lobatto S, Daha MR, Voetman AA, et al. Clearance of soluble aggregates of immunoblobulin G in healthy volunteers and chimpanzees. Clin Exp Immunol 1987; 68:133.

54. Schifferli JA, Ng YC, Estreicher J, Walport MJ. The clearance of tetanus toxoid/anti-tetanus toxoid immune complexes from the circulation of humans. Complement- and erythrocyte complement receptor 1-dependent mechanisms. J Immunol 1988; 140:899–904.

55. Davies KA, Peters AM, Beynon HLC, Walport MJ. Immune complex processing in patients with systemic lupus erythematos—in vivo imaging and clearance studies. J Clin Invest 1992; 90:2075–2083.

56. Davies KA, Erlendsson K, Beynon HLC, et al. Splenic uptake of immune complexes in man is complement-dependent. J Immunol 1993; 151:3866–3873.

57. Edberg JC, Kujala GA, Taylor RP. Rapid immune adherence reactivity of nascent, soluble antibody/DNA immune complexes in the circulation. J Immunol 1987; 139:1240.

58. Davies KA, Hird V, Stewart S, et al. A study of in vivo immune complex formation and clearance in man. J Immunol 1990; 144:4613–4620.

59. Brown DL, Lachmann PJ, Dacie JV. The in vivo behavior of complement-coated red cells: studies in C6-deficient, C3-depleted, and normal rabbits. Clin Exp Immunol 1970; 7:401–422.

60. Atkinson JP, Frank MM. Studies on the in vivo effects of antibody. Interaction of IgM antibody and complement in the immune clearance and destruction of erythrocytes in man. J Clin Invest 1974; 54:339–348.

61. Hughes-Jones NC, Mollison PL, Mollison PN. Removal of incompatible red cells by the spleen. Br J Haematol 1957; 3:125–133.

62. Mollison PL, Crome P, Hughes-Jones NC, Rochna E. Rate of removal from the circulation of red cells sensitised with different amounts of antibody. Br J Haematol 1965; 11:461–470.

63. Frank MM, Lawley TJ, Hamburger MI, Brown EJ. Immunoglobulin G Fc receptor-mediated clearance in autoimmune diseases. Ann Intern Med 1983; 98:206–218.

64. Smedsrod B, Pertoft H, Eggertsen G, Sundstrom C. Functional and morphological character-ization of cultures of Kupffer cells and liver endothelial cells prepared by means of density separation in Percoll, and selective substrate adherence. Cell Tissue Res 1985; 241(3):639–49.

65. Ross GD, Newman SL. Regulation of macrophage functions by complement, complement receptors, and IgG-Fc receptors. In: Bellanti JA, Herscowitz HB, eds. The Reticuloendothelial System, A Comprehensive Treatise, Vol. 6. New York: Plenum Publishing Corp., 1984:173–200.

66. Unkeless JC, Fleit H, Mellman IS. Structural aspects and heterogeneity of immunoglobulin Fc receptors. Adv Immunol 1981; 31:247–270.

67. Reist CJ, Wright JD, Labuguen RH, Taylor RP. Human IgG in immune complexes bound to human erythrocyte CR1 is recognized differently than human IgG bound to an erythrocyte surface antigen. J Immunol Methods 1993; 163:199–208.

68. Peters AM. Splenic blood flow and blood cell kinetics. Clin Haematol 1983; 12(2):421–447.

69. Weiss L. The Spleen. In: Weiss L, ed. Cell and Tissue Biology. 2nd ed. Baltimore: Urban and Schwarzenberg, 1988:517.

70. Robertson DA, Bullen AW, Hall R, Losowsky MS. Blood film appearances in the hyposplen-ism of coeliac disease. Br J Clin Pract 1983; 37:19–22.

71. Crocker SH, Eddy DO, Obenauf RN, Wismar BL, Lowery BD. Bacteremia: host specific lung clearance and pulmonary failure. J Trauma 1981; 21:215–220.

72. Wessels MR, Butko P, Ma M, Warren HB, Lage AL, Carroll MC. Studies of group B streptococcal infection in mice deficient in complement component C3 or C4 demonstrate an essential role for complement in both innate and acquired immunity. Proc Natl Acad Sci U S A 1995; 92:11490–11494.

73. Reid R, Prodeus AP, Khan W, Carroll MC. Natural antibody and complement are critical for endotoxin clerance from the circulation. Mol Immunol 1996; 33(1):78 (abstract).

74. Lynn WA, Cohen J. Adjunctive therapy for septic shock: a review of experimental approaches. Clin Infect Dis 1995; 20:143–158.

75. Seelen MA, Athanassiou P, Lynn WA, et al. The anti-lipid A monoclonal antibody E5 binds to rough gram-negative bacteria, fixes C3, and facilitates binding of bacterial immune complexes to both erythrocytes and monocytes. Immunology 1995; 84:653–661.

76. Tonoli M, Davies KA, Norsworthy PJ, Cohen J, Walport MJ. The anti-lipid antibody HA-1A binds to rough gram-negative bacteria, fixes complement and facilitates binding to erythrocyte CR1(CD35). Clin Exp Immunol 1993; 92:232–238.

77. Bowness P, Davies KA, Norsworthy PJ, et al. Hereditary C1q deficiency and systemic lupus erythematosus. QJ Med 1994; 87:455–464.

78. Ruddy S. Component deficiencies 3. The second component. Prog Allergy 1986; 39:250–267.

79. Botto M, Fong KY, So AK, et al. Homozygous hereditary C3 deficiency due to a partial gene deletion. Proc Natl Acad Sci USA 1992; 89:4957–4961.

80. Botto M, Walport MJ. Hereditary deficiency of C3 in animals and humans. Int Rev Immunol 1993; 10:37–50.

81. Vyse TJ, Spath PJ, Davies KA, et al. Hereditary complement factor I deficiency. QJ Med 1994; 87:385–401.

82. Fielder AH, Walport MJ, Batchelor JR, et al. Family study of the major histocompatibility complex in patients with systemic lupus erythematosus: importance of null alleles of C4A and C4B in determining disease susceptibility. Br Med J Clin Res 1983; 286:425–428.

83. Christiansen FT, Dawkins RL, Uko G, McCluskey J, Kay PH, Zilko PJ. Complement allotyp-ing in SLE: association with C4A null. Aust NZ J Med 1983; 13:483–488.

84. Howard PF, Hochberg MC, Bias WB, Arnett FC, Jr., McLean RH. Relationship between C4 null genes, HLA-D region antigens, and genetic susceptibility to systemic lupus erythematosus in Caucasian and black Americans. Am J Med 1986; 81:187–193.

85. Hartung K, Baur MP, Coldewey R, et al. Major histocompatibility complex haplotypes and complement C4 alleles in systemic lupus erythematosus. Results of a multicenter study. J Clin Invest 1992; 90:1346–1351.

86. Davies EJ, Snowden N, Hillarby MC, et al. Mannose-binding protein gene polymorphism in systemic lupus erythematosus. Arthritis Rheum 1995; 38:110–114.

87. Donaldson VH, Hess EV, McAdams AJ. Lupus-erythematosus-like disease in three unrelated women with hereditary angioneurotic edema [letter]. Ann Intern Med 1977; 86:312–313.

88. Brickman CM, Tsokos GC, Balow JE, et al. Immunoregulatory disorders associated with hereditary angioedema. I. Clinical manifestations of autoimmune disease. J Allergy Clin Immunol 77; 749–757.

89. Brickman CM, Tsokos GC, Chused TM, et al. Immunoregulatory disorders associated with hereditary angioedema. II. Serologic and cellular abnormalities. J Allergy Clin Immunol 77; 758–767.

90. Walport MJ, Davies KA, Botto M, et al. C3 nephritic factor and SLE. QJ Med 1994; 87:609–615.

91. Inai S, Akagaki Y, Moriyama T, et al. Inherited deficiencies of the late-acting complement components other than C9 found among healthy blood donors. Int Arch Allergy Appl Immunol 1989; 90:274–279.

92. Hassig A, Borel JF, Ammann P, Thoni M, Butler R. Essentielle hypokomplementamie. Pathol Microbiol 1964; 27:542.

93. Cork CL, Morris JM, Olson JL, Krakowka S, Winkelstein JA. Membranoproliferative glomer-ulonephritis in dogs with a genetically determined deficiency of the third component of complement. Clin Immunol Immunopathol 1991; 60:455–470.

94. Hogasen K, Jansen JH, Mollnes TE, Hovdenes J, Harboe M. Hereditary porcine membrano-proliferative glomerulonephritis type II is caused by factor H deficiency. J Clin Invest 1995; 95:1054–1061.

95. Fischer MB, Ma M, Goerg S, et al. Regulation of the B cell response to T-dependent antigens by classical pathway complement. J Immunol 1996; 157:549–556.

96. Matsumoto M, Fukada W, Goellner J, et al. Generation and characterisation of mice deficient for factor B. Mol Immunol 1996; 33(1):63–60.

97. Ahearn JM, Fischer MB, Croix D, et al. Disruption of the Cr2 locus results in a reduction in B-1a cells and in an impaired B cell response to T-dependent antigen. Immunity 1996; 4:251–262.

98. Goodnow CC, Cyster JG, Hartley SB, Bell SE, Cooke MP, Healy JI, Akkaraju S, Rathmell JC, Pogue SL, Shokat KP. Self-tolerance checkpoints in B lymphocyte development. Adv Immunol 1995; 375:279–368.

99. Takeuchi Y, Cosset FL, Lachmann PJ, Okada H, Weiss RA, Collins MK. Type C retrovirus inactivation by human complement is determined by both the viral genome and the producer cell. J Virol 1994; 68:8001–8007.

100. Rother RP, Fodor WL, Springhorn JP, et al. A novel mechanism of retrovirus inactivation in human serum mediated by anti-alpha-galactosyl natural antibody. J Exp Med 1995; 182:1345–1355.

101. Cornillet P, Philbert F, Kazatchkine MD, Cohen JH. Genomic determination of the CR1 (CD35) density polymorphism on erythrocytes using polymerase chain reaction amplification and HindIII restriction enzyme digestion. J Immunol Methods. 1991; 136(2): 193–7.

102. Moldenhauer F, David J, Fielder AHL, Lachmann PJ, Walport MJ. Inherited deficiency of erythrocyte complement receptor type 1 does not cause susceptibility to systemic lupus erythematosus. Arthritis Rheum 1987; 30:961–966.

103. Frank MM, Hamburger MI, Lawley TJ, Kimberly RP, Plotz PH. Defective reticuloendothelial system Fc-receptor function in systemic lupus erythematosus. N Engl J Med 1979; 300:518–523.

104. Hamburger MI, Lawley TJ, Kimberly RP, Plotz PH, Frank MM. A serial study of splenic reticuloendothelial sysyem Fc-receptor function in systemic lupus erythematosus. Arthritis Rheum 1982; 25:48.

105. Salmon JE, Brogle NL, Edberg JC, Kimberly RP: Allelic polymorphisms of human Fcγ receptor IIA and Fcγ receptor IIIB; independent mechanisms for differences in human phagocyte function. J Clin Invest 1992; 89: 1274–1281.

106. Salmon JE, Millard S, Schachter LA, et al. Fcγ RIIA alleles are heritable risk factors for lupus nephritis in African Americans. J Clin Invest 1996; 97:1348–1354.

107. Duits AJ, Bootsma H, Derksen RHWM, et al. Skewed distribution of IgG Fcγ receptor IIa is associated with renal disease in systemic lupus erythematosus patients. Arthritis Rheum 1995; 39:1832–1836.

108. Botto M, Theodoridis E, Thompson EM, et al. Fcγ RIIa polymorphism in systemic lupus erythematosus (SLE): no association with disease. Clin Exp Immunol 1996; 104:264–268.

109. Halma C, Breedveld FC, Daha MR, et al. Elimination of soluble ^{123}I-labeled aggregates of IgG in patients with systemic lupus erythematosus. Effect of serum IgG and numbers of erythrocyte complement receptor type 1. Arthritis Rheum 1991; 34:442–452.

110. Halma C, Daha MR, Camps JA, Evers Schouten JH, Pauwels EK, Van Es. Deficiency of complement component C3 is associated with accelerated removal of soluble 123I-labelled aggregates of IgG from the circulation. Clin Exp Immunol 1992; 90:394–400.

111. Cochrane CJ. Mediation of immunologic glomerular injury. Transplant Proc 1969; 1:949–956.

112. Henson PM, Cochrane CG. The effects of complement depletion on experimental tissue injury. Ann NY Acad Sci 1975; 256:426–440.

113. Sylvestre DL, Ravetch JV. Fc receptors initiate the Arthus reaction: redefining the inflammatory cascade. Science 1994; 265:1095–1098.

114. Hazenbos WLW, Gessner JE, Hofhuis FMA, et al. Impaired IgG depedent anaphylaxis and Arthus reaction in Fc gamma RIII (CD16) deficient mice. Immunity 1996; 5:181–188.

115. Ben-Efraim S, Cinader B. The role of complement in the passive cutaneous reaction of mice. J Exp Med 1964; 120:925–942.

116. Larsen GL, Mitchell BC, Henson PM. The pulmonary response of C5 sufficient and deficient mice to immune complexes. Am Rev Respir Dis 1981; 123:434–439.

117. Zhang Y, Ramos BF, Jakschik BA. Augmentation of reverse Arthus reaction by mast cells in mice. J Clin Invest 1991; 88:841–846.

118. Sylvestre DL, Ravetch JV. A dominant role for mast cell Fc receptors in the Arthus reaction. Immunity 1996; 5:387–390.

119. Bozic CR, Lu B, Hopken UE, Gerard C, Gerard NPR. Neurogenic amplification of immune complex inflammation. Science 1996; 273:1722–1725.

120. Rodwell JD, Tang LH, Schumaker VN. Antigen valence and Fc-localised secondary forces in antibody precipitation. Mol Immunol 1980; 17:1591–1597.

121. Wilson CB, Dixon FJ. Renal response to immunological injury. In: Brenner BM, Rector FC, eds. The Kidney. 4th ed. Philadelphia: W.B. Saunders, 1996:800–890.

122. Ng YC. C3 nephritic factor and membranoproliferative glonerulonephritis. In: Pusey CD, ed. Immunology of Renal Diseases. Dordrecht/Boston/London: Kluwer Academic Publishers, 1991:215–227.

123. Verroust PJ, Wilson CB, Dixon FJ. Lack of nephritogenicity of systemic activation of the alternative complement pathway. Kidney Int 1974; 6:157–169.

124. Simpson IJ, Moran J, Evans DJ, Peters DK. Prolonged complement activation in mice. Kidney Int 1978; 13:467–471.

125. Baker PJ, Adler S, Yang Y, Couser WG. Complement activation by heat-killed human kidney cells: formation, activity and stabilization of cell-bound C3 convertases. J Immunol 1984; 133:877–881.

126. Chesney RW, Oregan S, Guyda HJ, Drummond KN. Candida endocrinopathy syndrome with membranoproliferative glomerulonephritis: demonstration of glomerular candida antigen. Clin Nephrol 1976; 5:232–238.

127. Wisnieski JJ, Baer AN, Christensen J, et al. Hypocomplementemic urticarial vasculitis syndrome. Clinical and serologic findings in 18 patients. Medicine 1995; 74:24–41.

128. Wisnieski JJ, Jones SM. Comparison of autoantibodies to the collagen-like region of C1q in hypocomplementaemic urticarial vasculitis syndrome and systemic lupus erythematosus. J Immunol 1992; 148:1396–1403.

129. Uwatoko S, Gauthier VJ, Mannik M. Autoantibodies to the collagen-like region of C1q deposit in glomeruli via C1q immune deposits. Clin Immunol Immunopathol 1991; 61:268–273.

130. Halbwachs L, Leveille M, Lesavre P, Wattels S, Leibowitch J. Nephritic factor of the classical pathway of complement. Immunoglobulin autoantibody directed against the classical pathway C3 convertase enzyme. J Clin Invest 1980; 65:1249–1256.

131. Daha MR, Hazavoet HM, van Es LA, Katz A. Stabilization of the classical patway covertase C42 by a factor (F-42) isolated from sera of patients with SLE. Immunology 1980; 40:417–424.

132. Appel GB, Silva FG, Pirani CL. Renal involvement in systemic lupus erythematosus (SLE): a study of 56 patients emphasising histologic classification. Medicine 1978; 57:371–410.

133. Mannik M. Mechanisms of tissue deposition of immune complexes. J Rheumatol 1987; 14:35–42.

134. Van Damme BJC, Fleuren GJ, Bakker WW, Vernier RL, Hoedemaeker PJ. Experimental glomerulonephritis in the rat induced by antibodies to tubular antigens. IV. Fixed glomerular antigens in the pathogenesis of heterologous immune complex glomerulonephritis. Lab Invest 1978; 38:502–510.

135. Salant DJ, Belok S, Madaio MP, Couser WG. A new role complement in experimental membranous nephropathy in rats. J Clin Invest 1980; 66:1339–1350.

136. Kerjaschki D, Farquar MG. Immunocytochemical localisation of the Heymann nephritis antigen (GP330) in glomerular epithelial cells of normal Lewis rats. J Exp Med 1983; 157:667–685.

137. Camussi G, Brentjens JR, Noble B. Antibody-induced redistribution of Heymann's antigen on the surface of cultured glomerular visceral epithelial cells: possible role in the pathogenesis of Heymann glomerular nephritis. J Immunol 1985; 135:2409–2416.

138. Shoenfeld Y, Rauch J, Massicotte H, et al. Polyspecificity of monoclonal lupus autoantibodies produced by human–human hybridomas. N Engl J Med 1983; 308:414–420.

139. Madaio MP, Carlson J, Cataldo J, Ucci A, Milborini P, Pankewycz O. Murine monoclonal anti-DNA antibodies bind directly to glomerular antigens and form immune deposits. J Immunol 1987; 138(9):2883–2889.

140. Couser WG, Salant DJ. In-situ immune complex formation and glomerular injury. Kidney Int 1980; 17:1–13.

141. Agodoa LYC, Gauthier VJ, Mannik M. Precipitating antigen–antibody systems are required for the formation of sub-epithelial electron dense immune deposits in rat glomeruli. J Exp Med 1983; 158:1259–1271.

142. Izui S, Lambert PH, Miescher PA. In vitro demonstration of a particular affinity of glomerular basement membrane and collagen for DNA. A possible basis for a local formation of DNA-anti-DNA complexes in systemic lupus erythematosus. J Exp Med 1976; 144:428–443.

143. Ebling F, Hahn BH. Restricted subpopulations of DNA antibodies in kidneys of mice with systemic lupus. Comparison of antibodies in serum and renal eluates. Arthritis Rheum 1980; 23:392–403.

144. Dang H, Barbeck RJ. Comparison of anti-DNA antibodies from serum and kidney eluates of NZB X NZW F1 mice. J Clin Lab Immunol 1982; 9:139–145.

145. Couser WG, Salant DJ. Immunopathogenesis of glomerular capillary wall injury in nephrotic states. Contemp Issues Nephrol 1982; 9:47–83.

146. Mauer SM, Sutherland DER, Howard RJ. the glomerular mesangium. III. Acute immune mesangial injury: a new model of glomerulonephritis. J Exp Med 1973; 137:553–570.

147. Yamamoto T, Wilson CB. Antibody-induced mesangial damage: the model, functional alterations and effects of complement. Kidney Int 1986; 29:296 (abstract).
148. Matsuo S, Caldwell P, Brentjens J, Andres G. Nephrotoxic serum glomerulonephritis induced in the rabbit by anti-endothelial cell antibodies. Kidney Int 1985; 27:217 (abstract).
149. Brouet JC. Cryoglobulinaemias. Presse Med 1983; 12:2991–2996.
150. Pawlotsky JM, Dhumeaux D, Bago M. Hepatitis C virus in dermatology. A review. Arch Dermatol 1995; 131:1185–1193.
151. Dupin N, Chosidow O, Lunel F, et al. Essential mixed cryoglobulinemia. A comparative study of dermatologic manifestations in patients infected or noninfected with hepatitis C virus. Arch Dermatol 1995; 131:1124–1127.
152. Cacoub P, Fabiani FL, Musset L, et al. Mixed cryoglobulinemia and hepatitis C virus. Am J Med 1994; 96:124–132.
153. Galli M, Monti G, Invernizzi F, et al. Hepatitis B virus-related markers in secondary and in essential mixed cryoglobulinemias: a multicentric study of 596 cases. the Italian Group for he Study of Cryoglobulinemias (GISC). Ann Ital Med Int 1992; 7:209–214.
154. Wong VS, Egner W, Elsey T, Brown D, Alexander GJ. Incidence, character and clinical relevance of mixed cryoglobulinaemia in patients with chronic hepatitis C virus infection. Clin Exp Immunol 1996, 104(1):25–31.
155. Tanaka K, Aiyama T, Imai J, Morishita Y, Fukatsu T, Kakumu S. Serum cryoglobulin and chronic hepatitis C virus disease among Japanese patients. Am J Gastroenterol 1995; 90:1847–1852.
156. Maisch B. Autoreactive mechanisms in infective endocarditis. Springer Semin Immunopathol 1989; 11:439–456.
157. Petersdorf RG. Immune complexes in infective endocarditis [editorial]. N Engl J Med 1976; 295:1534–1535.
158. McKenzie PE, Hawke D, Woodroffe AJ, Thompson AJ, Seymour AE, Clarkson AR. Serum and tissue immune complexes in infective endocarditis. J Clin Lab Immunol 1980; 4:125–132.
159. Landoy Z, West TE, Vladutiu AO, Fitzpatrick JE. Evaluation of a Cordia-IC enzyme-linked immunosorbent assay kit for the detection of circulating immune complexes. J Clin Microbiol 1985; 22:279–282.
160. Williams RC, Jr., Kilpatrick K. Immunofluorescence studies of cardiac valves in infective endocarditis. Arch Intern Med 1985; 145:297–300.
161. Maisch B, Mayer E, Schubert U, Berg PA, Kochsiek K. Immune reactions in infective endocarditis. II. Relevance of circulating immune complexes, serum inhibition factors, lymphocytotoxic reactions, and antibody-dependent cellular cytotoxicity against cardiac target cells. Am Heart J 1983; 106:338–344.
162. Burton Kee J, Morgan Capner P, Mowbray JF. Nature of circulating immune complexes in infective endocarditis. J Clin Pathol 1980; 33:653–659.
163. Weetman AP, Matthews N, O'Hara SP, Amos N, Williams BD, Thomas JP. Meningococcal endocarditis with profound acquired hypocomplementaemia. J Infect 1985; 10:51–56.
164. Kerr MA, Wilton E, Naama JK, Whaley K. Circulating immune complexes associated with decreased complement-mediated inhibition of immune precipitation in sera from patients with bacterial endocarditis. Clin Exp Immunol 1986; 63:359–366.
165. Cochrane CG. Mechanisms involved in the deposition of immune complexes in tissues. J Exp Med 1971; 134:75–89.
166. Hagen EC, de Keizer RJ, Andrassy K, et al. Compassionate treatment of Wegener's granulomatosis with rabbit anti-thymocyte globulin. Clin Nephrol 1995; 43:351–359.
167. Tarkowski A, Andersson Gare B, Aurell M. Use of anti-thymocyte globulin in the management of refractory systemic autoimmune diseases. Scand J Rheumatol 1993; 22:261–266.
168. Bielory L, Gascon P, Lawley TJ, Young NS, Frank MM. Human serum sickness: a prospective analysis of 35 patients treated with equine anti-thymocyte globulin for bone marrow failure. Medicine 1988; 67:40–57.

169. McCann SR, Sullivan F, Reynolds M, Temperley IJ. Treatment of severe aplastic anaemia with anti-thymocyte globulin. Acta Haematol 1985; 74:144–147.
170. Lipkin DP, Reid CJ. Myocardial infarction: the first 24 hours. Br Med J 1988; 296:947–948.
171. Mason T. Proceedings of the Symposium on Intracoronary Thrombolysis in Acute Myocardial Infarction. Am Heart J 1981; 102:1123–1208.
172. McGrath KG, Patterson R. Anapylactic reactivity to streptokinase. JAMA 1984; 252:1314–1317.
173. Davies KA, Mathieson P, Winearls CG, Rees AJ, Walport MJ. Serum sickness and acute renal failure after streptokinase therapy for myocardial infarction. Clin Exp Immunol 1990; 80:83–88.
174. Totty WG, Romano T, Benian GM, Gilula LA, Sherman LA. Serum sickness following streptokinase therapy. AJR 1982; 138:143–144.
175. Alexopoulos D, Raine AEG, Cobbe SM. Serum sickness complicating intravenous streptokinase therapy in acute myocardial infarction. Eur Heart J 1984; 5:1010–1012.
176. Chandra RK, Joglekar SA, Tomas E. Penicillin allergy: anti-penicillin IgE antibodies and immediate hypersensitivity skin reactions employing major and minor determinants of penicillin. Arch Dis Child 1980; 55:857–860.
177. Whittingham S, Mackey IR. Adverse reactions to drugs: relationship to immunopathic disease. Med J Aust 1976; 1:486–8, 490–2.
178. Heckbert SR, Stryker WS, Coltin KL, Manson JE, Platt R. Serum sickness in children after antibiotic exposure: estimates of occurrence and morbidity in a health maintenance organization population. Am J Epidemiol 1990; 132:336–342.
179. Chopra R, Roberts J, Warrington RJ. Severe delayed-onset hypersensitivity reactions to amoxicillin in children [see comments]. Can Med Assoc J 1989; 140:921–923.
180. Brandslund I, Svehag SE, Teisner B, Hyltoft Petersen P. Activation of the complement system and accumulation of hemoglobin-haptoglobin complexes in plasma during an adverse reaction to penicillin treatment. Int Arch Allergy Appl Immunol 1983; 71:137–143.
181. Dirnhofer R, Sonnabend W, Sigrist T. [The enlarged diagnosis of the fatal penicillin accident. Immunehistologic demonstration of antigen-antibody complexes and of antibodies against the tubular basement membrane after administraiton of depot penicillin]. Schweiz Med Wochenschr 1978; 108:750–755.

21

C1 Inhibitor Gene and Hereditary Angioedema

ALVIN E. DAVIS III

Children's Hospital Research Foundation, University of Cincinnati
College of Medicine, Cincinnati, Ohio

I. HISTORICAL REVIEW

Although the disease now known as hereditary angioedema (HAE) was mentioned in earlier medical literature, Quincke and Osler (1,2), by virtue of their detailed, accurate descriptions of angioedema and its hereditary nature, are credited with the first descriptions of the disease. Quincke named the disease "angioneurotic edema" because of the assumption that the acute onset of the edema indicated a neurogenic mechanism. Although Quincke and others had recognized examples of symptoms in multiple family members (1), Osler, in his description of five generations of a family with the disease, accurately defined its dominant inheritance (2). In addition, he described the relatively common occurrence of laryngeal edema, recognized that abdominal symptoms were a manifestation of the disease, and correctly predicted the pathophysiology of the abdominal symptoms.

Lepow and his colleagues, during the course of studies that resulted in the isolation and characterization of the first component of complement, found that human serum contained a heat-labile factor that inhibited the esterolytic activity of C1 (3–5). They named this protein C1 esterase inhibitor, and subsequently achieved its partial purification (6,7). Shortly thereafter, Donaldson and Evans demonstrated that patients with HAE had significantly decreased serum levels of C1 inhibitor (C1 INH) (8). The previous year, Landerman et al. had shown that the serum of patients with HAE was deficient in kallikrein inhibitory capacity, although the fact that this was a result of C1 INH deficiency was not then appreciated (9). Taken together, these two observations indicated both that HAE was a result of C1 INH deficiency and that C1 INH was the primary plasma kallikrein inhibitor. Since that time, a great deal of information has accumulated related to the pathophysiology and molecular genetic basis of HAE, and the structure and function of C1 INH, and its gene.

II. C1 INHIBITOR GENE

A. Structure

C1 INH is encoded by a 17 kb single copy gene on chromosome 11 (11q11–q13.1) (10–12), and consists of eight exons separated by seven introns. The structure of the gene reveals no similarities in comparison with the genes encoding other related proteins (the

455

serpin superfamily of *serine proteinase inhibitors*; see Section V1). Several features of the gene are unusual and likely to be of some importance. First, its introns and flanking regions contain a relatively high density of Alu repetitive elements (10,11), which are the most common repetitive DNA sequences in the human genome (500,000–1,000,000 copies). They are transcribed by RNA polymerase III but are of unknown function. Alu repeats are relatively common sites of recombination that have resulted in deletions and duplications in a number of genes. Such deletions or duplications account for as many as 15–20% of individuals with HAE (see Section VI). The gene contains 17 complete Alu elements: 3 in intron 3, 7 in intron 4, 5 in intron 6, and 2 in intron 7 (11). Two additional complete elements are present, one each within the 5′ and 3′ flanking regions of the gene. Another partially sequenced element is present at the border of the sequence that has been determined 5′ to the gene (position −1121) and a partial element is present in intron 6.

The first exon of the C1 INH gene consists of only 38 nucleotides and encodes a portion of the 5′ untranslated region of the C1 INH mRNA. It is separated from exon 2 by a 424 base intron; this intron contains interferon- (IFN) responsive elements that are functional in vitro and that may play a role in IFN-γ-mediated induction of C1 INH synthesis (see Section II.B.). The second exon contains the translation initiation site and encodes the first 17 amino acids of the leader sequence. Intron 2 is approximately 1500 nucleotides in length and is of potential importance because it contains a region of purine/pyrimidine repeats that theoretically could form a Z DNA structure (a left-handed double helix). Such structures have been shown to form in vitro, and both negative and positive gene-regulatory effects have been suggested (13). Exons 3–8 contain the remainder of the protein coding sequence. The DNA encoding the reactive center sequence is within exon 8. The intron–exon junctions do not clearly delineate structural or functional domains, although all lie at the junctions of secondary structural elements.

B. Transcriptional Regulation and Synthesis

Although the liver is the source of the bulk of plasma C1 INH, a number of other cells, including fibroblasts, monocytes, macrophages, endothelial cells, amnionic epithelial cells, microglia, and perhaps other cells in the brain, are capable of C1 INH synthesis (14–19). Synthesis is stimulated by IFN-γ and, to a lesser extent, by several other cytokines including tumor necrosis factor-α (TNF-α), IFN-α, monocyte-colony stimulating factor (M-CSF), and interleukin 6 (IL-6) (15,20–25).

Synthesis of C1 INH by fibroblasts, endothelial cells, monocytes, and HepG2 hepatoma cells increases by approximately 4- to 20-fold in response to IFN-γ (15,23–26). The importance in vivo of C1 INH synthesis regulation by these cytokines remains unclear. Although C1 INH is a sensitive acute phase reactant, it does not respond to IL-1 in vitro and, compared with other acute inflammatory proteins, does not respond vigorously to IL-6. An initial study had suggested that treatment of colon cancer patients with IFN-γ resulted in a 1.5–2-fold enhancement of plasma C1 INH levels, but a subsequent study was unable to show an effect (27,28).

IFN-γ-induced synthesis of C1 INH is due primarily to an enhanced transcriptional rate, although in monocytes mRNA stabilization appears to play a role (26,29). IFN response elements are located in both the 5′ flanking region of the gene and in its first intron (29). In the 5′ region, there are four potential IFN-γ activated sequences (GAS) between nucleotides −738 and −80. The most proximal of these GAS elements (GAS4) (nucleotides -125 to -119), is the only one of the four responsive to IFN-γ (Zahedi et al., unpublished data). This induction, as expected, is mediated via STAT-1α. The interferon-responsive elements within the first intron consist of another GAS element that overlaps the first of two adjacent interferon-stimulated response elements (ISREs). This region mediates responsiveness to both IFN-γ and IFN-α (29; Zahedi et al., unpublished data).

Androgens or attenuated androgens are effective chronic preventive therapy for attacks of HAE (see Section V.C.) (30,31). Although this effect is assumed to result from increased synthesis, the mechanism that leads to the increased plasma Cl INH levels in treated patients is not clear. One in vitro study indicated that the androgen effect was on C1 INH synthesis (32), but others have been unable to demonstrate such an effect (33,34). The C1 INH gene contains a potential androgen response element at nucleotides -303 through -289, but functional activity of this element has not been demonstrated. The mechanism of the androgen effect in HAE, therefore, remains ill defined.

The C1 INH promoter does not contain a TATA element, which is unusual among the serpins, but not among the genes encoding other complement proteins. It does, however, contain a functional initiator element (CTCAGTCT at nucleotides -3 to $+5$) that is a member of the terminal deoxynucleotidyltransferase (TdT) family of initiators (consensus sequence CTCANTCT) (35,36). In this respect, it is unique among both the serpin and complement genes. Most initiator-driven genes are housekeeping genes or widely distributed cell surface receptors that tend to be developmentally regulated or differentially regulated during the cell cycle. Three other elements within the promoter region, a CAAT sequence at -61 to -58, a GC-rich sequence at -81 to -61, and a polypurine/polypyrimidine H-DNA segment at -48 to -17, also may play a role in promoter activity (11,29). The GC-rich segment appears to have a positive influence on transcription (29). Genes with TdT initiators usually do not contain a CAAT sequence, nor do they usually contain a GC-rich element, as do most other TATA-less genes. The C1 INH gene, therefore, combines elements from different families of initiator-driven genes; these may prove to be important in its transcriptional regulation.

III. C1 INHIBITOR STRUCTURE

C1 INH is a glycoprotein that consists of 478 amino acids and a 22 amino acid hydrophobic signal peptide. By sequence homology, C1 INH is a serpin (*serine proteinase inhibitor*), a large, diverse family of proteins found in animals, plants, and viruses. Most serpins, like C1 INH, are proteinase inhibitors, but some serve transport functions (e.g., thyroxin-binding globulin), or release biologically active peptides (e.g., angiotensinogen), while the function of others, such as ovalbumin, remains unknown. Homology among the serpins is restricted to the $\sim$380 carboxyl terminal amino acids, which is the proteinase inhibitor functional domain (Fig. 1). In addition, most serpins have an amino terminal domain that either confers a secondary function (such as the release of angiotensin by angiotensinogen) or modulates inhibitory activity (such as potentiation of antithrombin III activity by heparin). The C1 INH amino terminal domain is the longest among the serpins. Although it may modulate access to intact C1, its function remains incompletely defined.

C1 INH is approximately 26% carbohydrate by weight, and therefore is among the most heavily glycosylated plasma proteins (37–43). Its total peptide molecular weight is 52,869, while the carbohydrate increases its molecular weight to 71,100 (39,43). The apparent molecular weight observed on sodium dodecyl sulfate-polyacrylamide gel electro-

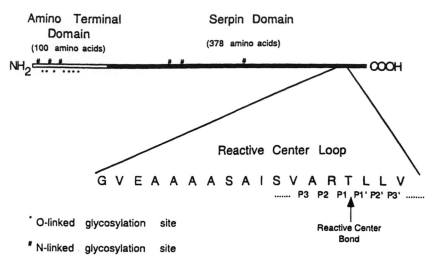

Figure 1 C1 inhibitor. The amino terminal heavily glycosylated domain does not have sequence homology with any other serpin. The carboxy terminal serpin domain retains the important structural elements required for protease inhibitor function. The amino acid sequence of the reactive center loop is indicated, as is the bond recognized by target protease.

phoresis (104,000) or analytical ultracentrifugation probably is an anomaly related to sequence characteristics and to the glycosylation pattern (37,38,41). The molecule contains six N-linked and seven O-linked oligosaccharides (39,43). All of the O-linked and three of the six N-linked sugars are within the amino terminal 100-residue nonserpin domain of the molecule (Fig. 1). No other serpin contains O-linked carbohydrate. It is presumed that this glycosylation pattern is responsible for the unusual two-domain appearance of C1 inhibitor on electron microscopy (44). One domain is globular, while the other, probably the amino terminal segment, is rodlike. This shape likely accounts for the lower than expected sedimentation coefficient (3.67S) and for the aberrantly high apparent molecular weight estimates on gel filtration (38,45). The serpin domain of C1 INH reveals approximately 20–25% identity with other inhibitor serpins. It has retained virtually all the highly conserved serpin sequence elements, and therefore also must share the three-dimensional structural elements that are common to the inhibitory serpins.

IV. BIOLOGICAL ROLE OF C1 INHIBITOR

A. Introduction: Serpin Function

Serpin inhibitory activity is dependent on the exposure of the reactive center within a peptide loop on the surface of the molecule. This reactive center loop is near the carboxyl terminus of the protein. The sequence of a portion of this loop mimics that of an ideal natural substrate of target proteases. However, when attacked by protease, rather than cleavage of the reactive center peptide bond, a tight enzyme-inhibitor complex, which may be a tetrahedral intermediate, is formed (46). The amino acid to the amino terminal side of the peptide bond recognized by target protease is the primary determinant of specificity and is termed the P1 residue (47). The amino acid on the carboxyl terminal side of the bond is the P1′ residue (Fig. 1). In the case of C1 INH, these residues are an Arg and a Thr, respectively (48). In each direction, the subsequent amino acids are numbered consecutively (P2, P3, P4, etc., toward the amino terminus and P2′, P3′, P4′, etc., toward the carboxy terminus). The reactive center loop overlies a five-stranded β-sheet (sheet A) that forms the prominent planar surface of the molecule (Fig. 2). Cleavage of this loop by nontarget proteases results in its insertion into sheet A as its fourth strand; β-sheet A then consists of six strands (49). This conformational rearrangement is accompanied by stabilization of the molecule, which can be demonstrated by enhanced resistance to heat or chemical denaturation (50–53) and by the expression of epitopes that are not detectable in the native molecule (54–56). This rearrangement can be mimicked by insertion of synthetic reactive center loop peptides into sheet A (57,58). These data, together with the analysis of several serpin-reactive center loop mutants (see Section VI) (59–63), and the crystallization of intact ovalbumin (a noninhibitory serpin) (64) and of intact antithrombin III dimers (65,66), have led to the concept that the reactive center loop is mobile and that insertion of the amino terminal portion of the loop into sheet A is required for inhibitory activity. Unfortunately, neither an intact, monomeric functional serpin nor a serpin-proteinase complex has been crystallized. Several important issues, therefore, remain ill-defined: Does reactive center loop insertion precede or is it induced by contact with protease? What is the degree of insertion of the reactive center loop of

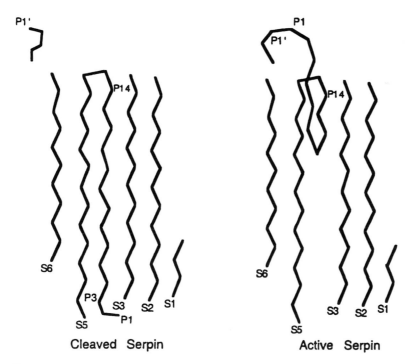

Cleaved Serpin   Active Serpin

Figure 2 Diagrammatic illustration of the structure of a serpin cleaved at P1-P1′ and of the hypothesized active serpin structure. For simplicity, only β sheet A and the reactive center loop are shown. In the active serpin molecule several residues of the hinge region of the reactive center loop are thought to be inserted into the cleft between strands 3 and 5 of β sheet A. Cleavage at the reactive center results in complete insertion of this strand resulting in the placement of the P1 and P1′ residues at opposite ends of the molecule.

a serpin in the protease-inhibitor complex? Is the reactive center peptide bond of a serpin in complex with protease cleaved or intact?

B. Complement System

C1 INH in vitro inactivates a number of proteases including C1r and C1s, the mannose-binding protein-associated serine protease (MASP), kallikrein, coagulation factors XIIa and XIa, plasmin, and tissue plasminogen activator (4,37,67–73). However, it plays biologically important roles primarily in regulation of the complement system (C1r and C1s) and of the contact system of kinin formation (factor XII and kallikrein). It may play a backup role in regulation of coagulation and fibrinolysis, but is less important in these systems. Its role in regulation of activation of the lectin pathway has not been analyzed.

C1 INH is the only plasma protease inhibitor that inactivates C1r and C1s (74,75). Activated C1r and C1s added to plasma complex only with C1 INH (74). In addition, the inhibition kinetics of C1r and C1s are identical in plasma and in purified systems (75). The rate of inhibition of C1r is significantly slower than that of C1s (2.8×10^3 $M^{-1}s^{-1}$ vs. 1.2–$6.0 \times 10^4 M^{-1}sec^{-1}$) (76,77). C1 INH does not prevent C1 activation by most immune complexes, although it can prevent activation by weak activators (78), and it prevents autoactivation of isolated C1 or C1r (79,80). This inhibition of activation likely is a result of efficient complex formation with the initial small amounts of activated C1r that are formed, thereby preventing activation of C1s and subsequent components (81,82). These differences in susceptibility are illustrated by two observations: in the presence of C1 INH, 8–10-fold more of a weak activator is required for C1 activation than in its absence (78); and, second, fluid phase isolated activated C1 is approximately 100-fold more sensitive to inactivation by C1 INH than is activated C1 bound to antibody sensitized sheep erythrocytes (83). With most immune complexes, therefore, C1 INH inactivates C1r and C1s after C1 activation and thereby limits consumption of the C1s substrates (C2 and C4). The reaction of C1 INH with activated C1 leads to the dissociation of the activated C1s-C1r-C1r-C1s tetramer from C1q as two C1 INH-C1r-C1s-C1 INH complexes (84,85). As with the fluid phase isolated proteases, C1s is more rapidly inhibited than is C1r. However, complex formation with C1r is the primary determinant of dissociation from C1q (86). After dissociation of C1r and C1s, the immune complex bound C1q then is able to to bind to its receptor(s) on leukocytes and other cells.

C. Contact System

In retrospect, the first evidence that C1 INH was involved in regulation of the contact system was the observation in 1962 that plasma from patients with HAE was deficient in kallikrein inhibitory capacity (Section I) (9). Although it soon became apparent that C1 INH could inhibit factor XIIa and kallikrein, its importance in contact system regulation was not initially clear because other inhibitors also inactivated these proteases. Several studies, based on a combination of kinetic analyses and quantitation of complex formation in plasma, indicated that C1 INH provided 42–84% of the plasma kallikrein inhibitory capacity (87–89). Similar experiments indicated that C1 INH provided as much as 90% of the plasma factor XIIa and XIIf inhibitory capacity (90,91). The majority of the additional inhibitory capacity toward kallikrein and factor XIIa is provided by α_2 macro-globulin, while α_2-antiplasmin is also involved in factor XIIf (β factor XIIa) inhibition. Other information that suggests that C1 INH is required for normal contact system regulation includes the detection of bradykinin in the plasma of patients with HAE and the role of C1 INH in protection from endotoxin shock associated with gram-negative bacterial sepsis (see Sections V.B. and VIII) (54,55,92,93).

V. HEREDITARY ANGIOEDEMA

A. Clinical and Laboratory Characteristics

HAE is characterized by recurrent acute episodes of localized edema of the skin and mucosa with a predilection to affect the extremities, face, larynx, and gastrointestinal tract (1,9,94–97) (Fig. 3). Edema involving the skin is nonpitting, does not itch and is not painful. An erythematous mottling of the skin similar to erythema marginatum also may develop in the presence or absence of typical episodes of swelling (2,9,94,97). Gastrointestinal tract involvement presents as acute, crampy abdominal pain that may be associated with nausea and vomiting and, less frequently, with diarrhea. Laryngeal edema is the most serious manifestation of the disease. Before effective preventive therapy was available,

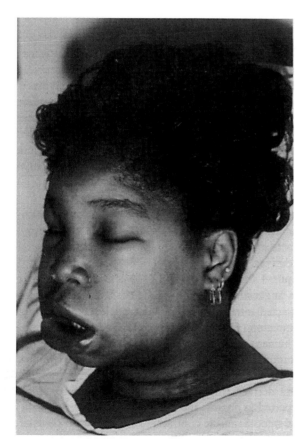

Figure 3 Edema of the face during an attack of angioedema. The edema is nonpitting, does not itch, and is not painful or erythematous. It is transient, typically resolving slowly after 24–72 h.

as many as 25–30% of patients died from laryngeal edema, although there was significant variation among different kindred (9,94–96,98–100). Attacks of edema may be precipitated by trauma, illness, or emotional distress, but also occur in the absence of any identifiable precipitating event. The edema usually lasts from 24 to 72 h before gradually resolving. Although onset of attacks may occur at virtually any age, most commonly they begin during childhood and the severity becomes worse during adolescence (94,95). For reasons that are not understood, the frequency and intensity of attacks tend to diminish during the fifth or sixth decades of life (94). There is a tendency toward an increased frequency of attacks during menstruation, and there is a dramatic decrease in frequency during the second and third trimesters of pregnancy (94,95,101). This observation is particularly interesting in view of the fact that C1 INH levels in women without HAE are somewhat reduced during pregnancy and during therapy with oral contraceptives (102–105). As discussed in Sections II.B. and V.C., androgen therapy results in a diminution in the frequency and severity of attacks and an increase in the plasma levels of C1 INH (30,31). Hormonal influences on disease expression, on C1 INH levels, and possibly on target protease levels obviously are complicated; the mechanisms responsible for these effects have not been elucidated.

B. Mediation of Symptoms

A number of studies over the years have implicated both the complement and contact systems in the generation of angioedema. Specifically, different studies have suggested that the mediator of symptoms is either a fragment of C2 with vascular permeability enhancing activity or is bradykinin. It, of course, is possible that both might be involved. The C1 activation that occurs during an attack of angioedema results in consumption, and diminished serum concentrations, of C2 and C4 (98,106,107). Activated C1 circulates in plasma during attacks of angioedema (106,108). The contact system also is activated during attacks, although direct evidence for this activation was more difficult to obtain (109–114). In addition, there is some evidence for activation of the fibrinolytic system during episodes of edema (109). It is, therefore, theoretically possible, that the mediator(s) of edema could be derived from activation of any of these systems.

Plasma obtained from patients with HAE during symptom-free periods, when incubated at 37°C, generated a factor that had both kininlike (smooth muscle contracting) and vascular permeability-enhancing activity when injected intradermally (115). Several studies suggested that this factor was derived from complement activation and suggested that C2 and C4 specifically were required for its generation (115–117). Several other observations, however, supported the suggestion that the mediator was derived from complement activation. C1s, when injected intradermally, induces angioedema with no itching, no pain, and no signs of inflammation (118–121). This response is greatly diminished or absent in both C2-deficient humans and guinea pigs (118,122). In the guinea pigs, the response develops after restoration of the C2 level (122). However, other studies presented evidence that suggested that a vasopermeability-enhancing factor was not derived from C2 (123,124). Second, a fragment derived from the carboxyl terminus of C2b by digestion with C1s and plasmin was reported to possess the same activity (125). Synthetic peptides based on this sequence induced smooth muscle contraction and enhanced vascular permeability in both guinea pig and human skin.

In addition to the contact system activation during episodes of edema, other direct evidence has supported the hypothesis that bradykinin is the mediator of edema. Curd et al., in an abstract in 1982, and Fields et al., in 1983, described experiments that suggested that bradykinin was generated during incubation of HAE plasma (124,126). More recently, using plasma immunodepleted of C1 INH, it was shown that vasopermeability-enhancing activity could not be generated in any contact system-deficient plasma (kallikrein, factor XII, or kininogen), but was readily generated in C2-deficient plasma (92). Furthermore, the vasopermeability-enhancing factor isolated from HAE plasma, by amino acid sequence analysis, was bradykinin (92). No other vasopermeability-enhancing peptide could be identified. Taken together, these data clearly indicate that bradykinin is generated in the plasma of individuals with HAE, and it very likely is a mediator of symptoms in the disease. These data alone, however, do not rule out participation of a C2-derived peptide. The synthetic C2 peptides clearly enhanced vascular permeability (125), and C2-deficient humans and guinea pigs do not respond to intradermal injection of C1s (118,122). However, the C2-derived peptides have not been demonstrated in vivo, and intradermal C1s injection may not duplicate the biological situation in patients with angioedema.

The analysis of a unique C1 INH mutant further strengthens the argument that bradykinin is the major mediator and that C2-derived peptides probably are not involved. Wisnieski et al. described a patient with systemic lupus erythematosus, chronically depressed C4 levels, and diminished C1 INH activity (127). Subsequent analyses showed that the responsible mutation was an Ala-443 → Val substitution, which is at the P2 position. This replacement resulted in alteration of target protease specificity such that inhibition of C1r and C1s activity was diminished approximately 10-fold (128) (Table 1). Subsequent studies have shown that this mutant inhibits kallikrein and factor XIIa normally (Zahedi, unpublished data). Lastly, neither the index case from this kindred nor any of the seven other family members with the same defect have ever had angioedema. This provides extremely strong evidence that complement system activation alone does not result in generation of a vascular permeability-enhancing peptide and is consistent with the hypothesis that bradykinin is the primary mediator of angioedema.

C. Therapy

In 1960, before it was discovered that C1 INH deficiency was responsible for HAE, methyltestosterone was found to prevent attacks of angioedema (31). Associated with this

Table 1 Dysfunctional C1 Inhibitor Proteins

Mutation	Functional defect
Ala 443 (P2) → Val	Decreased inhibition of C1r and C1s
	Normal inhibition of kallikrein and factor XIIa
Arg 444 (P1) → His, Cys, Ser, Leu	Nonrecognition of target proteases
Val 432 (P14) → Glu	Conversion to substrate
Ala 434 (P12) → Glu	Conversion to substrate
Ala 436 (P10) → Thr	Polymerization
Val 451 → Met	Polymerization
Phe 455 → Ser	Polymerization
Pro 476 → Ser	Polymerization
Lys 251 Deletion	Conversion to substrate
	Polymerization

reduction in number of episodes of edema was an increase in the plasma levels of C1 INH and C4 (129–131). Subsequently, Gelfand et al demonstrated that the attenuated androgen danazol had the same effects, while avoiding much of the virilizing and anabolic side effects of testosterone (30). Numerous studies have confirmed the effectiveness of danazol and shown similar effects with stanazolol (132–137). As discussed in Section II.B, it has been assumed that the mechanism of action of androgens is via enhanced C1 INH synthesis, but this remains unproven. Prior to the use of androgens, antifibrinolytic agents (tranexamic acid and ε-aminocaproic acid) frequently were used for preventive therapy, although they provided significant reductions in numbers of attacks in only about one-third of patients (100). They now are used rarely (e.g., in children, in order to avoid the use of androgens). Prevention of attacks, such as during dental manipulations, may be accomplished with relatively high doses of androgens (danazol, 600 mg/day or stanazolol, 6 mg/day) for 6 days before and 3 days after the procedure (100,138). The most effective therapy for serious acute attacks of angioedema, particularly those affecting the larynx or abdomen, is infusion of preparations of C1 INH (139–142). This approach might also be considered for prevention of attacks associated with dental or other surgical procedures (142).

VI. CONTRIBUTIONS FROM THE ANALYSIS OF C1 INHIBITOR MUTATIONS

A. Introduction

As expected from the dominant inheritance of HAE, individuals with the disease are heterozygous for mutations that result either in an absolute decrease in the quantity of circulating C1 INH protein or in the synthesis of a dysfunctional C1 INH together with decreased amounts of the normal protein. These have traditionally been referred to as type 1 and type 2, respectively. Molecular genetic analyses have made clear that a number of mutations result in the synthesis of abnormal proteins that may be degraded or retained intracellularly, or that may be secreted in small quantities. Because all individuals with the disease express one normal gene, small amounts of a dysfunctional protein may be extremely difficult to detect. These mutants, therefore, do not precisely fit the definition either for type 1 or type 2. However, operationally it is reasonable to differentiate type 1 from type 2 based on the absence or presence of a discrepancy between the antigenic and functional levels of C1 INH, with the understanding that some patients who technically might be considered type 2 rather than type 1 will be missed.

With two possible exceptions, the type of mutation that results in deficiency/dysfunction probably is not of clinical significance. These two exceptions are one large deletion, in which the abnormal transcript appears to inhibit transcription of the normal gene, and a small duplication, in which there appears to be inhibition of translation of the normal C1 INH transcript (143,144). Since HAE, with current therapy, is rarely a lethal disease, there is no indication for prenatal diagnosis. Diagnosis of the disease itself, with a combination of C1 INH protein and functional levels, C4 and C1q levels, is seldom difficult. Therefore, the information to be gained by the molecular genetic analysis of mutations in patients with deficiency relates primarily to potential contributions to defining the structural basis of C1 INH function and to understanding mechanisms of mutagenesis. The following discussion will organize the mutations that have been described in the C1

INH gene into three large groups: large deletions and duplications, small intraexonic deletions and duplications, and single base changes (Table 2).

B. Deletions and Duplications of One or More Exons

Among the 96 patients with HAE in whom the mutations are known, 22 have large deletions of one or more exons (Table 2) (145–152). Among those in whom the deletion or duplication has been sequenced, Alu repetitive elements were present at every recombination site. These repetitive elements have been associated with deletion in a number of genes in addition to C1 INH. In the case of C1 INH, because the Alu repeats in all instances have been oriented in the same direction, it is likely that the mechanism mediating these rearrangements is homologous recombination.

C. Intraexonic Deletions and Duplications

A number of small deletions and duplications contained completely within single exons have been described (Table 2) (152–159). Two groups of these are within DNA sequences that may be particularly susceptible to mutation (153,154). The first group consisted of two mutations within exon 8: a 33 nucleotide deletion of the region immediately preceding the reactive center Arg codon and a 20 nucleotide duplication that included the reactive center codon (154). This region contains a number of characteristics associated with

Table 2 Mutations in the C1 Inhibitor Gene

Mutations	Exon	# Kindred	References
Large deletions/duplications	—	22	145–152
Small deletions/duplications	2	1	159
	3	3	152,159
	4	3	152,159
	5	7	153,155,159
	6	3	152,159
	7 (junction intron 6)	2	159
	8	6	154,156–158
Single base changes	Promoter	2	159
	Intron 1	1	159
	2	2	159
	3	10	152,161,159
	4	2	152
	5	2	152,159
	6	7	152,159,160,162
	Intron 6	1	159
	7	6	152,159
	8 (RCL hinge)	7	60–62,152,164
	8 (P1 Arg substitutions)	27	59,163,152 165–170
	8 (C-terminal to RCL)	10	45,152,171,172

RCL, reactive center loop.

mutation, particularly recombination events. The sequence through this region forms a partial palindrome. Partial palindromes may form stem-loop structures and likely mediate both deletions/duplications and single base changes. The mechanism very likely involves interference with polymerase movement through the region, in addition to inappropriate mismatch repair within the stem of the structure. In this regard, within and near this segment of DNA that encodes the reactive center loop region, a number of single base changes, most of which result in dysfuncional proteins, have been described.

The second group of short deletions/duplications is within a short triplet repeat in exon 5 in which three different mutations (two deletions, one duplication) have been identified in 5 families (153,159). These mutations, like many other mutations within repetitive sequences, very likely are due to slipped mispairing, which results from an out of register reannealing of template and copied strands during replication. A 5′ slip, therefore, results in a duplication, while a 3′ slip results in a deletion. Nearly all of the short deletions/duplications have resulted in type 1 deficiency although one in frame deletion in the exon 5 triplet repeat segment has produced a particularly informative dysfunctional protein (153,155,160). This mutation results in deletion of Lys-251 in C1 inhibitor-Ta, which alters the sequence from Asn-Lys-Ile-Ser to Asn-Ile-Ser to create an N-glycosylation signal sequence (155). However, dysfunction results from the deletion itself rather than from the additional oligosaccharide group (see Section VI.D).

D. Single Base Changes

Single base changes have been observed throughout most of the coding sequence (Table 2), although the majority have been within exon 8 (45,59–62,152,159,161–173). There are at least two explanations for this localization. First, selection probably plays a role: the reactive center region is encoded within exon 8; therefore, in most studies it has been sequenced first. Second, two different mechanisms may be operative in creating a hypermutable region within exon 8. The reactive center Arg codon is CGC. The CpG dinucleotide is susceptible to mutation due to deamidation of methylated cytosine that converts it to a thymine. This may occur in the CG dinucleotide both in the coding strand and in the complementary strand. In the case of C1 INH this results in substitution of the reactive center Arg with either Cys or His. These make up the largest single group of mutations in C1 INH (Figs. 1, 2; Table 1). It is interesting that although there are several other CG dinucleotides within the C1 INH coding sequence, mutations have been found only at one of these (Arg472). This fact, together with the fact that 3 Ser and 2 Leu substitutions for Arg444 have been observed and the fact that a number of other mutations have occurred within the reactive center region, is consistent with the suggestion that other factors may influence the rate of mutation in this region. The single base changes in this region have resulted in the majority of dysfunctional C1 INH proteins that have been analyzed.

Analysis of these dysfunctional mutants has provided significant contributions to understanding the normal function of serpins. Dysfunctional C1 INH proteins may be classified into two broad groups: those that interfere with the serpin mechanism of action and those that interfere with target protease specificity. Mutations that disrupt the inhibitory mechanism interfere with the movement of mobile domains that is required for complex formation. These include mutations at the proximal and distal ends of the reactive center loop, and mutations that affect the stability of β sheet A. These mutations either convert the inhibitor to a substrate or induce multimerization. Those that interfere with target protease specificity usually have resulted from substitutions at the P1 residue, although one naturally occurring P2 mutant (which was discussed in Section V.B.), has been described. These mutations result in an inhibitor that, at least theoretically, remains capable of complex formation. In the case of C1 INH, only one P1 mutant has been shown to have acquired a new specificity. The P1 Arg → His mutant has acquired the ability to inhibit chymotrypsin (174). The best example of a P1 mutation with altered specificity is that of α_1-antitrypsin P1 Met → Arg (antithrombin Pittsburgh) which has acquired the ability to inhibit antithrombin III very efficiently (175).

Two mutations in the proximal end of the reactive center loop of C1 inhibitor, Ala 434 → Glu (P12) and Val 432 → Glu (P14) (Figs. 1, 2; Table 1), each convert the inhibitor to a substrate (60, 62) and as a result circulate in plasma in the cleaved form. Therefore, although recognized by protease, they are unable to form a stable complex and are cleaved between the P1 and P1′ residues. The side chains of the Glu residues at P12 and P14 probably can not be accommodated into sheet A during insertion of the reactive center loop. These mutants provide support for the hypothesis that insertion of the reactive center loop into sheet A, at least to the level of P12, is required for stable complex formation (49,57,64,176).

A number of mutations in serpins result in a tendency to polymerize. The first such C1 INH mutant was another reactive center loop mutant, Ala 436 → Thr, which is at the P10 position (Figs. 1, 2; Table 1). This substitution results in a nonreactive inhibitor that extensively multimerizes (61,62,165), as demonstrated by gel filtration, ultracentrifugation, nondenaturing electrophoresis, and electron microscopy. The mutant (both monomeric and multimeric forms) also expressed a neoepitope that normally is expressed only on the cleaved or on the protease-complexed form of the normal inhibitor (54–56,177). Another group of mutants that express this epitope and result in multimerization are those that affect the anchoring of the distal end of the reactive center loop. Three such mutants, two within s1C and one that is the third residue from the carboxyl terminus, have been described: Val 451 → Met, Phe 455 → Ser, and Pro 476 → Ser(45) (Table 1). Similar to the P10 mutation, these mutants also showed little complex formation or cleavage with target proteases. They also all are more stable to elevated temperature than is the native molecule, another property shared with the cleaved or complexed inhibitor. This also implies that these inhibitors have, at least partially, undergone the conformational changes that the normal inhibitor goes through during complex formation. It is likely that the P10 mutant and these carboxy terminal mutants adopt a conformation in which the reactive center loop is overinserted in β sheet A, presumably in a "locked" form, very much like the form present in the complex with protease. This overinsertion may result in a cleft in either β sheet A or C that can provide a site for interaction with the reactive center loop of another molecule with resultant multimer formation. This has been observed directly with the crystal structure of an intact antithrombin dimer in which the reactive center loop of one molecule is inserted into sheet C of another cleaved or latent-like molecule (65,66). It also is possible, particularly in the case of the P10 mutant in which the strands of sheet A may be "forced" apart by insertion of the P10 Thr, that polymerization via interaction with sheet A may take place.

One other C1 INH dysfunctional mutant with deletion of Lys-251 has been extensively analyzed, and is of interest because it shares characteristics with all of the above-described mutants and does not clearly fit into either category (155,160) (Table 1). Specifically, it did not complex with C1r, C1s or kallikrein but did inefficiently complex with β-factor XIIa. With each protease, however, 50–75% of the recombinant protein was susceptible to cleavage. It was not as thermostable as the P10 Ala → Thr or the carboxyl terminal mutants, but was more stable than the normal wild type protein. Variable proportions of the recombinant protein (20–40%) were multimerized; multimer formation was not enhanced at elevated temperature. The multimers expressed the neoepitope that is expressed on protease complexed normal C1 INH, but it was not detected on the monomeric mutant protein. This mutation appears to produce two populations of molecules, one of which multimerizes, expresses the neopepitopes and is not recognized by target proteases. This form very likely is characterized by loop overinsertion similar to the P10 and carboxyl terminal mutants. The other form is converted primarily to a substrate, more like the P12 and P14 reactive center loop mutants, but is, however, capable of inefficient complex formation. It exists only as a monomer and does not express the neoepitope.

Recently, several new C1 INH mutations have been identified, but their functional characterisics have not yet been defined. Several of these are within regions that also might be predicted to induce multimerization, via interference with the molecular movements that the inhibitor undergoes during complex formation (162,178). Most of the others are at highly conserved residues that might be expected to interfere with function or with folding, but will require structure–function analysis to define the mechanism by which they produce deficiency.

In summary, a number of mutations have been defined within the C1 INH gene, and the structural and functional consequences of many of these have been characterized. Among these mutants are examples of mutations that interfere with the mobile domains involved in the serpin conformational rearrangement that takes place during complex formation, mutations that interfere with target protease specificity and a variety of mutations that disrupt at other levels during protein synthesis or secretion. The functional analysis of C1 inhibitor mutant proteins has contributed to the current understanding of serpin function and has also helped us to define more completely the biological role of C1 inhibitor.

VII. ACQUIRED C1 INHIBITOR DEFICIENCY

Two types of acquired C1 INH deficiency that result in angioedema have been recognized. Type 1 acquired angioedema (AAE) was initially described in association with lymphoproliferative disorders and also has been observed with other malignancies (179–188). One study suggests that this association may result from depletion of C1 INH via extremely efficient complement activation by idiotype–antiidiotype immune complexes in which the antiidiotypic antibody is directed toward the idiotype of the monoclonal immunoglobulin that is circulating in plasma (in myelomas) or that is expressed only on the malignant B cell in other lymphoproliferative diseases (189). Type 2 AAE, on the other hand, occurs in association with diseases other than lymphoproliferative disorders or in the absence of any apparent associated disease (184,190,191). It is characterized by the presence of circulating autoantibodies directed toward C1 INH (190–199). These autoantibodies prevent the inactivation of target proteases by C1 INH. In most cases, the autoantibodies appear to mediate enhanced cleavage of C1 INH at its reactive center by the target protease (192,193,195,198–202). These antibodies, therefore, convert the inhibitor to a substrate, presumably by interference with the normal serpin conformational rearrangement that prevents stable complex formation. In those that have been analyzed, the antibodies appear to recognize epitopes within the reactive center loop (196–198). In some instances, the autoantibodies appear to interfere with complex formation without leading to C1 INH cleavage (M. Cicardi, personal communication), which suggests that the epitopes recognized by different autoantibodies may differ. None have been noted to destabilize a preformed protease-inhibitor complex (193,199).

The autoantibodies may be of any class and most are probably oligoclonal or monoclonal (192,195,196,198,202). It is interesting that several patients with autoantibodies to C1 INH have had readily detectable circulating monoclonal immunoglobulins (196,202). One of these had Waldenstrom's macroglobulinemia, while the others apparently have not developed clinically detectable lymphoproliferative disease (202). This, however, does suggest the possibility that type 1 and type 2 AAE may overlap, or that they may be variants of the same basic defect. Because of this, any patient with acquired C1 INH deficiency, with or without an autoantibody, should be monitored for the development of malignancy.

Clinically and biochemically, the two types of AAE are identical (with the exception of the presence of the anti-C1 INH autoantibody in type 2). Each has decreased functional C1 INH activity together with levels of C1 INH antigen that exceed the functional levels. This is due to the presence, in nearly all patients, of circulating nonfunctional C1 INH that has been cleaved at its reactive center (192,193,195). As in HAE, complement activation takes place secondary to the reduced C1 INH functional level, which results in decreased levels of C4 and C2. The C1q level is a valuable characteristic to help differentiate AAE from HAE. In AAE, but not in HAE, C1q serum levels are uniformly decreased. This decrease is understandable in type 1 AAE because C1q might be consumed by the efficient C1 activation induced by the antiidiotype–idiotype complexes (189). However, C1q is also virtually always decreased in type 2 AAE. In one example, it was clearly shown that the autoantibody–C1 INH complex did not induce C1 activation (192). The mechanism for this decrease in type 2 AAE, therefore, remains unexplained.

VIII. ROLE OF C1 INHIBITOR IN THE PATHOPHYSIOLOGY OF OTHER DISEASE STATES

C1 INH, by virtue of its regulation of contact system activation, very likely is important in protection from endotoxin shock associated with gram-negative bacterial sepsis. The contact and complement systems are activated during sepsis and septic shock. Furthermore, it is likely that contact system activation with generation of bradykinin plays an important role in mediation of the hypotension associated with septic shock, and may be involved in induction of cytokines that are released during sepsis. A number of studies over the past 25 years have provided evidence for this activation, have demonstrated complex formation between C1 INH and both kallikrein and factor XIIa during sepsis, and have shown that prevention of contact system activation attenuates the symptoms of septic shock (54,55,203–212). Intravenous infusion of C1 INH prevented the hypoxemia secondary to pulmonary dysfunction associated with contact system activation in dogs with *E. coli* endotoxin shock (213). Furthermore, preliminary studies have suggested that C1 INH may be useful in therapy of patients with septic shock or with the vascular leak syndrome associated with interleukin-2 therapy (214). It has recently been demonstrated that mice deficient in C4 or C3 are unable to clear endotoxin and are therefore highly susceptible to endotoxin shock (215). In addition, due to the excessive classical pathway activation induced by the endotoxin, C1 INH was depleted in these mice. Although it had no effect on endotoxin clearance, infusion of C1 INH protected the mice (M. C. Carroll, personal communication). These data also are consistent with the data indicating that contact system activation is important in the mediation of symptoms in septic shock and that excess C1 INH, by inhibition of contact system activation, may be protective.

REFERENCES

1. Quincke H. Uber akutes umschriebenes H autodem. Monatsschr Parkt Dermatol 1882; 1:129–131.
2. Osler W. Hereditary angio-neurotic oedema. Am J Med Sci 1888; 95:362–367.
3. Lepow I, Ratnoff O, Rosen F, Pillemer L. Observations on a proesterase associated with partially purified first component of complement (C1). Proc Soc Exp Biol Med 1956; 92:32–37.
4. Ratnoff O, Lepow I. Some properties of an esterase derived from preparations of the first component of complement. J Exp Med 1957; 106:327–343.
5. Lepow I, Ratnoff O, Levy L. Studies on the activation of a proesterase associated with partially purified first component of human complement. J Exp Med 1958; 107.
6. Levy L, Lepow I. Assay and properties of serum inhibitor of C'1 esterase. Proc Soc Exp Biol Med 1959; 101:608–611.
7. Pensky J, Levy L, Lepow I. Partial purification of a serum inhibitor of C'1 esterase. J Biol Chem 1961; 236:1674–1679.
8. Donaldson VH, Evans RR. A biochemical abnormality in hereditary angioneurotic edema. Am J Med 1963; 35:37–44.
9. Landerman NS, Webster ME, Becker EL, Ratcliffe HE. Hereditary angioneurotic edema. II. Deficiency of inhibitor for serum globulin permeability factor and/or plasma kallikrein. J Allergy 1962; 33:330–341.
10. Carter PE, Dunbar B, Fothergill JE. Genomic and cDNA cloning of the human C1 inhibitor. Intron-exon junctions and comparison with other serpins. Eur J Biochem 1988; 173:163–169.
11. Carter P, Duponchel C, Tosi M, Fothergill J. Complete nucleotide sequence of the gene for human C1 inhibitor with an unusually high density of Alu elements. Eur J Biochem 1991; 197:301–308.
12. Theriault A, Whaley K, McPhaden A, Boyd E, Connor J. Regional assignment of the human C1-inhibitor gene to 11q11–q13.1. Hum Genet 1989; 84:477–479.
13. Rich A. Speculation on the biological roles of left-handed Z-DNA. Ann NY Acad Sci 1994; 726:1–17.
14. Randazzo BP, Dattwyler RJ, Kaplan AP, Ghebrehiwet B. Synthesis of C1 inhibitor (C1INA) by a human monocyte-like cell line, U937. J Immunol 1985; 135:1313–1319.
15. Katz Y, Strunk R. Synthesis and regulation of C1 inhibitor in human skin fibroblasts. J Immunol 1989; 142:2041–5.
16. Yeung LA, Jones L, Hamilton AO, Whaley K. Complement-subcomponent-C1-inhibitor synthesis by human monocytes. Biochem J 1985; 226:199–205.
17. Bensa JC, Reboul A, Colomb MG. Biosynthesis in vitro of complement subcomponents C1q, C1s and C1 inhibitor by resting and stimulated human monocytes. Biochem J 1983; 216:385–392.
18. Katz Y, Gur S, Aladjem M, Strunk RC. Synthesis of complement proteins in amnion. J Clin Endocrinol Metab 1995; 80:2027–2032.
19. Walker DG, Yasuhara O, Patston PA, McGeer EG, McGeer PL. Complement C1 inhibitor is produced by brain tissue and is cleaved in Alzheimer disease. Brain Res 1995; 675:75–82.

20. Schmaier AH, Murray SC, Heda GD, et al. Synthesis and expression of C1 inhibitor by human umbilical vein endothelial cells. J Biol Chem 1989; 264:18173–18179.

21. Hamilton AO, Jones L, Morrison L, Whaley K. Modulation of monocyte complement synthesis by interferons. Biochem J 1987; 242:809–815.

22. Lotz M, Zuraw BL. Interferon-gamma is a major regulator of C1-inhibitor synthesis by human blood monocytes. J Immunol 1987; 139:3382–3387.

23. Schmidt B, Gyapay G, Valay M, Fust G. Human recombinant macrophage colony-stimulating factor (M-CSF) increases C1-esterase inhibitor (C1INH) synthesis by human monocytes. Immunology 1991; 74:677–9.

24. Zuraw B, Lotz M. Regulation of the hepatic synthesis of C1 inhibitor by the hepatocyte stimulating factors interleukin 6 and interferon gamma. J Biol Chem 1990; 265:12664–70.

25. Lappin D, Birnie G, Whaley K. Modulation by interferons of the expression of monocyte complement genes. Biochem J 1990; 268:387–92.

26. Lappin D, Guc D, Hill A, McShane T, Whaley K. Effect of interferon-gamma on complement gene expression in different cell types. Biochem J 1992; 281:437–42.

27. Gluszko P, Undas A, Amenta S, Szczeklik A, Schmaier AH. Administration of gamma interferon in human subjects decreases plasminogen activation and fibrinolysis without influencing C1 inhibitor. J Lab Clin Med 1994; 123:232–240.

28. Heda G, Mardente S, Weiner L, Schmaier A. Interferon gamma increases in vitro and in vivo expression of C1 inhibitor. Blood 1990; 75:2401–7.

29. Zahedi K, Prada A, Davis III AE. Transcriptional regulation of the C1 inhibitor gene by gamma interferon. J Biol Chem 1994; 269:9669–9674.

30. Gelfand J, Sherins R, Alling D, Frank M. Treatment of hereditary angioedema with danazol. Reversal of clinical and biochemical abnormalities. N Engl J Med 1976; 295:1444–84.

31. Spaulding WB. Methyltestosterone therapy for hereditary episodic edema (hereditary angioneurotic edema). Ann Intern Med 1960; 53:739–745.

32. Falus A, Feher K, Walcz E, et al. Hormonal regulation of complement biosynthesis in human cell lines. I. Androgens and gamma-interferon stimulate biosynthesis and gene expression of C1 inhibitor in human cell lines U937 and HepG2. Mol Immunol 1990; 27:191–5.

33. Alabdullah Ih, Sim RB, Sheil J, Greally JF. The effect of danazol on the production of C1 inhibitor in the guinea pig. Complement 1984; 1:27–35.

34. Lappin D, McPhaden A, Yap P, et al. Monocyte C1-inhibitor synthesis in patients with C1-inhibitor deficiency. Eur J Clin Invest 19:45–52 1989; 19:45–52.

35. Smale ST, Schmidt MC, Berk AJ, Baltimore D. Transcriptional activation by Sp1 as directed through TATA or initiator: specific requirements for mammalian transcription factor IID. Proc Natl Acad Sci USA 1990; 87:4509–4513.

36. Smale S, Baltimore D. The "initiator" as a transcription control element. Cell 1989; 57:103–113.

37. Harpel PC, Cooper NR. Studies on human plasma C1-inactivator-enzyme interactions. I. Mechanisms of interaction with C1s, plasmin and trypsin. J Clin Invest 1975; 55:593–604.

38. Haupt H, Heimburger N, Kranz T, Schwick HG. Ein beitrag zur isolierung und characterisierung des C1-inaktivators aus humanplasma. Eur J Biochem 1970; 17:254–261.

39. Bock SC, Skriver K, Nielsen E, et al. Human C1 inhibitor: primary structure, cDNA cloning, and chromosomal localization. Biochemistry 1986; 25:4292–4301.

40. Reboul A, Arlaud GJ, Sim RB, Colomb MG. A simplified procedure for the purification of C1-inactivator from human plasma. Interaction with complement subcomponents C1r and C1s. FEBS Lett 1977; 79:45–50.

41. Harrison RA. Human C1 inhibitor: improved isolation and preliminary structural characterization. Biochemistry 1983; 22:5001–5007.

42. Nilsson T, Wiman B. Purification and characterization of human C1-esterase inhibitor. Biochim Biophys Acta 1982; 705:271–276.

43. Perkins SJ, Smith KF, Amatayakul S, et al. Two-domain structure of the native and reactive centre cleaved forms of C1 inhibitor of human complement by neutron scattering. J Mol Biol 1990; 214:751–763.

44. Odermatt E, Berger H, Sano Y. Size and shape of human C1-inhibitor. FEBS Lett 1981; 131:283–285.

45. Eldering E, Verpy E, Roem D, Meo T, Tosi M. COOH-terminal substitutions in the serpin C1 inhibitor that cause loop overinsertion and subsequent multimerization. J Biol Chem 1995; 270:2579–2587.

46. Matheson N, van Halbeek H, Travis J. Evidence for a tetrahedral intermediate complex during serpin-proteinase interactions. J Biol Chem 1991; 266:13489–13491.

47. Schechter I, Berger A. On the active site of proteases. I. Papain. Biochem Biophys Res Commun 1967; 27:157–162.

48. Salvesen GS, Catanese JJ, Kress LF, Travis J. Primary structure of the reactive site of human C1-inhibitor. J Biol Chem 1985; 260:2432–2436.

49. Loebermann H, Tokuoka R, Deisenhofer J, Huber R. Human alpha1-proteinase inhibitor. Crystal structure analysis of two crystal modifications, molecular model and preliminary analysis of the implications for function. J Mol Biol 1984; 177:531–557.

50. Mast AE, Enghild JJ, Pizzo SV, Salvesen G. Analysis of the plasma elimination kinetics and conformational stabilities of native, proteinase-complexed, and reactive site cleaved serpins: comparison of alpha 1-proteinase inhibitor, alpha 1-antichymotrypsin, antithroombin III, alpha 2-antiplasmin, angiotensinogen, and ovalbumin. Biochemistry 1991; 30:1723–1730.

51. Pemberton PA, Harrison RA, Lachmann PJ, Carrell RW. The structural basis for neutrophil inactivation of C1 inhibitor. Biochem J 1989; 258:193–198.

52. Bruch M, Weiss V, Engel J. Plasma serine proteinase inhibitors (serpins) exhibit major conformational changes and a large increase in conformational stability upon cleavage at their reactive sites. J Biol Chem 1988; 263:16626–16630.

53. Batra PP, Sasa K, Ueki T, Takeda K. Circular dichroic study of conformational changes in ovalbumin induced by modification of sulhydryl groups and disulfide reduction. J Protein Chem 1989; 8:609–617.

54. Nuijens JH, Huijbregts CCM, Eerenberg-Belmer AJM, et al. Quantification of plasma factor XIIa-C1-inhibitor and kallikrein-C1-inhibitor complexes in sepsis. Blood 1988; 72:1841–1848.

55. Nuijens JH, Eerenberg-Belmer AJM, Huijbregts CCM, et al. Proteolytic inactivation of plasma C1 inhibitor in sepsis. J Clin Invest 1989; 84:443–450.

56. Agostini Ad, Patston PA, Marottoli V, Carrel S, Harpel PC, Schapira M. A common neoepitope is created when the reactive center of C1-inhibitoris cleaved by plasma kallikrein, activated factor XII fragment, C1 esterase, or neutrophil elastase. J Clin Invest 1988; 82:700–705.

57. Schulze AJ, Baumann U, Knof S, Jaeger E, Huber R, Laurell CB. Structural transition of alpha 1-antitrypsin by a peptide sequentially similar to beta-strand s4A. Eur J Biochem 1990; 194:51–56.

58. Schulze AJ, Frohnert PW, Engle RA, Huber R. Evidence for the extent of insertion of the active site loop of intact −1 proteinase inhibitor in -sheet A. Biochemistry 1992; 31:7560–7565.

59. Siddique Z, McPhaden AR, Whaley K. Type II hereditary angio-oedema associated with two mutations in one allele of the C1-inhibitor gene around the reactive-site coding region. Hum Hered 1992; 42:298–301.

60. Skriver K, Wikkoff WR, Patston PA, et al. Substrate properties of C1 inhibitor Ma (alanine 434 glutamic acid). Genetic and structural evidence suggesting that the P12-region contains critical determinants of serine protease inhibitor/substrate status. J Biol Chem 1991; 266:9216–9221.

61. Levy NJ, Ramesh N, Cicardi M, Harrison RA, Davis III AE. Type II hereditary angioneurotic edema that may result from a single nucleotide change in the codon for alanine-436 in the C1 inhibitor gene. Proc Natl Acad Sci USA 1990; 87:265–268.

62. Davis III AK, Aulak K, Parad RB, et al. C1 inhibitor hinge region mutations produce dysfunction by different mechanisms. Nature Genetics 1992; 1:354–358.

63. Schulze AJ, Huber R, Degryse E, Speck D, Bischoff R. Inhibitory activity and conformational transition of alpha 1-proteinase inhibitor variants. Eur J Biochem 1991; 202:1147–1155.

64. Carrell RW, Evans DL, Stein PK. Mobile reactive centre of serpins and the control of thrombosis. Nature 1991; 353:576–578.

65. Carrell R, Evans D, Stein P. Biological implications of a 3 A structure of dimeric antithrombin. Structure 1994; 2:257–270.

66. Schreuder HA, Boer Bd, Dijkema R, et al. The intact and cleaved human antithrombin III complex as a model for serpin-proteinase interactions. Struct Biol 1994; 1:48–54.

67. Schreiber AD, Kaplan AP, Austen KF. Inhibition by C1-INH of Hageman factor fragment activation of coagulation, fibrinolysis, and kinin generation. J Clin Invest 1973; 52:1402–1409.

68. Ratnoff O, Pensky J, Ogston D, Naff G. The inhibition of plasmin, plasma kallikrein, plasma permeability factor, and the C1'r subcomponent of complement by serum C1' esterase inhibitor. J Exp Med 1969; 129:315–331.

69. Gigli I, Mason JW, Colman RW, Austen KF. Interaction of plasma kallikrein with the C1 inhibitor. J Immunol 1970; 104:574–581.

70. Forbes C, Pensky J, Ratnoff O. Inhibition of activated Hageman factor and activated plasma thromboplastin antecedent by purified C1 inactivator. J Lab Clin Med 1970; 76:809–815.

71. Ranby M, Bergstorf N, Nilsson T. Enzymatic properties of one and two chain forms of tissue plasminogen activator. Thromb Res 1982; 27:175–184.

72. Matsushita M, Fujita T. Inhibition of mannose-binding protein-associated serine protease (MASP) by C1 inhibitor (C1 INH). Mol Immunol 1996; 33:44.

73. Wuillemin WA, Minnema M, Meijers JC, et al. Inactivation of factor XIa in human plasma assessed by measuring factor XIa-protease inhibitor complexes: major role for C1-inhibitor. Blood 1995; 85:1517–1526.

74. Sim RB, Reboul A, Arlaud GJ, Villiers CL, Colomb MG. Interaction of 125-labelled complement components C1r and C1s with protease inhibitors in plasma. FEBS Lett 1979; 97:111–115.

75. Ziccardi RJ. Activation of the early components of the classical complement pathway under physiological conditions. J Immunol 1981; 126:1768–1773.

76. Lennick M, Brew SA, Ingham KC. Kinetics of interaction of C1 inhibitor with complement C1s. Biochemistry 1986; 25:3890–3898.

77. Sim R, Arlaud G, Colomb M. Kinetics of reaction of human C1-inhibitor with the human complement system proteases C1r and C1s. Biochim Biophys Acta 1980; 612:433–449.

78. Doekes G, Es LAv, Daha MR. C1 inactivator: its efficiency as a regulator of classical complement pathway activation by soluble IgG aggregates. Immunology 1983; 49:215–222.

79. Ziccardi RJ. A new role for C1-inhibitor in homeostasis: control of activation of the first component of human complement. J Immunol 1982; 128:2505–2508.

80. Ziccardi RJ. Spontaneous activation of the first component of human complement (C1) by an intramolecular autocatalytic mechanism. J Immunol 1982; 128:2500–2504.

81. Tseng Y, Paan PH, Zavodszky P, Schumaker VN. Spontaneous activation of serum C1 in vitro. Role of C1 inhibitor. J Immunol 1991; 147:1884–1890.

82. Laurell A, Martensson U, Sjoholm A. C1 dissociation: spontaneous generation in human serum of a trimer complex containing C1 inactivator, activated C1r and zymogen C1s. J Immunol 1987; 139:4145–4151.

83. Tenner AJ, Frank MM. Activator-bound C1 is less susceptible to inactivation by C1 inhibition than is fluid-phase C1. J Immunol 1986; 137:625–630.

84. Laurell AB, Martensson U, Sjoholm AG. C1 subcomponent complexes in normal and pathological sera studied by crossed immunoelectrophoresis. Acta Pathol Microbiol Scand 1976; 84:455–464.

85. Ziccardi RJ, Cooper NR. Active disassembly of the first complement component C1 by C1-inhibitor. J Immunol 1979; 123:788–792.

86. Sim RB, Arlaud GJ, Colomb MG. C1 inhibitor dependent dissociation of human complement component C1 bound to immune complexes. Biochem J 1979; 179:449–457.

87. Schapira M, Scott CF, Colman RW. Contribution of plasma protease inhibitors to the inactivation of kallikrein in plasma. J Clin Invest 1982; 69:462–468.

88. Graaf Fvd, Koedam JA, Bouma BN. Inactivation of kallikrein in human plasma. J Clin Invest 1983; 71:149–158.

89. Harpel PC, Lewin MF, Kaplan AP. Distribution of plasma kallikrein between C1 inactivator and α2-macroglobulin in plasma utilizing a new assay for α2-macroglobulin-kallikrein complexes. J Biol Chem 1985; 260:4257–4263.

90. Agostini Ad, Lijnen HR, Pixley RA, Colman RW, Schapira M. Inactivation of factor XII active fragment in normal plasma. Predominant role of C1-inhibitor. J Clin Invest 1984; 73:1542–1549.

91. Pixley RA, Schapira M, Colman RW. The regulation of human factor XIIa by plasma proteinase inhibitors. J Biol Chem 1985; 260:1723–1729.

92. Shoemaker LR, Schurman SJ, Donaldson VH, Davis III AE. Hereditary angioneurotic edema: characterization of plasma kinin and vascular permeability-enhancing activities. Clin Exp Immunol 1994; 95:22–28.

93. Guerrero R, Velasco F, Rodriguez M, et al. Endotoxin-induced pulmonary dysfunction is prevented by C1-esterase inhibitor. J Clin Invest 1993; 91:2754–2760.

94. Donaldson VN, Rosen FS. Hereditary angioneurotic edema: a clinical survey. Pediatrics 1966; 37:1017–1027.

95. Frank M, Gelfand F, Atkinson J. Hereditary angioedema: the clinical syndrome and its management. Ann Intern Med 1976; 84:580–593.

96. Crowder JR, Crowder TR. Five generations of angioneurotic edema. Arch Intern Med 1971; 20:840–852.

97. Starr JC, Brasher GW. Erythema marginatum preceding hereditary angioedema. J Allergy Clin Immunol 1974; 53:352–355.

98. Austen KF, Sheffer AL. Detection of hereditary angioneurotic edema by demonstration of a profound reduction in the second component of human complement. N Engl J Med 1965; 272:649–656.

99. Hadjiyannaki K, Lachmann PJ. Hereditary angioedema: a review with particular reference to pathogenesis and treatment. Clin Allergy 1971; 1:221–233.

100. Agostoni A, Cicardi M. Hereditary and acquired C1-inhibitor deficiency: biological and clinical characteristics in 235 patients. Medicine 1992; 71:206–215.

101. Blohme G, Ysander K, Korsan-Bengsten K. Hereditary angioneurotic edema in three families. Acta Med Scand 1972; 191:209–219.

102. Ogston D, Walker J, Campbell DM. C1 inactivator level in pregnancy. Thrombosis Res 1981; 23:453–455.

103. Donaldson VN. Serum inhibitor of C′1 esterase in health and disease. J Lab Clin Med 1966; 68:369–382.

104. Amir J, Pensky J, Ratnoff OD. Plasma inhibition of activated plasma thromboplastin antecedent (factor XIa) in pregnancy. J Lab Clin Med 1972; 96:106–112.

105. Gordon EM, Ratnoff OD, Saito H, Donaldson VH, Pensky J, Jones PK. Rapid fibrinolysis, augmented Hageman factor (factor XII) titers, and decreased C1 esterase inhibitor titers in women taking oral contraceptives. J Lab Clin Med 1980; 96:762–769.

106. Donaldson VH, Rosen FS. Action of complement in hereditary angioneurotic edema: the role of C′1 esterase. J Clin Invest 1964; 43:2204–2213.

107. Carpenter CB, Ruddy S, Shehadeh IH, Muller-Eberhard HJ, Merrill JP, Austen KF. Complement metabolism in man: hypercatabolism of the fourth (C4) and third (C3) components

in patients with renal allograft rejection and hereditary angioedema (HAE). J Clin Invest 1969; 48:1495–1505.

108. Laurell AB, Lindegren J, Malmros I, Martensson HL. Enzymatic and immunochemical estimation of C1 esterase inhibitor in sera from patients with hereditary angioedema. Scand J Clin Lab Invest 1969; 24:221–225.

109. Cugno M, Hack CE, Boer JPd, Eerenberg AJ, Agostoni A, Cicardi M. Generation of plasmin during acute attacks of hereditary angioedema. J Lab Clin Med 1993; 121:38–43.

110. Kaplan AP, Silverberg M, Ghebrehiwet B, Atkins P, Zweiman B. Pathways of kinin formation and role in allergic diseases. Clin Immunol Immunopathol 1989; 50:S41–51.

111. Schapira M, Silver LD, Scott CF, et al. Prekallikrein activation and high-molecular-weight kininogen consumption in hereditary angioedema. N Engl J Med 1983; 308:1050–1053.

112. Kaufman N, Page JD, Pixley RA, Schein R, Schmaier AH, Colman RW. Alpha 2-macroglobulin-kallikrein complexes detect contact system activation in hereditary angioedema and human sepsis. Blood 1991; 77:2660–2667.

113. Lammle B, Zuraw BL, Heeb MJ, et al. Detection and quantitation of cleaved and uncleaved high molecular weight kininogen in plasma by ligand blotting with radiolabeled plasma prekallikrein or factor XI. Thromb Haemost 1988; 59:151–161.

114. Curd JG, L. J. Prograis J, Cochrane CG. Detection of active kallikrein in induced blister fluids of hereditary angioedema patients. J Exp Med 1980; 152:742–747.

115. Donaldson VH, Ratnoff OD, dias da Silva W, Rosen FS. Permeability-increasing activity in hereditary angioneurotic edema plasma. J Clin Invest 1969; 48:642–653.

116. Donaldson VH, Merler E, Rosen FS, Kretschmer KW, Lepow IH. A polypeptide kinin in hereditary angioneurotic edema plasma: role of complement in its formation. J Lab Clin Med 1970; 76:986.

117. Donaldson VH. Kinin formation in hereditary angioneurotic edema (HANE) plasma. Int Arch Allergy 1973; 45:206–209.

118. Klemperer MR, Donaldson VH, Rosen FS. Effect of C'1 esterase on vascular permeability in man: studies in normal and complement-deficient individuals and in patients with hereditary angioneurotic edema. J Clin Invest 1968; 47:604–611.

119. Davies GE, Lowe JS. A permeability factor released from guinea pig serum by antigen-antibody precipitates. Br J Exp Pathol 1960; 41:335–344.

120. Ratnoff OD, Lepow IH. Complement as a mediator of inflammation. Enhancement of vascular permeability by purified C'1 esterase. J Exp Med 1963; 118:681–698.

121. Andrews JM, Rosen FS, Silverberg SJ, Cory M, Schneeberger EE, Bing DE. Inhibition of C1s-induced vascular leakage in guinea pigs by substituted benzamidine and pyridinium compounds. J Immunol 1977; 118:466–471.

122. Strang CJ, Auerbach KS, Rosen FS. C1s-induced vascular permeability in C2-deficient guinea pigs. J Immunol 1986; 137:631–635.

123. Smith M, Kerr M. Cleavage of the second component of complement by plasma proteases: Implications in hereditary C1-inhibitor deficiency. Immunology 1985; 56:561–570.

124. Fields T, Ghebrewihet B, Kaplan A. Kinin formation in hereditaryangioedema plasma: evidence against kinin derivation from C2 and in support of spontaneous formation of bradykinin. J Allergy Clin Immunol 1983; 72:54–60.

125. Strang C, Cholin S, Spragg J, et al. Angioedema induced by a peptide derived from complement component C2. J Exp Med 1988; 168:1685–1698.

126. Curd JG, Yelvington M, Burridge N, et al. Generation of bradykinin during incubation of hereditary angioedema plasma. Mol Immunol 1982; 19:1365 (Abstract).

127. Wisnieski JJ, Knauss TC, Yike I, Dearborn DG, Narvy RL, Naff GB. Unique C1 inhibitor dysfunction in a kindred without angioedema. I. A mutant C1 inhibitor that inhibits C1s but not C1r2. J Immunol 1994; 152:3199–3209.

128. Zahedi R, Bissler JJ, Davis III AE, Andreadis C, Wisnieske JJ. Unique C1 inhibitor dysfunction in a kindred without angioedema. II. Identification of an Ala443-Val substitution and functional analysis of the recombinant mutant protein. J Clin Invest 1995; 95:1299–1305.

129. Davis PJ, Davis FB, Charache P. Long-term therapy of hereditary angioedema (HAE). Preventive management with fluoxymesterone and oxymetholone in severely affected males and females. Johns Hopkins Med J 1974; 135:391–398.

130. Rosse WF, Logue GL, Silverman HR, Frank MM. The effect of synthetic androgens in hereditary angioneurotic edema: alteration of C1 inhibitor and C4 levels. Trans Assoc Am Physicians 1976; 89:122–132.

131. Sheffer AL, Fearon DT, Austen KF. Methyltestosterone therapy in hereditary angioedema. Ann Intern Med 1977; 86:306–308.

132. Hauptmann G. Le traitement des deficits de l'inhibiter de la C1-esterase par le Danazol. Med Hyg 1978; 36:2569–2575.

133. Pitts JS, Donaldson VH, Forristal J, Wyatt RJ. Remissions induced in hereditary angioneurotic edema with an attenuated androgen (danazol): correlation between concentration of C1-inhibitor and the fourth and second components of complement. J Lab Clin Med 1978; 92:501–507.

134. Sheffer AL, Fearon DT, Austen KF. Clinical and biochemical effects of impeded androgen (oxymetholone) therapy of hereditary angioedema. J Allergy Clin Immunol 1979; 64:275–280.

135. Agostoni A, Cicardi M, Martignoni C, Bergamaschini L, Marasini B. Danazol and Stanazolol in long-term prophylactic treatment of hereditary angioedema. J Allergy Clin Immunol 1980; 65:75–79.

136. Sheffer AL, Fearon DT, Austen KF. Clinical and biochemical effects of stanazolol therapy for hereditary angioedema. J Allergy Clin Immunol 1981; 68:181–187.

137. Sheffer AL, Fearon DT, Austen KF. Hereditary angioedema: a decade of management with stanazolol. J Allergy Clin Immunol 1987; 80:855–860.

138. Atkinson JC, Frank MM. Oral manifestations and dental management of patients with hereditary angioedema. J Oral Pathol Med 1991; 20:139–142.

139. Bergamaschini L, Cicardi M, Tucci A, et al. C1 inhibitor concentrate in the therapy of hereditary angioedema. Allergy 1983; 38:81–84.

140. Gadek JE, Hosea SW, Gelfand JA, et al. Replacement therapy in hereditary angioedema: Successful treatment of acute episodes of angioedema with partly purified C1 inhibitor. N Engl J Med 1980; 302:542–546.

141. Sim TC, Grant JA. Hereditary angioedema: its diagnostic and management perspectives. Am J Med 1990; 88:656–664.

142. Waytes AT, Rosen FS, Frank MM. Treatment of hereditary angioedema with a vapor-heated C1 inhibitor concentrate. N Engl J Med 1996; 334:1630–1634.

143. Kramer J, Rosen F, Colten H, Rajezy K, Strunk R. Transinhibition of C1 inhibitor synthesis in type I hereditary angioneurotic edema. J Clin Invest 1993; 91:1258–62.

144. Ernst SC, Circolo A, Davis III AE, Gheesling-Mullis K, Fliesler M, Strunk RC. Impaired production of both normal and mutant C1 inhibitor proteins in type I hereditary angioedema with a duplication in exon 8. J Immunol 1996; 157:405–410.

145. Ariga T, Carter P, Davis III AE. Recombinations between Alu repeat sequences that result in partial deletions within the C1 inhibitor gene. Genomics 1990; 8:607–613.

146. Ariga T, Igarashi T, Ramesh N, Parad R, Cicardi M, Davis AI. Type I C1 inhibitor deficiency with a small mRNA resulting from deletion of one exon. J Clin Invest 1989; 83:1888–1893.

147. Stoppa-Lyonnet D, Carter PE, Meo T. Clusters of intragenic Alu repeats predispose the human C1 inhibitor locus to deleterious rearrangements. Proc Natl Acad Sci USA 1990; 87:1551–1555.

148. Cicardi M, Igarashi T, Kim MS, Frangi D, Agostoni A, Davis III AE. Restriction fragment length polymorphism of the C1 inhibitor gene in hereditary angioneurotic edema. J Clin Invest 1987; 80:1640–1643.

149. Stoppa-Lyonnet D, Duponchel C, Meo T, et al. Recombinational biases in the rearranged C1-inhibitor genes of hereditary angioedema patients. Am J Hum Genet 1991; 49:1055–1062.

150. McPhaden AR, Birnie GD, Whaley K. Restriction fragment length polymorphism analysis of the C1-inhibitor gene in hereditary C1-inhibitor deficiency. Clin Genet 1991; 39:161–171.

151. Ariga T, Hoshioka A, Kohno Y, Sakamaki T, Matsumoto S. A de novo deletion in the C1 inhibitor gene in a case of sporadic hereditary angioneurotic edema. Clin Immunol Immunopathol 1993; 69:103–105.

152. Bissler JJ, Aulak KS, Donaldson VH, et al. Molecular defects in hereditary angioneurotic edema. Proc Assoc Am Physicians 1997; 109:164–173.

153. Bissler JJ, Cicardi M, Donaldson VH, et al. A cluster of mutations within a short triplet repeat in the C1 inhibitor gene. Proc Natl Acad Sci USA 1994; 91:9622–9625.

154. Bissler JJ, Donaldson VH, Davis III AE. Contiguous deletion and duplication mutations resulting in type 1 hereditary angioneurotic edema. Hum Genet 1994; 9:265–269.

155. Parad RB, Kramer J, Strunk RC, Rosen FS, Davis III AE. Dysfunctional C1 inhibitor Ta: deletion of Lys-251 results in acquisition of an N-glycosylation site. Proc Natl Acad Sci USA 1990; 87:6786–6790.

156. Frangi D, Cicardi M, Sica A, Colotta F, Agostoni A, Davis III AE. Nonsense mutations affect C1 inhibitor messenger RNA levels in patients with type I hereditary angioneurotic edema. J Clin Invest 1991; 88:755–759.

157. Siddique Z, McPhaden AR, McCluskey D, Whaley K. C1-inhibitor gene nucleotide insertion causes type II hereditary angio-oedema. Hum Genet 1993; 92:189–190.

158. Siddique Z, McPhaden AR, McCluskey D, Whaley K. A single base deletion from the C1-inhibitor gene causes type I hereditary angio-oedema. Hum Hered 1992; 42:231–234.

159. Verpy E, Biasotto M, Brai M, Misiano G, Meo T, Tosi M. Exhaustive mutation scanning by fluorescence-assisted mismatch analysis discloses new genotype-phenotype correlations in angioedema. Am J Hum Genet 1996; 59:308–319.

160. Zahedi R, Aulak KS, Eldering E, Davis III AE. Characterization of C1 inhibitor-Ta: A dysfunctional C1 inhibitor with deletion of lysine-251. J Biol Chem 1996; 271:24307–24312.

161. Siddique Z, McPhaden AR, Lappin DF, Whaley K. An RNA splice site mutation in the C1-inhibitor gene causes type I hereditary angio-oedema. Hum Genet 1991; 88:231–232.

162. Stein P, Carrell R. What do dysfunctional serpins tell us about molecular mobility and disease? Struct Biol 1995; 2:96–113.

163. Siddique Z, McPhaden AR, Whaley K. Characterization of nucleotide sequence variants and disease-specific mutations involving the 3′ end of the C1-inhibitor gene in hereditary angio-oedema. Hum Hered 1995; 45:98–102.

164. Siddique ZM, McPhaden AR, Whaley K. Identification of type II hereditary angio-oedema (HAE) mutations. Clin Exp Immunol 1991; 85S:11 (abstract).

165. Aulak KS, Eldering E, Hack CE, et al. A hinge region mutation in C1-inhibitor (Ala436Thr) results in nonsubstrate-like behavior and in polymerization of the molecule. J Biol Chem 1993; 268:18088–18094.

166. Skriver K, Radziejewska E, Silbermann JA, Donaldson VH, Bock SC. CpG mutations in the reactive site of Human C1 inhibitor. J Biol Chem 1989; 264:3066–3071.

167. Donaldson VH, Bissler JJ. C1-inhibitors and their genes: an update. J Lab Clin Med 1992; 119:330–333.

168. Aulak KS, Pemberton PA, Rosen FS, Carrell RW, Lachmann PJ, Harrison RA. Dysfunctional C1-inhibitor(At), isolated from a type II hereditary-angio-oedema plasma, contains a P1 'reactive centre' (Arg444 → His) mutation. Biochem J 1988; 253:615–618.

169. Aulak KS, Harrison RA. Rapid and sensitive techniques for identification and analysis of 'reactive-centre' mutants of C1-inhibitor proteins contained in type II hereditary angio-oedema plasmas. 271 1990:565–569.

170. Aulak KS, Cicardi M, Harrison RA. Identification of a new P1 residue mutation (444Arg→Ser) in a dysfunctional C1 inhibitor protein contained in a type II hereditary angioedema plasma. FEBS Lett. 1990; 266:13–16.

171. Frangi D, Aulak KS, Cicardi M, Harrison RA, Davis AEI. A dysfunctional C1 inhibitor protein with a new reactive center mutation (Arg444-Leu). FEBS Lett 1992; 301:34–36.

172. Verpy E, Couture-Tosi Ed, Eldering E, et al. Crucial residues in the carboxy-terminal end of C1 inhibitor revealed by pathogenic mutants impaired in secretion or function. J Clin Invest, 1995; 95:350–359.

173. Siddique Z, McPhaden AR, Fothergill JE, Whaley K. A point mutation in the C1-inhibitor gene causes type I hereditary angio-oedema. Hum Hered 1993; 43:155–158.

174. Aulak KS, Davis III AE, Donaldson VH, Harrison RA. Chymotrypsin inhibitory activity of normal C1-inhibitor and P1 Arg to His mutant: evidence for the presence of overlapping reactive centres. Protein Sci 1992; 2:727–732.

175. Owen MC, Brennan SO, Lewis JH, Carrell RW. Mutation of antitrypsin to antithrombin. N Engl J Med 1983; 309:694–698.

176. Stein PE, Tewkesbury DA, Carrell RW. Ovalbumin and angiotensinogen lack serpin S-R conformational change. Biochem J 1989; 262:103–107.

177. de Smet BJ, de Boer J-P. Agterberg J, Rigter G, Bleeker WK, Hack CE. Clearance of human native, proteinase-complexed, and proteolytically inactivated C1-inhibitor in rats. Blood 1993; 81:56–61.

178. Stein P, Chothia C. Serpin tertiary structure transformation. J Mol Biol 1991; 221:99–102.

179. Caldwell JR, Ruddy S, Schur PH, Austen KF. Acquired C1 inhibitor deficiency in lymphosarcoma. Clin Immunol Immunopathol 1972; 1:39–52.

180. Day NK, Winfield JB, Gee T, Winchester R, Teshima H, Kunkel HG. Evidence for immune complexes involving anti-lymphocyte antibodies associated with hypocomplementemia in chronic lymphocytic leukaemia (CLL). Clin Exp Immunol 1976; 26:189–195.

181. Hauptmann G, Lang JM, North NL, Oberling F, Mayer G, Lachmann PJ. Acquired C1 inhibitor deficiencies in lymphoproliferative diseases with serum immunoglobulin abnormalities. Blut 1976; 32:195–206.

182. Schreiber AD, Zweiman B, Atkins P, et al. Acquired angioedema with lymphoproliferative disorder: association of C1 inhibitor deficiency with cellular abnormality. Blood 1976; 48:567–580.

183. Oberling F, Kauptmann G, Land GM, et al. Deficits acquis de l'inhibiteur de la C1 esterase au cours de syndromes lymphoides. Nouv Presse Med 1975; 4:2705–2708.

184. Gelfand JA, Boss GR, Conley CL, Reinhart R, Frank MM. Acquired C1 esterase inhibitor deficiency and angioedema: a review. Medicine 1979; 58:321–328.

185. Kondo M, Yokoe N, Nishibori H, et al. A case of secondary C1 inhibitor deficiency associated with benign monoclonal gammopathy and angioneurotic edema. Rinsho Ketsuki 1978; 19:1581–1587.

186. Hauptmann G, Petitjean F, Lang JM, Oberling F. Acquired C1 inhibitor deficiency in a case of lymphosarcoma of the spleen. Reversal of complement abnormalities after splenectomy. Clin Exp Immunol 1979; 37:523–531.

187. Feichtner JJ, Marx J, Walski KP, Schloessner LL. Acquired angioedema, autoimmune hemolytic anemia, and lymphoma: resolution after therapy. Clin Immunol Immunopathol 1980; 15:642–645.

188. Sheffer AL, Austen KF, Rosen FS, Fearon DT. Acquired deficiency of the inhibitor of the first component of complement: report of five additional cases with commentary on the syndrome. J Allergy Clin Immunol 1985; 75:640–646.

189. Geha RS, Quinti I, Austen KF, Cicardi M, Sheffer A, Rosen FS. Acquired C1-inhibitor deficiency associated with antiidiotypic antibody to monoclonal immunoglobulins. N Engl J Med 1985; 312:534–540.

190. Cohen SH, Koethe SM, Kozin F, Rodey G, Arkins JA, Fink JN. Acquired angioedema associated with rectal carcinoma and its response to danazol therapy. J Allergy Clin Immunol 1978; 62:217–221.

191. Cicardi M, Frangi D, Bergamaschini L, Gardinale M, Sacchi G, Agostoni A. Acquired C1 inhibitor deficiency with angioedema symptoms in a patient infected with *Echinococcus granulosus*. Complement 1985; 2:133–139.

192. Jackson J, Sim RB, Whelan A, Feighery C. An IgG autoantibody which inactivates C1-inhibitor. Nature 1986; 323:722–724.

193. Alsenz J, Bork K, Loos M. Autoantibody-mediated acquired deficiency of C1 inhibitor. N Engl J Med 1987; 316:1360–1366.

194. Frank MM, Malbran A, Simms H, et al. Acquired angioedema type II: a new autoimmune disease. Clin Res 1987; 35.

195. Malbran A, Hammer C, Frank MM, Fries LF. Acquired angioedema: observations on the mechanism of action of auto-antibodies directed against C1 esterase inhibitor. J Allergy Clin Immunol 1988; 81:1199–1204.

196. He S, Tsang S, North J, Chohan N, Sim RB. Epitope mapping of C1 inhibitor autoantibodies from patients with acquired C1 inhibitor deficiency. J Immunol 1996; 156:2009–2013.

197. Donaldson VH, Wagner CJ, Davis III AE. An autoantibody to C1-inhibitor recognizes the reactive center of the inhibitor. J Lab Clin Med 1996; 127:229–232.

198. Mandle R, Baron C, Roux E, et al. Acquired C1 inhibitor deficiency as a result of an autoantibody to the reactive center region of C1 inhibitor. J Immunol 1994; 152:4680–4685.

199. Donaldson VH, Bernstein DI, Wagner CJ, Mitchell BH, Scinto J, Bernstein IL. Angioneurotic edema with acquired C1-inhibitor deficiency and autoantibody to C1-inhibitor: response to plasmapheresis and cytotoxic therapy. J Lab Clin Med 1992; 119:397–406.

200. Zuraw BL, Altman LC. Acute consumption of C1 inhibitor in a patient with acquired C1-inhibitor deficiency syndrome. J Allergy Clin Immunol 1991; 88:908–918.

201. Boyar A, Zuraw BL, Beall G. Immunoabsorption in acquired angioedema: a therapeutic misadventure. Clin Immunol Immunopathol 1993; 66:181–183.

202. Cicardi M, Bisiani G, Cugno M, Spath P, Agostoni A. Autoimmune C1 inhibitor deficiency: report of eight patients. Am J Med 1993; 95:169–175.

203. Mason JW, Kleeberg U, Dolan P, Colman RW. Plasma kallikrein and Hageman factor in gram-negative bacteremia. Ann Intern Med 1970; 73:545–551.

204. Hirsch EF, Nakajima T, Oshima G, Erdos EG, Herman CM. Kinin system responses in sepsis after trauma in man. J Surg Res 1974; 17:147–153.

205. Robinson JA, Klodnycky ML, Loeb HS, Racic MR, Gunner RM. Endotoxin, prekallikrein, complement and systemic vascular resistance. Sequential measurements in man. Am J Med 1975; 59:61–67.

206. O'Donnell TF, Clowes GHA, Talamo RC, Colman RW. Kinin activation in the blood of patients with sepsis. Surg Gynecol Obstet 1976; 143:539–545.

207. Aasen AO, Smith-Erichsen N, Amundsen E. Plasma kallikrein–kinin system in septicemia. Arch Surg 1983; 118:343–346.

208. Kalter ES, Daha MR, Cate JWT, Verhoef J, Bouma BN. Activation and inhibition of Hageman factor-dependent pathways and the complement system in uncomplicated bacteremia or bacterial shock. J Infect Dis 1985; 151:1019–1027.

209. Martinez-Brotons F, Oncins JR, Mestres J, Amargos V, Reynaldo C. Plasma kallikrein-kinin system in pateints with uncomplicated sepsis and septic shock. Comparison with cardiogenic shock. Thromb Haemost 1987; 58.

210. Cadena RADL, Suffredini AF, Page JD, et al. Activation of the kallikrein–kinin system after endotoxin administration to normal human volunteers. Blood 1993; 81:3313–3317.

211. Pixley RA, Cadena RDL, Page JD, et al. The contact system contributes to hypotension but not disseminated intravascular coagulation in lethal bacteremia. In vivo use of a monoclonal anti-factor XII antibody to block contact activation in baboons. J Clin Invest 1993; 91:61–68.

212. Jansen PM, Pixley RA, Brouwer M, et al. Inhibition of factor XII in septic baboons attenuates the activation of complement and fibrinolytic systems and reduces the release of interleukin-6 and neutrophil elastase. Blood 1996; 87:2337–2344.

213. Guerrero R, Velasco F, Rodriguez M, et al. Endotoxin-induced pulmonary dysfunction is prevented by C1-esterase inhibitor. J Clin Invest 1992; 91:2754–2760.

214. Hack CE, Ogilvie AC, Eisele B, Jansen PM, Wagstaff J, Thijs LG. Initial studies on the administration of C1-esterase inhibitor to patients with septic shock or with a vascular leak syndrome induced by interleukin-2 therapy. Prog Clin Biol Res 1994; 388:335–357.

215. Prodeus AP, Fischer MB, Ma M, et al. Complement C3 and C4 deficient mice are highly susceptible to endotoxic shock. Mol Immunol 1996; 33:79 (abstract).

22

Paroxysmal Nocturnal Hemoglobinuria and Complement

WENDELL F. ROSSE
Duke University Medical Center, Durham, North Carolina

Paroxysmal nocturnal hemoglobinuria is an uncommon hematological disorder characterized by three major manifestations:

1. Hemolytic anemia and hemoglobinuria that is irregularly periodic, exacerbated at night, and highly variable in amount from patient to patient
2. Venous thrombosis, particularly of the veins of the abdomen and liver
3. Hematopoietic failure to a highly variable extent.

It was first reported in 1866 in a young tanner who had episodes of dark urine, particularly with infections (1). Other case studies followed, each suggesting a cause but offering no evidence for one (2). However, in 1913, Hijmans van den Bergh examined the red cells of a patient with the "hemoglobinuric crises" and found that they were hemolyzed when incubated in serum, either the patient's own or from an ABO-compatible donor, only when the mixture was acidified by "carbonic acid" (3). The hemolytic reactions of complement had been well described by Ehrlich (4,5) and Donath and Landsteiner (6), so it was natural for Hijmans van den Bergh to try to determine if it played a role in this "striking finding." He inactivated the complement of the serum by heating and noted that the reaction was abrogated but he could not revive the reaction by the addition of new serum as a source of complement. Precisely why he failed is not clear but it is likely that the added complement was in insufficient concentration to bring about the reaction.

Twenty-five years later, Ham and his associates essentially repeated the experiments of Hijmans van den Bergh with refined materials and demonstrated the lysis of the red cells of patients with PNH by normal serum when the pH was lowered by added acid (7–9). He was able to demonstrate convincingly that the hemolysis was due to activated complement, that only a portion of the cells were subject to lysis, and that the reaction apparently occurred in the absence of antibody, even though the cells were, in fact, more susceptible to lysis when complement was activated by isologous blood group antibodies.

Hemolysis of PNH red cells occurred in the patients own serum, although the reaction was sometimes less strong. When the alternative pathway of complement activation was proposed (10), the absence of antibody in this case was accounted for by the activation of the alternative pathway (11); during the warfare on the concept of an alternative activation, the lysis of PNH red cells was held up as being inexplicable by any other hypothesis. When the alternative pathway was revived, the role of its activation in the lysis of PNH red cell by acidified serum was affirmed (12).

I. QUANTITATIVE STUDIES OF COMPLEMENT LYSIS

When better techniques for analyzing the reactions of the components of complement more quantitatively became available, they were applied to the lysis of PNH erythrocytes (13,14). These studies quantified the abnormality of the cells and found that, as had been suspected, only a portion of the cells were abnormal in their susceptibility. There was nearly always present a population of cells that could not be differentiated from normal cells; these were termed PNH I cells. The characteristic cells required only 1/15th to 1/25th as much complement for an equal degree of lysis as the PNH I or as normal red cells. These were later called PNH III cells because some patients had cells of intermediate sensitivity to complement called PNH II cells (15,16). This classification was based on the characteristics of lysis by complement but was confirmed when other methods for characterizing the abnormalities in PNH became available (see below).

These studies as well as those of Yachnin (17) strongly suggested that the initial steps of the classical pathway were not altered on PNH red cells. This was confirmed when it was shown that the earliest abnormality that could be detected was the excessive deposition of C3 upon activation of either the classical or the alternative pathway (18,19). This was in contrast with the findings in a rare congenital disorder in which, based on in vitro data, susceptibility of the red cells to complement lysis had also been postulated: hereditary erythroblastic multinuclearity with a positive acidified serum test (HEMPAS) or congenital dyserythropoietic anemia type II (20,21). In this disorder, also characterized by lysis of the erythrocytes in acidified normal serum, the susceptibility to complement was found to reside in a more efficient activation of the early steps of the classical pathway (19,21). This is presumably related in some way to the underlying defect in these cells, which is the defective biosynthesis of the surface biantennary lactosaminylglycans due to the absence of an enzyme essential in the glycosylation steps of this molecule (22).

The studies on the PNH cells were refined by demonstrating that a given number C3bBb convertase complexes were capable of generating three to five times as much membrane-bound C3 on the abnormal cells (23) and that this did not appear to be due to abnormalities in the binding of factor B nor factor H (24). These studies suggested that the convertase was inactivated less readily on PNH than on normal cells and the studies of Nicholson-Weller et al. (25) and Pangburn et al. (26) demonstrated the absence of decay-accelerating factor on these cells (see Chap. 7).

The earlier detailed studies relating the amount of surface-bound C3 to the amount of lysis obtained indicated clearly that, in PNH cells, there was another step with increased efficiency since very much smaller amounts of C3 were bound for a given degree of lysis of these cells (19). The second defect was found to be due to the absence of regulators of the assembly of the polymeric C9 complex, the membrane inhibitor of reactive lysis (MIRL) (27) (see Chap. 7) and, less clearly defined, homologous restriction factor (HRF) or C8-binding protein (28,29).

The demonstration of the absence of these proteins has become the standard method for the detection of the abnormal red cells in PNH, since it is more precise and descriptive than the tests that depended upon lysis by complement. This is most conveniently done with monoclonal antibodies to CD59 (or less quantitatively with antibodies to CD55) and fluorescence activated cytometry (30–34). As shown in Figure 1, the proportion and the abnormality of the cells in PNH can be assessed by this means. The proportion of abnormal cells can vary from as little as 1–2% to 100% and the evidence of clinical hemolysis varies roughly with the proportion and abnormality of these cells.

Considerable evidence in vitro and in vivo has accumulated to indicate that the absence of these proteins accounts for the abnormal hemolysis of PNH cells. Wilcox and her associates demonstrated that hemolysis in acidified serum was increased when either DAF or MIRL was inhibited on normal cells but the effect of inhibition of both was more than additive, suggesting an interaction of the individual effects but the effect of inhibition of CD59 was the more important (35). The lysis of the cells by complement is roughly parallel to their content of the two proteins in that the PNH II cells described above have intermediate amounts of the two proteins on the surfaced (16,30,36). In vivo, the life span of the abnormal cells is much shorter than of the more nearly normal cells (37,38). PNH

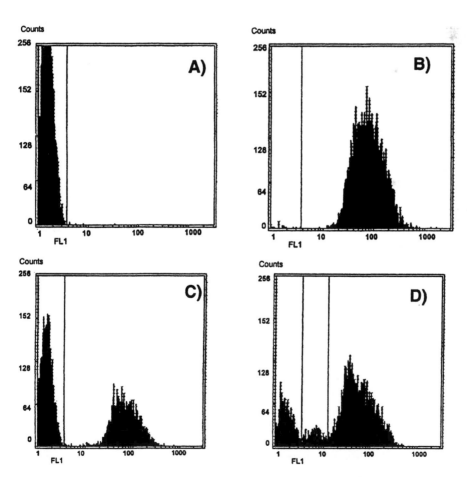

Figure 1 Analysis of erythrocytes by flow cytometry, using anti-CD59. (A) Isotype control. A nonreactive protein of the same isotype was used instead of the monoclonal antibody. (B) Normal erythrocytes. (C) PNH erythrocytes showing PNHIII cells (those similar to the negative control) and PNH I cells (those that are normal). (D) PNH erythrocytes showing PNH III, PNH I, and PNH II cells (those that are intermediate between the other populations).

III cells are lysed within the first 20 days of circulation compared to a normal 90 day survival for PNH I cells. PNH II cells in one patient had a survival of about 45 days compared with a normal survival of 90–120 days. Fujioka and Yamada also demonstrated an intermediate survival for these cells (38).

Most evidence suggests that the absence of CD59 is more important than the absence of CD55 in the abnormal lysis of PNH cells. Inhibition of CD59 by antibody results in greater lysis than inhibition of CD55 in quantitative assays of lysis (35,39). Congenital deficiency of CD59 results in cells markedly sensitive to the lytic action of complement and a hemolytic syndrome similar to that seen in PNH (40), whereas deficiency of CD55 (the so-called Inab phenotype) does not result in either (41,42).

In PNH, the peripheral blood granulocytes and platelets also lack CD55 and CD59 (43,44). This appears to make them more susceptible to lysis by complement in vitro (45,46), but both cells have a normal survival in vivo (47,48). Platelets are able to mobilize serum-based complement inhibitory proteins, particularly factor H, from internal stores when stimulated (49), which may in part replace the function of the absent CD55. However, both cellss are probably able to survive more nearly normally because they are able to remove nascent polymeric C9 complexes by vesiculation before they can permanently damage the cell (50,51); red cells are able to do this as well but much less efficiently (52).

This vesiculation process is not without its downside, however. The vesicles that are produced from platelets are unable to maintain acidic phospholipids on the internal leaflet of the plasma membrane; when phosphatidylserine is exposed to plasma, it provides a site for the generation of prothrombinase complexes that are able to activate prothrombin to thrombin (50,53–55). Since the abnormal platelets in PNH lack the inhibitor of polymeric C9 formation, more nascent membrane attack complexes are generated and hence more vesicles (56). The release of the vesicles from the platelet tends to "activate" the platelet surface and make it more easily able to aggregate (29). These reactions may be part of the reason that patients with PNH are exceptionally prone to venous thrombotic disease.

CD55 and CD59 were not the first proteins noted to be deficient on PNH cells. Two enzymes, leukocyte alkaline phosphatase (57,58) and erythrocyte acetylcholinesterase (AChE) (59), were both demonstrated to be deficient in a portion of the cells. It was further noted that the degree of deficiency of erythrocyte AChE corresponded to the degree of susceptibility to lysis by complement (60) and that the deficiency of the enzyme was due to a lack of surface protein expression (61).

The reason for the deficiency of all of these proteins came from the studies on the way in which they were attached to the membrane bilayer. Low found that surface-bound alkaline phosphatase could be removed by a bacterial enzyme, phosphatidylinositol-specific phospholipase C (PIPLC), which cleaved the phosphate from phosphatidylinositol but did not cleave peptide bonds. Furthermore, the enzyme had full activity after its release, suggesting that the protein structure had not been altered (62). The reason for this was that the protein had attached to the carboxyl end a complex glycolipid, ending in a phosphatidylinositol molecule inserted into the lipid bilayer (Fig. 2). The essential structure of this anchor has been preserved almost intact from earliest life forms and consists of the molecule of PI, a molecule of glucosamine, three molecules of mannose, and a molecule of phosphoethanolamine (ETN). This glycosylphosphatidylionositol (GPI) anchor is attached to the protein by an amide bond with the terminal ETN.

This anchor is synthesized in the endoplasmic reticulum by a series of steps that sequentially adds the saccharide moieties and finally the ethanolamine (63–65). It is added

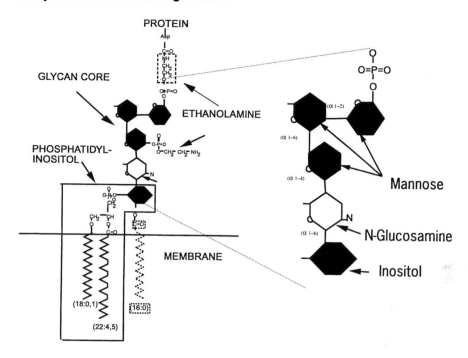

Figure 2 The structure of the glycosylphosphatidylinositol (GPI) anchor. The full anchor is shown on the left; the details of the glycan core are shown on the right.

to the protein posttranslationally by a transamidase that has not yet been characterized. The anchored protein is then processed in the Golgi apparatus and exported to the cell surface.

The deficiency from the cells of PNH of three proteins, all of which were attached to the membrane by the GPI, led to the conclusion that the anchor was either not synthesized or was too readily hydrolyzed by endogenous phospholipases. The former proved to be the case as it could be shown that the abnormal cells in PNH were not able to make the glycosylated intermediates necessary in the biosynthesis of the anchor. The defect appeared to be in the addition of N-acetylglucosamine to the molecule of PI (66–68). At least three gene products are needed to effect this: three murine cell lines (class A, C, and H) with this phenotype were able to complement one another, indicating that they had different defects in steps necessary to make this phenotype (69). Similar somatic cell fusion studies demonstrated that the abnormal cells in PNH in all cases did not complement the murine cells of class A, indicating that they bore the same defect (70–72).

Kinoshita and his associates were the first to isolate the gene that is defective in both class A cells and in the abnormal PNH cells by expression selection after transduction of defective cells from a patient with PNH (73). The cDNA obtained contained 4568 bp and an open reading frame that coded for a protein of 484 amino acids; in addition, there were 85 bp 5′ to the ORF and 3031 bp 3′ (74). To date, the protein has not been isolated or otherwise characterized and its exact role in GPI anchor synthesis is not known. However, the amino acid sequence derived from the sequence of the cDNA has considerable homology to the a family of glycosyltransferases, particularly near the amino terminus, suggesting that the pig-A protein is probably directly involved in transferring the sugar moiety to inositol.

The structure of the gene has also been elucidated. In consists of six exons, the first of which is not translated. The promoter region does not have tissue-specific sequences but does contain four CAAT boxes two AP-2 sequences and a CRE sequence (75). The gene is located on the short arm of the X chromosome in both humans and mice (73,76,77).

To date, about 100 defects have been identified in the *pig-A* gene in the hematopoietic cells of patients with PNH (73,78–91) (see Table 1). Many of these defects involve the insertion or deletion one or two to a few nucleotides, which nearly always results in a premature stop codon and, it is presumed, no usable gene product. Such insertions may also result in an alteration of the splicing signals or in an immediate stop signal. Only two genes were found with large deletions (31,92) and no abnormalities were reported in the promoter region. Thirty-five of the 98 known defects involve point mutations; about half of these result in a splicing abnormality or an immediate stop codon. Only 19 of 98 defects result in a missense mutation resulting in an abnormal protein; these are clustered in two regions of the 2nd exon that correspond in homology to conserved areas on other glycosyl transferases. Some of these defects have been identified in patients with cells that are partially deficient in CD59 (PNH II cells) and this has suggested that a small amount of the GPI anchor is made. On the other hand, in at least one patient with PNH II cells, the defects identified were the kind that would produce no protein.

Other point mutations result in an altered splice site (eight instances), usually with the elimination of an exon, or in the creation of a stop codon (nine instances). In these cases, no usable protein would be made.

Although most of the described alterations are unique, several have been found in more than one patient; in five instances two patients had cells with the same defect, and in two instances three patients had the same defect. Two other patients had a different defect at the same site. Furthermore, in several instances, a patient was found to have multiple abnormal clones; in two cases, four different defects were found in each patient (88,93).

Table 1 Identified Mutations in PNH in the *Pig-A* Gene by Category

	Total number	Duplicates	Triplicates
Point mutations			
Missense	19	2	1
Splice defect	8	1	1
Nonsense	8	2	
Nucleotide deletions or additions			
Frame shift	55	2	
Altered splicing	3	0	
Immediate stop	2	0	
In frame	1	0	
Large deletion	2	0	
Total	98	7	2

Source: From Ref. 137.

These findings suggest that the rate of somatic mutation in the *pig-A* gene may be very high indeed. It is possible that mutant clones are present in the bone marrow of many normal people but that the cells have such a disadvantage in proliferation that they remain undetectable. The mutant clone may have a proliferative advantage in a marrow affected by a suppressive influence as is seen in aplastic anemia and, under such circumstances, PNH appears.

II. EFFECT OF THE DEFECT

The presence of the defective gene in an hematopoietic cell results in a deficiency of all the proteins linked to the membrane by the GPI anchor. To date, at least 19 proteins have been shown to be deficient on the abnormal PNH cells (see Table 2). Many of these are receptors or counterligands of immunological proteins. Some, such as the FcγRIII and LFA-3 (CD48) may be expressed because the transmembrane form of the protein also is synthesized.

Table 2 Proteins Known to Be Absent on Hematopoietic Cells in PNH

Name	Other names	Function	References
CD55	Decay accelerating factor (DAF)	Down-regulation of C3 convertase	25,26
CD59	Membrane inhibitor of reactive lysis (MIRL), HRF 20, protectin, MACIF, etc.	Down-regulation of membrane attack complex	27
	C8 binding protein, homologous restriction protein (HRP)	Same as CD59	28,123
CD16a	FcγReceptor III	Binding to IgG	124
	Urokinase receptor (UPAR)	Binds urokinase (plasminogen activator)	125
CD14	Endotoxin-binding protein receptor	Binds endotoxin-binding protein	126
	Folate receptor	Binds and internalizes folate	127
CD58	Leukocyte function antigen-3, LFA-3	Binds CD2, etc.	128
CD48	Blast-1	Adhesion-activation protein	32
CDw52	CAMPATH-1	Activates through CD2 system	129
CDw108	JMH-bearing protein	Possible activation antigen	130,131
CD24	Heat-stable antigen (HSA), nectadrin	Binds P-selectin	33,132
CD66		CEA family of adhesion proteins	133
CD67		Related to CD66 family	33
	Gy^{a}hHy/Do protein		134
p50–80			33
	Acetylcholinesterase	Cleaves acetylcholine	59,60
	Leukocyte alkaline phosphatase	A phosphatase	57
CD78	5′ecto nucleotidase	Cleaves nucleotides	135

The absence of these proteins can be easily quantitatively assessed by flow cytometry, using specific monoclonal antibodies and the absence of an expected protein on an hematopoietic cell is taken as evidence of the presence of a PNH defect. As this technique is easier and more reliable than the techniques dependent on complement lysis (see above), it has begun to be the standard method of diagnosis of the disorder (30–32,34,94,95).

The defective *pig-A* gene apparently arises in very early hematopoietic precursors since a population of the earliest identifiable progenitor cells (CD34$^+$ CD38$^-$) of the PNH marrow lack the GPI-linked proteins (96). The defect is seen in all progeny from the hematopoietic precursor, including red cell neutrophils, eosinophils, monocytes, and lymphocytes but the proportion of cells in the abnormal population is greatly variable in a given patient. In general, the proportion of abnormal granulocytes, monocytes, and platelets is higher than that of abnormal red cells because their survival in the circulation is no different from the normal clone whereas the abnormal red cells have a much shorter life span than the cell of the normal clone. The proportion of abnormal lymphocytes varies greatly (97–98) but is usually lower than the proportion of the abnormal cells in the other cell lines; in many instances, only very small populations of lymphocytes may be found. These discrepancies may be due to the fact that the turnover rate for lymphocytes is very much less than for the other cells. Lymphocytes are long-lived and abnormal lymphocytes may be found long after the PNH cells in other cell lines have disappeared (99,100).

III. CAN THE SYMPTOMS OF PNH BE EXPLAINED BY THE ABSENCE OF GPI-LINKED PROTEINS?

PNH is a protean disease and has a variety of symptoms and manifestations that should be explained by the defect characteristic of the syndrome. This has proven both easy and difficult to do.

Certainly, the intravascular hemolysis of the red cells is, as discussed above, easily explained by the absence of the membrane regulators of complement, CD55 and CD59. The degree of hemolysis in a given patient is roughly parallel to the proportion and abnormality of the cells lacking these proteins. When hemolysis occurs, the abnormal cells that are specifically hemolyzed. Hemolytic episodes are triggered by events that activate complement (e.g., infections, trauma, incompatible blood transfusions, etc.). All of these facts support the relationship between the deficiency of the proteins and the clinical manifestation.

As explained above, the thrombosis seen in PNH may in part be due to the abnormal activation of platelets because of the defective downregulation of the formation of the membrane attack complex. In addition, the receptor for urokinase (UPAR) is missing from monocytes. It is postulated that, after clotting has occurred, monocytes infiltrate the clot and urokinase bound to UPAR is able to activate plasminogen to plasmin, which in turn digests fibrin; the absence of this function because of the absence of UPAR would result in the persistence of the clots. At any event, the incidence of venous thrombosis is very high (about 40% of patients) in European and American series (100,101) but much less in Asiatic series (102,103). It is clear that other factors play a role in the hypercoaguable state.

The third major manifestation of PNH is a relative or absolute diminution in hematopoiesis. This is manifest in the association of PNH and aplastic anemia, first noted by Dacie and his associates (104,105). PNH often develops in patients presenting with aplastic anemia (102,106,107), particularly when treated with antithymocyte globulin (108–110), and many patients with PNH develop bone marrow failure during the course of their disease (100,101).

It is possible that the defect renders the abnormal cell unable to proliferate but this is difficult to match with the fact that these cells begin with one abnormal cell and come to dominate the marrow. Lymphocytes and monocytes are important regulators of hematopoiesis and it is possible that the GPI-defective accessory cells "overregulate" proliferation, but there is not a clear relationship between their numbers and the occurrence of aplastic anemia. Furthermore, it is difficult to see how the process could begin since they would not be present from the start.

The most reasonable hypothesis suggests that the development of PNH requires, in addition to the defect in the *pig-A* gene, a suppressive effect on the marrow, similar to or the same as that seen in aplastic anemia, where it is often thought to be due to autoimmune processes (111–113). This would imply that the GPI-defective progenitors were somewhat less susceptible to this influence, perhaps because they lack a receptor for a suppressive cytokine or a counterreceptor for a suppressive cell. If the suppressive influence were sufficiently great, both normal and abnormal clones would be suppressed. As the influence was decreased by treatment, the PNH clone(s) would have a growth advantage and could come to dominate the marrow. When the aplastic influence went away completely, the normal clone would again have the advantage and would come to dominate the marrow, as happens in about 1/3 of patients having the disease over 10 years (100,101). More work is needed to understand the hematopoietic defect in PNH and its relationship to aplastic anemia.

Although many of the proteins missing on PNH cells are involved in immunological reactions, a clinical immunological deficiency is not apparent. This may be due to the fact that some of the missing proteins (e.g., LFA-3 and FcγIIIa) are backed up by almost identical proteins held in place by the usual transmembrane hydrophobic sequence (114,115). Furthermore, they may be backed up by similar molecules as the function of FcγIIIa is taken up by FcγII. Probing the function of the abnormal lymphocytes has not revealed any major problems (97,101,116).

IV. TREATMENT

To date, the treatment of PNH is primarily the treatment of symptoms by empirical means. No attempt has been made to modify specifically the reactions of complement although an experiment of nature, the congenital absence of C9 in a patient with PNH, has shown that at least the hemolytic manifestations of the disease could be modified (117). Prednisone in high dosages modifies the activation of complement and this may account for the fact that hemolysis can be diminished in some patients by its use (118,119). The hematopoietic deficiency can be relieved to a greater or lesser extent by the use of antithymocyte globulin, as is used in aplastic anemia, but the population of abnormal cells may increase as a result. The only definitive cure for PNH currently available is bone marrow transplantation (120,121). In one famous case, the PNH population disappeared spontaneously after infusion of the syngeneic marrow even without conditioning (122).

In some respects, PNH is an ideal candidate for cure by gene therapy. The cell to be altered is available, the gene is isolated, the effects could be easily monitored, and so on. However, much more needs to be learned about the technique of gene therapy itself and about the abnormal hematopoiesis in PNH before gene therapy can become a reality.

REFERENCES

1. Gull WW. A case of intermittent haematinuria, with remarks. Guys Hosp Rep 1866; 12:381.
2. Strubing P. Paroxysmale Hämoglobinurie. Dtsch Med Wochenschr 1882; 8:1.
3. Hijmans van den Bergh AA. Ictère hemolytique avec crises hemoglobinunques. Fragilité globulaire. Rev Méd 1911; 31:63.
4. Ehrlich P. Uber paroxysmale Hämoglobinurie. Z Klin Med 1891; 3:383.
5. Ehrlich P. Uber paroxysmale Hämoglobinurie. In: Farbenalalytische Untersuchungen zur Histologie und Klinik des Blutes. Berlin: August Hischwald, 1891; 110.
6. Donath J, Landsteiner K. Uber paroxysmale Hämoglobinurie. München Med Wochenschr 1904; 51:1590.
7. Ham TH, Dingle JH. Studies on destruction of red blood cells. II. Chronic hemolytic anemia with paroxysmal nocturnal hemoglobinuria: certain immunological aspects of the hemolytic mechanism with special reference to serum complement. J Clin Invest 1938; 18:657.
8. Ham TH. Chronic hemolytic anemia with paroxysmal nocturnal hemoglobinuria. A study of the mechanism of hemolysis in relation to acid-base equilibrium. N Engl J Med 1938; 217:915.
9. Ham TH. Studies on the destruction of red blood cells. I Chronic hemolytic anemia with paroxysmal nocturnal hemoglobinuria: an investigation of the mechanism of hemolysis with observations on five cases. Arch Intern Med 1939; 64:1271.
10. Pillemer L, Blum L, Lepow IH, Ross OA, Todd EA, Wardlaw AC. The properdin system and immunity: I. Demonstration and isolation of a new serum protein, properdin, and its role in immune phenomena. Science 1954; 129:279.
11. Hinz CJ jr, Jordan WS, Pillemer LT. The properdin system and immunity. IV. The hemolysis of erythrocytes from patients with paroxysmal nocturnal hemoglobinuria. J Clin Invest 1956; 35:453.
12. Gotze O, Muller-Eberhard HJ. Paroxysmal nocturnal hemoglobinuria. Hemolysis initiated by the C3 activator system. N Engl J Med 1972; 286:180.
13. Rosse WF, Dacie JV. Immune lysis of normal human and paroxysmal nocturnal hemoglobinuria red blood cells. I. The sensitivity of PNH red cells to lysis by complement and specific antibody. J Clin Invest 1966; 45:736.
14. Rosse WF, Dacie JV. Immune lysis of normal human and paroxysmal nocturnal hemoglobinuria (PNH) red blood cells. II. The role of complement components in the increased sensitivity of PNH red cells to immune lysis. J Clin Invest 1966; 45:749.
15. Rosse WF, Adams JP, Thorpe AM. The population of cells in paroxysmal nocturnal haemoglobinuria of intermediate sensitivity to complement lysis: significance and mechanism of increased immune lysis. Br J Haematol 1974; 28:181.
16. Rosse WF, Hoffman S, Campbell M, Borowitz M, Moore JO, Parker CJ. The erythrocytes in paroxysmal nocturnal haemoglobinuria of intermediate sensitivity to complement basis. Br J Haematol 1991; 79:99.
17. Yachnin S. The hemolysis of red cells from patients with paroxysmal nocturnal hemoglobinuria by paritally purified supcomponents of the third complement component. J Clin Invest 1965; 44:1534.
18. Logue GL, Rosse WF, Adams JP. Mechanisms of immune lysis of red blood cells in vitro. I. Paroxysmal nocturnal hemoglobinuria cells. J Clin Invest 1973; 52:1129.
19. Rosse WF, Logue GL, Adams J, Crookston JH. Mechanisms of immune lysis of the red cells in hereditary erythroblastic multinuclearity with a positive acidified serum test and paroxysmal nocturnal hemoglobinuria. J Clin Invest 1974; 53:31.
20. Verwilghen RL, Lewis SM, Dacie JV, Crookston JH, Crookston M. HEMPAS. Congenital dyserythropoietic anemia (Type II). Q J Med 1973; 42:257.
21. Crookston JH, Crookston MC, Rosse WF. Red-cell abnormalities in HEMPAS (hereditary erythroblastic multinuclearity with a positive acidified-serum test). Br J Haematol 1972; 23P(Supp):83–91.

22. Fukuda MN. HEMPAS disease: genetic defect of glycosylation. Glycobiology 1990; 1:9.

23. Parker CJ, Baker PJ, Rosse WF. Increased enzymatic activity of the alternative pathway convertase when bound to the erythrocytes of paroxysmal nocturnal hemoglobinuria. J Clin Invest 1982; 69:337.

24. Parker CJ, Baker PJ, Rosse WF. Comparison of binding characteristics of factors B and H to C3b on normal and paroxysmal nocturnal hemoglobinuria erythrocytes. J Immunol 1983; 131:2484.

25. Nicholson-Weller A, March JP, Rosenfeld SI, Austen KF. Affected erythrocytes of patients with paroxysmal nocturnal hemoglobinuria are deficient in the complement regulatory protein, decay accelerating factor. Proc Natl Acad Sci USA 1983; 80:5430.

26. Pangburn MK, Schreiber RD, Muller-Eberhard HJ. Deficiency of an erythrocyte membrane protein with complement regulator activity in paroxysmal nocturnal hemoglobinuria. Proc Natl Acad Sci USA 1983; 80:5430.

27. Holguin MH, Frederick LR, Bernshaw NJ, Wilcox LA, Parker CJ. Isolation and characterization of a membrane protein from normal human erythrocytes that inhibits reactive lysis of the erythrocytes of paroxysmal nocturnal hemoglobinuria. J Clin Invest 1989; 84:7.

28. Zalman LS, Wood LM, Frank MM, Muller-Eberhard HJ. Deficiency of the homologous restriction factor in paroxysmal nocturnal hemoglobinuria. J Exp Med 1987; 165:572.

29. Blaas P, Berger B, Weber S, Peter HH, Hansch GM. Paroxysmal nocturnal hemoglobinuria. Enhanced stimulation of platelets by the terminal complement components is related to the lack of C8bp in the membrane. J Immunol 1988; 140:3045.

30. Hall S, Rosse WF. The use of monoclonal antibodies and flow cytometry in the diagnosis of paroxysmal nocturnal hemoglobinuria. Blood 1996; 87:5332.

31. Fletcher A, Bryant JA, Gardner B, Judson PA, Spring FA, Parsons SF, Mallinson G, Anstee DJ. New monoclonal antibodies in CD59: use for the analysis of peripheral blood cells from paroxysmal nocturnal haemoglobinuria (PNH) patients and for the quantitation of CD59 on normal and decay accelerating factor (DAF)-deficient erythrocytes. Immunology 1992; 75:507.

32. Schubert J, Alvarado M, Uciechowski P, Zielinska Skowronek M, Freund M, Vogt H, Schmidt RE. Diagnosis of paroxysmal nocturnal haemoglobinuria using immunophenotyping of peripheral blood cells. Br J Haematol 1991; 79:487.

33. van der Schoot CE, Huizinga TW, van't Veer-Korthof ET, Wijmans R, Pinkster J, von dem Borne AE. Deficiency of glycosyl-phosphatidylinositol-linked membrane glycoproteins of leukocytes in paroxysmal nocturnal hemoglobinuria; description of a new diagnostic cytofluorometric assay. Blood 1990; 76:1853.

34. Shichishima T, Terasawa T, Saitoh Y, Hashimoto C, Ohto H, Maruyama A. Diagnosis of paroxysmal nocturnal haemoglobinuria by phenotypic analysis of erthrocytes using two-color flow cytometry with monoclonal antibodies to DAF and CD59/MACIF. Br J Haematol 1993; 85:378.

35. Wilcox LA, Ezzell JL, Bernshaw NJ, Parker CJ. Molecular basis of the enhanced susceptibility of the erythrocytes of paroxysmal nocturnal hemoglobinuria to hemolysis in acidified serum. Blood 1991; 78:820.

36. Shichishima T, Terasawa T, Hashimoto C, Ohto H, Uchida T, Maruyama Y. Heterogenous expression of decay accelerating factor and CD59/membrane attack complex inhibition factor on paroxysmal nocturnal haemoglobinuria (PNH) erythrocytes. Br J Haematol 1991; 78:545.

37. Rosse WF. The life-span of complement-sensitive and -insensitive red cells in paroxysmal nocturnal hemoglobinuria. Blood 1971; 37:556.

38. Fujioka S, Yamada T. Longer in vivo survival of CD59- and decay-accelerating factor-almost normal positive and partly positive erythrocytes in paroxysmal nocturnal hemoglobinuria as compared with negative erythrocytes: a demonstration by differential centrifugation and flow cytometry. Blood 1992; 79:1842.

39. Jackson GH, Noble RS, Maung ZT, Main J, Smith SR, Reid MM. Severe haemolysis and renal failure in a patient with paroxysmal nocturnal haemoglobinuria. J Clin Pathol 1992; 45:176.

40. Yamashina M, Ueda E, Kinoshita T, Takami T, Ojima A, Ono H, Tanaka H, Kondo N, Orii T, Okada N, Okada H, Inoue K, Kitani T. Inherited complete deficiency of 20-kilodalton homologous restriction factor (CD59) as a cause of paroxysmal nocturnal hemoglobinuria. N Engl J Med 1990; 323:1184.

41. Telen MJ, Green AM. The Inab phenotype: characterization of the membrane protein and complement regulatory defect. Blood 1989; 74:437.

42. Merry AH, Rawlinson VI, Uchikawa M, Daha MR, Sim RB. Studies on the sensitivity to complement-mediated lysis of erythrocytes (Inab phenotype) with a deficiency of DAF (decay accelerating factor). Br J Haematol 1989; 73:248.

43. Nicholson-Weller A, Spicer DB, Austen KF. Deficiency of the complement regulatory protein "decay accelerating factor," on membranes of granulocytes, monocytes, and platelets in paroxysmal nocturnal hemoglobinuria. N Engl J Med 1983; 312:1091.

44. Kinoshita T, Medof ME, Silber R, Nussenzweig V. Distribution of decay accelerating factor in the peripheral blood of normal individuals and patients with paroxysmal nocturnal hemoglobinuria. J Exp Med 1985; 162:75.

45. Aster RH, Enright SE. A platelet and granulocyte membrane defect in paroxysmal nocturnal hemoglobinuria: Usefulness for the detection of platelet antibodies. J Clin Invest 1969; 48:1199.

46. Stern M, Rosse WF. Two populations of granulocytes in paroxysmal nocturnal hemoglobinuria. Blood 1979; 53:928.

47. Brubaker L, Essig LJ, Mengel CE. Neutrophil life span in paroxysmal nocturnal hemoglobinuria. Blood 1977; 50:657.

48. Devine DV, Siegel RS, Rosse WF. Interactions of the platelets in paroxysmal nocturnal hemoglobinuria with complement. Relationship to defects in the regulation of complement and to platelet survival in vivo. J Clin Invest 1987; 79:131.

49. Devine DV, Rosse WF. Regulation of the activity of platelet-bound C3 convertase of the alternative pathway of complement by platelet factor H. Proc Natl Acad Sci USA 1987; 84:5873.

50. Sims PJ, Faioni EM, Wiedmer T, Shattil SJ. Complement proteins C5b-9 cause release of membrane vesicles from the platelet surface that are enriched in the membrane receptor for coagulation factor Va and express prothrombinase activity. J Biol Chem 1988; 263:18205.

51. Morgan BP, Dankert JR, Esser AF. Recovery of human neutrophils from complement attack: removal of the membrane attack complex by endocytosis and exocytosis. J Immunol 1987; 138:246.

52. Iida K, Whitlow MB, Nussenzweig V. Membrane vesiculation protects erythrocytes from destruction by complement. Medicine 1991.

53. Van der Meer BW, Fugate RD, Sims PJ. Complement proteins C5b-9 induce transbilayer migration of membrane phospholipids. Biophys J 1989; 56:935.

54. Chang CP, Zhao J, Wiedmer T, Sims PJ. Contribution of platelet microparticle formation and granule secretion to the transmembrane migration of phosphatidylserine. J Biol Chem 1993; 268:7171.

55. Gilbert GE, Sims PJ, Wiedmer T, Furie B, Furie BC, Shattil SJ. Platelet-derived microparticles express high affinity receptors for factor VIII. J Biol Chem 1991; 266:17261.

56. Wiedmer T, Hall SE, Ortel TL, Kane WH, Rosse WF, Sims PJ. Complement-induced vesiculation and exposure of membrane prothrombinase sites in platelets of paroxysmal nocturnal hemoglobinuria. Blood 1993; 82:1192.

57. Beck WS, Valentine WN. Biochemical studies on leucocytes. II. Phosphatase activity in chronic lymphatic leukemia, acute leukemia, and miscellaneous hematologic conditions. J Lab Clin Med 1951; 38:245.

58. Lewis SM, Dacie JV. Neutrophil (leucocyte) alkaline phosphatase in paroxysmal nocturnal haemoglobinuria. Br J Haematol 1965; 11:549.

59. Auditore JV, Hartmann RC, Flexner JM, Balchum OJ. The erythrocyte acetylcholinesterase enzyme in paroxysmal nocturnal hemoglobinuria. Arch Pathol 1960; 69:534.

60. Kunstling TR, Rosse WF. Erythrocyte acetylcholinesterase deficiency in paroxysmal nocturnal hemoglobinuria (PNH). A comparison of the complement-sensitive and insensitive populations. Blood 1969; 33:607.

61. Chow FL, Telen MJ, Rosse WF. The acetylcholinesterase defect in paroxysmal nocturnal hemoglobinuria: evidence that the enzyme is absent from the cell membrane. Blood 1985; 66:940.

62. Low MG, Finean JB. Release of alkaline phosphatase from membranes by a phosphatidylinositol-specific phospholipase C. Biochem J 1977; 167:281.

63. Cross GAM. Glycolipid anchoring of plasma membrane proteins. Annu Rev Cell Biol 1990; 6:1.

64. Ferguson MAJ, Williams AF. Cell-surface anchoring of proteins via glycosylphosphatidylinositol structures. Ann Rev Biochem 1988; 57:285.

65. Englund PT. The structure and biosynthesis of glycosyl-phosphatidylinositol protein anchors. Ann Rev Biochem 1993; 62:121.

66. Takahashi M, Takeda J, Hirose S, Hyman R, Inoue N, Miyata T, Ueda E, Kitani T, Medof ME, Kinoshita T. Deficient biosynthesis of N-acetylglucosaminyl-phosphatidylinositol, the first intermediate of glycosyl phosphatidylinositol anchor biosynthesis, in cell lines established from patients with paroxysmal nocturnal hemoglobinuria. J Exp Med 1993; 177:517.

67. Hillmen P, Bessler M, Mason PJ, Watkins WM, Luzatto L. Specific defect in N-acetylglucosamine incorporation in the biosynthesis of the glycosylphosphatidylinositol anchor in cloned cell lines from patients with paroxysmal nocturnal hemoglobinuria. Proc Natl Acad Sci USA 1993; 90:5272.

68. Hirose S, Ravi L, Prince GM, Rosenfeld MG, Silber R, Andresen SW, Hazra SV, Medof ME. Synthesis of mannosylglucosaminylinositol phospholipids in normal but not paroxysmal nocturnal hemoglobinuria cells. Proc Natl Acad Sci USA 1992; 89:6025.

69. Hyman R. Somatic genetic analysis of the expression of cell surface molecules. Trends Genet 1988; 4:5.

70. Hillmen P, Bessler M, Crawford DH, Luzzatto L. Production and characterization of lymphoblastoid cell lines with the paroxysmal nocturnal hemoglobinuria phenotype. Blood 1993; 81:193.

71. Ueda E, Nishimura J, Kitani T, Nasu K, Kageyama T, Kim YU, Takeda J, Kinoshita T. Deficient surface expression of glycosylphosphatidylinositol-anchored proteins in B cell lines established from patients with paroxysmal nocturnal hemoglobinuria. Int Immunol 1992; 4:1263.

72. Norris J, Hall S, Ware RE, Kamitani T, Chang H-M, Yeh ETH, Rosse WF. Glycosylphosphatidylinositol anchor synthesis in paroxysmal nocturnal hemoglobinuria: partial or complete defect in an early step. Blood 1994; 83:816.

73. Takeda J, Miyata T, Kawagoe K, Iida Y, Endo Y, Fujita T, Takahashi M, Kitani T, Kinoshita T. Deficiency of the GPI anchor caused by a somatic mutation of the PIG-A gene in paroxysmal nocturnal hemoglobinuria. Cell 1993; 73:703.

74. Miyata T, Takeda J, Iida Y, Yamada N, Inoue N, Takahashi M, Maeda K, Kitani T, Kinoshita T. The cloning of PIG-A, a component in the early step of GPI-anchor biosynthesis. Science 1993; 259:1318.

75. Iida Y, Takeda J, Miyata T, Inoue N, Nishimura J, Kitani T, Maeda K, Kinoshita T. Characterization of genomic PIG-A gene: a gene for GPI-anchor biosynthesis and paroxysmal nocturnal hemoglobinuria. Blood 1994; 83:3126.

76. Bessler M, Hillmen P, Longo L, Luzzatto L, Mason PJ. Genomic organization of the X-linked gene (PIG-A) that is mutated in paroxysmal nocturnal haemoglobinuria and of a related autosomal pseudogene mapped to 12q21. Hum Mol Genet 1994; 3:751.

77. Ware RE, Howard TA, Kamitani T, Chang H-M, Yeh ETH, Seldin MF. Chromosomal assignment of genes involved in glycosylphosphatidylinositol anchor biosynthesis: implications for the pathogenesis of paroxysmal nocturnal hemoglobinuria. Blood 1994; 83:3753.

78. Miyata T, Yamada N, Iida Y, Nishimura J, Takeda J, Kitani T, Kinoshita T. Abnormalities of PIG-A transcripts in granulocytes from patients with paroxysmal nocturnal hemoglobinuria. N Engl J Med 1994; 330:249.

79. Bessler M, Mason PJ, Hillmen P, Miyata T, Yameda N, Takeda J, Luzzatto L, Kinoshita T. Paroxysmal nocturnal hemoglobinuria (PNH) is caused by somatic mutations in the PIG-A gene. EMBO J 1994; 13:110.

80. Bessler M, Mason P, Hillmen P, Luzzatto L. Somatic mutations and cellular selection in paroxysmal nocturnal haemoglobinuria. Lancet 1994; 343:951.

81. Bessler M, Mason PJ, Hillmen P, Luzzatto L. Mutations in the PIG-A gene causing partial deficiency of GPI-linked surface proteins (PNH II) in patients with paroxysmal nocturnal haemoglobinuria. B J Haematol 1994; 87:863.

82. Nafa K, Mason PJ, Hillmen P, Luzzatto L, Bessler M. Mutations in the PIG-A gene causing paroxysmal nocturnal hemoglobinuria are mainly of the frameshift type. Blood 1995; 86:4650.

83. Ware RE, Rosse WF, Howard TA. Mutations within the Pig-a gene in patients with paroxysmal nocturnal hemoglobinuria. Blood 1994; 83:2418.

84. Stafford HA, Nagarajan S, Weinberg JB, Medof ME. PIG-A, DAF and proto-oncogene expression in paroxysmal nocturnal haemoglobinuria-associated acute myelogenous leukaemia blasts. Br J Haematol 1995; 89:72.

85. Yamada N, Miyata T, Maeda K, Kitani T, Takeda J, Kinoshita T. Somatic mutations of the PIG-A gene found in Japanese patients with paroxysmal nocturnal hemoglobinuria. Blood 1995; 85:885.

86. Pramoonjago P, Wanachiwanawin W, Chinprasertsak S, Pattanapanayasat K, Takeda J, Kinoshita T. Somatic mutations of PIG-A in Thai patients with paroxysmal nocturnal hemoglobinuria: somatic mutations of PIG-A in Thai patients with paroxysmal nocturnal hemoglobinuria. Blood 1995; 86:1736.

87. Ostendorf T, Nischan C, Schubert J, Grussenmeyer T, Scholz C, Zielinska-Skowronek M, Schmidt RE. Heterogeneous PIG-A mutations in different cell lineages in paroxysmal nocturnal hemoglobinuria. Blood 1995; 85:1640.

88. Endo M, Ware RE, Vreeke TM, Singh SP, Howard TA, Tomita A, Holguin MH, Parker CJ. Molecular basis of the heterogeneity of expression of glycosyl phosphatidylinositol anchored proteins in paroxysmal nocturnal hemoglobinuria. Blood 1996; 87:2546.

89. Nagarajan S, Brodsky RA, Young NS, Medof ME. Genetic defects underlying paroxysmal nocturnal hemoglobinuria that arises out of aplastic anemia. Blood 1995; 86:4656.

90. Savoia A, Ianzano L, Lunardi C, De Sandre G, Carotenuto M, Musto P, Zelante L. Identification of three novel mutations in the PIG-A gene in paroxysmal nocturnal haemoglobinuria (PNH) patients. Hum Genet 1996; 97:45.

91. Nishimura J, Inoue N, Azenishi Y, Hirota T, Akaogi T, Shibano M, Kawagoe K, Ueda E, Machii T, Takeda J, Kinoshita T, Kitani T. Analysis of *pig-A* gene in a patient who developed reciprocal translocation of chromosome 12 and paroxysmal nocturnal hemoglobinuria during follow-up of aplastic anemia. Am J Hematol 1996; 51:229.

92. Huang AT, Mold NG, Zhang SF. Antithymocyte globulin stimulates human hematopoietic progenitor cells. Proc Natl Acad Sci USA 1987; 84:5942.

93. Nishimura J, Inoue N, Wada H, Ueda E, Pramoonjago P, Hirota T, Machii T, Kageyama T, Kanamaru A, Takeda J, Kinoshita T, Kitani T. A patient with paroxysmal nocturnal hemoglobinuria bearing four independent PIG-A mutant clones. Blood 1997; 89:3470.

94. Plesner T, Hansen NE, Carlsen K. Estimation of PI-bound proteins on blood cells from PNH patients by quantitative flow cytometry. Br J Haematol 1990; 75:585.

95. Kwong YL, Lee CP, Chan TK, Chan LC. Flow cytometric measurement of glycosylphosphatidyl-inositol-linked surface proteins on blood cells of patients with paroxysmal nocturnal hemoglobinuria. Am J Clin Pathol 1994; 102:30.

96. Leon WMM, Terstappen L, Nguyen M, Huang S, Lazarus H, Medof ME. Defective and normal hematopoietic stem cells in paroxysmal nocturnal hemoglobinuria. Br J Haematol 1993; 84:504.

97. Tseng JE, Hall SE, Howard TA, Ware RE. Phenotypic and functional analysis of lymphocytes in paroxysmal nocturnal hemoglobinuria. Am J Hematol 1995; 50:244.

98. Nagakura S, Nakakuma H, Horikawa K, Hidaka M, Kagimoto T, Kawakita M, Tomita M, Takatsuki K. Expression of decay-accelerating factor and CD59 in lymphocyte subsets of health individuals and paroxysmal nocturnal hemoglobinuria patients. Am J Hematol 1993; 43:14.

99. Jankovic S, Kraguljac N, Basara N, Donfrid M, Petrovic M. Paroxysmal nocturnal hemoglobinuria: golden standards vs. modern technologies [letter]. Am J Hematol 1995; 50:66.

100. Hillmen P, Lewis SM, Bessler M, Luzzatto L, Dacie JV. Natural history of paroxysmal nocturnal hemoglobinuria. N Engl J Med 1995; 333:1253.

101. Socie G, Mary J, De Gramont A, Rio B, Leporrier M, Rose C, Heudier P, Rochant H, Cahn J, Gluckman E. Paroxysmal nocturnal haemoglobinuria: long term follow-up and prognostic factors. Lancet 1996; 348:573.

102. Kruatrachue M, Wasi P, Nanakorn S. Paroxysmal nocturnal haemoglobinuria in Thailand with special reference to an association with aplastic anemia. B J Haematol 1978; 39:267.

103. Dunn P, Shih LY, Liaw SJ. Paroxysmal nocturnal hemoglobinuria: analysis of 40 cases. J Formos Med Assoc 1991; 90:831.

104. Dacie JV, Lewis SM. Paroxysmal nocturnal haemoglobinuria: variation in clinical severity and association with bone marrow hypoplasia. Br J Haematol 1961; 7:442.

105. Lewis SM, Dacie JV. The aplastic anaemia-paroxysmal nocturnal haemoglobinuria syndrome. Br J Haematol 1967; 13:236.

106. Rosse WF. Paroxysmal nocturnal haemoglobinuria in aplastic anaemia. Clin Haematol 1978; 7:541.

107. Kruatrachue M, Na-Nakorn S. Transient paroxysmal nocturnal hemoglobinuria during the course of aplastic anemia. J Med Assoc Thai 1974; 57:427.

108. Nissen C, Moser Y, dalle Carbonare V, Gratwohl A, Speck B. Complete recovery of marrow function after treatment with anti-lymphocyte globulin is associated with high, whereas early failure and development of paroxysmal nocturnal haemoglobinuria are associated with low endogenous G-CSA-release. Br J Haematol 1989; 72:573.

109. de Planque MM, Bacigalupo A, Wursch A, Hows JM, Devergie A, Frickhofen N. Brand A, Nissen C. Long-term follow-up of severe aplastic anaemia patients treated with antithymocyte globulin. Severe Aplastic Anaemia Working Party of the European Cooperative Group for Bone Marrow Transplantation (EBMT). Br J Haematol 1989; 73:121.

110. Schubert J, Vogt HG, Zielinska Skowronek, Freund M, Kaltwasser JP, Hoelzer D, Schmidt RE. Development of the glycosylphosphatidylinositol-anchoring defect characteristic for paroxysmal nocturnal hemoglobinuria in patients with aplastic anemia. Blood 1994; 83:2323.

111. Maciejewski JP, Hibbs JR, Anderson S, Katevas P, Young NS. Bone marrow and peripheral blood lymphocyte phenotype in patients with bone marrow failure. Exp Hematol 1994; 22:1102.

112. Frickhofen N, Liu JM, Young NS. Etiologic mechanisms of hematopoietic failure. [Review]. Am J Pediatr Hematol Oncol 1990; 12:385.

113. Baranski BG, Young NS. Autoimmune aspects of aplastic anemia. [Review]. In Vivo 1988; 2:91.

114. Dustin ML, Selvaraj P, Mattaliano RJ, Springer TA. Anchoring mechanisms for LFA-3 cell adhesion glycoprotein at membrane surface. Nature 1988; 329:846.

115. Kurosaki T, Ravetch JV. A single amino acid in the glycosyl phosphatidylinositol attachment domain determines the membrane topology of Fc gamma III. Nature 1989; 342:805.

116. Schubert J, Uciechowski P, Zielinska-Skowronek M, Tietjen C, Leo R, Schmidt RE. Differences in activation of normal and glycosylphosphatidylinositol-negative lymphocytes derived from patients with paroxysmal nocturnal hemoglobinuria. J Immunol 1992; 148:3814.

117. Yonemura Y, Kawakita M, Koito A, Kawaguchi T, Nakakuma H, Kagimoto T, Schichishima T, Terasawa T, Akagaki Y, Inai S. Paroxysmal nocturnal haemoglobinuria with coexisting deficiency of the ninth component of complement: lack of massive haemolytic attack. Br J Haematol 1990; 74:108.

118. Firkin F, Goldberg H, Firkin BG. Glucocorticoid management of paroxysmal nocturnal hemoglobinuria. Aust Ann Med 1968; 17:127.

119. Rosse WF. Treatment of paroxysmal nocturnal hemoglobinuria. Blood 1982; 60:20.

120. Kawahara K, Witherspoon RP, Storb R. Marrow transplantation for paroxysmal nocturnal hemoglobinuria. Am J Hematol 1992; 39:283.

121. Antin JR, Ginsburg D, Smith BR, Nathan DG, Orkin SH, Rappeport JM. Bone marrow transplantation for paroxysmal nocturnal hemoglobinuria: eradication of the PNH clone and documentation of complete lymphohematopoietic engraftment. Blood 1985; 66:1247.

122. Fefer A, Freeman H, Storb R, Hill J, Singer J, Edwards A, Thomas ED. Paroxysmal nocturnal hemoglobinuria and marrow failure treated by infusion of marrow from an identical twin. Ann Intern Med 1976; 84:692.

123. Hänsch GM, Schoenermark S, Roelcke D. Paroxysmal nocturnal hemoglobinuria type III. Lack of an erythrocyte membrane protein restricting the lysis of C5b-9. J Clin Invest 1987; 80:7.

124. Selvaraj P, Rosse WF, Silber R, Springer TA. The major Fc receptor in blood has a phosphatidylinositol anchor and is deficient in paroxysmal nocturnal haemoglobinuria. Nature 1988; 333:565.

125. Ploug M, Plesner T, Ronne E, Ellis V, Hoyer Hansen G, Hansen NE, Dano K. The receptor for urokinase-type plasminogen activator is deficient on peripheral blood leukocytes in patients with paroxysmal nocturnal hemoglobinuria. Blood 1992; 79:1447.

126. Simmons DL, Tan S, Tenen DG, Nicholson-Weller A, Seed B. Monocyte antigen CD14 is a phospholipid anchored membrane protein. Blood 1989; 73:284.

127. Antony AC. The biological chemistry of folate receptors. Blood 1992; 79:2807.

128. Selvaraj P, Dustin ML, Silber R, Low MG, Springer TA. Deficiency of lymphocyte function-associated antigens 3 (LFA-3) in paroxysmal nocturnal hemoglobinuria. Functional correlates and evidence for a phosphatidylinositol membrane anchor. J Exp Med 1987; 166:1011.

129. Nagakura S, Kawagauchi T, Horikawa K, Hidaka M, Iwamoto N, Takasuki K, Nakakuma H. A deficiency of CDw52 (Campath-1 antigen) of paroxysmal nocturnal hemoglobinuria lymphocytes. Blood 1993; 82:3790.

130. Bobolis KA, Moulds JJ, Telen MJ. Isolation of the JMH antigen on a novel phosphatidylinositol-linked human membrane protein. Blood 1992; 79:1574.

131. Mudad R, Rao N, Angelisova P, Horejsi V, Telen MJ. Evidence that CDw108 membrane protein bears the JMH blood group antigen. Transfusion 1995; 35:566.

132. Sammar M, Aigner S, Hubbe M, Schirrmacher V, Schachner M, Vestweber D, Altevogt P. Heat-stable antigen (CD24) as ligand for mouse P-selectin. Int Immunol 1994; 6:1027.

133. Mayne KM, Pulford K, Jones M, Micklem K, Nagel G, van der Schoot CE, Mason DY. Antibody By114 is selective for the 90 kD PI-linked component of the CD66 antigen; a new reagent for the study of paroxysmal nocturnal haemoglobinuria. Br J Haematol 1993; 83:30.

134. Rao N, Udani M, Nelson J, Reid ME, Telen MJ. Investigations using a novel monoclonal antibody to the glycosylphosphatidylinositol-anchored protein that carries Gregory, Holley, and Dombrock blood group antigens. Transfusion 1995; 35:459.

135. Misumi Y, Ogata S, Ohkubo K, Hirose S, Ikehara Y. Primary structure of human placental 5'-nucleotidase and identification of the glycolipid anchor in the mature form. Eur J Biochem 1990; 181:563.
136. Rosse WF. Paroxysmal nocturnal hemoglobinuria as a molecular disease. Medicine (in press) 1997; 76:63.

23

Complement System in Central Nervous System Disorders

MOON L. SHIN, HOREA RUS, and FLORIN NICULESCU

University of Maryland at Baltimore, School of Medicine, Baltimore, Maryland

I. INTRODUCTION

Complement activation constitutes an effective host defense mechanism during early infection by generating effectors involved in cell death and immune/inflammatory responses. Activation of early-acting proteins of the complement cascade generates proteolytic peptides with inflammatory and opsonic activities. Activation of late-acting proteins results in sequential assembly of terminal complement complexes (TCC), which include C5b-7, C5b-8, and C5b-9 in the membrane. C5b-8 and C5b-9 are pore-forming complexes with cytotoxic activity. As it occurs outside of the central nervous system (CNS), complement activation is expected to generate inflammatory and cytotoxic effectors in the CNS affected by immune and inflammatory disorders. Cells of the CNS such as neurons, astrocytes, microglia, or oligodendrocytes, however, may respond to the complement effectors in a cell-specific manner. Futhermore, breakdown of the bloody–brain barrier (BBB) and/or glia cell activation by cytokines will likely cause transient increase in complement proteins within the CNS, where the constitutive complement levels are very low. Therefore, it is important to understand the molecular and functional consequences of complement activation affecting different types of cells involved in specific CNS diseases, which include multiple sclerosis, various encephalitis, Alzheimer's disease, Parkinson's disease, and stroke.

In the past, our laboratory has been focused to study the effect of TCC on immune-mediated demyelination by exploring the mechanisms of TCC generation within the CNS and the effects of TCC on myelin and the myelin-producing oligodendrocytes. At present, we are beginning to understand the membrane signaling pathways initiated by TCC, in part, due to the rapid progress made to elucidate the molecular, biochemical, and cellular mechanisms involved in signaling, in general. In the absence of cell death, TCC have been shown to stimulate various biological activities in target cells, through diverse membrane signaling. These include increased cytosolic Ca^{2+} and protein kinase C activity, generation of cAMP, and lipid-derived signal messengers such as sn-1,2-diacylglycerol and ceramide. TCC also activate heterotrimeric G proteins of the Gi/Go subfamily, and the downstream kinases ERK1 and JNK. Thus, it is also critical to understand the signaling mechanisms responsible for the specific CNS disorders mediated by complement.

II. COMPLEMENT PROTEINS IN THE CENTRAL NERVOUS TISSUE

Proteins of the complement system in blood may enter the CNS compartment when the BBB is disturbed under pathological conditions, which include inflammatory, infectious, and vascular CNS disorders. Very small amounts of complement proteins are also found in human cerebrospinal fluid (CSF) in the absence of any damage to BBB and they are produced locally by the cells of the CNS. Individual complement components in normal CSF have been measured by using the hemolytic functional assay (Table 1) (1). The functional activity of individual components is not stable in normal CSF even at $-70°C$ and the spontaneous decay can be prevented by adding gelatin during storage (1). Total CSF complement activity is about 0.23% (1/450) of the serum level, while individual titers are variable, ranging from 0.15% for C1, to 1.34% for C7, of the corresponding serum level. Glial cells of the CNS are able to express some of the complement genes constitutively. Complement genes are also inducible in glial cells by inflammatory stimuli, such as cytokines, LPS, and viruses. Primary rodent astrocytes can synthesize in vitro many components of the classical and the alternative pathway proteins, including C2, C3, C4, C5–C9, factor B, and regulatory proteins factors H and I, C4bp, S-protein, and clusterin (2–8). Astrocytes also express complement membrane inhibitors DAF, MCP, and CD59 (9), in addition to CR1, CR2, and C5a receptor, but not CR3 (10,11). There is very little information on complement protein synthesis in microglia, oligodendrocytes, neurons, and CNS endothelial cells.

Expression of complement genes and protein secretion studied in primary astrocytes and astrocytoma-derived cell lines are markedly upregulated in response to various stimuli. Enhanced expression of the transcripts and proteins induced by proinflammatory cytokines or LPS is much more rapid in primary astrocytes occurring within 10 h, compared to the 24–48 h requirement to obtain similar effects in astrocytoma cell lines (2–4). Complement protein synthesis, specifically C3, is markedly enhanced in astrocytes by TNFα, IL-1β, and IL-8, whereas other proinflammatory cytokines IL-1α and IL-6 are ineffective (3). In

Table 1 Complement Hemolytic Activities in CSF

Hemolytic activities	CSF (n = 7) (mean ± SD)		NHS	NHS/CSF ratio
Total complement (CH50 u/ml)	1.26 ±	0.29	550	436
C1	78.0 ±	18.7[a]	51,300[a]	658
C4	368	± 180	66,000	179
C2	3.72 ±	0.91	683	184
C3	63.5 ±	11.0	17,300	272
C5	222	± 42.8	116,000	523
C6	237	± 79.5	114,000	481
C7	1262	± 269	94,100	74.5
C8	111	± 32.7	61,500	554
C9	107	± 19.2	26,200	245

NHS, pooled normal human serum.
[a] Site-forming units per milliliter.
Source: From Ref. 1.

addition, IFN-γ, which is unable to upregulate C3 in macrophages and hepatocytes (12), is remarkably effective in inducing enhanced C3 expression in astrocytes and astrocytoma cell lines (3,4). The C3 and other complement protein expression is also enhanced by LPS, which is mediated, in part, by inducing cytokines (3). Newcastle disease virus is also capable of inducing C3, which requires PKC activities unlike the PKC-independent C3 induction mediated by cytokines (3). Pretreatment of astrocytes with TGF-β1 for 2 h abolished the enhancing effect of C3 synthesis by TNFα, IL-1β, and IFN-γ and the inhibition persisted at least for 72h (13). These data indicate that significant upregulation of endogenous synthesis of complement proteins by the glial cells can occur during infectious, inflammatory, and immune-mediated diseases involving the CNS and TGF-β1 may act as a regulatory cytokine to inhibit the amplification of protein synthesis in situ.

III. COMPLEMENT SYNTHESIS IN DEMYELINATION DISORDERS

A. Introduction

Multiple sclerosis (MS) represents a major prototype of demyelinating diseases of the CNS in human. MS is considered as an immune-mediated disease in which myelin and the myelin-producing oligodendrocytes (OLG) are the targets of autoimmune attack. The mechanisms governing myelin breakdown and OLG cell death are still not clearly understood. Experimental evidence indicate that myelin proteins act as autoantigens in perpetuating the immune response (14). Encephalitogenic antigen presentation and generation of chemotactic signal within the CNS together with adhesion molecules expressed or upregulated in cerebrovascular endothelium are thought to be essential requirements for antigen-specific CD4+ T cells to accumulate and initiate the characteristic inflammation. Subsequent myelin membrane destruction, known as primary demyelination, may occur following activation of antigen-independent effectors, including macrophages, cytotoxic T cells, and their products, in addition to the complement system (14). T cells reactive to antigenic determinants of myelin basic proteins (MBP) are found in patients with MS, and T cells carrying rearranged T-cell receptor with MBP reactivity are present within the MS lesion with higher frequency than in T cells present in other CNS inflammatory lesions (15). Antimyelin antibodies produced in patients following the development of cellular immune response can elicit antibody-mediated myelin destruction by activating complement in the CNS with damaged BBB. In fact, antibodies to myelin proteins like MBP and myelin oligodendrocyte glycoproteins (MOG) have been detected in MS patients (16,17). Complement may also participate in myelin damage in the absence of myelin-specific antibodies, since both myelin and OLG directly activate the classical pathway of complement in vitro (18). While it remains to be determined whether all of the complement proteins are constitutively synthesized in the CNS, significant complement activation by myelin or OLG may not occur in the absence of BBB damage, because activated complement proteins or complexes are not detected in normal brains.

The role of complement in immune-mediated inflammatory demyelination has been studied extensively during the last decade. In antibody-mediated demyelination, the requirement of complement activation has been unequivocally demonstrated in CNS tissue explant models (19,20), using serum from patients with MS, antibodies to myelin, or myelin proteins (18–21). The requirement of complement activation in demyelination has also been demonstrated in in vivo system, experimental allergic encephalitis (EAE), an animal model for MS induced by immunization with antigenic myelin proteins and peptides (22,23). Activation of complement has been shown to play a critical role even in EAE induced by adaptive transfer of antigen-specific T cells in animals in which antimyelin antibodies are not generated (23).

In following section, we will review experimental evidence derived from in vitro and in vivo studies and studies in MS patients that implicate an active role of complement activation and assembly of terminal complement complexes (TCC) involved in myelin destruction.

B. In Vitro Demyelination by Activation of Terminal Complement Complexes

The requirement of humoral factors in demyelination is studied in vitro by using myelinated CNS explant cultures, prepared by culturing tissue slices of neonatal cerebellum or spinal cord until most axons are myelinated (19,20). Earlier studies showed that myelinated explants treated with serum from MS patients or EAE animals, as well as antimyelin antibodies undergo extensive vesicular fragmentation of myelin sheets and this process requires the presence of fresh serum. The in vitro demyelination requires IgG and IgM isotypes of antibodies and fresh serum as a source of complement, suggesting an involvement of membrane attack complex of complement in myelin membrane damage. To study the role of membrane attack complex of complement in antibody-mediated demyelination, myelinated rat cerebellar explants were incubated with rabbit IgM against guinea pig spinal cord in the presence of C8-deficient human serum (C8D) with or without C8 reconstitution (21). Activation of complement up to C7 failed to cause significant myelin vesiculation, whereas addition of C8 to C8D to form C5b-9 induced extensive myelin vesiculation when examined 20 h later. Removal of antibody and complement after 2 h failed to reduce myelin vesiculation (21), suggesting the biochemical changes required for demyelination are initiated by C5b-9 within 2h. Although isolated myelin and OLG can activate C1 and generate C5b-9 in vitro (24–29), a topic to be discussed further in this chapter, antibodies to spinal cord, myelin, or to galactocerebroside (GC) appear to be required for complement to induce significant demyelination in explant cultures. To achieve in vitro demyelination, which is identified as massive myelin vesiculation, the effector requirement may differ from those required for in vivo demyelination. To induce myelin vesiculation in the explants may require unusually large number of C5b-9 assembly in the absence of activated macrophages, which may function as a potent in vivo effector by phagocytosing myelin that has been opsonized and damaged by complement attack. In fact, consumption of serum complement by myelin can be increased 50–100-fold in the presence of antimyelin antibody (Fig. 1a). Extensive demyelination of CNS explants induced by antibody and complement is not associated with extensive OLG cell death, since active myelin synthesis takes place 12 h following demyelination. This was shown by a twofold increase in membrane lipid synthesis over the control in myelin membrane fractions prepared from explant cultures labeled with [^{14}C]oleic acid for 4 days after demyelination (Liu and Shin, unpublished observation).

C. Effect of Complement Activation on Myelin and Oligodendrocytes

Mechanisms of demyelination mediated by terminal complement complexes are explored in vitro using isolated myelin and primary cultures of OLG.

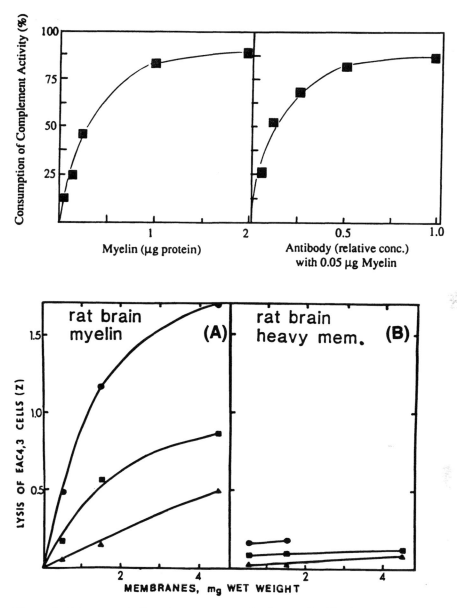

Figure 1 Upper panel: Complement consumption by myelin. Varying concentrations of myelin purified from adult human spinal cord were incubated with diluted human serum for 45 min at 37°C. Myelin was centrifuged and the supernatants were assayed for the residual complement activity on sheep erythrocytes sensitized with antibody (left panel). Right panel shows identical experiments performed with 0.05 μg myelin previously incubated with rabbit antiserum against human myelin. Consumption of serum complement is expressed as percentage consumed from the hemolytic activity of the serum incubated in buffer without myelin as 100%. Lower panel: C1 activation by CNS myelin. Myelin membranes (A) and heavy membranes (B) from adult rat brains were tested for C1 activation. Membranes were incubated with various dilutions of C2-deficient serum as a source of C1 for 45 min and at 37°C. Membranes were washed and mixed with sheep erythrocytes (1.5×10^7) carrying C4b and C3b but not C1 and C2 (EAC4,3) for 15 min at 30°C. Cells were further incubated with C2 for 10 min, then lysed with excess C3 and C5–C9. Although myelin binds and activates C1, no detectable C1 activity was observed with the nonmyelin membranes. C2-D serum dilutions used: ●, 1:1,000; ■ 1:3,000; ▲, 1:9,000. Z value represents the average number of lytic sites per cell. (From Ref. 24.)

1. Activation of Complement by Myelin and Oligodendrocytes

When myelin purified from adult human spinal cord and rat or rabbit brains was incubated with fresh serum, consumption of total hemolytic activity and complement components, C3 cleavage, and C5b-9 assembly occurred in the absence of antibody (21,24–26), Complement activation by CNS myelin is mediated by activation of C1 (24,25,27) (Fig. 1B). The C1-activating molecules are not fully characterized. When myelin proteins separated by sodium dodecyl sulfate–polyacrylamide gel electrophoresis (SDS-PAGE), are transferred onto nitrocellulose membranes, and the membranes exposed to C1q and reacted with anti-C1q IgG, two sets of immunoreactive bands are found, migrating as 58–56 and 46–45 kDa (27). Upper bands representing Wolfgram 2 doublets (?CNPase) are also stained immunochemically when incubated with normal human serum, followed by anti-C3 IgG. There is no evidence indicating that the immunoreactive lower bands also activate C1. Biological significance of complement activation by myelin is speculative. In view of the finding that complement components, especially C1, C5, C6, and C8 in normal CSF, are very low (1), but glial cells are capable of producing most if not all of the complement proteins in response to inflammatory cytokines and bacterial or viral infection (3–5), The increase in complement in the CNS may occur in inflammation, infection and vascular injury by regional complement synthesis and/or influx of serum. Under such condition, complement activation by myelin and OLG may have a significant biological consequences.

Primary oligodendrocytes isolated from rat brain can activate complement through the classical pathway, as in the case of myelin. The activation takes place in heterologous as well as homologous complement, and leads to the assembly of C5b-9 in OLG in the absence of antibody (28,29)(Fig. 2). It is significant to note that differentiated oligodendro-

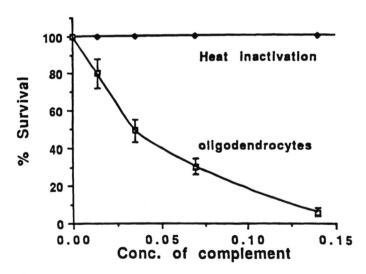

Figure 2 Activation of complement by oligodendrocytes and its effect on OLG survival. Oligodendrocytes exposed to complement in the absence of additional antibodies were lysed, but cells were not lysed by heat-inactivated complement. The ED_{50} for oligodendrocytes occurred at a concentration of 0.03 (1.0 = undiluted Buxted rabbit complement). Data points represent the mean ± SEM of three experiments, in each of which triplicate determinations were made. (From Ref. 29.)

cytes are susceptible to the lysis by homologous and also by heterologous complement, whereas perinatal O-2A progenitor, type 1 and 2 astrocytes, are resistant to the complement-mediated lysis (28,29).

2. Effects of Terminal Complement Complex Assembly on Myelin

Immunologically mediated demyelination in vivo first manifests as separation of myelin lamellae as a result of loss of myelin compaction. This process is followed by loss of myelin proteins, especially myelin-associated glycoprotein (MAG) and MBP (30–33). Loss of MBP, proteolipid protein (PLP), in CNS myelin and P0 and PLP in peripheral nervous system (PNS) myelin have significant implications since these proteins are the major structural proteins essential for myelin membrane compaction by forming homoligands. Therefore, loss of structural integrity of myelin by complement-induced hydrolysis of MBP and P0 would further enhance the vulnerability of myelin to the damage caused by macrophages and macrophage-derived enzymes (33,34). The appearance of macrophages and macrophages containing phagocytosed myelin still showing immunoreactive MBP that is observed in very early and active MS lesions is highly significant (35). Macrophages remaining in resolving and older lesions may still show myelin figures containing no longer immunoreactive MBP (36). These data collectively indicate that the opsonization of myelin by C3b/iC3b and myelin attack by C5b-9 are synergistic with the effector functions of macrophages in achieving demyelination.

To study the mechanisms of complement-mediated myelin damage, myelin protein hydrolysis was studied in detail using resealed, multilayered myelin vesicles prepared from human myelin (37). Treatment of myelin vesicles with C5b-8 or C5b-9 induced a similar degree of Ca^{2+}-dependent MBP hydrolysis, as assessed by SDS-PAGE and densitometric quantitation of MBP fragments (37)(Table 2). The PNS myelin treated with complement produced P0 hydrolysis in a similar manner to those of CNS MBP hydrolysis (38)(Table 2). About 1/3 of MBP hydrolysis inducible by C5b-9 was due to the effect of C5b-7, which did not require Ca^2. When a synthetic neutral protease inhibitor E64 was added before sealing myelin, Ca^{2+}-dependent MBP hydrolysis induced by C5b-9 was abolished (Table 2). The finding indicates that Ca^{2+} influx through C5b-8/C5b-9 pores in myelin can cause MBP and P0 hydrolysis through activation of Ca^{2+}-dependent neutral proteases (18,37). Hydrolysis of MBP in myelin was also induced by large granular lymphocyte granules containing perforin and granzymes. The enzymatic activity to hydrolyze MBP was found to be predominantly in granzyme A and by tumor necrosis factor (38,39). In addition, neutral proteases such as cathepsin A derived from macrophages also induce myelin protein hydrolysis in unsealed myelin and this process is enhanced in the presence of complement activation (34). It should also be considered that C5b-7, C5b-8, and C5b-9 can cause proteolysis of myelin proteins and this process can be enhanced by C5b-9 channels allowing the entry of other proteolytic enzymes released from macrophages and glial cells in situ.

The number and size of C5b-9 channels, which affect the outcome of complement attack on myelin, are regulated by the complement-regulatory proteins expressed on myelin. Human CNS and PNS myelin are deficient in DAF (CD55) and MCP (CD46), where as they express CD59 (40) (Fig. 3). Blocking CD59 with neutralizing anti-CD59 IgG increased poly C9 formation by fivefold over the level of untreated human myelin after exposure to NHS (40). Thus, complement activation on myelin is likely to be enhanced at the level of C3 and C5 cleavage due to the absence of DAF and MCP, whereas

Table 2 Hydrolysis of Myelin Proteins by TCC is Inhibited by E64 (Expoxyxuccinyllecucylamido Butane), a Neutral Protease Inhibitor

Area under MBP peak

	C7D-HS	C7D-HS + C7	% hydrolysis by TCC
1	2.81 ± 0.025	2.28 ± 0.025	18.9
2 Me$_2$SO	12.39 ± 0.72	10.32 ± 0.09	17.0
2 E64/Me$_2$SO	12.72 ± 0.45	13.11 ± 0.7	0.0

Area under PO peak

	C5b6	C5b-9	% hydrolysis by TCC
1	67.3 ± 4.4	47.8 ± 2.9	28.9
2 E64/Me$_2$SO	65.7 ± 1.3	61.7 ± 3.5	6.1
2 EGTA	64.6 ± 2.1	63.6 ± 2.4	1.5

Resealed CNS (top) or PNS (bottom) myelin vesicles were made in 0.02 mM Ca^{2+} (top, 1, bottom, 1), 0.02 mM Ca^{2+}/0.05% Me$_2$SO (top, 2), 0.02 mM Ca^{2+}/100μ ME 64 dissolved in 0.05% Me$_2$SO (top, 3, bottom, 2), and 0.1 mM EGTA (bottom, 3). CNS myelin in triplicate was incubated for 30 min at 37°C with C5b6 complex or with C5b6 plus C7, C8, and C9 for 30 min at 37°C (bottom). The remaining MBP or P0 in myelin was assessed by SDS-PAGE and densitometric analysis of the Coomassie blue-stained MBP and P0 bands. The percentage TCC-mediated breakdown of MBP and P0 was estimated using the values of C7D-HS- or C5b6-treated vesicles as 100% for CNS and PNS myelin, respectively.
Source: From Ref. 18.

the number of C5b-9 assembly in myelin and the size of C5b-9 channels are restricted by CD59, as in other cells (40).

3. Effects of Terminal Complement Complex Assembly on Oligodendrocytes

A decrease in surviving OLG in chronic MS plaques has been well documented. However, OLG in early MS lesion display proliferative and remyelinating activity (41). The regenerating activity of OLG in MS is considered as transient, since denuded axons remyelinated by OLG show incomplete myelination and remyelinated tissues become new targets for immune attack (42). Remyelination can also be achieved by OLG derived from de novo differentiation of adult O-2A cells, the OLG progenitors that persist in adult CNS (41,42). Oligodendrocytes and O-2A progenitors are both susceptible to lysis by C5b-9, even when complement is activated directly without OLG-specific antibody (28,29). The cause of lytic susceptibility of OLG to both heterologous and homologous complement is unknown. Incorporation of human CD59 in rat OLG substantially increased the survival from human complement attack and this protection was reversed by anti-CD59 antibody (44). In contrast to rat OLG, human OLG that express CD59 are shown to be more resistant to lysis by human serum (45). This latter finding is in agreement with the presence of CD59 in human CNS and PNS myelin (40), produced by OLG and Schwann cells, respectively. Therefore, quantitative studies of complement regulatory protein expression such as CD59, DAF, MCP, and CR1 on OLG, myelin, and other CNS cells are required to evaluate the relative lytic susceptibility to C5b-9 and also to the nonlethal effects of C5b-9.

Interaction of TCC with the plasma membranes activates multiple signaling pathways. All of the C5b-7, C5b-8, and C5b-9 complexes, collectively referred to as TCC,

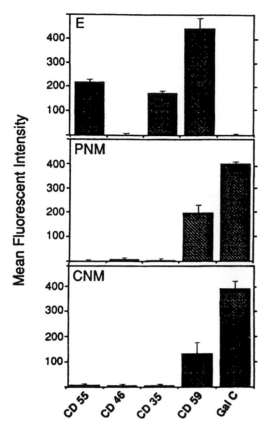

Figure 3 Relative expression of complement-regulatory proteins on membrane vesicles from human myelin and human erythrocytes. Central nerve myelin (CNM) and periphral nerve myelin (PNM) from human myelin membrane were prepared by sealing the purified myelin membrane. Vesicles smaller than erythrocytes were discarded by centrifugation method. Membrane vesicles of human erythrocyte ghost (E) were also prepared and resealed. Vesicles were stained and analyzed by FACS. The specific shift in mean fluorescence intensity on FACS analysis for CD55 (DAF), CD46 (MCP), CD35 (CRI), CD59, or galactocerebroside is presented as a histogram. Data represent the specific fluorescent after substraction of the value of an irrelevant isotype Ab. Data for each membrane preparation are expressed as mean ± SD values (n=4). The PNM and CNM expressed only CD59 and a myelin marker galactocerebroside, whereas erythrocyte membranes expressed CD55, CD35, and CD59, but not galactocerebroside. (From Ref. 40.)

are able to activate trimeric G-proteins (46), and generate DAG and ceramide (47). The effect of TCC, not observed at the stage of C5b6 formation, reaches the maximum at the stage of C5b-9 assembly. Activation of PKC, which occurs in response to C5b-8 and C5b-9, is in part, mediated by Ca^{2+} influx (48–50) and this signal pathway is responsible for arachidonic acid mobilization (49,51). Studies on signaling pathways by which sublytic C5b-9 induces functional and molecular changes in OLG have been limited. The effects of Ca^{2+} influx and PKC activation during sublytic C5b-9 attack have been studied with primary rat OLG and also in a C6 glioma-OLG hybrid cell line (52,53). OLG prelabled with [^{14}C]arachidonic acid and treated with anti-GC and C6D-serum reconstituted with sublytic C6 produced leukotriene E_4, leukotriene B_4, and 15-hydroxyeicosatetraenoic acid, as determined by thin layer chromatography and high-performance liquid chromatography (HPLC) (52). When OLG cell death and leukotriene B_4 production were examined as a function of C5b-9 numbers, leukotriene B_4 released in response to a sublytic dose of C5b-9 was about 500pg/5 $\times$ 10^5 cells, whereas less than 200pg was produced by either four or eight times more C5b-9, which induced 50 and 60% cell death, respectively (Fig. 4) (53). Therefore, the arachidonic acid-derived inflammatory mediators are produced by surviving OLG following C5b-9 attack. Arachidonic acid mobilization induced by C5b-9 in OLG is PKC-dependent, and requires Ca^{2+}, and this process is inhibited by Pertussis toxin. The data indicate that the PKC activation is mediated by two signal messengers: a significant Ca^{2+} influx through C5b-9 channels (48) and DAG generated by C5b-7, C5b-8, and C5b-9 through activation of Pertussis toxin-sensitive G proteins, as shown in human B lymphoblastoid cell line (46,47). The lipid-derived inflammatory mediators produced by OLG may have a significant implication by amplifying the inflammatory cascade.

In addition to the generation of inflammatory mediators, sublytic complement attack also induces the repair process of OLG by eliminating through shedding the potentially lethal C5b-9 complexes from the plasma membrane, as shown in many cell types (54–56). We have also found that the surviving OLG following complement attack express markedly reduced levels of myelin protein mRNAs, especially those encoding MBP and PLP, but not a minor myelin protein CNPase or β-actin (57)(Fig. 5a). The complement effect on myelin mRNAs appears as early as 1h, reaches the maximum at 3h, and is detected at 24h. The expression of MBP and PLP mRNA was similarly reduced in rat OLG exposed to serum complement derived from human or rat (57,58). Such quantitatively similar

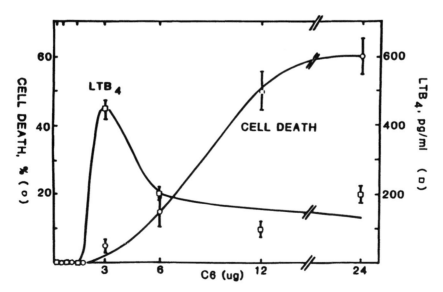

Figure 4 Dose–response of leukotriene B_4(LTB$_4$) from oligodendrocytes and cell death by C5b-9. Oligondendrocytes (OLG) (5 $\times$ 10^5 cells) were treated with C6-deficient serum (C6D) plus varying doses of C6 for 1 h at 37°C. Specific cytolysis of OLG (○) and release of LTB$_4$(□) were determined by vital dye uptake and radioimmunoassay, respectively. The LTB$_4$ released by C6D was subtracted to give the TCC-specific release. (From Ref. 52.)

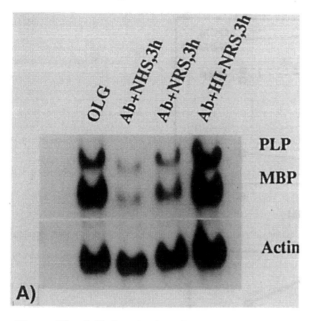

Figure 5A Sublytic activation of rat and human serum complement reduced PLP and MBP mRNA expression in rat OLG. Primary rat OLG cultured in defined serum-free medium were incubated with anti-GC Ab, then with 1/10 dilutions of normal human serum (NHS) or rat serum (NRS) on heat-inactivated rat serum (HI-NRS) for 3 h at 37°C. Total RNA was isolated and PLP and MBP mRNA expression was determined by Northern blot analysis. Expression of β-actin mRNA was used as a control. (From Ref. 58.)

effects were also seen in TCC-mediated signaling of DAG generation and activation of G proteins in human B cell lines with or without the expression of homologous complement restriction proteins DAF and CD59 (46,47). Therefore, the mechanisms of TCC-mediated signaling in homologous and heterologous system differ from the cell death pathway induced by TCC; all of the TCC complexes can elicit G-protein initiated membrane signaling, whereas cell death is primarily affected by the C5b-9 channel, its pore size and Ca^{2+} influx (see review in 59). The use of C7D serum to determine the role of TCC showed that MBP and PLP mRNA downregulation was achieved only when C7D-serum was reconstituted with C7 to from C5b-9 and this effect was not affected by a RNA-polymerase II inhibitor, α-amanitin (57)(Fig. 5b). These data indicate that C5b-9 enhances selective myelin mRNA degradation by destabilizing otherwise stable mRNAs. Limited investigation of signaling required for the enhanced myelin mRNA decay showed that the PLP mRNA downregulation was influenced by Ca^{2+} influx and the MBP mRNA decay was sensitive to cAMP and cGMP-dependent protein kinases inhibitors (57). At present, the effect of TCC on myelin gene transcription has not been explored. Concomitant with downregulation of myelin genes, complement activation on OLG induces expression of protooncogenes c-jun, c-fos and jun D, and increases AP-1 DNA-binding activity (58). Since these protooncogenes are important regulatory promoters of cell cycle entry and cell cycle progression, whether C5b-9 can induce OLG to reenter the cell cycle through protooncogene activation has been examined. DNA synthesis in OLG is significantly increased in response to anti-GC and NHS, as well as in OLG treated with sublytic C5b-

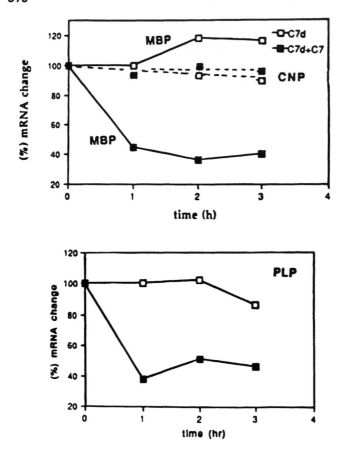

Figure 5B   C5b-9 induces enhanced mRNA degradation encoding PLP and MBP in oligodendrocytes. In the presence of 5 μg/ml transcriptional inhibitor α-amanitin, antibody-sensitized rat oligodendrocytes were incubated with human C7D or C7D plus a sublytic dose of C7 for 1, 2, and 3 h at
37°C. The remaining myelin proteins mRNA encoding in the presence of α-amanitin were evaluated
by Northern blot analysis. The density ratios were obtained using β-actin mRNA and expressed as
the percentage decrease from 0 h, which was identical to 1 h incubation in C7D. Cyclic nucleotide
phosphodiesterase (CNP) mRNA was not significantly changed, as determined by CNP mRNA to
β-actin ratio. (From Ref. 57.)

9 assembled with purified proteins (58) (Fig. 6a). Oligodendrocytes differentiated in vitro
for 3 days are resting cells in G1/G0 phase, and induction into S-phase entry occurs
between 10–12 h with the S phase activity sustaining at least for 24 h. Anti-GC antibody
alone or preactivated C5b-9 had no effect. The DNA synthesis induced by serum is further
increased in the presence of TCC assembly. The role of c-jun on DNA synthesis was
assessed by pretreating OLG with antisense c-jun oligonucleotide. Antisense c-jun, but
not sense c-jun oligonucleotide, completely abolished the thymidine incorporation induced
by complement activation as well as that induced by the serum (58) (Fig. 6b). These
findings indicate that C5b-9 assembly induces the cell cycle in OLG to enter the S phase
in a c-jun dependent pathway. The promoter/enhancer of genes such as thymidine kinase,
histone H3.2, and proliferating cell nuclear antigen, all involved in G1-S transition phase,

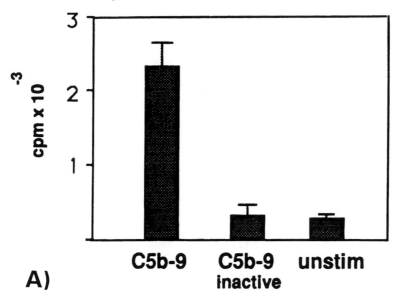

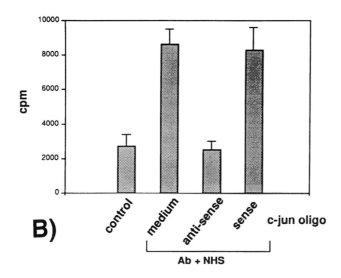

Figure 6   DNA synthesis in OLG induced by C5b-9. (A) OLG were incubated 18 h in the presence of [^{3}H]thymidine with C5b-9 formed by sequential addition of purified C5b6, C7, C8, and C9 or with previously inactivated C5b-9. (B) OLG were preincubated for 4 h with 20 μM antisense c-jun (anti-sense), sense c-jun oligonucleotides (sense), or medium alone. Cells were then sensitized with anti-GC antibodies, and treated with normal human serum for 18 h, an incubation time previously determined by kinetic experiments, in the presence of [^{3}H]thymidine. Treatment with antibody alone did not increase the thymidine uptake. Results represent the mean ± SEM from three separate experiments performed in triplicates (From Ref. 58.)

are known to have AP-1-binding sites (60,61). Although OLG have been considered "terminally differentiated cells" incapable of mitotic division, active DNA synthesis has been observed in cells that remain attached to the axons in lesions of CNS trauma (62,63). Stimulation of OLG to enter the S phase by C5b-9 is associated with cell cycle—associated kinase activation. cdc2 and cdk4 kinases, important for the G1 progression and G1/S transition, respectively, are increased in OLG following C5b-9 assembly in mid G1 phase for cdc2 and in late G1 and G1/S transition phase for Cdk4 activity (58) (Fig. 7). Despite the S phase entry, proliferation of OLG has not been observed following complement attack. Instead, we have found that sublytic C5b-9 prevents OLG from apoptosis in cultures. Oligodendrocytes cultured in defined medium undergo spontaneously apoptosis even in the presence of trophic factors (64,65). The nuclei of 52 ± 0.5% of OLG grown in defined medium for 72 h, were positive for apoptosis, as determined by TUNEL method, whereas treatment of OLG with C5b-9 for 18 h reduced the apoptotic cells to 33 ± 2.5% cells with apoptotic changes (Fig. 8). Similar results were obtained with OLG treated with anti-GC and NHS or HI-NHS (Table 3) (58). Thus, stimulation of OLG by C5b-9 appears to inhibit the apoptotic signals or produce trophic factors for OLG. PDGF, a trophic factor for OLG, is induced by C5b-9 (66). Protooncogene expression, enhanced myelin protein mRNA decay, and cell cycle entry from G0/G1 to S phase in OLG indicate

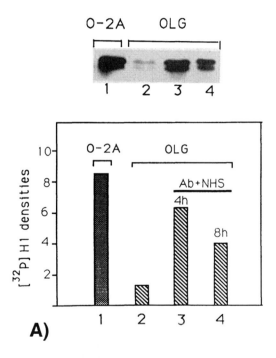

Figure 7A The effects of sublytic complement activation on cdc2 activity in OLG. The cdc2 activities in OLG following complement activation. O-2A cells were cultured in growth medium (lane 1) or OLG-defined medium (lane 2) for 72 h. Cells grown in OLG-defined medium were sensitized, then treated with NHS for 4 and 8 h (lanes 3, 4). Cells were lysed and immunoprecipitated with anti-cdc2 IgG. The kinase activity of the immunoprecipitated complexes was determined using histone H1 as a substrate.

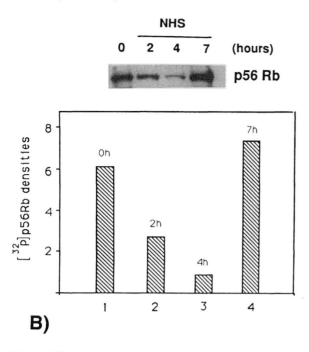

Figure 7B The effects of sublytic complement activation on cdk4 activity in OLG. Unstimulated (lane 1) or Ab-sensitized OLG treated with NHS for 2, 3, and 7 h (lanes, 2–4) were lysed. The lysates were immunoprecipitated with anti-cdk4 IgG and the precipitates assayed for cdk4 kinase activity using the recombinant truncated form of Rb protein (p56Rb) as a substrate. The autoradiogram of labeled Rb protein bands and the scan densities are presented. (From Ref. 58.)

that OLG surviving complement attack are progenitor-like cells that may have the capacity to myelinate when inflammation subsides.

The TCC signaling responsible for the cell cycle entry has been explored. Because of the critical role of c-jun for cell cycle activation (67) the c-Jun NH_2-terminal kinase (JNK) activity was examined in OLG following TCC attack (Fig. 9). JNK, also known as stress activated protein kinase (SAPK), is activated by variety of extracellular stimuli, which include heat shock, ultraviolet (UV) irradiation, tumor necrosis factor (TNF)α, interleukin (IL)1β, or lipopolysaccharides (LPS) (68). JNK activates c-Jun by phosphorylation of the c-Jun NH_2-terminal domain, thus increasing transcription of protooncogenes such as c-jun and c-fos. JNK activity is transiently induced by purified C5b-9, with a peak at 20 min (Fig. 9). The increase in JNK activity is associated with transient increase in AP-1 DNA-binding activity, and a return to the basal level at 60 min (58).

D. Role of the Complement System in Demyelination In Vivo

Mechanisms of immune-mediated demyelination have been studied mostly in experimental allergic encephalitis (EAE), an in vivo model for MS. EAE is induced by active immunization of rodent and rabbit with spinal cord myelin, or encephalitogenic myelin proteins and peptides (14). EAE is also induced by transfer of MHC-compatible T cells from EAE

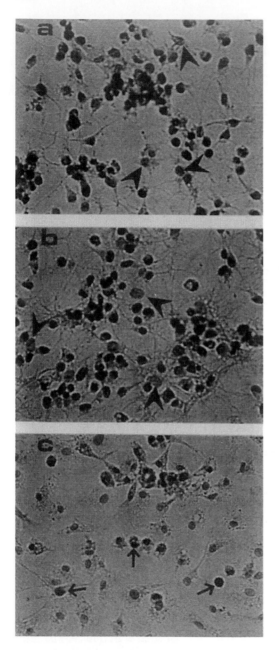

Figure 8 Effect of TCC on apoptosis of OLG. OLG were grown on plastic slides for 72 h in defined medium. Unstimulated OLG (a) or antibody-sensitized cells were treated with 1/10 dilution of HI-NHS (b) or NHS (c) for 18h. After fixation for 10 min in buffered formalin, apoptosis was assessed by staining the cells using the Apop Tag kit. The positive nuclei were counted and expressed as a percentage of total nuclei counted. Arrowheads indicate negative nuclei in (a) and (b); arrows show positive nuclei in (c). (From Ref. 58.)

Table 3 Sublytic Complement Attack Reduces Apoptotic Cell Death in Oligodendrocytes[a]

	Medium	HI-NHS	NHS
% NUCLEI STAINED	61 ± 0.7	62 ± 1.7	33 ± 1.7
	Medium	C5b6	C5b-9
% NUCLEI STAINED	52 ± 0.5	55 ± 4.9	33 ± 2.1

[a] OLG differentiated in defined medium for 72 h were sensitized with anti-GC Ab, then incubated with 1/10 dilutions of NHS or HI-NHS (at 56 °C for 45 min to inactivate complement) for 18 h. In addition, unsensitized OLG were incubated with C5b6 or C5b6 with C7, C8 and C9 to form C5b-9 complexes, under identical conditions.
Apoptotic cells were assessed by staining the cells on plastic slides using the Apoptag kit (Oncor, Gaithersburg). Minimum 500 nuclei per assay were counted in two separate experiments and the results are expressed as mean percentage nuclei stained ± SEM. Spontaneous apoptosis of OLG was reduced by 46% and 37% when cells were treated with sublytic NHS and C5b-9 respectively.
Source: From Ref. 58.

animals or MBP or PLP peptide-specific CD4+ T cell lines or clones (69–71). Although the kinetics and degree of illness depend on experimental protocols and animal species, tail weakness, ataxia, and hind limb paralysis developed within 7–21 days after initiation of the experiment. Clinical signs occurring early or in the hyperacute state of EAE can be due to tissue edema and early perivascular inflammatory cell infiltrate associated with breakdown of BBB, and may not be due to demyelination. Although antimyelin antibodies are detected in EAE induced by active immunization, antibodies do not appear to be significant factors in the hyperacute form of MBP-induced EAE (20,71). However, humoral factors such as complement and antibodies are implicated in demyelination in chronic relapsing EAE, as shown by the ability of the serum from rats with chronic relapsing EAE to induce complement-dependent demyelination (20,71). Unequivocal evidence of demyelination may require histological evaluation.

The effects of complement in EAE were evaluated by depletion of serum complement with cobra venom factor (CVF). CVF is a cobra C3b analog that can bind to factor B to

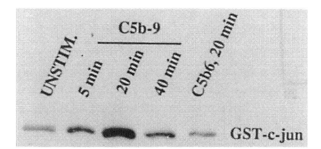

Figure 9 JNK1 activation induced by TCC. OLG cultured for 72h in defined medium (UNSTIM) were exposed to C5b-9 or C5b6 for the indicated time periods. Cells were lysed and kinase activity was determined on the anti-JNK IgG immunoprecipitates using GST-c-jun79 as a substrate. Similar results were obtained in three independent experiments. (From Ref. 58.)

form a stable C3b,Bb enzyme, not susceptible to degradation by mammalian factors H and I. Systemic injection of CVF, therefore, depletes serum C3 and abolishes the total serum complement activity. Clinical signs noted during hyperacute phase of EAE, which may represent tissue edema associated with BBB breakdown, are not affected by CVF (22,72–75). A single injection of CVF into guinea pig or rat can maintain relatively low C3 level for less than 10 days and a single CVF injection can delay the onset of paralysis and decrease the mortality without affecting the CNS inflammation (22,74,75). Treatment of Lewis rats with CVF completely suppressed the monophasic clinical activity at 10–12 days after transfer of MBP-specific T cells, an EAE model induced by T cells in which antibody response is not present. (23) (Fig. 10). CVF treatment does not always produce unequivocal results, even in experiments in which antibodies have been implicated in disease development activity and disease severity. Since CVF depletes the complement by activating the alternative pathway, CVF injection preceding the disease induction may affect the outcome of the disease, since CVF inject is associated with generation of biologically active complement peptides. A better method to block complement activation appears to be the use of soluble form of CR1 (sCR1), which inhibits the cascades of the classical and alternative pathway by inactivating the C3 convertase. Systemic use of sCR1 markedly reduced the inflammatory tissue injury of myocardial infarction, graft rejection, and adult respiratory distress syndrome in animal models (76–78). When administered

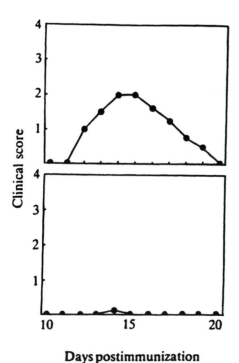

Days postimmunization

Figure 10 Influence of CVF treatment on the clinical course in animal rat with EAE. EAE was induced with purified MBP in Lewis rats. Animals were injected intraperitoneally on day 10 with either Tris/saline (upper panel, n = 8) or CVF (1 μg/g body weight; lower panel, n = 10). In no case was the SEM greater than 20% of the mean clinical score for the control animals between days 10 and 17 after injection. (From Ref. 23.)

daily for 6 days, the disease activity in rats with severe EAE induced by MBP immunization was markedly suppressed (79). Treatment with sCR1 also produced effective suppression of EAE disease activity, even in the presence of additional anti-MOG IgG injected into rats immunized with MBP (79). The suppression in these animals was associated with significant reduction of inflammation, near total absence of demyelination, and reduced deposition of C1, C3, and C9 in the CNS tissue (79). Thus sCR1 offers a better and less toxic method to inhibit in vivo complement activation and to evaluate the role of complement.

In MS, unequivocal evidence indicating the complement system as a demyelinating effector remains to be established. Determination of early-acting complement components in serum and CSF in patients with MS failed to show any significant pattern. Low C1, C3 and C4 activity (80) and normal to higher levels of C3 and C4 (81) have been reported in serum or CSF of patients with MS with acute exacerbating or chronic progressive illness. In contrast, the CSF titers of late-acting C5-C9 proteins and their activation product SC5b-9 revealed decreased C9 and increased SC5b-9 (82–84). The low levels of C9 have been correlated with disease activity, indicating C9 consumption during active demyelination (82,83). The presence of SC5b-9 in CSF of patients with MS and higher titers of SC5b-9 in CSF compared to the corresponding serum SC5b-9 have been observed (84). Since normal CSF is devoid of SC5b-9, the findings indicate an activation of complement within the CNS compartment. Deposition of C9 and mC5b-9 in autopsy brains from patients with MS is associated with capillary endothelial cells within the MS plaques and also in the adjacent white matter (85). These findings suggest that complement activation up to C9 takes place in brains of patients with MS in the presence of BBB breakdown (86).

Extensive studies, as described above, indicate that activation of complement in the presence or absence of antimyelin antibodies may affect the outcome of demyelination through multiple mechanisms. Assembly of TCC on myelin and OLG can induce myelin vesiculation and OLG cell death. Chemotactic factors and opsonic fragments derived from complement activation may enhance myelin–macrophage interaction and synergically affect macrophage-mediated myelin removal. On the other hand, sublytic TCC induce cellular changes in OLG that may be critical for cell survival and to gain myelinating potential.

IV. INVOLVEMENT OF COMPLEMENT IN POSTSTROKE SYNDROME

In patients with subarachnoid hemorrhage, cerebral vasospasm is one of the critical factors affecting morbidity and mortality. Involvement of complement has been suggested by the presence of activated complement components in the CSF and in the vessel wall (87,88), the ability of aged erythrocytes to activate complement, and the requirement of aged erythrocytes to induce late onset vasospasm in porcine models (89). In addition, cerebral vasospasm can be ameliorated by a synthetic protease inhibitor FUT-175, which inhibits C1 esterase activity in rabbit models and in humans (90). Although the mechanisms of complement activation by aged erythrocytes and contribution of complement in vasospasm are not well understood, evidence indicates that erythrocytes in CSF for 2–3 days can be lysed in a complement-mediated manner and the oxyhemoglobin and free radicals produced by hemolysis are thought to act as vascular spasmogens responsible for delayed cerebral vasospasm in poststroke syndrome. Recently, the questions of whether activation of complement by aged erythrocytes generates C5b-9 complexes and whether C5b-9 can induce conductance changes in vascular smooth muscle cells have been examined using a patch clamp technique. Freshly isolated smooth muscle cells from rat basilar artery were monitored for conductance changes in the presence of rat serum with autologous erythrocytes previously aged in CSF. In the absence of antibodies to erythrocytes, the steady-state conductance for aged erythrocytes and autologous serum ($30.8+18.2$ nS) was over 30-fold higher than fresh cells in autologous serum ($0.89+0.44$ nS). This effect was not observed with heat-inactivated serum or in the presence of Mg^{2+}EGTA (91). The conductance changes in muscle cells are due to the bystander assembly of C5b-9 as a result of complement activation by CSF-aged erythrocytes. This is shown by the ability of supernatants of the aged erythrocyte or zymogen incubated with autologous serum, or supernatants of zymogen incubated with human C8D+C8 or C9D+C9 to induce the conductance changes, but not by C8D or C9D alone (91). Although an increase in cytosolic Ca^{2+} and activation of Ca^{2+}-dependent kinases have been suggested to cause smooth muscle contraction, studies are needed to delineate the mechanisms by which CSF-aged erythrocytes activate the alternative complement pathway, the way C5b-9 complexes are assembled, and the biological effects of C5b-7, C5b-8, and C5b-9 in vascular smooth muscle cells in a bystander model.

V. COMPLEMENT SYSTEM IN DEGENERATIVE DISORDERS

A. Alzheimer's Disease

Alzheimer's disease (AD), occurring in the later decades of life, is a progressive dementia characterized by diffuse deterioration of cognitive mental function, especially the memory processes. The brains affected by this disorder are characterized by the presence of senile plaques consist of neurofibrillary tangles, interstitial deposition of β-amyloid in the brain tissue and cerebral blood vessels, and other proteins that are poorly defined (92). Neuronal loss is also a significant feature of AD (92). The β-amyloid of the Alzheimer plaque is βA4 amyloid of approximately 4.2 kDa peptides derived from a cleavage of the amyloid precursor protein (APP). APP is synthesized as seven alternatively spliced forms of the APP gene and the neuronal splicing form lacks the Kunitz-type protease inhibitor domain (93). In several types of familial Alzheimer's disease, point mutations involving exon 17 of the APP have been shown to associate with the disease. Importance of the mutation in exon 17 in disease induction and the tissue changes associated with the disease has been demonstrated in transgenic mice overexpressing the three most common alternatively spliced forms of APP. In these mice β amyloid deposition in predicted regions of the brain occurred in association with aberrant dendritic processes and altered expression of synaptic proteins occurring about 9 months after birth (94).

A possible role of complement in Alzheimer's disease was first suggested when the senile plaques were found to contain complement proteins, proinflammatory cytokines, and MHC class II proteins, similar to those seen in inflammatory CNS lesions. Eikelenbson and Stom were the first to demonstrate the presence of C1q, C3, and C4 together with immunoglobulins in all senile plaques (95). Early-acting complement proteins are also present at the lesions where dystrophic neurites and neurofibrillary tangles are present (96). It is interesting to note that deposition of C5b-9 is also associated with dystrophic neurites, neurofibrillary tangles, and β-AP deposits in Alzheimer's disease brains (97,98).

Deposition of clusterin and vitronectin, which inhibit cytolytic C5b-9 activity, has been found in areas of amyloid deposition in the absence of C5b-9 (99,100). A soluble form of β-amyloid detected in CSF is complexed with clusterin, suggesting that clusterin may able to maintain the solubility of β-amyloid and prevent C5b-9 formation (101). These findings clearly indicate in situ activation of complement and a possible role in the cellular and tissue changes associated with Alzheimer's disease.

Subsequent studies showed that β-amyloid, peptides of 39–43 amino acids, activate the classical pathway of complement in vitro by direct C1 activation, through binding to a region within the collagen-like domain of C1q (102) (Fig. 11). Synthetic peptides of βAP1–42 and βAP1–40 are also potent activators of complement, as determined by consumption of serum complement hemolytic activity and C4. The βAP1–42 is signifi-

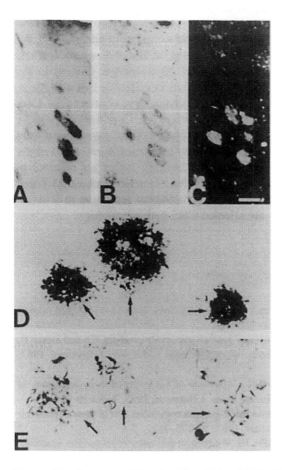

Figure 11 Immunostaining for C1q, C4d, and C5b-9 in Alzheimer's disease brain. (A–C) Serial 50 μm thick sections from the superior frontal gyrus of an Alzheimer's brain show immunohistochemical colocalization of C1q (A), C4d (B), and thioflavin S-positive senile plaques (C). The C4d (D) and C5b-9 immunoreactivities (E) are shown in serial sections from hippocampus of Alzheimer's brain. Note that although the same plaques are labeled, different elements within the plaque are stained. This is the expected result, since C5b-9 (but not C4d) requires cell membranes to insert (From Ref. 98.)

cantly more effective than βAP1–40 in C1q binding and subsequent complement activation, a property possibly related to the lower solubility of the βAP1–42. In the CSF of patients with Alzheimer's disease, the level of C1q was lower than that of control CSF, and the low C1q level was correlated with diminished cognitive capacity, memory, and concentration (103). Neurons, the terminally differentiated postmitotic cells, are likely to be exposed to complement attack as bystander targets when complement is activated by β-amyloid peptides.

B. Role of Complement in Other Neurodegenerative Disorders

Complement protein deposition has been observed in neurodegenerative diseases other than Alzheimer's disease. In amyotrophic lateral sclerosis (ALS), clusters of degenerating axons are stained for C3d and C4d (104). These C3 and C4 activation products are also found on OLG (104). Since deposition of C3d and C4d does not occur in normal CNS, the presence of these peptides suggests complement activation at the site of damaged neurites.

Parkinson's disease is characterized by the loss of dopaminergic neurons in the substantia nigra and the existence of Lewy bodies, which may be related to neural damage. Immunohistological studies showed that the involved substantia nigra contains C3d, C4d, C7, and C9 (105), in the absence of C1q, factor B, or properdin. Complement proteins and their fragments are not detected in axonal spheroid bodies of the nigrostriatal tract (105). The findings suggest that complement activation may take place in substantia nigra, which may not require activation of C1q or factor B. Detailed studies are required to determine whether complement is activated in situ in CNS disorders such as ALS and Parkinsons' disease, and the cause and conditions of complement activation in order to begin to study the role of complement on the affected CNS pathophysiology.

REFERENCES

1. Sano Y. Studies on the complement system in cerebrospinal fluid. Acta Med Univ Kagoshima 1985; 27:1.
2. Levi-Strauss M, Mallat M. Primary cultures of murine astrocytes produce C3 and factor B, two components of the alternative pathway of complement activation. J Immunol 1987; 139:2361–2366.
3. Rus HG, Kim LM, Niculescu FI, Shin ML. Induction of C3 expression in astrocytes is regulated by cytokines and Newcastle disease virus. J Immunol 1992; 148:928–933.
4. Barnum SR, Jones JL, Benveniste EN. Interferon-gamma regulation of C3 gene expression in human astroglioma cells. J Neuroimmunol 1992; 38:275–282.
5. Barnum SR, Ishii Y, Agrawal A, Volanakis JE. Production and interferon-gamma-mediated regulation of complement component C2 and factors B and D by the astroglioma cell line U105-MG. Biochem J 1992; 287:595–601.
6. Wu E, Brosnan CF, Raine CS. SP-40,40, immunoreactivity in inflammatory CNS lesions displaying astrocyte/oligodendrocyte interactions. J Neuropathol Exp Neurol 1993; 52:129–134.
7. Barnum SR. Biosynthesis and regulation of complement by cells of the central nervous system. In: Cruse JM, Lewis RI, eds. Complement Today. Complement Profiles. Basel: Karger, 1993:76–95.

8. Gasque P, Fontaine M, Morgan BP. Complement expression in human brain. Biosynthesis of terminal pathway components and regulators in human glial cells and cell lines. J Immunol 1995; 154:4726–4733.

9. Yang C, Jones JL, Barnum SR. Expression of decay-accelerating factor (CD55), membrane cofactor protein (CD46) and CD59 in the human astroglioma cell line, D54-MG, and primary rat astrocytes. J Neuroimmunol 1993; 47:123–132.

10. Gasque P, Chan P, Fontaine M, Ischenko A, Lamacz M, Gotze O, Morgan BP. Identification and characterization of the complement C5a anaphylatoxin receptor on human astrocytes. J Immunol 1995; 155:4882–4889.

11. Gasque P, Chan P, Mauger C, Schouft MT, Singhrao S, Dierich MP, Morgan BP, Fontaine M. Identification and characterization of complement C3 receptors on human astrocytes. J Immunol 1996; 156:2247–2255.

12. Volanakis JE. Transcriptional regulation of complement genes. Annu Rev Immunol 1995; 13:277–305.

13. Barnum SR, Jones JL. Transforming growth factor-beta 1 inhibits inflammatory cytokine-induced C3 gene expression in astrocytes. J Immunol 1994; 152:765–773.

14. Martin R, McFarland HF, McFarlin DE. Immunological aspects of demyelinating diseases. Annu Rev Immunol 1992; 10:153–187.

15. Allegretta M, Nicklas JA, Sriram S, Albertini RJ. T cells responsive to myelin basic protein in patients with multiple sclerosis. Science 1990; 247:718–721.

16. Warren KG, Catz I. Autoantibodies to myelin basic protein within multiple sclerosis central nervous system tissue. J Neurol Sci 1993; 115:169–176.

17. Xiao BG, Linington C, Link H. Antibodies to myelin-oligodendrocyte glycoprotein in cerebro-spinal fluid from patients with multiple sclerosis and controls. J Neuroimmunol 1991; 31:91–96.

18. Shin ML, Koski CL. The complement system in demyelination. In: Martenson RE, ed. Myelin: Biology and Chemistry. Boca Raton: CRC Press, 1992:801–831.

19. Bornstein MB, Crain SM. Functional studies of cultured brain tissues as related to "demyelinative disorders." Science 1965; 148:1242.

20. Seil FJ. Tissue culture studies of demyelinating disease: a critical review. Annu Neurol 1977; 2:345–355.

21. Liu WT, Vanguri P, Shin ML. Studies on demyelination in vitro: the requirement of membrane attack components of the complement system. J Immunol 1983; 131:778–782.

22. Morariu MA, Dalmasso AP. Experimental allergic encephalomyelitis in cobra venom factor-treated and C4-deficient guinea pigs. Ann Neurol 1978; 4:427.

23. Linington C, Morgan BP, Scolding NJ, Wilkins P, Piddlesden S, Compston DA. The role of complement in the pathogenesis of experimental allergic encephalomyelitis. Brain 1989; 112:895–911.

24. Vanguri P, Koski CL, Silverman B, Shin ML. Complement activation by isolated myelin: activation of the classical pathway in the absence of myelin-specific antibodies. Proc Natl Acad Sci USA 1982; 79:3290–3294.

25. Cyong JC, Witkin SS, Rieger B, Barbarese E, Good RA, Day NK. Antibody-independent complement activation by myelin via the classical complement pathway. J Exp Med 1982; 155:587–598.

26. Silverman BA, Carney DF, Johnston CA, Vanguri P, Shin ML. Isolation of membrane attack complex of complement from myelin membranes treated with serum complement. J Neurochem 1984; 42:1024–1029.

27. Vanguri P, Shin ML. Activation of complement by myelin: identification of C1-binding proteins of human myelin from central nervous tissue. J Neurochem 1986; 46:1535–1541.

28. Scolding NJ, Morgan BP, Houston A, Campbell AK, Linington C, Compston DA. Normal rat serum cytotoxicity against syngeneic oligodendrocytes. Complement activation and attack in the absence of anti-myelin antibodies. J Neurol Sci 1989; 89:289–300.

29. Wren DR, Noble M. Oligodendrocytes and oligodendrocyte/type-2 astrocyte progenitor cells of adult rats are specifically susceptible to the lytic effects of complement in absence of antibody. Proc Natl Acad Sci USA 1989; 86:9025–9029.

30. Raine CS, Bornstein MB. Experimental allergic encephalomyelitis: an ultrastructural study of experimental demyelination in vitro. J Neuropathol Exp Neurol 1970; 29:177–191.

31. Lampert P. Electron microscopic studies on ordinary and hyperacute experimental allergic encephalomyelitis. Acta Neuropathol 1967; 9:99–126.

32. Whitaker JN. The distribution of myelin basic protein in central nervous system lesions of multiple sclerosis and acute experimental allergic encephalomyelitis. Ann Neurol 1978; 3:291–298.

33. Cammer W, Bloom BR, Norton WT, Gordon S. Degradation of basic protein in myelin by neutral proteases secreted by stimulated macrophages: a possible mechanism of inflammatory demyelination. Proc Natl Acad Sci USA 1978; 75:1554–1558.

34. Cammer W, Brosnan CF, Basile C, Bloom BR, Norton WT. Complement potentiates the degradation of myelin proteins by plasmin: implications for a mechanism of inflammatory demyelination. Brain Res 1986; 364:91–101.

35. Prineas JW, Graham JS. Multiple sclerosis: capping of surface immunoglobulin G on macrophages engaged in myelin breakdown. Ann Neurol 1981; 10:149–158.

36. Prineas JW. The neuropathology of multiple sclerosis. In: Vinken PJ, Bruyn GW, Klawans HL, eds. Handbook of Clinical Neurology. Amsterdam: Elsevier Science Publishers BV, 1985:213–257.

37. Vanguri P, Shin ML. Hydrolysis of myelin basic protein in human myelin by terminal complement complexes. J Biol Chem 1988; 263:7228–7234.

38. Selmaj KW, Raine CS. Tumor necrosis factor mediates myelin and oligodendrocyte damage in vitro. Ann Neurol 1988; 23:339–346.

39. Vanguri P, Lee E, Henkart P, Shin ML. Hydrolysis of myelin basic protein in myelin membranes by granzymes of large granular lymphocytes. J Immunol 1993; 150:2431–2439.

40. Koski CL, Estep AE, Sawant-Mane S, Shin ML, Highbarger L, Hansch GM. Complement regulatory molecules on human myelin and glial cells: differential expression affects the deposition of activated complement proteins. J Neurochem 1996; 66:303–312.

41. Prineas JW, Kwon EE, Goldenberg PZ, Ilyas AA, Quarles RH, Benjamins JA, Sprinkle TJ. Multiple sclerosis. Oligodendrocyte proliferation and differentiation in fresh lesions. Lab Invest 1989; 61:489–503.

42. Raine CS, Wu E. Multiple sclerosis: remyelination in acute lesions. J Neuropathol Exp Neurol 1993; 52:199–204.

43. Prineas JW, Barnard RO, Kwon EE, Sharer LR, Cho ES. Multiple sclerosis: remyelination of nascent lesions. Ann Neurol 1993; 33:137–151.

44. Wing MG, Zajicek J, Seilly DJ, Compston DA, Lachmann PJ. Oligodendrocytes lack glycolipid anchored proteins which protect them against complement lysis. Restoration of resistance to lysis by incorporation of CD59. Immunology 1992; 76:140–145.

45. Zajicek J, Wing M, Skepper J, Compston A. Human oligodendrocytes are not sensitive to complement. A study of CD59 expression in the human central nervous system. Lab Invest 1995; 73:128–138.

46. Niculescu F, Rus H, Shin ML. Receptor-independent activation of guanine nucleotide-binding regulatory proteins by terminal complement complexes. J Biol Chem 1994; 269:4417–4423.

47. Niculescu F, Rus H, Shin S, Lang T, Shin ML. Generation of diacylglycerol and ceramide during homologous complement activation. J Immunol 1993; 150:214–224.

48. Carney DF, Lang TJ, Shin ML. Multiple signal messengers generated by terminal complement complexes and their role in terminal complement complex elimination. J Immunol 1990; 145:623–629.

49. Seeger W, Suttorp N, Hellwig A, Bhakdi S. Noncytolytic terminal complement complexes may serve as calcium gates to elicit leuotriene B4 generation in human polymorphonuclear leukocytes. J Immunol 1986; 137:1286–1293.

50. Wiedmer T, Ando B, Sims PJ. Complement C5b-9-stimulated platelet secretion is associated with a Ca^{2+}-initiated activation of cellular protein kinases. J Biol Chem 1987; 262:13674–13681.

51. Imagawa DK, Osifchin NE, Paznekas WA, Shin ML, Mayer MM. Consequences of cell membrane attack by complement: release of arachidonate and formation of inflammatory derivatives. Proc Natl Acad Sci USA 1983; 80:6647–6651.

52. Shirazi Y, Imagawa DK, Shin ML. Release of leukotriene B_4 from sublethally injured oligodendrocytes by terminal complement complexes. J Neurochem 1987; 48:271–278.

53. Shirazi Y, McMorris FA, Shin ML. Arachidonic acid mobilization and phosphoinositide turnover by the terminal complement complex, C5b-9, in rat oligodendrocyte $\times$ C_6 glioma cell hybrids. J Immunol 1989; 142:4385–4391.

54. Shin ML, Carney DF. Cytotoxic action and other metabolic consequences of terminal complement proteins. Prog Allergy 1988; 4:44.

55. Morgan BP. Complement membrane attack on nucleated cells: resistance, recovery and nonlethal effects. Biochem J 1989; 264:1.

56. Scolding NJ, Morgan BP, Houston WA, Linington C, Campbell AK, Compston DA. Vesicular removal by oligodendrocytes of membrane attack complexes formed by activated complement. Nature 1989; 339:620–622.

57. Shirazi Y, Rus HG, Macklin WB, Shin ML. Enhanced degradation of messenger RNA encoding myelin proteins by terminal complement complexes in oligodendrocytes. J Immunol 1993; 150:4581–4590.

58. Rus HG, Niculescu F, Shin ML. Sublytic complement attack induces cell cycle in oligodendrocytes S-phase induction is dependent on c-jun activation. J Immunol 1996; 156:4892–4900.

59. Shin ML, Rus HG, Niculescu FI. Membrane attack by complement: assembly and biology of terminal complement complexes. In: Lee AG, ed. Biomembranes, Vol. 5. JAI Press, 1996:119–146.

60. Carter R, Cosenza SC, Pena A, Lipson K, Soprano DR, Soprano KJ. A potential role for c-jun in cell cycle progression through late G1 and S. Oncogene 1991; 6:229–235.

61. Naeve GS, Sharma A, Lee AS. Identification of a 10-base pair protein binding site in the promoter of the hamster H3.2 gene required for the S phase dependent increase in transcription and its interaction with a Jun-like nuclear factor. Cell Growth Diff 1992; 3:919–928.

62. Ludwin SK. Proliferation of mature oligodendrocytes after trauma to the central nervous system. Nature 1984; 308:274–275.

63. Ludwin SK, Bakker DA. Can oligodendrocytes attached to myelin proliferate? J Neurosci 1988; 8:1239–1244.

64. Barres BA, Schmid R, Sendnter M, Raff MC. Multiple extracellular signals are required for long-term oligodendrocyte survival. Development 1993; 118:283–295.

65. Raff MC, Barres BA, Burne JF, Coles HS, Ishizaki Y, Jacobson MD. Programmed cell death and the control of cell survival: lessons from the nervous system. Science 1993; 262:695–700.

66. Benzaquen LR, Nicholson-Weller A, Halperin JA. Terminal complement proteins C5b-9 release basic fibroblast growth factor and platelet-derived growth factor from endothelial cells. J Exp Med 1994; 179:985–992.

67. Karin M. The regulation of AP-1 activity by mitogen-activated protein kinases. J Biol Chem 1995; 270:16483–16486.

68. Coso OA, Chiariello M, Kalinec G, Kyriakis JM, Woodgett J, Gutkind JS. Transforming G protein-coupled receptors potentially activate JNK (SAPK). Evidence for a divergence from the tyrosine kinase signaling pathway. J Biol Chem 1995; 270:5620–5624.

69. Bernard CC, Carnegie PR. Experimental autoimmune encephalomyelitis in mice: immunologic response to mouse spinal cord and myelin basic proteins. J Immunol 1975; 114:1537–1540.

70. Whitham RH, Bourdette DN, Hashim GA, Herndon RM, Ilg RC, Vandenbark AA, Offner H. Lymphocytes from SJL/J mice immunized with spinal cord respond selectively to a

peptide of proteolipid protein and transfer relapsing demyelinating experimental autoimmune encephalomyelitis. J Immunol 1991; 146:101–107.

71. Satoh J, Sakai K, Endoh M, Koike F, Kunishita T, Namikawa T, Yamamura T, Tabira T. Experimental allergic encephalomyelitis mediated by murine encephalitogenic T cell lines specific for myelin proteolipid apoprotein. J Immunol 1987; 138:179–184.

72. Lassmann H, Brunner C, Bradl M, Linington C. Experimental allergic encephalomyelitis: the balance between encephalitogenic T lymphocytes and demyelinating antibodies determines size and structure of demyelinated lesions. Acta Neuropathol 1988; 75:566–576.

73. Lassmann H, Kitz K, Wisniewski HM. In vivo effect of sera from animals with chronic relapsing experimental allergic encephalomyelitis on central and peripheral myelin. Acta Neuropathol 1981; 55:297–306.

74. Levine S, Cochrane CG, Carpenter CB, Behan PO. Allergic encephalomyelitis: effect of complement depletion with cobra venom. Proc Soc Exp Biol Med 1971; 138:285–289.

75. Pabst H, Day NK, Gewurz H, Good RA. Prevention of experimental allergic encephalomyelitis with cobra venom factor. Proc Soc Exp Biol Med 1971; 136:555–560.

76. Weisman HF, Bartow T, Leppo MK, Marsh HC, Jr., Carson GR, Concino MF, Boyle MP, Roux KH, Weisfeldt ML, Fearon DT. Soluble human complement receptor type 1: in vivo inhibitor of complement suppressing post-ischemic myocardial inflammation and necrosis. Science 1990; 249:146–151.

77. Pruitt SK, Baldwin WM, 3d, Marsh HC, Jr., Lin SS, Yeh CG, Bollinger RR. The effect of soluble complement receptor type 1 on hyperacute xenograft rejection. Transplantation 1991; 52:868–873.

78. Mulligan MS, Yeh CG, Rudolph AR, Ward PA. Protective effects of soluble CR1 in complement- and neutrophil-mediated tissue injury. J Immunol 1992; 148:1479–1485.

79. Piddlesden SJ, Storch MK, Hibbs M, Freeman AM, Lassmann H, Morgan BP. Soluble recombinant complement receptor 1 inhibits inflammation and demyelination in antibody-mediated demyelinating experimental allergic encephalomyelitis. J Immunol 1994; 152:5477–5484.

80. Kuwert E, Noll K, Firnhaber W. Komplement system and Liquor Cerebrospinalis. 3. Das Verhalten von Gesamt-C′ und C′1-C′4 in serum und Liquor von patienten mit multiple sklerose. Z Immunitaetsforsch 1968; 135:462–480.

81. Link H. Complement factors in multiple sclerosis. Acta Neurol Scand 1972; 48:521–528.

82. Morgan BP, Campbell AK, Compston DA. Terminal component of complement (C9) in cerebrospinal fluid of patients with multiple sclerosis. Lancet 1984; 2:251–254.

83. Compston DA, Morgan BP, Oleesky D, Fifield R, Campbell AK. Cerebrospinal fluid C9 in demyelinating disease. Neurology 1986; 36:1503–1506.

84. Sanders ME, Alexander EL, Koski CL, Shin ML, Sano Y, Frank MM, Joiner KA. Terminal complement complexes (SC5b-9) in cerebrospinal fluid in autoimmune nervous system diseases. Ann NY Acad Sci 1988; 540:387–388.

85. Compston DA, Morgan BP, Campbell AK, Wilkins P, Cole G, Thomas ND, Jasani B. Immunocytochemical localization of the terminal complement complex in multiple sclerosis. Neuropathol Appl Neurobiol 1989; 15:307–316.

86. Ffrench-Constant C. Pathogenesis of multiple sclerosis. Lancet 1994; 343:271–275.

87. Kasuya H, Shimizu T. Activated complement components C3a and C4a in cerebrospinal fluid and plasma following subarachnoid hemorrhage. J Neurosurg 1989; 71:741–746.

88. Niculescu F, Rus HG, Vlaicu R. Immunohistochemical localization of C5b-9, S-protein, C3d and apolipoprotein B in human arterial tissues with atherosclerosis. Atherosclerosis 1987; 65:1–11.

89. Findlay JM, Macdonald RL, Weir BK. Current concepts of pathophysiology and management of cerebral vasospasm following aneurysmal subarachnoid hemorrhage. Cerebrovasc Brain Metabol Rev 1991; 3:336–361.

90. Inagi R, Miyata T, Maeda K, Sugiyama S, Miyama A, Nakashima I. FUT-175 as a potent inhibitor of C5/C3 convertase activity for production of C5a and C3a. Immunol Lett 1991; 27:49–52.

91. Park CC, Shin ML, Simard JM. The complement membrane attack complex and the bystander effect in cerebral vasospasm. J. Neurosurg 1997; 87:294–300.

92. Banati RB, Beyreuther K. Alzheimer's disease. In: Kettenmann H, Ranson BR, eds. Neuroglia. New York: Oxford University Press, 1995:1027–1043.

93. Selkoe DJ. Normal and abnormal biology of the beta-amyloid precursor protein. Annu Rev Neurosci 1994; 17:489–517.

94. Games D, Adams D, Alessandrini R, Barbour R, Berthelette P, Blackwell C, Carr T, Clemens J, Donaldson T, Gillespie F, et al. Alzheimer-type neuropathology in transgenic mice overexpressing V717F beta-amyloid precursor protein. Nature 1995; 373:523–527.

95. Eikelenboom P, Stam FC. Immunoglobulins and complement factors in senile plaques. An immunoperoxidase study. Acta Neuropathol 1982; 57:239–242.

96. Ishii T, Haga S. Immuno-electron-microscopic localization of complements in amyloid fibrils of senile plaques. Acta Neuropathol 1984; 63:296–300.

97. McGeer PL, Akiyama H, Itagaki S, McGeer EG. Activation of the classical complement pathway in brain tissue of Alzheimer patients. Neurosci Lett 1989; 107:341–346.

98. Rogers J, Cooper NR, Webster S, Schultz J, McGeer PL, Styren SD, Civin WH, Brachova L, Bradt B, Ward P, Lieberburg I. Complement activation by beta-amyloid in Alzheimer disease. Proc Natl Acad Sci USA 1992; 89:10016–10020.

99. McGeer PL, Kawamata T, Walker DG. Distribution of clusterin in Alzheimer brain tissue. Brain Res 1992; 579:337–341.

100. Akiyama H, Kawamata T, Dedhar S, McGeer PL. Immunohistochemical localization of vitronectin, its receptor and beta-3 integrin in Alzheimer brain tissue. J Neuroimmunol 1991; 32:19–28.

101. Ghiso J, Matsubara E, Koudinov A, Choi-Miura NH, Tomita M, Wisniewski T, Frangione B. The cerebrospinal-fluid soluble form of Alzheimer's amyioid beta is complexed to SP-40,40 (apolipoprotein J), an inhibitor of the complement membrane-attack complex. Biochem J 1993; 293:27–30.

102. Jiang H, Burdick D, Glabe CG, Cotman CW, Tenner AJ. beta-Amyloid activates complement by binding to a specific region of the collagen-like domain of the C1q A chain. J Immunol 1994; 152:5050–5059.

103. Smyth MD, Cribbs DH, Tenner AJ, Shankle WR, Dick M, Kesslak JP, Cotman CW. Decreased levels of C1q in cerebrospinal fluid of living Alzheimer patients correlate with disease state. Neurobiol Aging 1994; 15:609–614.

104. Kawamata T, Akiyama H, Yamada T, McGeer PL. Immunologic reactions in amyotrophic lateral sclerosis brain and spinal cord tissue. Am J Pathol 1992; 140:691–707.

105. Yamada T, McGeer PL, McGeer EG. Lewy bodies in Parkinson's disease are recognized by antibodies to complement proteins. Acta Neuropathol 1992; 84:100–104.

24

Development of Clinically Useful Agents to Control Complement-Mediated Tissue Damage

ERIC WAGNER and MICHAEL M. FRANK
Duke University Medical Center, Durham, North Carolina

I. INTRODUCTION

The complement system includes more than 20 proteins, each acting at a specific step in the complement cascade (1). Some molecules are involved directly in the continuing process of complement activation whereas others serve as regulators. Extensive information has accumulated about the structure and amino acid composition of complement proteins over the years. One might have expected the development of clinically useful agents that control complement activation. However, most efforts aimed at the development of such agents have begun only recently. The reasons for this are manifold. First, the precise role of the complement system in immune-mediated diseases in which tissue damage is observed has been unclear. Second, the points of possible intervention in the complement cascade are numerous and it was unclear which were the most fruitful areas of development. Third, inhibition of complement might increase the danger of infection in the drug recipient. In addition, the number of individuals trained in this area of research is limited. Thus, the number of clinically useful agents designed to control complement-mediated tissue damage is, at the present time, quite small.

The development of complement-inhibitory agents acting at individual steps in the complement cascade seems reasonable, since individuals with single complement protein deficiencies often are symptom-free from the deficiency for a long period of time. The array of human diseases in which complement inhibitors could be of benefit is broad (2). It includes renal, rheumatological, neurological, dermatological, and hematological illnesses, to name a few. Furthermore, there is a growing number of conditions in which complement-mediated tissue damage is believed to be involved. This chapter will review the current state of knowledge concerning agents with anticomplement activity used in vivo and their potential clinical usefulness.

II. DESIRABLE CHARACTERISTICS OF A USEFUL COMPLEMENT INHIBITOR

An appropriate complement inhibitor must have properties that render it potent yet safe to use in humans. Complement is believed to be critical in the control of infections through

527

direct pathogen lysis or, more importantly, through phagocytosis following opsonization. Thus, the ideal complement inhibitor should not interfere with the ability of complement to control infections. However, a high-potency inhibitor should limit the formation of the C3 convertase of both the classical and the alternative pathways. If this were the case, the C5 convertase would not form and consequently neither C5a nor the membrane attack complex would be generated. One might suppose that severe inflammation would then be prevented. Whether it is possible to limit inflammation but not inhibit the antimicrobial functions of complement is unclear. It is presumed that this type of process occurs during the course of an antimicrobial response. Factors H and I fail to mediate the destruction of C3b when it is at a protected site on the bacterial surface. However, they downregulate complement function when C3b is bound to host tissue. Since C3 convertase inhibition may lead to increased susceptibility to infections, the use of late-acting component inhibitors might prove more useful. However, such inhibitors would not block C3a and C5a generation and these might induce severe inflammation. Specific inhibitors of C3a and C5a are being developed at the present time. Designing inhibitors of specific complement proteins and peptides will certainly allow a better understanding of the function of each of the peptides in the production of inflammation, so that the tailoring of appropriate complement inhibitors will become possible.

III. COBRA VENOM FACTOR

Although venoms from animal species such as spiders (3), tropical ants (4), ticks (5), and bees (6) have been shown to possess anticomplementary activity, snake-related venoms have been more extensively studied. It is noteworthy that a variety of different strains of snake's venoms are able to lower complement activity in human and other mammalian sera (7). However, we focus on the most widely utilized venom with complement-inhibiting activity: that obtained from *Naja naja*.

Nearly a century ago, Flexner and Noguchi at the Rockefeller University noted the presence of a factor with anticomplement activity in cobra venom (8). Given the incomplete understanding of the complement system of that day, it was impossible for them to understand the mechanism of action of cobra venom factor (CVF). In the last decades however, major progress has been made so that more details are known about CVF. CVF is a C3-like polypeptide that activates the alternative pathway through its reversible association with factor B upon cleavage by factor D (9). The CVFBb complex serves as a C3 convertase capable of activating C3 and C5. However, it should be noted that CVF from the *Naja naja* cobra is efficient at cleaving both C3 and C5, whereas that of the *Naja haje* cobra is considerably less efficient at activating C5 in the fluid phase, so that CVF from *Naja haje* does not deplete serum of late-acting components (10). One important characteristic of CVF is that, when complexed with the high-molecular-cleavage fragment of factor B (Bb), it is resistant to mammalian inactivators such as factors H and I (11), making it a very potent complement activator.

Cobra venom factor has been widely used to study the importance of complement proteins in several immune-mediated diseases, the evolution of the complement system, and the development of inhibitors of the Bb subunit (12). The use of CVF in animals leads to massive complement activation. It has been shown to induce pulmonary microvascular endothelium injury as well as leakage of plasma proteins into a number of tissues (13). Still, the lack of extensive tissue injury following injection of CVF, due to the rapid inactivation of complement split products, is striking to those who work with this agent. It is an attractive agent for the study of the contribution of complement to tissue pathology.

When injected into an animal, CVF reduces the complement titers to less than 5% of the normal values; the effect lasts 4–6 days. CVF, a highly immunogenic compound, is then inactivated by anti-CVF-specific antibodies that form in the recipient animal, allowing for a restoration of complement activity (14). CVF has been shown in many experimental models to inhibit or downregulate tissue injury, thus providing evidence for the importance of the complement system in the development of tissue damage. Some of the models studied include hyperacute xenograft rejection (15), Forssman shock (16), IgA-mediated renal inflammation (17), immune complex-mediated vasculitis (18), and experimental allergic encephalomyelitis (model for multiple sclerosis) (19). Although CVF has been used extensively in the past and is still used to examine the role of complement in experimental animal models of disease, animal strains with complement deficiencies are more helpful for the study of the role of isolated complement components. In addition, genetically engineered mice that lack a single complement component (C3, C4 and factor B knock-out mice) will certainly prove useful in the understanding of the involvement of complement in various situations (20).

CVF has no direct application in human beings. It is strongly antigenic and its effect lasts only until an antibody response has been generated This agent causes massive activation of the complement system through the alternative pathway. There is a high likelihood that anaphylatoxins such as C3a and C5a will generate undesirable side effects in patients. Moreover, activation blockade rather than massive activation is the desired effect. However, CVF perhaps could prove useful in anticancer therapies if conjugated to tumor-specific antibodies. In this form, it might target complement activation directly to the affected tissue and recruit more complement receptor-positive immune cells (21).

IV. REGULATORS OF COMPLEMENT ACTIVATION

To control inadvertant complement activation that could lead to autologous tissue damage, many regulatory molecules exist that function to downregulate nonspecific complement activation. Among these molecules are the members of the activation regulators of complement (RCA) family, which, in humans, are all encoded on the short arm of chromosome 1 (22). Included in this family are two plasma proteins, factor H and C4-binding protein, and four membrane-anchored proteins: complement receptors types 1 (CR1) and 2 (CR2), decay-accelerating factor (DAF), and membrane cofactor protein (MCP). As reviewed elsewhere in this volume, these molecules share a basic structure of repeated 60 amino acid modules or "short consensus repeats" (SCR). Depending on the regulator protein, the number of these repeating units will vary (22). CR1, DAF, and MCP, all prepared using genetic engineering techniques, have been examined for their potential usefulness as therapeutic agents.

A. Complement Receptor Type 1

Complement receptor type 1 (CR1) is a 205 kDa protein with C3b- and C4b-binding activity. It contains 30 SCRs. Twenty-eight of these SCRs are organized in repeating units of seven SCRs termed long homologous repeats (LHR) (23). Thus, this molecule is composed of four LHRs (A through D) followed by two additional SCRs: a hydrophobic transmembrane domain and a 43kDa cytoplasmic tail. Binding regions of this cell surface receptor to complement components have been determined to reside in the first two SCRs of LHR-A for C4b and in the two first SCRs of LHR-B and LHR-C for C3b (24). As discussed elsewhere in this volume, there exist four different allotypes of CR1 with duplications or deletion of individual LHRs. CR1 functions as a cofactor for factor I-mediated cleavage of C3b and C4b (22). It also possesses decay-accelerating activity toward both the classical and the alternative pathway C3/C5 convertases (25). Because of its elongated structure, CR1 has complement-regulatory activity not only on the surface of the cell that expresses it but also on a variety of other surfaces such as immune complexes and neighboring cells. CR1 is expressed on a variety of cell types including erythrocytes, neutrophils, monocytes, B lymphocytes, eosinophils, a subpopulation of T lymphocytes, follicular dendritic cells, glomerular podocytes, and peripheral nerve fibers.

Because of its high potency in inhibiting complement activation at the level of both the C3 and C5 convertases, a soluble form of CR1 has been produced by genetic engineering that was shown to inhibit activation of both the classical and alternative pathways at concentrations 100 times lower than physiological concentrations of factor H and C4-binding protein (26). It was also shown to be able to bind to C3b and to serve as a cofactor for factor I-mediated cleavage of C3b. Because of its high molecular weight, this molecule has to be given parenterally and has a short half-life in vivo. However, efforts are presently directed at producing smaller molecules with better bioavailability and longer in vivo half-lives (23). Still, sCR1 was shown to be a very potent agent for the control of complement activation in a variety of experimental models. Indeed, sCR1 treatment of cynomolgous monkeys allowed prolongation of pig heart xenograft survival from 1 h to 48–90 h, thus interfering with the hyperacute rejection phenomenon, mediated by the action of natural antibodies and complement (27). In a guinea pig-to-rat cardiac xenograft model, sCR1 prolonged organ survival from about 20 min to 747 min (28). In a cardiac allograft model in which rats were presensitized, sCR1 prolonged graft survival from 3 to 32 h (29). In another antibody-mediated tissue damage disease model involving complement, sCR1 was shown to inhibit vasculitis in the reversed passive Arthus reaction using a rat model (30) and alveolitis in a pulmonary Arthus model (31). In these latter two models, an actively immunized animal is challenged with the antigen by injection in the skin (classical Arthus reaction), by injecting antibody intradermally with the antigen administered systemically (reversed passive Arthus reaction) or by breathing of an aerosol containing the antigen (pulmonary Arthus reaction). Precipitating antibodies then activate complement at the site of antigen introduction and induce extensive tissue damage through vasculitis (classical Arthus reaction; classical and alternative pathways involved) or alveolitis (pulmonary Arthus reaction; alternative pathway involved). Also, sCR1 was demonstrated to have a potent effect on antibody-mediated experimental allergic encephalomyelitis (32). In this rat model of multiple sclerosis, sCR1 reduced inflammation and myelin damage.

A series of antibody-independent diseases in which complement plays an active role have also been studied in relation to the effect of sCR1. Reperfusion injury leads to tissue damage after a period of ischemia followed by reperfusion. This tissue injury is mediated by local inflammation attendant upon complement activation induced by the damaged tissue and by the release of toxic oxygen radicals. Reperfusion injury to the myocardial tissue in rats (26,33,34), the intestine in rats (35), and the rat liver (36) was reduced significantly by using sCR1, proving the major role of complement in this process. Thermal and physical traumas are both associated with acute inflammation and complement activation. sCR1 was shown in rat models to reduce lung and skin damage caused by thermal injury (31) and to reduce neutrophil accumulation in the brains of rats subjected to head injury (37). It is noteworthy that sCR1 is now in clinical trials examining its effect in severely burned patients (2). Furthermore, sCR1 proved useful in other models in which complement activation plays a pivotal role such as pulmonary damage following cardiopulmonary bypass surgery (38), complement-mediated proliferative glomerulone-phritis (39), and in preventing complement and granulocyte activation induced by dialysis membranes (40,41). Since CR1 inhibits complement activation at the level of the C3/C5 convertases and is a cofactor for C3b cleavage, there is a concern about the ability of the treated patient to fight infections. In vitro and in vivo, it was shown that sCR1 inhibits the phagocytosis of *Streptococcus pneumoniae* and even the phagocytosis of preopsonized particles. Host defense was markedly reduced in rats treated with sCR1 and injected with *Streptococcus pneumoniae* and *Pseudomonas aeruginosa* (42). Although sCR1 is a very promising agent in the control of complement-mediated diseases, the potential risk of infection must be taken into account.

B. Decay Accelerating Factor

Decay accelerating factor (DAF) is a 70 kDa glycoprotein expressed at the surface of all circulating cells, vascular endothelial cells, and epithelial cells (22). It inserts into cell membranes through a glycosyl–phosphatidylinositol anchor, so that purified DAF can insert easily into cell membranes of heterologous erythrocytes (43). As its name implies, DAF causes the dissociation of both the classical and alternative pathway C3/C5 convertases (22). It is not a cofactor for factor I-mediated cleavage of C3b. DAF binds C4b and C3b only weakly but the affinity is greatly enhanced when these molecules are part of a convertase. One disadvantage in the use of DAF as a complement-inhibitory agent is that it does not lead to irreversible inactivation of C3b and C4b (44). The classical pathway C3 convertase decay activity was recently localized in SCRs 2 and 3 whereas that of the alternative pathway was observed in SCRs 2, 3 and 4 (45). A soluble form of DAF (sDAF) was produced and tested for its ability to inhibit complement activation. Both in vitro and in vivo using a reversed passive Arthus reaction model, sDAF was shown to be potent in guinea pigs (46). However, the most promising use of DAF in human disease will undoubtedly be in the generation of transgenic pigs that express human complement regulatory proteins, used as donor organs in human transplantation. This will be discussed later.

C. Membrane Cofactor Protein

Membrane cofactor protein (MCP) is a glycoprotein expressed on all circulating cells except erythrocytes, on hemopoietic cell lines, epithelial cells, endothelial cells, fibroblasts, spermatozoa, and placental trophoblasts (22). It functions as a cofactor for factor I-mediated cleavage of C3b but has no decay-accelerating activity for the C3 convertases (47). MCP binds to C4b but only with weak avidity, such that cofactor activity for its cleavage is less than that of C3b. Although it cannot insert spontaneously in cell membranes such as DAF, purified MCP, in fluid-phase assays of C3b cleavage by factor I, maintains a cofactor activity 50 times greater than that of factor H (22). However, the primary role of MCP is to inhibit C3/C5 convertases on a cell surface. Four different isotypes (BC1, BC2, C1, C2) each composed of four SCRs, exist. The BC isoforms are more potent in binding C4b, thus inhibiting more efficiently the classical pathway C3 convertase (48). MCP is able to inhibit irreversibly C3b and C4b and can recycle to inhibit multiple C3b and C4b molecules. However, it is monovalent and has a relatively weak affinity for its natural substrates, so that most authors believe that its usefulness as a soluble inhibitor in diseases is uncertain (23). Nevertheless, one recent report stated that a soluble form of MCP (sMCP) is potent in reducing inflammatory infiltration and edema associated with the reverse passive Arthus reaction in rats. (49). When used in an vitro model of complement-mediated cell lysis, sMCP achieved better results when in combination with sDAF (49). There is interest in using molecular techniques to combine MCP with other regulatory proteins to enhance its activity. As for DAF, the most potent use of MCP alone may well reside in its cell-bound form, when incorporated into pig organs aimed at human transplantation (see below).

V. INHIBITORS OF ANAPHYLATOXINS

As reviewed in Chapter 11, the complement activation cleavage peptides, C4a, C3a and C5a (the anaphylatoxins) have important biologic activity and are attractive targets for therapeutic intervention. Antibodies to these molecules have potent effects in vitro and in vivo and specific antagonists to the anaphylatoxins and their receptors have been developed. In vivo administration of a polyclonal antibody to $C5a_{desarg}$ proved efficient in reducing the C5a plasma levels in primates in which sepsis was induced by injection of *E. coli* (50) and prevented death from adult respiratory distress syndrome in septic primates (51) Monoclonal antibodies to C5a decreased IL-6 synthesis in a pig septic shock model (52) and reduced infarct size in a pig model of ischemia-reperfusion myocardial injury (53). A polyclonal antibody to a synthetic N-terminal peptide from C5aR blocked zymosan-induced chemotaxis and intracellular enzyme release from human neutrophils and IL-6 and IL-8 production in human monocytes (54). Potent monoclonal antibodies to this receptor are available (55, 56) and antagonists of C5a receptor binding are being synthesized and tested both in vitro and in vivo. An antagonist termed L-156, 602, isolated from *Streptomyces* sp. A1502, inhibited delayed-type hypersensitivity reactions in mice (57), as well as concanavalin A-induced inflammation in a murine model (58). Furthermore, several synthetic peptides derived from the N-terminal region of C5a have been shown to lack agonist activity but still bind the C5a receptor, thereby inhibiting C5a effects in vitro (59, 60).

VI. INHIBITORS OF THE MEMBRANE ATTACK COMPLEX: MEMBRANE INHIBITOR OF REACTIVE LYSIS

Membrane inhibitor of reactive lysis (CD59) is a small protein (18–20 kDa) expressed on all circulating cells, glomerular podocytes, epithelial cells, endothelial cells, and spermatozoa (22). Like DAF, it is anchored onto the cell surface via a glycosyl-phosphatidylinositol intermediate. Not only is it a cell surface molecule but it also exists in a soluble form in tears, sweat, saliva, breast milk, blood plasma, amniotic fluid, and seminal plasma (22). CD59 interferes with the late assembly of the membrane attack complex by binding to the alpha chain of C8 and to the b domain of C9 (61). A recombinant soluble form of

CD59 was produced that inhibits hemolysis (62), but its use in experimental models of disease has not yet been tested. As is the case with DAF and MCP, its mechanism of action is believed to be maximal on the surface on which it is expressed The main application of CD59 thus far has been in transgenic pigs to be used in human transplantation. In antitumor therapy, it has been suggested that the generation of bifunctional antibodies that recognize both CD59 and a tumor-specific antigen could help in reducing tumor cell resistance to complement attack (22).

VII. ANTIBODIES TO COMPLEMENT PROTEINS

Since blockade of the early complement components may lead to infectious complications and C5a generation may induce severe inflammation, investigators have used monoclonal antibodies to C5 to block complement activation efficiently. In vitro perfusion studies suggested that anti-C5 monoclonal antibody was potent in inhibiting hyperacute rejection of porcine organs alone (63) and in combination with an anti-C8 antibody (64). The development of more sophisticated recombinant antibody fragments could lead to use in human disease (65,66). Blocking C5 activity might prove to be a key in some diseases in which complement activation induces tissue damage.

C5a is known for its high potency in recruiting neutrophils, causing neutrophil aggregation and embolization in acute inflammation. In a model of myocardial infarction in pigs, Amsterdam et al. showed that an antibody to C5a was able to inhibit neutrophil cytotoxic activity (67). Antibodies reacting with the C5a receptor on neutrophils and monocytes were likewise shown to block cell activation effectively (68). Their usefulness in in vivo cases in which complement activation is seen awaits further testing.

VIII. DRUGS THAT INHIBIT COMPLEMENT ACTIVATION

As reviewed extensively by von Zabern elsewhere (69), a wide variety of pharmacological drugs with basic anticoagulant, anti-inflammatory, antimicrobial, and other properties have the ability to interfere with the complement cascade. However, most of these compounds are toxic or are poor complement inhibitors (70). Nevertheless, since precise information is becoming available on the interaction of complement peptides, it should be possible to obtain precise inhibition of various steps in the complement cascade. Although under current development (C3-binding peptide, for example; 71), no such agent is yet available. Some drugs are worth discussing because of the interest they generate.

A. Anticoagulants

1. Heparin

Heparin, the widely used anticoagulant, has been known for years to inhibit complement activation. Heparin is a polyanionic mucopolysaccharide. This agent is able to inhibit the alternative pathway C3 convertase complex formation by blocking the association between C3b and factor B (72,73). Heparin has also been reported to bind to the C1q collagenous stalk, thereby inactivating C1 (74,75). This molecule can also upregulate the activity of factor H (76). In a guinea pig model, heparin proved to be potent in interfering with complement activation induced by cobra venom factor (77). Although the anticomplementary activity of heparin is well studied in vitro, little information is available in in vivo settings (78). It should also be noted that protamine-heparin complexes have been thought to activate complement in much the same way that complement is activated by antigen–antibody complexes (78). Again, most of the experiments have been performed in vitro and there is little in vivo data available (79,80). A number of naturally occurring mucopolysaccharides such as chondroitin sulfate and dermatan sulfate are also known for their complement-inhibiting properties. For more complete details, the reader is referred to an excellent review on the subject (81).

2. Nafamstat mesilate

Another potentially exciting agent is the protease inhibitor nafamstat mesilate (FUT-175) that has been synthesized by the Fujita Pharmaceutical Company. This compound was originally developed as a potent anticoagulant (82,83). In addition, it was shown to possess complement-inhibiting properties. Its mechanism of action appears to reside in the inhibition of C4a, C3a, and C5a generation through action on the C3/C5 convertases at μmolar concentrations (84,85) and in the inhibition of C1r and C1s as well (86). FUT-175 was investigated for its potency in inhibiting complement in various disease models and was shown to be effective. For example, it was reported to inhibit complement activation upon extracorporeal circulation during cardiopulmonary bypass surgery (87), to reduce adjuvant-induced arthritis lesions in a rat model (88), and to be more efficient than dexamethasone in the treatment of lupus nephritis in mice (89). Recently, FUT-175 was demonstrated to inhibit the alternative pathway factor B and to prolong discordant xenograft survival by a factor of 3 in a guinea pig-to-rat combination (90). Nevertheless, it has been available for years and is being applied to human illness slowly if at all, suggesting that it is more toxic than the literature implies.

B. Natural Products

A fungal metabolite isolated from *Stachybotrys complementi*, K76 monocarboxylic acid (K76COOH) has been isolated and shown to possess complement inhibitory activity in both the classical and the alternative pathways (91). Its mode of action would appear to be inhibition at the level of C5 activation (92). In vivo, K76COOH was able to interfere with several complement-mediated pathological experimental models such as passive cutaneous anaphylaxis, nephrotoxic nephritis, Forssman shock, and lupus nephritis (93). In combination with FUT-175, this agent proved to be potent in prolonging guinea pig-to-rat cardiac xenograft survival (90). Its usefulness in clinical trials has not yet been assessed.

In a search for new compounds that might be potent inhibitors of complement activation, natural products are being tested. To name a few, sulfated polysaccharides isolated from brown seaweed are reported to have inhibitory activity on both the classical and the alternative pathways by acting at several sites. They inhibit C3 convertases by blocking C1 activation, C4 cleavage, binding of Factor B, and they interfere with the stabilizing role of properdin (94). A component extracted from a Chinese medicinal herb (ephedra) demonstrated inhibitory activity in both the classical and alternative pathways, the sites of action being at the level of C2 and C9 for the classical pathway but unknown for the alternative pathway (95). It is likely that the future will yield additional discoveries of agents derived from natural sources that are potent inhibitors of complement activation.

C. Glucocorticoids

In a number of settings, glucocorticoids have been considered as anticomplementary agents. For example, it has been suggested that, in some patients with paroxysmal nocturnal hemoglobinuria (PNH), high-dose prednisone limits alternative pathway-mediated cell damage (96). Such complement-mediated tissue damage is not highly susceptible to glucocorticoid therapy and it may be that the effects of glucocorticoids are indirect rather than directly acting on the complement system. There have been a limited number of experiments examining this issue.

In guinea pigs, it has been shown that high-dose glucocorticoid therapy lowers the level of C3 and other complement components except C1 and C9 (97,98). Direct studies of turnover performed some years ago demonstrated that the decrease in C3 levels was related to both decreased synthesis and increased degradation (98,99). Other in vitro studies using cell cultures demonstrated that glucocorticoids such as dexamethasone induced decreased synthesis of C3 and factor B whereas synthesis of factor H was increased, suggesting a possible mechanism of action of its immunosuppressive effect (100,101). Although the effects of high-dose glucocorticoids were striking, the required doses were so high that they are unlikely to be useful clinically.

D. C1 Inhibitor

As reviewed elsewhere in this volume, C1 inhibitor is a 105 kDA plasma protein that inhibits classical pathway activation through interaction with activated C1r and C1s (1). C1 inhibitor is reported to slow C1 activation and to destroy C1 activity once the C1 is activated. It would seem reasonable that a high concentration of C1 inhibitor might be a potent inhibitor of the classical pathway in a variety of models. Indeed, treatment with C1 inhibitor abrogated complement activation onto the surface of porcine endothelial cells subjected to contact with human serum (102). Using a feline model of myocardium reperfusion injury following a period of ischemia, C1 inhibitor was shown to reduce neutrophil infiltration and maintain endothelial cell function (103). This provides data that classical pathway activation may be crucial in reperfusion injury of organs. Concentrated vapor-heated C1 inhibitor was recently used in patients with hereditary angioedema, both for prevention and treatment of acute attacks (104). This treatment regimen resulted in C4 and C1 inhibitor levels close to normal and was effective at preventing and inhibiting acute attacks. The major limitation in the extensive use of C1 inhibitor is the difficulty in producing pharmacologically useful amounts of the protein at reasonable costs. However, methods have been published that may allow production of appreciable amounts of this protein (104,105).

E. Androgens

In hereditary angioedema (HAE), the use of anabolic steroids such as danazol has proven to be highly effective (106). Danazol appears to upregulate C1 inhibitor synthesis, bringing its plasma concentration toward normal (107). Most patients with hereditary angioedema have a single defective C1 inhibitor gene leading to 1/3 to 1/2 of the normal level of circulating protein. Treatment with danazol increases the plasma C1 inhibitor level. It has recently been proposed that the mechanism of action of danazol in humans includes increased C4 synthesis due to its anabolic effect, leading to improved complement function with increased immune complex clearance. However, the data to support this hypothesis are still incomplete. The minor increase in C1 inhibitor levels seen with some androgens might result from a decrease in utilization (108). Although danazol causes an increase in C1 inhibitor levels, the effect is not great enough to downregulate complement function. Methylated androgens are required to achieve the C1 inhibitor increase and testosterone administered subcutaneously does not have this effect. As our knowledge of the biochemical basis of androgen-induced augmentation of complement protein synthesis evolves, it may become possible to develop more potent agents that could prove useful. Since increasing C1 inhibitor levels by two or three times above normal downregulates complement function, it might have many applications.

IX. PLASMAPHERESIS

Plasmapheresis has been used to remove pathological antibodies from the circulation (109,110) and, to some extent, complement proteins as well. One advantage of plasmapheresis is that it is possible to remove a high proportion of IgM antibodies since 70–80% of the total amount is in the intravascular space. Since IgG is distributed throughout the extracellular compartment and is not confined to the intravascular space, it cannot be removed as easily. Repeated plasmaphereses can reduce the IgG level by two-thirds over a period of days, as it reequilibrates with the intravascular space between each procedure. A rapid return of both IgM and IgG after plasmapheresis is usually observed, due to rapid synthesis by B cells (111). For this reason, many have advocated the use of cytotoxic agents that destroy rapidly dividing cells, including the B lymphocyte population (110,112).

The effective removal of complement components by plasmapheresis is difficult. In theory, a large molecule like C1 can be removed. However, the rate of synthesis of most complement proteins is about 2%/h in resting state. They behave as acute phase proteins in an inflammatory state and the rate of synthesis increases markedly. Because of the rapid turnover, effective removal is difficult or impossible and this is not an effective approach to therapy.

X. INTRAVENOUS IMMUNOGLOBULIN
PREPARATIONS

Although not the product of recombinant technology, pooled human IgG (IVIg) preparations may prove useful in some complement-related diseases. Some years ago, using IgG-sensitized pneumococci, it was shown that up to 30% of C3 deposited on the bacterial surface after exposure to a source of complement was bound to the IgG and not to the bacterial surface (113). This suggested that IgG acts as a preferential acceptor of C3 molecules. Since then, extensive work by Carroll and Pangburn has supported this point and the site at which C3 binds to IgG has been identified (114). The interaction between C3 and IgG greatly promotes complement-mediated effector functions. For example, by engaging two receptors on the surface of phagocytic cells, C3 bound to IgG increases substantially the opsonization potential of IgG (115,116). C3 bound to IgG was also shown to be resistant to factors H and I-mediated cleavage (117) but not to CR1-mediated cleavage with factor I (118).

IVIg is currently used in a number of autoimmune and inflammatory diseases that include, among others, idiopathic thrombocytopenic purpura (ITP), Kawasaki's disease, Guillain-Barré syndrome, and myasthenia gravis (119). The proposed effects of IVIg include idiotype–anti-idiotype interactions, blockade of Fc receptors on phagocytic cells, modulation of cytokine production, blockade of T and B cell proliferation, and selection of immune repertoires and diversion of complement activation from target cells (120, 121). However, we will focus here on the effect of IVIg on complement activation and binding to targets.

In in vivo experimental models, IVIg was proven to be a very potent agent in inhibiting complement binding onto target surfaces. Using the Forssman shock model, Basta et al. showed survival of guinea pigs treated with high doses of IVIg (122). Forssman shock is a cataclysmic reaction that takes place in guinea pigs after intravenous injection of rabbit antisheep erythrocyte antiserum. The Forssman antigen is a ceramide pentasaccharide that is expressed in species including the sheep and guinea pig but not in others, including the rabbit. Thus, injection of rabbit IgG antibodies directed against the Forssman antigen into guinea pigs causes a rapid pulmonary shock leading to death within minutes. This reaction is mediated by the binding of anti-Forssman antibodies to the pulmonary endothelium, one of the first vascular beds encountered by the antibody when injected intravenously. Rapid complement activation leads to pulmonary damage and death. The reaction requires an intact classical pathway and represents an excellent model for the study of complement-inhibiting agents. Complement binding to target tissue and subsequent tissue damage was markedly reduced by IVIg without affecting C3 and C4 serum levels. The action of IVIg appears to be mainly on the classical pathway, suggesting that IVIg-treated individuals might have the ability to control infectious agents through the action of the alternative pathway.

In a guinea pig model, the clearance of IgM-sensitized erythrocytes was decreased but the effect was modest (123). In a pig-to baboon cardiac xenograft model, Magee and collaborators noted extented organ survival of up to 10 days with the use of IVIg, as compared to minutes in controls (124). As will be discussed below, xenotransplantation is followed by hyperacute rejection, a phenomenon that occurs rapidly upon restoration of the blood flow. Hyperacute rejection is mediated by natural antibodies and complement.

In humans, the effect of IVIg has also been investigated to some extent in situations in which complement is activated. Thus, treatment of patients with dermatomyositis with a high dose of IVIg inhibited C3b and C5b-9 deposition on endomysial capillaries and reduced in vitro C3 uptake onto IgG-coated human erythrocytes without affecting serum complement levels (125). IVIg was also able to reduce C3 binding to erythrocytes in autoimmune hemolytic anemia and affect in vitro erythrocyte acid lysis in patients with paroxysmal nocturnal hemoglobinuria (126).

The mechanism through which IVIg inhibits complement binding to target cell surfaces remains unclear. It would appear that the Fc portion of IgG is responsible for the effect seen (127,128). Some have postulated that IVIg acts as an acceptor for C1 on the target surface, removing the C1 and preventing further complement activation (128,129). However, since IgA is effective at preventing complement binding to antibody-coated cells (130,131), although it does not bind C1 efficiently, this does not appear to be the principal action. Inhibition of C4 binding may be more important than inhibition of the binding of C3 (131). It is interesting that Miletic et al. (131) showed that IgA and IgM were far more potent at inhibiting complement activation on antibody-coated surfaces than is IgG. The molecular basis of this observation is currently under study but these molecules represent potentially effective therapeutic agents. IVIg represents a very potent complement-inhibiting agent that is widely available and may be useful in several diseases in the future.

XI. GENERATION OF TRANSGENIC ANIMALS EXPRESSING HUMAN COMPLEMENT REGULATORY MOLECULES

One of the most challenging areas in the field of transplantation is the use of animal organs to overcome the critical shortage of human organs available. Indeed, with the high success rate of human allotransplantation, the number of patients on a waiting list for organ donation has increased remarkably because of the limited number of donors compared to that of potential recipients (132). For a number of reasons including ethics, cost, ease of breeding, and potential infectious agent transmission, many in the field have turned to the pig as a potential donor for human transplantation rather than the primate. However, vascularized organs from porcine origin, when implanted into humans or nonhuman primates, undergo a very rapid rejection reaction termed hyperacute rejection. This reaction is mediated by natural antibodies reacting with a carbohydrate highly expressed on pig endothelial cells lining the organ's blood vessels (133,134). Antibody binding leads to complement activation. Upon activation of complement through the classical pathway, endothelial cells are physiologically modified and have procoagulant activity, which results in thrombosis, interstitial edema, and necrosis (135). Hyperacute rejection is the first barrier to the widespread use of porcine organs in humans.

   Since complement activation plays a major role in the pathophysiology of discordant (phylogenetically disparate species) xenograft hyperacute rejection (136), efforts aimed at blocking complement activation have been investigated. As mentioned above, cobra venom factor, sCR1, C1 inhibitor, FUT-175, and IVIg have been successfully used to prolong xenograft survival in a number of experimental models, both in vitro and in vivo. However, the susceptibility of porcine endothelial cells to complement attack is believed to be in part due to the failure of the complement control proteins on the pig endothelium within the grafted organ to control complement-mediated damage by the recipient's complement (136). It is known that porcine complement-regulatory molecules on the surface of porcine endothelial cells do not protect from human complement-induced damage. The control proteins show homologous restriction, meaning that they are far more effective against homologous complement. For this reason, efforts are presently directed at the production of pigs that express human complement regulatory molecules at the surface of their cells through genetic manipulation (137,138). To inhibit deleterious complement activation at its surface, a pig cell should be able to block both early and later steps in the cascade. DAF, MCP, and CD59 have been suggested as the molecules to transfer into pig cells. As reviewed elsewhere in this volume, DAF dissociates C3/C5 convertases, MCP acts as a cofactor for factor I-mediated cleavage of C3b and CD59 (protectin) interferes with the formation of the membrane attack complex at the level of C8 and C9. These molecules, when inserted into pig cells, induced protection against complement-mediated injury to both cells and tissues (139–142). Using pig-to-baboon cardiac transplantation models, it was recently shown that hearts expressing both human DAF and

CD59 demonstrated organ survival of up to 30 h, as compared to minutes for nontransgenic pig organs (143). Molecular engineering and gene therapy with chimeric complement regulatory proteins such as DAF-CD59 may prove useful in the generation of transgenic pigs and in the treatment of diseases with complement regulatory molecule deficiencies through gene therapy (144). We will certainly see the introduction of transgenic porcine organs into the transplantation field in the next few years, given the rapid growth of knowledge in xenotransplantation.

XII. CONCLUSION

As reviewed in this chapter, the number of agents presently used in human beings for complement system regulation is quite limited. As we learn more about the exact role of complement in various diseases and about their tight physiological control, it will be easier to tailor appropriate agents that can be used safely in patients. Already, several agents are being evaluated and one of them (sCR1) is in the first phase of clinical trials in severely burned patients. It is important to keep in mind that the ideal complement-inhibiting agent should be potent at diverting complement activation from surfaces of organs involved in tissue damage without affecting the normal function of the complement system. With the current available technology and the extended knowledge on complement protein's precise function in relation to structure and amino acid content, the number of complement inhibitors that will have potential use in the clinical arena should increase substantially in the next few years.

REFERENCES

1. Frank MM, Fries LF. Complement. In: Paul WE, ed. Fundamental Immunology. New York: Raven Press, 1989:679–701.
2. Morgan BP. Physiology and pathophysiology of complement: progress and trends. Crit Rev Clin Lab Sci 1995; 32:265–298.
3. Rees RS, O'Leary JP, King LE. The pathogenesis of loxocelism following brown recluse spider venom. J Surg Res 1983:35:1–10.
4. Schultz DR, Loos M, Bub F, Arnold PI. Differentiation of hemolytically active fluid-phase and cell-bound human C1q by an ant-venom-derived polysaccharide. J Immunol 1980; 124:1251–1257.
5. Berenberg JL, Ward PA, Soneshine DE. Tick-bite injury: mediation by a complement-derived chemotactic factor. J Immunol 1972; 109:451–456.
6. Gencheva G, Shkenderov SV. Inhibition of complement activity by certain bee venom components. Doklady Bolgarskoi Akademii 1986; 359:137–139.
7. Eggersten G, Fohlman J, Sjöquist J. In vitro studies on complement inactivation by snake venoms. Toxicon 1980; 18:87–96.
8. Flexner S, Noguchi H. Snake venom in relation to hemolysis, bacteriolysis, and toxicity. J Exp Med 1903; 6:277–301.
9. Vogel CW, Müller-Eberhard HJ. The cobra venom factor-dependent C3 convertase of human complement. J Biol Chem 1982; 257:8292–8299.
10. von Zabern I, Hinsh B, Przyklenk H, Schmidt G, Vogt W. Comparison of *Naja n. naja* and *Naja h. haje* cobra venom factors: correlation between binding affinity for the fifth component of complement and mediation of its cleavage. Immunobiology 1980; 157:499–514.

11. Lachman PJ, Halbwachs L. The influence of C3b inactivator (KAF) concentration on the ability of serum to support complement activation. Clin Exp Immunol 1975; 21:109–114.

12. von Zabern I. Effects of venoms of different animal species on the complement system. In: Sim RB, ed. Activators and Inhibitors of Complement. Dordrecht, The Netherlands: Kluwer Academic Publishers, 1993:127–135.

13. Till GO, Johnson KJ, Kunkel R, Ward PA. Intravascular activation of complement and acute lung injury. Dependency on neutrophils and toxic oxygen metabolites. J Clin Invest 1982; 69:1126–1135.

14. Pepys MB. Role of complement in the induction of immunological responses. Transplant Rev 1976; 32:92–120.

15. Leventhal JR, Dalmasso AP, Cromwell JW, Platt JL, Manivel CJ, Bolman RM III, Matas AJ. Prolongation of cardiac xenograft survival by depletion of complement. Transplantation 1993; 55:857–866.

16. Nelson RA. A new concept of immunosuppression in hypersensitivity reactions and in transplantation immunity. Surv Ophthalmol 1966; 11:498–505.

17. Stad RK, van Gijlswijk-Janssen DJ, van Es LA, Daha MR. Complement depletion abolishes IgA-mediated glomerular inflammation in the rat. Exp Nephrol 1994; 2:182–189.

18. Henson PM, Cochrane CG. Acute immune complex disease in rabbits. The role of complement and of a leukocyte-dependent release of vasoactive amines from platelets. J Exp Med 1971; 133:554–571.

19. Pabst H, Day NK, Gewurz H, et al. Prevention of experimental allergic encephalomyelitis with cobra venom factor. Proc Soc Exp Biol Med 1971; 136:555–560.

20. Frank MM. Animal models for complement deficiencies. J Clin Immunol 1995; 15 (6 Suppl):113S–121.

21. Juhl H, Sievers M, Baltzer K, Helmig F, Wolf H, Brenner W, Kalthoff H. A monoclonal antibody-cobra venom factor conjugate increases the tumor-specific uptake of a 99mTc-labeled anti-carcinoembryonic antigen antibody by a two-step approach. Cancer Res 1995; 55 (23 Suppl):5749s–5755.

22. Morgan BP, Meri S. Membrane proteins that protect against complement lysis. Semin Immunopathol 1994; 15:369–396.

23. Kalli KR, Hsu P, Fearon DT. Therapeutic uses of recombinant complement protein inhibitors. Semin Immunopathol 1994; 15:417–431.

24. Klickstein LB, Bartow TJ, Miletic V, Rabson LD, Smith JA, Fearon DT. Identification of distinct C3b and C4b recognition sites in the human C3b/C4b receptor (CR1, CD35) by deletion mutagenesis. J Exp Med 1988; 168:1699–1717.

25. Fearon DT. Cellular receptors for fragments of the third component of complement. Immunol Today 1984; 5:105–110.

26. Weisman HF, Bartow T, Leppo MK, et al. Soluble human complement receptor type 1: in vivo inhibitor of complement suppressing post-ischemic myocardial inflammation and necrosis. Science 1990; 249:146–151.

27. Pruitt SK, Kirk AD, Bollinger RR, et al. The effect of soluble complement receptor type 1 on hyperacute rejection of porcine xenografts. Transplantation 1994; 57:363–370.

28. Pruitt SK, Baldwin WM III, Marsh HC Jr, Lin SS, Yeh CG, Bollinger RR. The effect of soluble complement receptor type 1 on hyperacute xenograft rejection. Transplantation 1991; 52:868–873.

29. Pruitt SK, Bollinger RR, The effect of soluble complement receptor type 1 on hyperacute allograft rejection. J Surg Res 1991; 50:350–355.

30. Yeh CG, Marsh HC Jr, Carson GR, et al. Recombinant soluble complement receptor type 1 inhibits inflammation in the reversed passive arthus reaction in rats. J Immunol 1991; 146:250–256.

31. Mulligan MS, Yeh CG, Rudolph AR, Ward PA. Protective effects of soluble CR1 in complement- and neutrophil-mediated tissue injury. J Immunol 1992; 148:1479–1485.

32. Piddlesden SJ, Storch, MK, Hibbs M, Freeman AM, Lassman H, Morgan BP. Soluble recombinant complement receptor type 1 inhibits inflammation and demyelination in antibody-mediated demyelinating experimental allergic encephalomyelitis. J Immunol 1994; 152:5477–5484.

33. Shandelya SM, Kuppusamy P, Herskowitz A, Weisfeld ML, Zweier JL. Soluble complement receptor type 1 inhibits the complement pathway and prevents contractile failure in the postischemic heart. Evidence that complement activation is required for neutrophil-mediated reperfusion injury. Circulation 1993; 88:2812–2826.

34. Smith EF III, Griswold DE, Egan JW, Hillegass LM, Smith RA, Hibbs MJ, Gagnon RC. Reduction of myocardial reperfusion injury with human soluble complement receptor type 1 (BRL 55730). Eur J Pharmacol 1993; 236:477–481.

35. Hill J, Lindsay TF, Ortiz F, Yeh CG, Hechtman HB, Moore FD Jr. Soluble complement receptor type 1 ameliorates the local and remote organ injury after intestinal ischemia-reperfusion in the rat. J Immunol 1992; 149:1723–1728.

36. Chavez-Cartaya RE, DeSola GP, Wright L, Jamieson NV, White DW. Regulation of the complement cascade by soluble complement receptor type 1. Protective effect in experimental liver ischemia and reperfusion. Transplantation 1995; 59:1047–1052.

37. Kaczorowski SL, Schiding JK, Toth CA, Kochanek PM. Effect of soluble complement receptor-1 on neutrophil accumulation after traumatic brain injury in rats. J Cereb Blood Flow Metabol 1995; 15:860–864.

38. Gillinov AM, DeValeria PA, Winkelstein JA, et al. Complement inhibition with soluble complement receptor type 1 in cardiopulmonary bypass. Ann Thorac Surg 1993; 55:619–624.

39. Couser WG, Johnson RJ, Young BA, Yeh CG, Toth CA, Rudolph AR. The effects of soluble compement receptor type 1 on complement-mediated experimental glomerulonephritis. J Am Soc Nephrol 1995; 5:1888–1894.

40. Cheung AK, Parker CJ, Honholt M. Soluble complement receptor type 1 inhibits complement activation induced by hemodialysis membranes in vitro. Kidney Int 1994; 46:1680–1687.

41. Himmelfarb J, McMonagle E, Holbrook D, Toth C. Soluble complement receptor 1 inhibits both complement and granulocyte activation during ex vivo hemodialysis. J Lab Clin Med 1995; 126:392–400.

42. Swift AJ, Collins TS, Bugelski P, Winkelstein JA. Soluble complement receptor type 1 inhibits complement-mediated host defense. Clin Diagn Lab Immunol 1994; 1:585–589.

43. Medof ME, Kinoshita T, Nussenweig V. Inhibition of complement activation on the surface of cells after incorporation of decay-accelerating factor (DAF) into their membranes. J Exp Med 1984; 160:1558–1578.

44. Pangburn MK, Reduced activity of DAF on complement enzymes bound to alternative pathway activators. Similarity with Factor H. Immunology 1990; 71:598–600.

45. Brodbeck WG, Liu D, Sperry J, Mold C, Medof ME. Localization of classical and alternative pathway regulatory activity within the decay-accelerating factor. J Immunol 1996; 156:2528–2533.

46. Moran P, Beasley H, Gorrell A, et al. Human recombinant soluble decay accelerating factor inhibits complement activation in vitro and in vivo. J Immunol 1992; 149:1736–1743.

47. Seya T, Turner J, Atkinson JP. Purification and characterization of a membrane protein (gp 45–70) which is a cofactor for cleavage for C3b and C4b. J Exp Med 1986; 163:837–855.

48. Liszewski MK, Atkinson JP. Membrane cofactor protein (MCP; CD46). Isoforms differ in protection against the classical pathway of complement. J Immunol 1996; 156:4415–4421.

49. Christiansen D, Milland J, Thorley BR, McKenzie IFC, Loveland BE. A functional analysis of recombinant soluble CD46 in vivo and a comparison with recombinant soluble forms of CD55 and CD35 in vitro. Eur J Immunol 1996; 26:578–585.

50. Hangen DH, Stevens JH, Satoh PS, Hall EW, O'Hanley PT, Raffin TA. Complement levels in septic primates treated with anti-C5a antibodies. J Surg Res 1989; 46:195–199.

51. Stevens JH, O'Hanley P, Shapiro JM, Mihm FG, Satoh PS, Collins JA, Raffin TA. Effects of anti-C5a antibodies on the adult respiratory distress syndrome in septic primates. J Clin Invest 1986; 77:1812–1816.

52. Hopken U, Mohr M, Struber A, Montz H. Burchardi H, Gotze O, Opperman M. Inhibiton of interleukin-6 synthesis in an animal model of septic shock by anti-C5a monoclonal antibodies. Eur J Immunol 1996; 26:1103–1109.

53. Amsterdam EA, Stahl GL, Pan HL, Rendig SV, Fletcher MP, Longhurst JC. Limitation of reperfusion injury by a monoclonal antibody to C5a during myocardial infarction in pigs. Am J Physiol 1995; 268:H448–457.

54. Morgan EL, Ember JA, Sanderson SD, Scholz W, Buchner R, Ye RD, Hugli TE. Anti-C5a receptor antibodies. Characterization of neutralizing antibodies specific for a peptide, C5aR-(9-29), derived from the predicted amino-terminal sequence of the human C5a receptor. J. Immunol 1993; 151:377–188.

55. Watanabe H, Kuraya M, Kasukawa R, Yanagisawa H, Yanagisawa M, Fujita T. Analysis of C5a receptor by monoclonal antibody. J Immunol Methods 1995; 185:19–29.

56. Elsner J, Oppermannn M, Kapp A. Detection of C5a receptors on human eosinophils and inhibition of eosinophil effector functions by anti-C5a receptor (CD88) antibodies. Eur J Immunol 1996: 26:1560–1564.

57. Tsuji RF, Uramoto M, Koshino H, Tsuji NM, Magae J, Nagai K, Yamasaki. Preferential suppression of delayed-type hypersensitivity by L-156, 602, a C5a receptor antagonist. Biosci Biotechnol Biochem 1992: 56: 1686–1689.

58. Tsuji RF, Magae J, Nagai K, Yamasaki M. Effects of L-156, 602, a C5a receptor antagonist, on mouse experimental models of inflammation. Biosci Biotechnol Biochem 1992; 56:2034–2036.

59. Kaneko Y, Okada N, Baranyi L, Azuma T, Okada H. Antagonistic peptides against human anaphylatoxin C5a. Immunology 1995; 86:149–154.

60. Konteatis ZD, Siciliano SJ, Van Riper G, et al. Development of C5a receptor antagonists. Differential loss of functional responses. J Immunol 1994; 153:4200–4205.

61. Ninomiya N, Sims PJ. The human complement regulatory protein CD59 binds to the alpha chain of C8 and the "b" domain of C9. J Biol Chem 1992; 267:13675–13680.

62. Sugita Y, Ito K, Shiozuka K, Suzuki H, Gushima H, Tomita M, Masuho Y. Recombinant soluble CD59 inhibits reactive haemolysis with complement. Immunology 1994; 82:34–41.

63. Kroshus TJ, Rollins SA, Dalmasso AP, Elliott EA, Matis LA, Squinto SP, Bolman RM III. Complement inhibition with an anti-C5 monoclonal antibody prevents acute cardiac tissue injury in an ex vivo model of pig-to-human xenotransplantation. Transplantation 1995; 60:1194–1202.

64. Rollins SA, Matis LA, Springhorn JP, Setter E, Wolff DW. Monoclonal antibodies directed against human C5 and C8 block complement-mediated damage of xenogeneic cells and organs. Transplantation 1995; 60:1284–1292.

65. Evans MJ, Rollins SA, Wolff DW, et al. In vitro and in vivo inhibition of complement activity by a single-chain Fv fragment recognizing human C5. Mol Immunol 1995; 32:1183–1195.

66. Matis LA, Rollins SA. Complement-specific antibodies: designing novel anti-inflammatories. Nat Med 1995; 1:839–842.

67. Amsterdam EA, Stahl GL, Pan HL, Rendig SV, Fletcher MP, Longhurst JC. Limitation of reperfusion injury by a monoclonal antibody to C5a during myocardial infarction in pigs. Am J Physiol 1995; 268:H448–H457.

68. Morgan EL, Ember JA, Sanderson SD, Scholz W, Buchner R, Ye RD, Hugli TE. Anti-C5a receptor antibodies. Characterization of neutralizing antibodies specific for a peptide, C5aR-(9–29), derived from the predicted amino-terminal sequence of the human C5a receptor. J Immunol 1993; 151:377–388.

69. von Zabern I. Drugs and low molecular weight compounds affecting the complement system. In: Sim RB, ed. Activators and Inhibitors of Complement. Dordrecht, The Netherlands: Kluwer Academic Publications, 1993: 137–148.

70. Asghar SS. Pharmacological manipulation of the complement system. Pharmacol Rev 1984; 36:223–244.

71. Sahu A, Kay BK, Lambris JD. Inhibition of complement by a C3-binding peptide isolated from a phage-displayed random peptide library. Mol Immunol 1996; 33 (Suppl. 1):61.

72. Weiler JM, Yurt RW, Fearon DT, Austen KF. Modulation of the amplification convertase of complement, C3bBb, by native and commercial heparin. J Exp Med 1978; 147:409–421.

73. Maillet F, Kazatchkine MD, Glotz D, Fisher E, Rowe M. Heparin prevents formation of the human C3 amplification convertase by inhibiting the binding site for B on C3b. Mol Immunol 1983; 20:1401–1404.

74. Almeda S, Rosenberg RD, Bing DH. The binding properties of human complement component C1q. Interaction with mucopolysaccharides. J Biol Chem 1983; 258:785–791.

75. McKay EJ, Laurell AB, Martensson K, Sjöholm AG. Activation of C1, the first component of complement, the generation of C1r-C1s and C1 inactivator complexes in normal serum by heparin affinity chromatography. Mol Immunol 1981; 18:349–357.

76. Boakle RJ, Caughman GB, Vesely J, Medgyesi G, Fudenberg HH. Potentiation of factor H by heparin: a rate-limiting mechanism for inhibition of the alternative pathway. Mol Immunol 1983; 20:1157–1164.

77. Weiler JM, Edens RE, Linhardt RJ, Kapelanski DP. Heparin and modified heparin inhibit complement activation in vivo. J Immunol 1992; 148:3210–3215.

78. Rent R, Ertel N, Eisenstein R, Gewurz H. Complement activation by interaction of polyanions and polycations. I. Heparin-protamine induced consumption of complement. J Immunol 1975; 114:120–124.

79. Fehr J, Rohr H. In vivo complement activation by polyanion-polycation complexes: evidence that C5a is generated intravascularly during heparin-protamine interaction. Clin Immunol Immunopathol 1983; 29:7–14.

80. Cavarocchi NC, Schaff HV, Orszulak TA, Homburger HA, Schnell WA Jr, Pluth JR. Evidence for complement activation by protamine-heparin interaction after cardiopulmonary bypass. Surgery 1985; 98:525–531.

81. von Zabern I. Action of polyionic substances on the complement system. In: Sim RB, ed. Activators and Inhibitors of Complement. Dordrecht, The Netherlands: Kluwer Academic Publishers, 1993:149–165.

82. Hitomi Y, Ikari N, Fujii S. Inhibitory effect of a new synthetic protease inhibitor (FUT-175) on the coagulation system. Haemostasis 1985; 15:164–168.

83. Hosokawa S, Oyamaguchi A, Yoshida O. Clinical evaluation of nafamstat mesilate (FUT-175). A new anticoagulant for plasmapheresis. ASAIO J 1982; 38:59–60.

84. Sinagi R, Miyata T, Maeda K, Sugiyama S, Miyama A, Nakashima I. FUT-175 as a potent inhibitor of C5/C3 convertase activity for production of C5a and C3a. Immunol Lett 1991; 27:49–52.

85. Issekutz AC, Roland DM, Patrick RA. The effect of FUT-175 (nafamstat mesilate) on C3a, C4a and C5a generation in vitro and inflammatory reactions in vivo. Int J Immunopharmacol 1990; 12:1–9.

86. Fujii S, Hitomi Y. New synthetic inhibitors of C1r, C1 esterase, thrombin plasmin kallikrein and trypsin. Biochim Biophys Acta 1981; 661:342–345.

87. Miyamato Y, Matsuda H, Kawashima Y. Deleterious effects of complement activation on the lungs during extracorporeal circulation and its inhibition by FUT-175. J Biomater Appl 1989; 4:56–68.

88. Ino Y, Sato T, Koshiyama Y, Suzuki K, Oda M, Iwaki M. Effects of FUT-175, a novel synthetic protease inhibitor, on the development of adjuvant arthritis in rats and some biological reactions dependent on complement activation. Gen Pharmacol 1987; 18:513–516.

89. Ikehara S, Shimamura K, Aoyama T, Fujii S, Hamashima Y. Effect of FUT-175, a new synthetic protease inhibitor, on the development of lupus nephritis in (NZB X NZW) F1 mice. Immunology 1985; 55:595–600.

90. Miyagawa S, Shirakura R, Matsumiya G, et al. Prolongation of discordant xenograft survival with anticomplement reagents K76COOH and FUT-175. Transplantation 1993; 55:709–713.

91. Miyazaki W, Tamaoka H, Shinohara M, et al. Complement inhibitor produced by Stachybotrys complementi nov. sp. K-76, a new species of fungi imperfecti. Microbiol Immunol 1980; 24:1091–1108.

92. Hong K, Kinoshita T, Miyazaki W, Izawa T, Inoue K. An anticomplementary agent, K-76 monocarboxylic acid: its site and mecahnism of inhibition of the complement activation cascade. J Immunol 1979; 122:2418–2423.

93. Miyazaki W, Izawa T, Nakano R, Shinohara M, Hing K, Kinoshita T, Inoue K. Effects of K-76 monocarboxylic acid, an anticomplementary agent, on various in vivo immunological reactions and on experimental glomerulonephritis. Complement 1984; 1:134–146.

94. Blondin C, Fisher E, Boisson-Vidal C, Kazatchkine MD, Jozefonvicz J. Inhibition of complement activation by natural sulfated polysaccharides (fucans) from brown seaweed. Mol Immunol 1994; 31:247–253.

95. Ling M, Piddlesden SJ, Morgan BP. A component of the medicinal herb ephedra blocks activation in the classical and alternative pathways of complement. Clin Exp Immunol 1995; 102:582–588.

96. Firkin F, Goldberg H, Firkin BG. Glucocorticoid management of PNH. Aust Ann Med 1968; 17:127–134.

97. Atkinson JP, Frank MM. Effect of cortisone therapy on serum complement components. J Immunol 1973; 111:1061–1066.

98. Atkinson JP, Shin H, Frank MM. Metabolic behavior of C3 in normal, C4-deficient (C4D) and cortisone-treated guinea pigs. J Immunol 1974; 113:1085–1092.

99. Pennington JE, Matthews WJ Jr, Marino JT Jr, Colten HR. Cyclophosphamide and cortisone acetate inhibit complement biosynthesis by guinea pig bronchoalveolar macrophages. J Immunol 1979; 123:1318–1321.

100. Munoz-Canoves P, Tack BF, Vik DP. Analysis of complement factor H mRNA expression: dexamethasone and IFN-gamma increase the level of H in L cells. Biochemistry 1989; 28:9891–9897.

101. Lemercier C, Julen N, Coulpier M, Dauchel H, Ozanne D, Fontaine M, Ripoche J. Differential modulation by glucocorticoids of alternative complement protein secretion in cells of the monocyte/macrophage lineage. Eur J Immunol 1992; 22:909–915.

102. Dalmasso AP, Platt JL. Prevention of complement-mediated activation of xenogeneic endothelial cells in an in vitro model of xenograft hyperacute rejection by C1 inhibitor. Transplantation 1993; 56:1171–1176.

103. Buerke M, Murohara T, Lefer AM. Cardioprotective effects of a C1 esterase inhibitor in myocardial ischemia and reperfusion. Circulation 1995; 91:393–402.

104. Waytes AT, Rosen FS, Frank MM. Treatment of angioedema with a vapor-heated C1 inhibitor concentrate. N Engl J Med 1996; 334:1630–1634.

105. Poulle M, Burnouf-Radosevich M, Burnouf T. Large-scale preparation of highly purified human C1 inhibitor for therapeutic use. Blood Coagul Fibrinolysis 1994; 5:543–549.

106. Gelfand JA, Sherins RJ, Alling AW, Frank MM. Treatment of hereditary angioedema with danazol. N Engl J Med 1976; 295:1444–1448.

107. Al-Abdullah IH, Sim RB, Sheil J, Greally JF. The effect of danazol on the production of C1 inhibitor in the guinea pig. Complement 1984; 1:27–35.

108. Fabiani JE, Paulin P, Simkin G, Leoni J, Palombarani S, Squinquera L. Hereditary angioedema: therapeutic effect of danazol on C4 and C1 esterase inhibitors. Ann Allergy 1990; 64:388–392.

109. Erickson RW, Franklin WA, Emlen W. Treatment of hemorrhagic lupus pneumonitis with plasmapheresis. Semin Arthritis Rheum 1994; 24:114–123.

110. Lockwood CM, Boulton-Jones JM, Lowenthal RM, Simpson IJ, Peters DK. Recovery from Goodpasture's syndrome after immunosuppressive therapy and plasmapheresis. Br Med J 1975; 2:252–254.

111. Euler HH, Krey U, Schroder O, Loffler H. Membrane plasmapheresis technique in rats. Confirmation of antibody rebound. J Immunol Methods 1985; 84:313–319.

112. Dau PC, Callahan J, Parker R, Golbus. Immunologic effects of plasmapheresis synchronized with pulse cyclophosphamide in systemic lupus erythematosus. J Rheumatol 1991; 18:270–276.

113. Brown EJ, Berger M, Joiner KA, Frank MM. Classical complement pathway activation by antipneumococcal antibodies leads to covalent binding of C3b to antibody molecules. Infect Immun 1983; 42:594–598.

114. Sahu A, Pangburn MK. Covalent attachment of human complement C3 to IgG. Identification of the amino acid residue involved in ester linkage formation. J Biol Chem 1994; 269:28997–29002.

115. Malbran A, Frank MM, Fries LF. Interactions of monomeric IgG bearing covalently bound C3b with polymorphonuclear leukocytes. Immunology 1987; 61:15–20.

116. Fries LF, Siwik SA, Malbran A, Frank MM. Phagocytosis of target particles bearing C3b-IgG covalent complexes by human monocytes and polymorphonuclear leukocytes. Immunology 1987; 62:45–51.

117. Fries LF, Gaither TA, Hammer CH, Frank MM. C3b covalently bound to IgG demonstrates a reduced rate of inactivation by factors H and I. J Exp Med 1984; 160:1640–1655.

118. Fries LF, Prince GM, Gaither TA, Frank MM. Factor I co-factor activity of CR1 overcomes the protective effect of IgG on covalently bound C3b residues. J Immunol 1985; 135:2673–2679.

119. Dwyer JM. Manipulating the immune system with immune globulin. N Engl J Med 1992; 326:107–116.

120. Frank MM, Basta M, Fries LF. The effects of intravenous immune globulin on complement-dependent immune damage of cells and tissues. Clin Immunol Immunopathol 1992; 62:S82–86.

121. Mouthon L, Kaveri SV, Spalter SH, Lacroix-Desmazes S, Lefranc C, Desai R, Kazatchkine MD. Mechanism of action of intravenous immune globulin in immune-mediated diseases. Clin Exp Immunol 1996; 104 (Suppl. 1):3–9.

122. Basta, Kirsbom P, Frank MM, Fries LF. Mechanism of therapeutic effect of high-dose intravenous immunoglobulin. Attenuation of acute, complement-dependent immune damage in a guinea pig model. J Clin Invest 1989; 84:1974–1981.

123. Basta M, Langlois PF, Marques M, Frank MM, Fries LF. High-dose immunoglobulin modifies complement-mediated in vivo clearance. Blood 1989; 74:326–333.

124. Magee JC, Collins BH, Harland RC, Lindman BJ, Bollinger RR, Frank MM, Platt JL. Immunoglobulin prevents complement-mediated hyperacute rejection in swine-to-primate xenotransplantation. J Clin Invest 1995; 96:2404–2412.

125. Basta M, Dalakas MC. High-dose intravenous immunoglobulin exerts its beneficial effect in patients with dermatomyositis by blocking endomysial deposition of activated complement fragments. J Clin Invest 1994; 94:1729–1735.

126. Basta M. Modulation of complement-mediated immune damage by intravenous immune globulin. Clin Exp Immunol 1996; 104 (Suppl. 1):21–25.

127. Miletic VD, Frank MM. Complement-immunoglobulin interactions. Curr Opin Immunol 1995; 7:41–47.

128. Mollnes TE, Høgasen K, Hoaas BF, Michaelsen TE, Garred P, Harboe M. Inhibition of complement-mediated red cell lysis by immunoglobulins is dependent on the Ig isotype and its C1 binding properties. Scand J Immunol 1995; 41:449–456.

129. Qi M, Schifferli JA. Inhibition of complement activation by intravenous immunoglobulins. Arthritis Rheum 1995; 38:146.

130. Russel-Jones GJ, Ey PL, Reynolds BL. The ability of IgA to inhibit the complement-mediated lysis of target red blood cells sensitized with IgG antibody. Mol Immunol 1980; 17:1173–1180.

131. Miletic VD, Hester CG, Frank MM. Regulation of complement activity by immunoglobulin. I. Effect of immunoglobulin isotype on C4 uptake on antibody-sensitized sheep erythrocytes and solid phase immune complexes. J Immunol 1996; 156:749–757.
132. Steele DJR, Auchincloss H Jr. Xenotransplantation. Annu Rev Med 1995; 46:345–360.
133. Platt JL, Lindman BJ, Chen H, Spitalnik SL, Bach FH. Endothelial cell antigens recognized by xenoreactive antibodies. Transplantation 1990; 50:817–822.
134. Vaughan HA, McKenzie IFC, Sandrin MS. Biochemical studies of pig xenoantigens detected by naturally occurring human natural antibodies and the galactose α (1–3) galactose reactive lectin. Transplantation 1995; 59:102–109.
135. Pratt JL, Vercelotti GM, Dalmasso AP, Matas AJ, Bolman RM, Najarian JS, Bach FH. Transplantation of discordant xenografts: a review of progress. Immunol Today 1990; 11:450–456.
136. Dalmasso AP. The complement system in xenotransplantation. Immunopharmacology 1992; 24:149–160.
137. Platt JL, Logan JS. Use of transgenic animals in xenotransplantation. Transplant Rev 1996; 10:69–77.
138. Cozzi E, White DJG. The generation of transgenic pigs as potential organ donors for humans. Nat Med 1995; 1:964–966.
139. Miyagawa S, Shirakura R, Matsumiya G, et al. Test for ability of decay-accelerating factor (DAF, CD55) and CD59 to alleviate complement-mediated damage of xenoerythrocytes. Scand J Immunol 1993; 38:37–44.
140. Fodor WL, Williams BL, Matis LA, et al. Expression of a functional human complement inhibitor in a transgenic pig as a model for the prevention of xenogeneic hyperacute organ rejection. Proc Natl Acad USA 1994; 91:1153–1157.
141. Diamond LE, McCurry KR, Martin MJ, McClellan SB, Oldham ER, Platt JL, Logan JS. Characterization of transgenic pigs expressing functionally active human CD59 on cardiac endothelium. Transplantation 1996; 61:1241–1249.
142. Miyagawa S, Mikata S, Shirakura R, et al. C5b-8 step lysis of swine endothelial cells by human complement and functional feature of transfected CD59. Scand J Immunol 1996, 43:361–366.
143. McCurry KR, Kooyman DL, Alvarado CG, et al. Human complement regulatory proteins protect swine-to-primate cardiac xenografts from humoral injury. Nat Med 1995; 1:423–427.
144. Fodor WL, Rollins SA. Guilmette ED, Setter E, Squinto SP. A novel bifunctional chimeric complement inhibitor that regulates C3 convertase and formation of the membrane attack complex. J Immunol 1995; 155:4135–4138.

25

Autoimmune Hemolytic Anemia

ALAN D. SCHREIBER
University of Pennsylvania School of Medicine, Philadelphia, Pennsylvania

Immunological mechanisms play a significant role in the pathophysiology of many disease processes. However, there are relatively few disorders for which it is possible to gain a detailed understanding of the mechanisms of immune damage in humans. Autoimmune hemolytic anemia is of particular interest in this regard, as it is possible to define many of the immunopathological processes that occur in this disease in molecular and cellular terms. Autoimmune hemolytic anemia represents a group of disorders in which individuals produce antibodies directed toward one or more of their own erythrocyte membrane antigens. This leads to destruction of the antibody-coated erythrocytes by tissue macrophages.

In this chapter we will discuss the underlying mechanisms responsible for the immune clearance of red blood cells by antibodies. We will then discuss briefly the clinical syndrome of paroxysmal nocturnal hemoglobinuria (PNH), a complement-mediated hemolytic anemia characterized by intravascular hemolysis due to a red cell membrane defect. We contrast the clinical findings to those in autoimmune hemolytic anemia in which extravascular destruction of red blood cells predominates. Finally, we discuss drug-induced immune hemolytic anemia.

The most effective way to approach autoimmune hemolytic anemia is to determine which class of antibody is responsible for the hemolysis. In general, there are two major classes of antierythrocyte antibodies that produce hemolysis in humans: IgG and IgM. The pattern of red blood cell clearance, the site of organ sequestration, the response to therapy, and the prognosis all relate to the class of antierythrocyte antibody involved.

I. PATHOPHYSIOLOGY OF IMMUNE HEMOLYSIS

A. IgG-Induced Immune Hemolytic Anemia

Some years ago, an experimental model of immune hemolytic anemia was established in the guinea pig to examine the pathophysiology of erythrocyte destruction by antibodies (1,2). As with human erythrocytes, guinea pig erythrocytes are relatively resistant to the lytic action of complement, and their hemolysis, which is mediated by antibody and complement, is primarily extravascular. Each of the factors important in erythrocyte destruction defined in this model has been found to be of importance in the disease as it occurs in humans. An understanding of this experimental model provides a clearer understanding of many aspects of the human disease. IgG and IgM anti-guinea-pig erythrocyte antibodies were used to sensitize chromium 51-radiolabeled guinea pig erythrocytes. The radiolabeled, antibody-coated erythrocytes were then injected intravenously into guinea pigs and the rate and pattern of clearance as well as the site of organ sequestration of the antibody-sensitized cells were determined.

The number of antibody molecules on the erythrocytic surface was quantitated by both radiolabeling the antibody to assess directly the number of antibody molecules bound to the red cells and by using a sensitive complement fixation assay. With the latter test, antibody per erythrocyte could be expressed in terms of the number of complement or C1- (the first component of complement) activating sites generated by the antibody. A single molecule of IgM antibody bound to an erythrocyte binds and activates a single molecule of C1 to initiate the classical complement pathway. In the case of IgG antibodies, two molecules of the IgG antibody need to be in close proximity to one another on the eythrocyte surface in order for C1 binding and initiation of the classical pathway to occur. With antigens widely distributed on the erythrocyte surface, such as the antigens recognized by most antierythrocyte antibodies, many hundreds or thousands of IgG antibody molecules must be deposited on the erythrocyte membrane before two bind sufficiently close to one another to permit complement activation.

IgG-sensitized erythrocytes are removed progressively from the circulation and sequestered predominantly in the spleen (Fig. 1). Erythrocyte survival is determined by the number of antibody molecules per cell; increasing the number of IgG molecules per cell progressively increased the splenic sequestration of these cells.

IgG-coated erythrocytes are cleared from the circulation in an accelerated fashion even in the absence of complement activation. This was evident from the studies with IgG-coated erythrocytes performed in guinea pigs deficient either in the fourth (C4) or

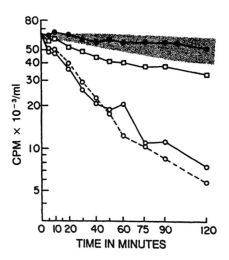

Figure 1 Survival of chromium 51 (^{51}Cr)-labeled guinea pig erythrocytes coated with IgG antibody in normal (open circles) and C4-deficient (open squares) guinea pigs. The survival of IgG-coated erythrocytes in C3-depleted guinea pigs was similar to that observed in C4-deficient guinea pigs. The closed circles represent the survival of ^{51}Cr-unsensitized erythrocytes. (Shaded area, 95% confidence limits.)

third (C3) component of complement (see Fig. 1). Complement-independent clearance of IgG-coated erythrocytes was predominantly by macrophages in the spleen, and a rather large number of antibody molecules per cell was required.

These studies indicated the importance of complement in accelerating the clearance of IgG-coated red cells. C4-deficient guinea pigs have a complete block in their classical complement pathway and complement is not activated beyond the C1 step. A comparison of C4-deficient and normal animals allowed for the assessment of the role of antibody compared with the role of antibody plus complement in altering erythrocyte survival. In addition, we depleted guinea pigs of the third component of complement (C3), as well as the later-acting complement components by treating the animals with cobra venom factor. In animals genetically deficient in C4 or depleted of C3 by cobra venom factor, the complement activation sequence does not proceed through C3, and erythrocytes do not become coated with C3 in vivo. As shown in Figure 1, IgG-coated cells are cleared much more rapidly in normal than in C4-deficient animals. The defect in the clearance of IgG-coated erythrocytes in both C4-deficient and C3-depleted animals resides in the failure of C3 to bind to the erythrocyte surface. The similar survival of IgG-coated erythrocytes in C4-deficient and C3-depleted guinea pigs suggests that the classical, rather than the alternative, complement pathway is of prime importance in the clearance of IgG-coated erythrocytes.

Thus, these studies demonstrated that IgG-coated erythrocytes are cleared predominantly in the spleen regardless of whether complement activation occurs. When very large amounts of IgG are bound to the erythrocytes, the liver becomes the predominant organ of clearance. In vitro studies have shown that macrophages of the reticuloendothelial system have several classes of surface receptors for the Fc domain of IgG antibodies (Fcγ receptors). These receptors are responsible for the binding and phagocytosis of IgG-coated erythrocytes. One of the Fcγ receptor isoforms is a high-affinity receptor present on macrophages and monocytes, FcγRI. There are also two low-affinity receptors on macrophages FcγRIIA and FcγRIIIA (3–6). Fcγ receptors appear responsible, at least in part, for the clearance of IgG-coated cells, since they are not inhibited as efficiently by plasma concentrations of IgG. Erythrocytes coated with multiple IgG molecules interact with macrophages with multiple Fcγ receptors, leading to the binding of the erythrocytes to the macrophage surface which in turn induces phagocytosis.

Macrophages can alter IgG- and/or C3b-coated erythrocytes in a manner that causes the red blood cells to form microspherocytes (4,13). These spherocytes are less able to pass through the splenic cords and sinuses and, therefore, have a decreased survival. Their presence in the circulation is an indication of immune hemolysis. Macrophages also have receptors, designated CR1 and CR2, for the activated third component of complement, which recognize the C3b and iC3b forms of C3b, respectively, and which are capable of binding C3b-coated erythrocytes. The receptors for the various C3 fragments do not recognize native C3; they only recognize fragments of C3 after C3 has undergone activation. Therefore they are capable of efficient function in the presence of normal plasma concentrations of C3. Fcγ receptors and C3b receptors can interact synergistically in their binding of IgG and C3b-coated cells and therefore the clearance of erythrocytes coated with IgG and C3b is greater than of those coated with IgG alone.

B. IgM-Induced Immune Hemolytic Anemia

When erythrocytes are coated with IgM antibody and injected intravenously into guinea pigs, the pattern of clearance and site of organ sequestration are different from those of

IgG-coated erythrocytes (Fig. 2). IgM-coated cells are cleared rapidly within the liver rather than the spleen. Erythrocyte survival is proportional to the number of IgM molecules per red blood cell.

There is an absolute requirement for complement for the clearance of IgM-coated cells. This was determined by examining the erythrocyte survival of IgM-coated cells in C4-deficient and C3-depleted guinea pigs. IgM-coated erythrocytes survive normally in complement-deficient animals, even when agglutinating concentrations of IgM antibody are employed. In vitro studies showed that macrophages did not bind IgM-coated erythrocytes in the absence of complement. This is because macrophages do not have receptors for the Fc domain of IgM antibodies, in contrast to their abundant receptors for the Fc domain of IgG antibodies. Activation of the complement sequence by IgM results in the deposition of C3b on the erythrocyte surface. Erythrocyte-bound C3b and iC3b leads to an interaction with hepatic macrophage C3b and iC3b receptors. This interaction with complement is responsible for the clearance of IgM-coated erythrocytes. Thus, IgM-coated erythrocytes require complement for their clearance.

IgM- and C3b-coated erythrocytes are rapidly sequestered within the liver. Subsequently, they are either phagocytosed and destroyed or they are released from their hepatic macrophage C3 receptor attachment site back into the circulation where they then survive normally, even though they still are coated with IgM and antigenically detectable C3. Extensive in vitro and in vivo studies indicate that this release of IgM- and C3-coated erythrocytes from the macrophage C3 receptor attachment site is not due to elution of the antibody from the surface. Rather, the C3b/iC3b inactivator system, which involves several circulating plasma proteins including factor I and factor H, causes the release of C3-coated erythrocytes from the macrophage C3b and iC3b receptor attachment sites (1,7). These released C3-coated cells have on their surface an antigenically altered form of C3 (C3d) that is no longer strongly bound by the macrophage C3b/C3bi receptors. These C3d-coated erythrocytes then survive normally. Increasing the concentration of

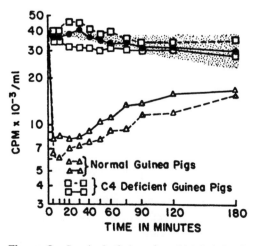

Figure 2 Survival of chromium 51-labeled guinea pig erythrocytes coated with IgM antibody in normal (open triangles) and C4-deficient (open squares) guinea pigs. The survival of IgM-coated erythrocytes in C3-depleted guinea pigs was similar to that observed in C4-deficient guinea pigs. (Shaded area, 95% confidence limits.)

IgM per erythrocyte accelerates the sequestration by the liver macrophages and also decreases the number of erythrocytes released from the hepatic macrophage receptor binding sites. Pretreatment of IgM- and C3-coated erythrocytes with a source of serum C3 inactivator system proteins alters the erythrocyte cell-bound C3 and improves erythrocyte survival.

Thus, these studies demonstrated that the two major classes of antibody that cause autoimmune hemolytic anemia, IgG and IgM, differ markedly in their biological effects. IgG-coated erythrocytes are cleared predominantly in the spleen, whereas IgM-coated erythrocytes are sequestered predominantly within the liver. Splenic macrophage Fc receptors and C3 receptors are responsible for the clearance of IgG-coated cells. IgG-coated erythrocytes do not require complement for their clearance. However, complement accelerates the clearance of IgG-coated erythrocytes in the spleen. Blood flow in the spleen is slower with closer contact between sinusoidal macrophage and circulating red blood cells. This facilitates IgG-mediated splenic macrophage clearance.

The pattern of clearance of IgM-coated erythrocytes is entirely different from that of IgG-coated cells. IgM-coated cells are cleared rapidly by the hepatic macrophage C3 receptors. The clearance is entirely complement dependent and in the absence of complement activation these cells survive normally. The C3 inactivator system serves as an important control mechanism for the clearance of IgM-coated cells, mediating the release of IgM- and C3-coated cells from the their hepatic macrophage C3 receptor attachment sites. Furthermore, exposure of IgM- and C3-coated erythrocytes to C3 inactivator system proteins can attenuate the clearance of these C3-coated cells by hepatic macrophages.

II. CLINICAL FEATURES

A. IgG-Induced Autoimmune Hemolytic Anemia

Autoimmune hemolytic anemia is most commonly caused by IgG antibodies (8,9). The antigen to which the IgG antibody is directed is usually one of the Rh erythrocyte antigens, although often its precise specificity is not easily defined. This antibody usually has its maximal activity at 37° C and thus this entity has been termed warm antibody-induced hemolytic anemia.

IgG-induced immune hemolytic anemia can occur without an apparent underlying disease (idiopathic autoimmune hemolytic anemia); however, it can also occur with an underlying immunoproliferative disorder, either malignant or nonmalignant, such as chronic lymphocytic leukemia, non-Hodgkin's lymphoma, and systemic lupus erythematosus. Certain patients with immunodeficiency states such as agammaglobulinemia can develop autoimmune hemolytic anemia as well. In rare cases, IgG-induced immune hemolytic anemia has also been observed in patients with an underlying malignant disease that is not an immunoproliferative disorder (Table 1). Such malignant disorders include ovarian tumors and myelofibrosis with myeloid hyperplasia. Additionally, bacterial infections, such as tuberculosis; viral infections, such as cytomegalovirus disease; and chronic inflammatory conditions, such as ulcerative colitis, have been described as associated conditions. The incidence of idiopathic IgG-induced autoimmune hemolytic anemia varies among different series. However, overall approximately half of the patients with IgG-induced immune hemolysis do not have a detectable underlying disease at the time of diagnosis. The other half have an underlying disease, such as those mentioned above, or have a drug-induced immune hemolytic anemia (10). In both the "idiopathic" disease and that

Table 1   Diseases associated with autoimmune hemolytic anemia

Infections
    Viral infections, especially respiratory infections
    Infectious mononucleosis and cytomegalovirus
    Mycoplasma, especially *M. pneumoniae*
    Tuberculosis

Disorders
    Systemic lupus erythematosus
    Rheumatoid arthritis
    Thyroid disorders
    Ulcerative colitis
    Chronic active hepatitis

Immunodeficiency syndromes
    X-linked agammaglobulinemia
    Dysgammaglobulinemia
    Common variable hypogammaglobulinemia
    IgA deficiency
    Wiskott-Aldrich syndrome

Malignancies
    Non-Hodgkin's lymphoma
    Hodgkin's disease
    Acute lymphocytic leukemia
    Carcinoma
    Thymoma
    Ovarian cysts and tumors

associated with an underlying immunoproliferative disorder, some patients have immune thrombocytopenia (ITP) in conjunction with IgG-induced autoimmune hemolytic anemia (Evan's syndrome). In addition, patients have been described with immune hemolytic anemia, immune thrombocytopenia, and immune granulocytopenia with antibodies directed toward erythrocytes, platelets, and granulocytes (12). It is not clear whether such IgG antibodies directed against each blood cell line recognize a common blood cell antigen or represent antibodies with different specificities.

In IgG-induced autoimmune hemolytic anemia, many IgG molecules on the erythrocyte surface are needed to bind and activate a single molecule of C1, the first component of complement, because two IgG molecules in close proximity to each other (a doublet) are required. Once C1 is bound and activated, C4 and C2 activation occurs in a manner similar to that described for IgM antibody (see below), and C3 convertase is formed. C3 cleavage results and C3b is deposited on the erythrocyte surface. Macrophages within the reticuloendothelial system have receptors not only for C3b but also for the Fc fragment of IgG as well (Fcγ receptors). These macrophage Fcγ receptors bind IgG-coated erythrocytes and mediate spherocyte formation or phagocytosis. Thus, patients who have IgG on the erythrocyte surface in insufficient numbers or distributed in such a way to be unable to cause C1 binding and activation still have a substantial decrease in erythrocyte survival. However, once sufficient IgG is present on the erythrocyte surface so that C1 activation occurs, erythrocyte clearance is further accelerated. In such a circumstance, clearance is due to the macrophage Fcγ receptors and the macrophage C3b/C3bi receptors. These receptors interact synergistically to induce the binding of erythrocytes coated with IgG and C3b/C3bi IgG-coated erythrocytes are cleared progressively from the circulation, primarily in the spleen, and hemolysis is almost always extravascular.

B. IgM-Induced Autoimmune Hemolytic Anemia

In humans, IgM-induced autoimmune hemolytic anemia is caused by an IgM antibody that reacts most efficiently with erythocytes in the cold (15,16). Thus, this disorder has also been called cold hemagglutinin disease. The IgM antibody in cold hemagglutinin disease is usually directed against the I antigen or related antigens on the human erythrocyte membrane. As with all IgM antibodies, agglutinating activity is particularly efficient because of the multiple antigen-combining sites on the IgM molecule. In this disorder, the IgM antibody has a particular affinity for its red cell antigen in the cold (0–10°C) and the affinity is lower at higher temperatures. Like warm antibody (i.e., IgG-mediated) autoimmune hemolytic anemia, cold hemagglutinin disease can be classified into those cases considered primary or idiopathic or those associated with an underlying disease (secondary).

Chronic cold hemagglutinin disease is due to a clonal expansion of lymphocytes that produce a monoclonal antibody that recognizes a polysaccharide antigen on red cells termed I or i. The most common form of chronic cold hemagglutinin disease is the primary or idiopathic form. This is usually a disease of older persons, with a peak incidence in the 50s and 60s in some series (17). Most often it presents as fatigue, anemia, and occasionally jaundice in an elderly individual, but it may be associated with the development of acrocyanosis due to sludging of blood in peripheral vessels on exposure to cold or with acute hemolysis. This disease is associated with the presence of a monoclonal IgM antibody, usually exhibiting a high cold agglutinin titer (>1:1000). This IgM antibody binds to erythrocytes avidly in the cold but shows no binding activity at 37° C. In most, but not all, patients the antibody is of the κ light chain type and has specificity for the I antigen present on the erythrocytes of most adults. The I antigenic determinants are closely related to the ABO core antigenic determinants. Although present on the erythrocytes of almost all persons, the antigenic groupings recognized by the antibody develop during childhood and are not present on blood taken from the umbilical vein of the newborn. Thus, operationally, I specificity is established by the ability of the antibody to agglutinate the blood of almost all adults, but an inability to agglutinate the erythrocytes of newborns. Although the monoclonal antibody responsible for the development of the cold hemagglutinin syndrome presumably reflects the expansion of a single clone of cells, patients with this condition do not develop the symptom complex associated with multiple myeloma or Waldenstrom's macroglobulinemia. The monoclonal antibody appears to represent a highly restricted clonal response to the I antigen. Although each patient usually has only a single antibody with a single amino acid sequence, the antibodies among patients virtually always differ. Nevertheless, these antibodies tend to share idiotypic determinants consistent with their uniform recognition of the I antigen.

Secondary cold hemagglutinin disease or IgM-induced immune hemolytic anemia is most commonly associated with an underlying mycoplasma infection, particularly *Mycoplasma pneumoniae*, in which antibody with typical anti-I specificity is produced. However, it may also occur with other infections, such as infectious mononucleosis, cytomegalovirus, and mumps. With infectious mononucleosis anti-i (antibody to an antigen related to I, but present on cord blood cells) cold agglutinins are produced, but overt hemolysis is unusual. Under most circumstances with an underlying infection the cold agglutinin (IgM antibody) is polyclonal, that is, immunochemically heterogeneous.

Cold hemagglutinin disease can also be seen in patients with an underlying immunoproliferative disorder, such as chronic lymphocytic leukemia and non-Hodgkin's lymphoma, or an underlying connective tissue disease such as systemic lupus erythematosus (18). As in idiopathic cold hemagglutinin disease, patients with an underlying malignant immunoproliferative disorder, such as one of the non-Hodgkin's lymphomas, have a cold agglutinin that is commonly monoclonal or of restricted heterogeneity (oligoclonal). Waldenstrom's macroglobulinemia, a variant of multiple myeloma and one of the B-cell immunoproliferative disorders, is also at times associated with the formation of IgM antibody against red blood cells. Anti-i, often with λ light chains, may be seen in more malignant lymphocytic neoplasias.

It is unclear why patients with an underlying infection such as *M. pneumoniae* produce anti-red-cell (anti-I) antibodies. Older studies suggested cross-antigenicity between the mycoplasma cell wall and the human red blood cell membrane (19,20); however, these data are tenuous.

The plasma of healthy adults and children contains low levels of IgM antierythrocyte antibodies, that is, low levels of IgM cold agglutinins. In rare cases, cold-reacting autoantibodies have been observed with specificity directed against red blood cell antigens other than I or i, that is, the P and the PR antigens. Also IgA cold agglutinins have been observed rarely.

The reason for the preferential reaction of cold agglutinin with the human red blood cell membrane in the cold is not completely understood. Most cold agglutinins have no measurable activity above 30°C. Although it has been postulated that either the antibody or the antigen may undergo a structural change on exposure to cold, most data suggest that the antigen on the erythrocyte surface is altered in the cold. This may represent a cold-dependent conformational change in the antigen recognized by the antibody-combining site or a cold-induced change in the erythrocyte surface that increases antigen availability. When intact erythrocytes are studied, IgM anti-I interactions occur only in the cold. However, reactivity at 37°C is noted when the I antigen is isolated from the erythrocyte membrane.

As in all patients with autoimmune hemolytic anemia, erythrocyte survival is generally proportional to the amount of antibody on the erythrocyte surface. In cold hemagglutinin disease, the extent of hemolysis is a function of the titer of the antibody (cold agglutinin titer), the thermal amplitude of the IgM antibody (the highest temperature at which the antibody is active), and the level of the circulating control proteins of the C3 inactivator system.

The factors that govern the survival of antibody- and complement-coated erythrocytes in humans are much the same as factors governing the clearance of these cells in animals. In cold hemagglutinin disease, the IgM antibody in the circulation of patients with the disease interacts with the erythrocyte surface, when the cells circulate to areas below body temperatures, and activates the early steps of the classical complement pathway (21,22). Once C1, the first component of complement is bound to the IgM molecule and activated, it sequentially binds and activates the fourth and second components of complement. The first of these two steps takes place at temperatures as low as 0°C. When the cells return to body temperature, activation proceeds, even though the cold agglutinin antibody can dissociate from the erythrocyte. The C3 convertase (C142) generated cleaves C3 into two antigenic fragments, one of which, C3b (and iC3b), binds to the erythrocyte surface. At this step there is considerable amplification of the IgM effect with a single C142 classical pathway C3 convertase capable of cleaving many C3 molecules and depositing many C3b molecules on the erythrocyte surface. In some cases the complement sequence of reactions may be completed with resulting hemolysis, but this is unusual because of the presence of membrane-bound proteins that restrict complement action. These C3b/C3bi-coated erythrocytes are recognized by the hepatic macrophage complement receptors. The macrophage C3b and iC3b receptors bind, sphere, and may mediate phagocytosis of the C3b-coated erythrocytes (23–25). Extravascular sequestration usually predominates in patients with this disease. In humans, as in the guinea pig model, there are no receptors on macrophages capable of interacting with IgM-coated cells in the absence of complement; thus, in the absence of an intact classical complement pathway, through activation of C3, IgM-coated red cells have a normal survival.

In humans, clearance of IgM-plus-complement-coated cells has been shown to be very rapid and takes place primarily in the liver (2,26). The human erythrocyte membrane, in contrast to the sheep erythrocyte membrane, is relatively resistant to the lytic action of complement. However, when large numbers of IgM molecules are present on the erythrocyte surface sufficient terminal complement components (C5–C9) are occasionally generated to lyse the erythrocytes in the intravascular space.

Control proteins involved in the C3 inactivator system are particularly important in cold hemagglutinin disease, because cell destruction is mediated entirely by C3 and the later complement components. Thus the level of the C3 inactivator proteins in plasma is thought to play an important role in determining hemolysis by regulating the number of active C3 fragments on the cell surface. The C3-coated erythrocytes interacting with C3 inactivator system proteins are degraded to C3dg or C3d. The C3dg- or C3d-coated erythrocytes are not bound by the macrophage C3 receptors and have a normal survival (1,27–28,41). Thus the presence of C3- (C3dg or C3d) coated erythrocytes in cold hemagglutinin disease explains the earlier observations of a normal erythrocyte survival in patients who still have C3, as detected by the Coombs' antiglobulin test, on their erythrocyte membranes (29).

The thermal amplitude of the IgM cold agglutinin is important in determining the extent of hemolysis in cold hemagglutinin disease. At a relatively low level of cold agglutinin sensitization, patients with higher thermal amplitude antibodies (those antibodies that possess activity at temperatures approaching 37°C) may still have considerable hemolysis. Such patients have been described as having a low-titer cold hemagglutinin syndrome with a high thermal amplitude antibody. The correct diagnosis in such patients is important because they appear to respond to glucocorticoid therapy in a manner different from the usual patient with high-titer cold hemagglutinin disease (24). Furthermore, some unusual patients have an IgG cold agglutinin. The presence of such an IgG antibody is potentially important since it appears to indicate responsiveness to treatment with steroids or splenectomy (26).

III. GENERAL FEATURES

There appears to be little genetic predisposition to the development of autoimmune hemolytic anemia (30). The occasional rare familial association of cases may be secondary to the familial predisposition to systemic lupus erythematosus or a similar underlying connective tissue disease. Thus, there are patients with autoimmune hemolytic anemia who have a family history of other autoimmune diseases, such as autoimmune thrombocytopenia, rheumatoid arthritis, and glomerulonephritis.

Autoimmune hemolytic anemia is not an uncommon disease. In large centers 15–30 cases are seen yearly, with an annual incidence of approximately 1:75,000–80,000 persons in the general population (31). As with any disease that may require careful serological study for diagnosis, the level of sophistication and diagnostic capability of the institution influence the reported incidence. Nevertheless, autoimmune hemolytic anemia occurs considerably less commonly than does autoimmune thrombocytopenia.

Autoimmune hemolytic anemia caused by either IgG or IgM antibody does not appear to be more prevalent in any particular racial group and can affect persons of any age. There is a general impression that autoimmune hemolytic anemia occurs more commonly in females, although in most series the incidence is roughly equivalent between genders. An increased incidence in females may be due to the increased incidence of systemic lupus erythematosus in women. Although warm antibody (IgG-induced) immune hemolytic anemia can occur at any age, there appears to be a peak incidence in the 50-year-old age group. In contrast, idiopathic cold hemagglutinin disease is a disease predominantly of the elderly.

The peak incidence of autoimmune hemolytic anemia in childhood is in the first 4 years of life. Children older than 10 years at onset are most likely to have a chronic course and most likely to have an underlying disorder. In a study of the prevalence of the disease in childhood, the incidence in those less than 20 years old was slightly less than 0.2:100,000 (32). In contrast to the situation in adults, in the reported series in children there is a male preponderance (33–38).

Patients with autoimmune hemolytic anemia vary considerably in their mode of clinical presentation, which may be either indolent or fulminant. In general, the course of autoimmune hemolytic anemia is more acute in children than it is in adults, often ending in complete resolution of the disease. The fall in hemoglobin may occur over a period of hours to days, with resolution of the disease often within 3 months.

The Donath-Landersteiner cold homolysin is an unusual IgG antibody with anti-P specificity that was originally noted in cases of congenital or acquired syphilis (15). The disease it causes is termed paroxysmal cold hemoglobinuria. Hemolysis in this syndrome most commonly occurs intravascularly, after the antibody has passed through an erythrocyte attachment phase at the lower temperatures of the peripheral circulation. The intravascular hemolysis is due to the unusual complement-activating efficiency of this IgG antibody. As its name implies, this antibody is associated with cold hemoglobinuria. This antibody, although uncommon, is most frequently found in children with viral infections (39–40). Hemolysis, although sometimes severe, is usually mild, and tends to resolve as the infection clears.

Mortality in the pediatric age group has ranged from 9 to 29% (33–39,42). Death during the acute stage is usually due to severe anemia or to hemorrhage from associated thrombocytopenia. Mortality in the chronic cases or in adults is higher and usually occurs because of an underlying serious disorder, such as Hodgkin's disease or non-Hodgkin's lymphoma or as a complication of therapy. Fatal sepsis has, of course, been observed following splenectomy (36).

IV. CLINICAL AND LABORATORY FINDINGS

Many of the symptoms of autoimmune hemolytic anemia, such as weakness, malaise, and light-headedness, are caused by the presence of anemia. Patients who have underlying cardiovascular disease may have significant dypsnea on exertion and peripheral edema, as well as angina pectoris. If hemolysis is significant, mild jaundice may be noted, particularly in the presence of hepatic dysfunction. In addition, patients with an underlying disease often have the symptoms associated with that disease, for example, fever and weight loss with an underlying malignant disease or joint symptoms secondary to an underlying systemic vasculitis. Physical findings are also generally referable to the underlying disease. For example, in patients with an underlying non-Hodgkin's lymphoma, hepatosplenomegaly and lymphadenopathy are common. Mild splenomegaly may be present in patients with severe autoimmune hemolytic anemia. Massive splenomegaly suggests an underlying disorder such as lymphoma. Other signs that may result from the anemic state include those caused by congestive heart failure (edema, ascites, or pulmonary congestion). Severe jaundice is uncommon.

Thus the common presenting symptoms are pallor, jaundice, dark urine, abdominal pain, and fever. Pallor may precede the appearance of jaundice. The clinical status depends on the rapidity of the hemolysis and the severity of the anemia. In mild cases fatigue may be the only symptom. In severe cases the patient may appear acutely ill or even moribund, with tachycardia, tachypnea, signs of hypoxia, and even cardiovascular collapse. In severe IgM-induced cold hemagglutinin disease the skin may have a livedo reticularis pattern and the patient may demonstrate acrocyanosis on exposure to the cold.

Laboratory data reveal the presence of anemia and, if bone marrow function is adequate, reticulocytosis. Diagnosis rests on the presence of anemia, reticulocytosis, and a positive result on direct Coombs' test. Examination of the peripheral blood smear may show spherocytes, polychromasia, nucleated red blood cells, and erythrophagocytosis. Rosetting of red cells around white cells may be visible in a buffy coat preparation.

Agglutination of the red cells may be evident in cold agglutinin disease. In severe cases macroagglutination is visible on the microscope slide or in a capillary tube. The white cell count is usually normal or elevated. Autoimmune hemolysis is also associated with thrombocytopenia and/or leukopenia in a small number of patients. Indirect hyperbilirubinemia is common. The positive result on direct Coombs' test, however, alerts the clinician to the correct diagnosis.

Reticulocytopenia may be observed, especially in children, in the first days of the anemia. In a small percentage of patients the reticulocytopenia may persist for weeks to months (44–46). Bone marrow aspiration usually shows erythroid hyperplasia, but hypoplasia is present in a few patients (46). Autoantibodies directed against early erythroid precursors are believed to be responsible for the reticulocytopenia in some patients (46). However, antibody directed at a blood cell antigen present primarily on reticulocytes is a theoretical possibility, but not proved.

The diagnosis of autoimmune hemolytic anemia is most effectively established by directly examining the patient's circulating red blood cells for the presence of antibody and/or complement components on their surface. This is most easily done by performing a direct Coombs' antiglobulin test. In this test the patient's red blood cells are made to interact with a rabbit or goat antihuman serum globulin reagent and agglutination of the patient's red blood cells is assessed. It is also possible to use antibody to human immunoglobulin or complement components as a more specific test reagent. In this case, agglutination induced by anti-IgG (a γ Coombs' test) indicates the presence of IgG on the surface of the red blood cells, whereas agglutination with an anti-C3 or anti-C4 (a non-γ Coombs' test) is used to test for the presence of C4 and C3. In IgG-induced hemolytic anemia, IgG or IgG plus complement components are found on the surface of erythrocytes. Therefore, such patients usually have a positive result in the γ Coombs' test, but may have a negative result on non-γ Coombs' test as well. In IgM-induced hemolytic anemia (cold hemagglutinin disease), IgG is not found on the red cells, and the IgM cold agglutinin, because of its low affinity for red cell antigens at 370°C, is not found either. In contrast, C3, stably bound at 37°C, is detected on the red cell membrane. Therefore, in cold hemagglutinin disease, usually, only a positive result in the non-γ (C3) Coombs' test is observed. In rare cases, patients with IgG-induced immune hemolysis have levels of IgG per erythrocyte undetectable by the standards Coombs' test, which requires the presence of hundreds of molecules of IgG on the erythrocyte surface for the result to be positive. When this phenomenon was originally described, the small amounts of red cell-bound IgG antibody were detected with a complex antiglobulin consumption test (47–48). However, now, a Coombs' test using radiolabeled anti-IgG, which is 10 times more sensitive than the standard Coombs' test, also may be used to detect the antibody (49).

Thus, testing with Coombs' antisera shows several patterns of reactivity (42). The red cells may be coated with IgG in the presence or absence of detectable complement (warm antibody IgG-mediated autoimmune hemolytic anemia) or with complement protein alone (IgM-induced hemolysis, i.e., cold hemagglutinin disease). IgM is rarely detected as well. In one large series of patients, IgG with or without complement was found on the red cells in 85–95% of patients with chronic disease, but in fewer (approximately 30%) of those with acute disease (35,42). Cold agglutinins (IgM-induced autoimmune hemolytic anemia) or the coating of red blood cells with complement alone were more common in the acute disease. Early studies suggested that the finding of IgG plus complement suggested a more guarded prognosis; however, it is now believed that it is not possible to predict chronicity or severity of autoimmune hemolytic anemia from the Coombs' testing pattern.

A cold agglutinin titer is also diagnostically helpful. This test is performed by examining the patient's plasma for agglutinating activity at 0°C directed against normal ABO-compatible erythrocytes containing the I antigen. The cold agglutinin titer is the highest dilution of antibody that still agglutinates normal red blood cells in the cold. Most patients with immune hemolysis secondary to cold hemagglutin disease have cold agglutinin titers greater than 1:1000.

V. THERAPY

In many patients with IgG- or IgM-induced immune hemolytic anemia, no therapeutic intervention is necessary, since the hemolysis is mild. If an underlying disease is present, control of this disease often brings the hemolytic anemia under control as well. However, if the patient is having significant anemia secondary to hemolysis, therapeutic intervention is in order.

A. Glucocorticoids

We have studied the effect of glucocorticoids and other steroid hormones on the clearance of IgG- and IgG-coated erythrocytes (8,24,25,50,51). We observed that pretreatment of guinea pigs with glucocorticoids impairs the splenic clearance of IgG-coated erythrocytes. Pretreatment is necessary to observe this effect. Not all animals or individuals respond to steroids equally well, although the vast majority are steroid responsive. Glucocorticoids actually decrease the surface expression of splenic macrophage Fcγ receptors, probably by decreasing Fcγ receptor transcription.

Patients with IgG antibody-mediated autoimmune hemolytic anemia or immune thrombocytopenic purpura (ITP) treated with glucocorticoids often respond within days of the onset of therapy. At the time of response, the cells remain antibody coated and there may be no decrease in antibody synthesis. Furthermore, it has been observed that some patients with IgG-mediated destruction of erythrocytes and platelets remain in clinical remission on steroid therapy, even when their cells remain antibody coated. These observations suggest that glucocorticoids affect the clearance mechanisms in humans. The data also suggest that high doses of glucocorticoids may be effective in improving red blood cell (RBC) survival in some patients with IgM-indirect immune hemolytic anemia whose RBCs are coated with limited amounts of IgM and C3. This observation led to studies in which patients were identified with a low-titer IgM- (cold hemagglutinin) induced immune hemolytic anemia, whose cells were coated with limited amounts of C3. These patients were observed to respond to corticosteroids. However, very high concentrations of glucocorticoids were required to impair the clearance of IgM- and C3 coated cells in these patients.

More recently we examined the capacity of other steroids and their analogues to modulate the clearance of IgG-coated erythrocytes by splenic macrophages (50–51). We observed that estradiol, in contrast to cortisol, enhances the clearance of IgG-coated erythrocytes by splenic macrophages in a dose-dependent manner. On the other hand, estradiol does not alter the splenic macrophage clearance of heat-altered erythrocytes or the hepatic macrophage clearance of IgM- and C3b-coated erythrocytes. This suggests that the effect of estradiol is on the splenic macrophage Fcγ receptors responsible for the clearance of IgG- coated cells. These studies suggested that the macrophage Fcγ receptors may be modulated in vivo by hormonal mechanisms and were supported by studies demonstrating that splenic macrophages isolated from estradiol-treated animals exhibited remarkably enhanced Fcγ receptor, but not C3 receptor expression, when compared with control animals. These data may explain the alteration in the clinical status of patients with immune hemolytic anemia and immune thrombocytopenia during changes in hormonal states, such as pregnancy. During pregnancy estrogen levels rise to a level similar to that necessary to accelerate the clearance of IgG-coated erythrocytes. During pregnancy the course of IgG-induced autoimmune hemolytic anemia is likewise known to accelerate.

Patients with IgG-induced immune hemolytic anemia respond, in general, to glucocorticoid therapy in dosages equivalent to 1–2 mg of prednisone per kilogram of body weight a day. These drugs are believed to decrease hemolysis in IgG-induced hemolytic anemia by three major mechanisms (52,53). First, they decrease the production of the abnormal IgG antibody. This is a common effect, is gradual, and can be expected to produce a gradual decrease in the strength of the Coombs' test result and a rise in hemoglobin within 2–6 weeks. Second, glucocorticoids are reported to be associated with a fall in the amount of antibody detected by the direct Coombs' test and a rise in the amount detected by the indirect Coomb's test, as if they induced a decrease in antibody affinity. This is probably an uncommon effect of glucocorticoid therapy. Third, glucocorticoids have been shown in vitro and in vivo to interfere with the macrophage $Fc\gamma$ receptors responsible for the erythrocyte clearance from the circulation (25,50–53). The effect is to improve erythrocyte survival despite the continued prescence of IgG on the erythrocyte surface. Thus, the Coombs' test in some patients may remain positive in the face of an improved erythrocyte survival and rising hemoglobin. This effect of glucocorticoids may be rapid and may be responsible for the rise in hemoglobin noted in some patients to occur with 1–4 days of glucocorticoid therapy. However, in a number of animal studies it was shown that glucocorticoids have no effect on erythrocyte survival until therapy has been continued for 5–7 days. Most patients will respond to glucocorticoid therapy within 2–3 weeks. Although 4–6 weeks of therapy may be required for a response to be evident, in many of these delayed responders further therapy will be needed.

Approximately 60–80% of patients have an initial response to high-dose glucocorticoids. In many patients with acute autoimmune hemolytic anemia and in a small proportion of patients with chronic autoimmune hemolytic anemia the steroids can be tapered and stopped with the patient remaining in remission. Some patients have control of their hemolytic process on continued low- to medium-dose steroid therapy. For the patients who are steroid dependent, the initial and long-term side effects of these drugs must be considered. These include exacerbation of diabetes and hypertension, electrolyte imbalance, cataracts, increased appetite and weight gain, moonlike facies, osteoporosis, myopathy, and increased susceptibility to infection. The severity of these side effects relates both to duration of therapy and to dosage. Splenectomy should be considered in patients who are steroid unresponsive or require more than 10–20 mg prednisone per day or substantial dosages of steroid every other day for maintenance. Each patient requires individual evaluation of underlying diseases, surgical risk, extent of anemia, and steroid intolerance. In some patients the prescence of a mild hemolytic anemia may be preferable to splenectomy or other treatment options. The initial goal of therapy is to return the patient to normal hematological values and nontoxic levels of glucocorticoid therapy. However, in some patients, a modified goal of improvement in hemolysis to a clinically asymptomatic state with minimum glucocorticoid side effects is more realistic.

Glucocorticoids are not usually effective in cold hemagglutinin disease (16,53). This is probably due to the fact that patients with this condition generally have large amounts of IgM anti-erythrocyte antibody and large numbers of C3 molecules deposited on their red cells. Furthermore, macrophage C3b receptors, in contrast to $Fc\gamma$ receptors, are less responsive to glucocortcoid therapy. In addition, some of the hemolysis may be intravascular and glucocorticoids do not inhibit complement-mediated cell lysis. A few patients with a low-titer cold hemagglutinin disease syndrome, in which the antierythrocyte antibody has activity at temperatures approaching 37C, do respond to steroid therapy. In addition, the few patients described with an IgG cold agglutinin apppear to be both steroid and splenectomy responsive (26). Patients with cold hemagglutinin disease respond best to the avoidance of cold and control of their underlying disease. In many patients hemolytic anemia is mild.

B. Splenectomy

The spleen with its resident macrophages is the major site for sequestration of IgG-coated blood cells in humans as in animals. This appears to be due to the unique circulatory pathways in the spleen whereby hemoconcentration occurs in the splenic cords and erythrocytes make their way through fine fenestrations between macrophages. This results in intimate contact between macrophages (with their membrane Fcγ receptors) and IgG-coated blood cells, possibly in the presence of a minimal amount of plasma IgG.

The effect of splenectomy on the clearance of antibody- and complement-coated erythrocytes was also studied in the experimental model. Splenectomy markedly decreases the sequestration of IgG-sensitized cells. However, as the antibody concentration is increased, splenectomy became less effective in preventing the clearance of IgG-coated cells, since the liver became the dominant organ in erythrocyte clearance. Splenectomy does not alter the clearance of IgM-coated cells.

Removal of this major site of red cell destruction is an effective therapeutic strategy in IgG-induced immune hemolytic anemia. The response rate to splenectomy is approximately 50–70%; however, the vast majority of the responses are partial remissions. Before glucocorticoid therapy became available for the treatment of autoimmune hemolytic anemia, splenectomy was performed routinely. Remissions were common, but the patient usually relapsed. Presumably, as the sensitized erythrocytes continued to circulate, they bound more and more antibody. They finally achieved a degree of sensitization at which the liver was able to mediate clearance. Probably those patients who are least responsive to splenectomy are those whose erythrocytes are coated with large amounts of IgG. In this circumstance the liver plays a larger role in clearance. The partial remissions that occur with splenectomy are often quite helpful: they result in a lessening of the hemolytic rate, with a rise in the hemoglobin value, and/or allow a reduction in the amount of glucocorticoid needed to control the hemolytic anemia. Because of the increased risk of sepsis (36), patients should be carefully selected. Patients who are unresponsive to steroids, require moderate to high maintenance doses, or have developed glucocorticoid intolerance can be considered for splenectomy. Cr-labeled red cell kinetic studies are probably not helpful since the procedure is time-consuming, expensive, and not a reliable indicator of response to splenectomy in most cases.

A second effect of splenectomy also has been suggested in autoimmune hemolytic anemia and shown to be important in autoimmune thrombocytopenia. Splenectomy may lead to a decrease in the production of the IgG antierythrocyte antibody, since the spleen contains a large B-cell pool.

Splenectomy, like glucocorticoid therapy, is usually not effective in patients with cold hemagglutinin disease because IgM-coated erythrocytes are cleared predominantly in the liver. An occasional case in which a patient with an apparent IgM-induced hemolytic anemia responded to splenectomy has been reported. This may be due to decreased production of IgM antibody by the spleen in these few patients or to the presence of an IgG cold agglutinin (26). Immunization with pneumococcal vaccine should be performed prior to splenectomy to decrease the likelihood of postsplenectomy pneumococcal infection.

C. Immunosuppressive Agents

Several immunosuppressive agents have been used in the treatment of immune hemolytic anemia. The drugs most commonly used include the thiopurines (6-mercaptopurine, azathioprine, and thioguanine) and alkylating agents (cyclophosphamide and chlorambucil). Immunosuppressive agents act to decrease the production of antibody, and therefore it generally takes at least 2 weeks before any therapeutic result is observed. A reasonable clinical trial consists of 3–4 months of therapy. These drugs are rarely needed in the treatment of childhood autoimmune hemolytic anemia.

Patients are selected for immunosuppressive therapy when a clinically unacceptable degree of hemolytic anemia persists following corticosteroid and splenectomy treatment. They may also be corticosteroid resistant or intolerant and a poor surgical risk for splenectomy. Clinical benefit has been noted in about 50% of patients. Although the side effects of these agents are not considered here, the use of alkylating agents, such as cyclophoshamide, may also have a long-term potential for increasing the incidence of malignancy, particularly acute leukemia. Such side effects require that the clinical indications for an immunosuppressive trial be strong and that patient's exposure to the drug be limited.

Immunosuppressive therapy has been effective therapy in cold hemagglutinin disease. Alkylating agents (cyclophosphamide or chlorambucil) have been used and appear to have a beneficial effect in up to 50–60% of patients.

D. Transfusion

The majority of patients with autoimmune hemolytic anemia do not require transfusion therapy because the anemia has developed gradually and physiological compensation has occurred (54). However, occassional patients experience acute and/or severe anemia and require transfusions for support until other treatment reduces the hemolysis. Transfusion therapy is complicated by the fact that the blood bank may be unable to find any "compatible" blood. This usually is due to the presence of an autoantibody directed at a core component of the Rh locus, which is present on the erythrocytes of essentially all potential donors, regardless of Rh subtype. The usual recommendation is for the blood bank to identify the most compatible units of blood of the patient's own major blood group and Rh type and to transfuse the patient with the most compatible units available. With this approach, it is unlikely that the donor blood will have a dramatically shortened red blood cell survival.

E. Miscellaneous Therapy

Intravenous gamma globulin, which has been used extensively in the treatment of ITP, may be effective in patients with autoimmune hemolytic anemia, probably by interfering with the clearance of the IgG-coated cells. Treatment regimens vary from 400 mg/kg/day for 5 days to 2 g/kg, with additional treatment as needed to maintain the effect. Currently data are incomplete, but gamma globulin seems considerably less effective in autoimmune hemolytic anemia than in ITP (55). Since autoimmune hemolytic anemia is usually very transient, prolonged treatment is rarely necessary.

Plasmapheresis or exchange transfusion has been used in patients with severe IgG-induced immune hemolytic anemia, but has met with limited success, possibly because more than half of the IgG is extravascular and the plasma contains only small amounts of the antibody (most of the antibody being on the red blood cell surface). However, plasmapheresis has been effective in IgM-induced hemolytic anemia (cold agglutinin disease), since IgM is a high-molecular-weight molecule that remains predominantly within the intravascular space and at 37°C most of the IgM is in the plasma fraction. Plasmapheresis is only useful as short-term therapy, but it may be lifesaving in the rare patient with severe uncontrollable hemolysis.

Other measures that have been used effectively in some patients with IgG-induced immune hemolysis are vincristine, vinblastine infusions, and hormonal therapy. For example, there has been great interest in the use of the synthetic weak or impeded androgen danazol (56). Because of the limited side effects (limited masculinizing effects, mild weight gain), danazol is an additional agent for use in some patients with IgG-induced immune hemolytic anemia. The results of these agents in IgM-induced hemolysis suggest that it is ineffective.

VI. IMMUNE PANCYTOPENIA

Evan's syndrome refers to autoimmune hemolytic anemia accompanied by thrombocytopenia (11). It occurs in a small percentage of adults and children with acute autoimmune hemolytic anemia. In an even smaller percentage of patients it is also associated with marked neutropenia. Autoimmune hemolytic anemia in the presence of thrombocytopenia and/or neutropenia is more commonly associated with a chronic or relapsing course. Many patients have associated disorders, such as chronic lymphadenopathy or dysgammaglobulinemia. Some patients are hematologically normal between relapses, which may involve depressions in any of the three cell lines. Usually glucocorticoid therapy is effective in controlling the acute episodes and is not needed between relapses. However, some patients have persistent immune cytopenia and require prolonged steroid treatment or more aggressive therapy. Splenectomy may result in improvement, but the risk of infection is probably higher in children and adults with pancytopenia than in those with autoimmune hemolytic anemia alone and relapses are more common (11,57–64).

Antibodies directed against red cells, leukocytes, and platelets were demonstrated in some patients with immune pancytopenia (58,65). Suppresion of hematopoietic cell maturation by T cells has been observed as well as circulating autoantibodies (57).

VII. PAROXYSMAL NOCTURNAL HEMOGLOBINURIA

Paroxysmal nocturnal hemoglobinuria (PNH) is an acquired disorder initially thought to consist of paroxysms of intravascular hemolysis causing nocturnal hemoglobinuria (66,67). It is considered in detail elsewhere. It is now recognized that chronic intravascular hemolysis is the more frequent clinical presentation. PNH is a primary bone marrow disorder that affects not only the red cell lineage but also the platelet, leukocyte, and pluripotent hematopoietic stem cell lines. It is believed to be a disorder of stem cells of a clonal nature (68–69) and can arise from or evolve into other dysplastic bone marrow diseases, including aplastic anemia, sideroblastic anemia, and myelofibrosis. In rare cases, PNH may also evolve into acute leukemia. Recently it has been shown that patients have a somatic mutation for a protein (phosphatidylinositol [PI] glycan class A) important in the pathway that controls the formation of the phosphatidylinositol anchor of several membrane proteins including complement control proteins (70).

PNH is often a disease of young adults, but it can occur in any age group and in individuals of either gender. Chronic intravascular hemolysis of varying severity is the most common presentation. The severity of the hemolysis and the degree of hemoglobinuria depend on the number of circulating abnormal red cells and the degree of expression of the membrane abnormality among these cells. Two to three populations of abnormal red cells, termed PNH type I, II, and III cells, may be present simultaneously and differ in their lytic susceptibility. Patients commonly have iron deficiency anemia as well because of the large amount of iron lost in the urine during intravascular hemolysis with persistent hemoglobinuria and hemosiderinuria. Other frequent clinical complaints include abdominal, back, and musculoskeletal pain. Such pain may be associated with intravascular hemolysis and hemoglobinuria, or it may be ischemic, secondary to the complication of venous thrombosis of major or minor vessels. Thromboses of the hepatic veins (Budd-Chiari syndrome) and of portal, splenic, mesenteric, cerebral, and other veins may occur and are common causes of death. Acute intestinal infarction requiring surgical resection has been reported and thrombotic episodes may require anticoagulant therapy (70–72). Platelets and leukocytes also appear to have unusual susceptibility to lysis, and thrombocytopenia or granulocytopenia or both may be the initial manifestation(s) of the disease and be commonly present. The bone marrow is usually hyperplastic but may be hypocellular, consistent with aplastic anemia. The clinical course is variable and depends on the occurrence of the life-threatening complications of progressive bone marrow disease or venous thrombosis. PNH should be considered in everyone with aplastic anemia (73). In general, patients are not predisposed to the development of infection. At least half the patients live for many years.

A. Pathogenesis

These patients have an unusual sensitivity of their erythrocytes and often granulocytes and platelets to the lytic action of complement. Activation of complement by either the classical or alternative pathway results in the deposition of larger numbers of C3 molecules on the PNH blood cell surface than on normal cells. The excessive binding of C3 to blood cells in PNH is due to more efficient alternative pathway C3-convertase activity on the cell surface (74). The surface of a PNH erythrocyte is a better acceptor for C3 than is the surface of a normal cell. This results in greater activation of the terminal complement components C5–C9, causing more cell lysis than with normal cells. Furthermore, type II PNH cells are more effectively damaged by the C5b–C9 complex generated on the erythrocyte surface (75,76) because the C5b–C9 lytic complex penetrates the PNH cell membrane more efficiently than the normal cell membrane. These patients lack the complement regulatory proteins present on the membranes of all normal blood cells, causing their increased susceptibility to complement lysis.

Many patients with PNH have several populations of abnormal erythrocytes. The complement lysis sensitivity test, which examines the susceptibility of antibody-sensitized erythrocytes to complement-mediated lysis, can be used to define the various PNH cell populations. PNH type II cells have a moderate increase in susceptibility to complement attack. These erythrocytes appear to have markedly decreased levels of DAF, but do not have the membrane deficit that leads to sensitivity to attack by the C5b complex. PNH type III cells are highly susceptible to complement attack. They appear to lack phosphatidylinositol-linked control proteins completely.

As noted, the platelets and leukocytes in PNH are also abnormally sensitive to complement-mediated lysis and this abnormality is likely to have the same cause (77,67). This may relate to the pathogenesis of the venous thromboses.

B. Therapy

Hemolysis is controlled in a proportion of patients with prednisone therapy. A dose of 15–40 mg every other day has been reported to decrease the rate of hemolysis in some adult patients (72), but a response is by no means certain. During acute episodes a higher dosage given daily for a short period may help to control the hemolysis. In patients with anemia, androgens, including the anabolic steroid danazol, may be effective (72,56). Bone marrow transplantation has been successful in some patients, but in general the treatment of PNH has been unsatisfactory.

VIII. DRUG-INDUCED IMMUNE HEMOLYSIS

Drug-induced immune hemolytic anemia may be classified into three primary pathophysiological entities. The clinical signs and symptoms are identical to those of autoimmune hemolytic anemia. Patients may present with chronic hemolytic anemia or occasionally with catastrophic intravascular hemolysis (quinidine type). The diagnosis is established primarily by history and in vitro assay.

A. α-Methyldopa Type

α-Methyldopa type and its derivatives (such as levodopa) produce a clinical syndrome virtually identical to IgG-induced immune hemolytic anemia (8,78). This is the most common type of drug-induced immune hemolytic anemia. The mechanisms of the IgG antibody formation are poorly understood. This drug stimulates production IgG warm-reactive antibodies with anti-Rh specifity; it may also inhibit the splenic macrophage clearance of the IgG-coated cells. A primary mode of action of the drug in this disorder may be an alteration of immunoregulation, allowing B-lymphocytes that produce Rh antibodies to escape from suppression. It is not believed that complement plays a critical role.

As stated, may patients receiving α-methyldopa therapy develop a positive result on Coombs' test (both direct and indirect) for IgG, but few patients develop significant hemolysis (8). It appears that the level of IgG per erythrocyte accounts at least in part for this observation, since those patients with the highest amount of erythrocyte-associated IgG appear to have the most significant hemolysis. A second feature, in the author's view, that may explain the high incidence of Coombs' positivity without hemolysis in this syndrome, is a low-affinity antibody. The striking finding that almost all patients have antibody present in their plasma, as well as on the erythrocytic surface, contrasts with the finding in most other patients with IgG-induced autoimmune hemolytic anemia, in which a positive result on indirect Coombs' test (plasma antibody) is less common. Second, the IgG antierythrocyte antibody appears to be easily elutable from the erythrocyte surface (78). These observations suggest that α-methyldopa-induced IgG anti-erythrocyte antibody may be an antibody having low affinity for its erythrocyte Rh antigen. This may partially explain its lack of efficacy in producing hemolysis.

B. Hapten Type

The hapten type of drug-induced immune hemolysis classicalally develops in patients exposed to high doses of penicillin. A portion of the penicillin molecule or its active metabolites combines with the erythrocyte surface, acting as a hapten. This induces an antibody response directed against the penicillin-coated erythrocyte membrane. This is usually an IgG response and complement activation is common. The erythrocytes become coated with IgG and often with C3. This syndrome rarely develops unless patients have received 10–20 million units of penicillin a day. The diagnosis can be established by incubating the patient's serum with donor erythrocytes preincubated with penicillin. The deposition of IgG antibody will occur only in the presence of penicillin and can be detected with the Coombs' test.

C. Quinidine Type

The quinidine type of autoimmune hemolytic anemia usually occurs with quinidine, but has been reported with quinine, stibophen, chlorpromazine, and sulfonamides (79). Commonly called an innocent bystander reaction, it is thought to be due to an antibody directed against quinidine having a low affinity for the red cell surface. Presumably the drug binds weakly to the cell glycoprotein. The antibody recognizes the complex (80) and this interaction results in activation of the classical complement pathway and deposition of C3 on the erythrocyte surface. It is believed that the immune complex transiently adheres to the red blood cell surface, activates complement, and then dissociates. With quinidine it has been shown that an IgM antiquinidine antibody appears to be involved. The diagnosis can be established in vitro by examining the complement deposition on donor erythrocytes by patient serum that occurs only in the presence of the drug, for example, quinidine. The Coombs' test is employed to detect the complement depositition on the erythrocyte surface.

Nonspecific coating of the erythrocyte surface has been observed with the cephalosporin antibiotics such as cephalothin. Cephalothin becomes bound to the erythrocyte membrane and causes the red blood cell to be coated by many plasma proteins. The Coombs' test result is positive. Hemolytic anemia does not occur. Cephalothin, however, can cause hemolytic anemia by acting as a hapten by a mechanism similar to that of penicillin.

In all these drug-induced processes, patients respond to withdrawal of the offending drug. If necessary a brief course of corticosteroid therapy can be administered effectively.

Many autoimmune or drug-related hemolytic anemias are accompanied by thrombocytopenia and/or neutropenia as a result of similar pathophysiologic processes. Postinfectious ITP may also result from similar mechanisms. The role of complement in antibody-mediated destruction of platelets and/or neutrophils seems to be analogous to its role in erythrocyte destruction. Thus, at low levels of antibody, complement accelerates clearance by the reticuloendothelial system, while at high levels of antibody, complement may cause direct intravascular cell lysis.

REFERENCES

1.   Schreiber AD, Frank MM. Role of antibody and complement in the immune clearance and destruction of erythrocytes. II. Molecular nature of IgG and IgM complement-fixing sites and effects of their interaction with serum. J Clin Invest 1972; 51:563.
2.   Schreiber AD, Frank MM. Role of antibody and complement in the immune clearance and destruction of erythrocytes. I. In vivo effects of the IgG and IgM complement-fixing sites. J Clin Invest 1972; 51:575.
3.   Ravetch JV, et al., Fc receptors. Annu Rev Immunol 1991; 9:457.
4.   Schreiber AD, et al. The immunobiology of human Fcγ receptors on hematopoietic cells and tissue macrophages. Clin Immunol Immunopathol 1992; 62:566.

5. McKenzie SE, Schreiber AD. Biologic advances and clinical applications of Fc receptors for IgG. Curr Opin Hematol 1994; 1:45–52.

6. Indik ZK, Park J-G, Schreiber S, Schreiber AD. The molecular dissection of Fcγ mediated phagocytosis. Blood 1995; 96:4389–4399.

7. Screiber AD, McDermott PL. Effect of C3b inactivator on monocyte bound C3 coated erythrocytes. Blood 1978; 52:896.

8. Dacie JV, Worlledge SM. Autoimmune haemolytic anemia. Prog Hematol 1969; 6:82.

9. Pirofsky B. Clinical aspects of autoimmune hemolytic anemia. Semin Hematol 1976; 13:251.

10. Worledge SM. Immune drug-induced hemolytic anemias. Semin Hematol 1973; 10:327.

11. Evans RS, et al. Primary thrombocytopenia porpura and acquired hemolytic anemia: evidence of a common etiology. Arch Intern Med 1951; 87:48.

12. Cines DB, August DS, Schreiber AD. Personal communication.

13. Leddy JP. Immunological aspects of red cell injury in man. Semin Hematol 1966; 3:48.

14. LoBuglio AF, Cotran RS, Jandl JH. Red cells coated with immunogloguclin G: binding and sphering by mononuclear cells in man. Science 1967; 158:1582.

15. Landsteiner K. Ueber der Beziehungen Zwischen dem Blutserum und der Köperzellen. Munch Med Wochenschr 1903; 50:812.

16. Pruzanski MD. Biologic activity of cold-reacting autoantibodies. N Engl J Med 1977; 297:538.

17. Schubotke H. The cold hemagglutinin disease. Semin Hematol 1966; 3:27.

18. Friedman D, et al. The role of clonal selection in the pathogenesis of autoreactive human B cell lymphoma. J Exp Med 1991; 174:525.

19. Costea N, Yahulus V, Heller P. Experimental production of cold agglutinin in rabbits. Blood 1965; 25:323.

20. Lind K. Production of cold agglutinins in rabbits induced by *Mycoplasma pneumoniae*, *Listeria monocytogenes* and *Streptococcus M60*. Acta Pathol Microbiol Scand 1973; 81:487.

21. Borsos T, Rapp HJ. Complement fixation on cell surfaces by 19S and 7S antibodies. Science 1965; 105:505.

22. Ruddy S, Gigli J, Austen KF. Complement biology in man. N Engl J Med 1972; 287:489.

23. Hurbner H, et al. Human monocytes: distant receptor sites for the third component of complement and for immunoglobulijn G. Science 1962; 162:1281.

24. Schreiber AD, Herskovitz B, Goldwein M. Low titer cold hemagglutinin disease: mechanisms of hemolysis and response to corticosteroids. N Engl J Med 1977; 296:1490.

25. Schreiber AD, et al. The effect of corticosteroids on the human monocyte and complement receptors. J Clin Invest 1975; 56:1189.

26. Silberstein LE, Berkman EM, Schreiber AD. Cold hemagglutinin disease associated with IgG cold reactive antibody. Ann Intern Med 1987; 106:238.

27. Atkinson JP, Frank MM. Studies on the in vivo effects of antibody: interaction of IgM antibody and complement in the immune clearance and destruction of erythrocytes in man. J Clin Invest 1974; 54:339.

28. Jaffe CS, Atkinson JP, Frank MM. The role of complement in the clearance of cold agglutinin sensitized erythrocytes in man. J Clin Invest 1976; 58:942.

29. Evans RS, Turner E, Bingham M. Chronic hemolytic anemia due to cold agglutinins. J Clin Invest 1967; 46:1461.

30. Pirofsky B. Hereditary aspects of autoimmune hemolytic anemia; a restrospective analysis. Vox Sang 1968; 14:334.

31. Swisher SN. Acquired hemolytic disease. Postgrad Med 1966; 40:378.

32. Sohol RH, Hewitt S, Stamps BK. Autoimmune haemolysis: an 18-year study of 865 cases referred to a regional transfusion centre. Br Med J 1981; 282:2033.

33. Buchanan GR, Boxer LA, Nathan DG. The acute and transient nature of idiopathic immune hemolytic anemia in childhood. J Pediatr 1976; 88:780.

34. Carapella deLuca E, et al. Auto-immune haemolytic anemia in childhood. Follow-up on 29 cases. Vox Sang 1979; 36:13.

35. Habibi B, et al. Autoimmune hemolytic anemia in children. A review of 80 cases. Am J Med 1974; 56:61.
36. Heisel MA, Ortega JA. Factors influencing prognosis in childhood autoimmune hemolytic anemia. Am J Pediatr Hematol Oncol 1983; 5:147.
37. Zuelzer WW, et al. Autoimmune hemolytic anemia. Natural history and viral–immunologic interactions in childhood. Am J Med 1970; 49:80.
38. Zupanska B, et al. Autoimmune haemolytic anaemia in children. Br J Haematol 1976; 34:511.
39. Johnson HE, Brostrom K, Madsen M. Paroxysmal cold haemoglobinuria in children: 3 cases encountered within a period of 7 months. Scand J Haematol 1978; 20:413.
40. Rausen AR, et al. Compatible transfusions therapy for paroxysmal cold hemoglobinuria. Pediatrics 1974; 55:275.
41. Herskovitz B, et al. Effect of cytocholorin B on human monocyte binding and sphering of IgG coated human erythrocytes. Blood 1977; 49:289.
42. Lalaezari P. Serologic profile in autoimmune hemolytic disease: pathophysiologic and clinical interpretations. Semin Hematol 1976; 13:291.
43. Gelfand EW, et al. Buffy-coat observations and red-cell antibodies in acquired hemolytic anemia. N Engl J Med 1971; 284:1250.
44. Conley CL, et al. Autoimmune hemolytic anemia with reticulocytopenia and erythroid marrow. N Engl J Med 1982; 306:281.
45. Greenberg J, et al. Prolonged reticulocytopenia in autoimmune hemolytic anemia in childhood. J Pediatr 1980; 97:784.
46. Wolach B, et al. Transient Donath-Landsteiner haemolygic anaemia. Br J Haematol 1981; 48:425.
47. Gilliland BC. Coombs-negative hemolytic anemia. Semin Hematol 1976; 13:267.
48. Gilliland BC, Baxter E, Evans RS. Red-cell antibodies in acquired hemolytic anemia with negative antiglobulin serum tests. N Engl J Med 1971; 285:252.
49. Cines DB, Schreiber AD. Immune thrombocytopenia: use of a Coombs' antiblobulin test to detect IgG and C3 on platelets. N Engl J Med 1979; 300:106.
50. Friedman D, Nettl F, Schreiber AD. Effect of estradiol and steroid analogues on the clearance of IgG coted erythrocyhtes. J Clin Invest 1985; 75:162.
51. Ruiz P, et al. In vivo glucocorticoid modulation of guinea pig splenic macrophage Fcγ receptors. J Clin Invest 1991; 88:148.
52. Atkinson JP, Schreiber AD, Frank MM. Effects of corticosteroids and splenectomy on the immune clearance and destruction of erythrocytes. J Clin Invest 1975; 52:1509.
53. Schreiber AD. Clinical immunology of the corticosteroids. Prog Clin Immunol 1977; 3:103.
54. Rosenfield RE, Jagathambal. Transfusion therapy for autoimmune hemolytic anemia. Semin Hematol 1976; 13:311.
55. Bussel JB, Cunningham-Rundles C, Hilgartner MW. Intravenous treatment of autoimmune hemolytic anemia with gammaglobulin. Submitted for publication.
56. Schreiber AD, et al. Effect of danazol therapy in immune thrombocytopenic purpura. N Engl J Med 1987; 310:503.
57. Daneshbod-Skibba G, et al. Immune pancytopenia. Br J Haematol 1979; 43:7.
58. Fagioli E. Platelet and leukocyte antibodies in autoimmune hemolytic anemia. Acta Haematol 1976; 56:97.
59. Hansen OP, Sorensen CH, Astrup L. Evan's syndrome in IgA deficiency. Scand J Haematol 1982; 29:265.
60. Miller BA, Beardsley DS. Autoimmune pancytopenia of childhood associated with multisystem disease manifestations. J Pediatr 1983; 103:877.
61. Pegels JG, et al. The Evans syndrome: characterization of the responsibile autoantibodies. Br J Haematol 1982; 51:445.
62. Pui C-H, Wilimas J, Wang W. Evans syndrome in childhood. J Pediatr 1980; 97:754.

63. Richard KA, Robinson RJ, Worlledge SM. Acute acquired haemolytic anemia assoociated with polyagglutination. Arch Dis Child 1969; 44:102.
64. Robbins JB, Skinner RG, Pearson HA. Autoimmune hemolytic anemia in a child with congenital X-linked hypogammaglobulinemia. N Engl J Med 1969; 280:75.
65. Petz LD. Transfusion in special situations. Autoimmune haemolytic anemia. Human Pathol 1983; 14:252.
66. May JE, Rosse W, Frank MM. Paroxysmal nocturnal hemoblobinuria. Alternate-complement-pathway-mediated lysis induced by magnesium. N Engl J Med 1973; 289:705.
67. Schreiber AD. Paroxysmal nocturnal hemoglobinuria. N Engl J Med 1983; 309:723.
68. Dessyrris EN, et al. Increased sensitivity to complement of erythroid and myeloid progenitors in paroxysmal nocturnal hemoglobinuria. N Engl J Med 1983; 309:690.
69. Rotoli B, Robledo R, Luzzatto L. Decreased number of circulating BFU-Es in paroxysmal nocturnal hemoglobinuria. Blood 1982; 60:157.
70. Fran K MM, et al. The role of complement in defense against bacterial disease. Baillieres Clin Immunol Allergy 1988; 2:335.
71. Takeda J, et al. Deficiency in the GPI anchor caused by a somatic mutation of the PIG-A gene in paroxysmal nocturnal hemoglobin urea. Cell 1993; 73:703.
72. Rosse WF. Treatment of paroxysmal nocturnal hemoglobinuria. Blood 1982; 60:20.
73. Conrad ME, Barton JC. The aplastic anemia–paroxysmal nocturnal hemoglobinuria syndrome. Am J Hematol 1979; 7:61.
74. Parker CJ, Baker PJ, Rosse WF. Increased enzymatic activity of the alternative pathway convertase when bound to the erythrocytes of paroxysmal nocturnal hemoglobinuria. J Clin Invest 1982; 69:337.
75. Packman CH, et al. Complement lysis of human erythrocytes: differing susceptibility of two types of paroxysmal nocturnal hemoglobinuria cells to C5b-9. J Clin Invest 1979; 64:428.
76. Roualt TA, et al. Differences in the terminal steps of complement lysis of normal and paroxysmal nocturnal hemoglobinuria red cells. Blood 1968; 51:325.
77. Aster RH, Enright SE. A platelet and granulocyte membrane defect in paroxysmal nocturnal hemoglobinuria: usefulness for the detection of platelet antibodies. J Clin Invest 1969; 48:1199.
78. Worlledge SM, Carstairs KC, Dacie JV. Autoimmune hemolytic anemia associated with α-methyldopa therapy. Lancet 1966; 2:135.
79. Petz LD, Fudenberg HH. Immunologic mechanisms in drug induced cytopenias. Prog Haematol 1975; 9:185.
80. Habibi B, et al. Les antigènes de groupes sanguins peuvent être les cibles des conflits immunoallergiques medicamenteux à affinité. CR Acad Sci III 1983; 296:693.

26

Complement and Glomerular Disease

CLARK WEST

University of Cincinnati College of Medicine, and Children's Hospital
Medical Center, Cincinnati, Ohio

I. INTRODUCTION

Evidence of activation of the complement system is abundant in the glomerulonephritides. Activation can occur both in the renal glomerulus, as evidenced by the glomerular deposition of complement proteins, and in the circulation, as evidenced in some nephritides by abnormal serum levels of complement components. Although some have proposed that complement activation in the glomerulus is responsible for the perturbation of circulating complement (1), it is more likely that in most diseases complement activation in the glomerulus has a minimal, if any, effect on serum complement levels.

Although evidence of complement activation is abundant, its role in producing the glomerular inflammation has not in all diseases been established. In the inflamed glomerulus, a number of other inflammatory mediators have been found or have the potential to be present. These include numerous cytokines, eicosanoids, prostacyclines, proteolytic enzymes, and reactive oxygen metabolites. The interrelationships of these mediators and their relative importance in human glomerular disease have not been completely elucidated. It is, however, increasingly clear that in several nephritides activation of the complement system is the event initiating the inflammation. Glomerular cells, often as bystander targets, respond by proliferating and by releasing some or all of the above mediators. Complement was first identified as directly involved in an experimental nephritis in 1964 when Unanue et al. (2) showed that depletion of complement would prevent the nephritis produced by heterologous antiglomerular basement membrane (GBM) antibody. We now know that the glomerular inflammation in that model is produced by polymorphonuclear leukocytes attracted to the area by chemoattractants, principally C5a, and maintained at the site by adhesion molecules (3). Later it was shown that in the rat complement is essential for Heymann nephritis (4) and for a mesangioproliferative nephritis produced by antithymocyte serum (5).

In the human nephritides, evidence of complement involvement is derived, first, by analogies to experimental nephritides and, second, by the circumstantial evidence, which is itemized in Table 1. In most cases, of all the listed nephritides complement components and, often, immunoglobulins are present in the glomeruli. In a number there may be circulating material perturbing the complement system. In most of these diseases C3 is a prominent constituent of the glomerular deposit. However, it may be absent in a minority

Table 1 Frequency of IgG, IgA, C3, and C4 in Glomerular Deposits and of Perturbation of Circulating Complement in the Glomerulonephritides

	Composition of glomerular deposits with respect to					Incidence of complement perturbation (%)	Complement-reactive material in circulation
	Biopsies (n)	C3 (%)	C4 (%)	IgG (%)	IgA (%)		
Acute post-streptococcal[a]	42	100	0	75	0	90	not identified
MPGN type I[a]	18	100	75	90	0	≈70	imm. complexes, NF$_t$
MPGN type II[a]	12	100	22	8	0	≈80	NF$_a$
MPGN type III[a]	18	100	0	50	0	≈80	NF$_t$
SLE (WHO class II-V)[a]	37	100	64	100	68	100	Imm. complexes
IgA nephropathy (6)	1949	85	10	57	100	0	None
Henoch Schoenlein (7)	65	100	0	40	100	≈10	? Cryo-like protein
Membranous nephropathy (8)	75	70	42	100	17	0	None

[a] Data from first biopsies of children to age 21 years from author's clinic.

of patients with IgA nephropathy, Henoch-Schoenlein purpura, and membranous nephropathy. Glomerular C4 is most frequent in systemic lupus erythematosus (SLE) and membranoproliferative glomerulonephritis (MPGN) type I, two diseases in which immune complexes deposited from the circulation are known or assumed to be basic to pathogenesis. In the circulation, the immune complexes produce the hypocomplementemia characterizing these diseases (9). On the other hand, in most of the cases of membranoproliferative glomerulonephritis, the hypocomplementemia is produced by circulating autoantibodies known as nephritic factors.

It should be noted that in a number of diseases other than those in Table 1, C3 and immunoglobulin may be found in the glomerulus but their significance with respect to pathogenesis is unclear. Thus, IgG and C3 may be found in the glomeruli in polyarteritis nodosa, the hypocomplementemic vasculitis syndrome, and in cryoglobulinemia. IgG and IgM accompanied by C1q may be found in some cases of mesangial proliferative glomerulonephritis and focal glomerulosclerosis. In many of these, the immunoglobulin and complement components may be trapped in the tissue or nonspecifically adherent to damaged cells. Because complement is not intimately involved in these diseases, they will not be covered in this review.

II. CIRCULATING COMPLEMENT REACTIVE FACTORS IN THE GLOMERULONEPHRITIDES

Material in the circulation reactive with complement and producing distinctive complement profiles falls into three categories: immune complexes, nephritic factors, and complement reactive immunoglobulins.

A. Immune Complexes

Immune complexes activating the classical pathway and lowering levels of complement components (9) are considered to be basic to membranoproliferative glomerulonephritis (MPGN) type I, the nephritis often accompanying systemic lupus erythematosus (SLE) and that occurring with chronic bacteremia. In all three diseases, the complement profile is characterized by reduced levels of C3, properdin, and usually one or more early components (10,11), the latter constituting distinct evidence of classical pathway activation.

Circulating immune complexes not only alter the level of components of the complement system but also are themselves profoundly altered by complement. The deposition of C4b and C3b on a complex, a consequence of its activation of the classical pathway, reduces its size and increases its solubility (12–14). More important is that the C4b and C3b serve as ligands for complement receptor-1 (CR-1) found on erythrocytes and leukocytes. By these ligands, complexes formed in vivo adhere to (immune adherence), and are transported by, cells. Red cells predominate in this transport because of their greater numbers. Complexes so bound are subsequently either released into the plasma to bind to receptors on lymphocytes or stripped from the red cell by macrophages.

Release of the complex into the plasma follows conversion of the CR-1 bound C3b to iC3b and subsequently to C3c and C3dg (15). This conversion is mediated by factor I with CR-1 as cofactor. As a cofactor, CR-1 is unique in that the end product of its interaction with factor I is degradation of C3b to C3dg. Following release of the immune complex from the erythrocyte, the complex-bound C3dg is converted to C3d by plasma proteases (15), allowing the binding of the complex to CR-2 on lymphocytes.

Stripping of the complex occurs as the cells pass through the spleen and liver. The immune complex and the CR-1 are stripped from the cell by fixed macrophages (14). If the patient is forming immune complexes in abundance, as in SLE, cold agglutinin disease, and Sjögren's syndrome, the CR-1/erythrocyte can be markedly decreased (16). The decrease in CR-1/erythrocyte together with the lowered levels of C3 and C4 in the plasma make disposal by this mechanism less efficient. Complexes failing to adhere to erythrocytes remain in the fluid phase and deposit in various organs including the renal glomerulus. Absence of this disposal system, as in patients with homozygous deficiencies of subunits of C1, C2, and C4, greatly increases the risk for immune complex disease (17). Even a partial deficiency of C4 increases the risk (18). Why these patients often develop discoid lupus and nonrenal systemic lupus rather than nephritis (19) is not clear.

It is of interest that the immune complexes adhering to red cells via C3b are able to activate the classical pathway. Some of the fluid phase C3b resulting from this activation fixes to the red cell by its metastable binding site in proximity to the complex (16). The C3b is subsequently degraded to iC3b and then to C3dg. The C3dg is not lost with passage of the cell through liver or spleen. As a result, in active lupus, the CR-1/erythrocyte and C3dg/erythrocyte are inversely related. A high C3dg with a low CR-1 indicates that complexes had adhered and were subsequently stripped from the cells.

The number of CR-1/erythrocyte appears to be inherited by a multigenic mechanism. There is, however, no evidence that a low CR-1/erythrocyte predisposes to SLE (20).

B. Nephritic Factors

1. Nephritic Factor of the Amplification Loop

A circulating factor in patients with MPGN, which, in vitro, activated C3 was designated the C3 nephritic factor or C3NeF by Spitzer et al in 1969 (21). Subsequently, C3NeF was found to be an IgG autoantibody (22) directed at the activated factor B found on the C3b-dependent convertase, C3bBb (23). It both slowed intrinsic decay of the convertase (24) and inhibited factor H-mediated extrinsic decay (25). Cell-bound C3b,Bb stabilized with C3NeF has a half-life of 52 min compared to 3 min for unstabilized convertase (23). This nephritic factor increases the turnover of the C3b amplification loop without activating terminal components or involving classical components. Thus, despite a very low C3 level, the catabolic rate of C5 is normal (26). The low C3 is often the only abnormality in the complement profile; occasionally the levels of properdin and factor B may be slightly depressed (27). This nephritic factor, which was later designated the nephritic factor of the amplification loop (NF_a), is found in patients with MPGN type II and with partial lipodystrophy. It is commonly demonstrated by quantitating C3c in mixtures of normal and nephritic serum incubated for 30 min at 37°C using crossed immunoelectrophoresis (28). In similar mixtures, it can also be quantitated by the loss of the B antigen of C3, which occurs when C3 is activated in the fluid phase (29). Another method is the demonstration by hemolytic methods of the ability of nephritic serum to stabilize convertase on erythrocytes (30).

2.   Nephritic Factor of the Terminal Pathway

The cause of the hypocomplementemia found in patients with MPGN type III was not known until Mollnes (31) and Clardy (32) found that in mixtures containing type III serum, little C3 conversion can be demonstrated after 30 min incubation but conversion is marked after 3 or 4 h of incubation. Clardy (32) and subsequently Tanuma (33) showed that this "slow" nephritic factor differs from that found in MPGN type II; it would activate C5 and C9 in vitro and that conversion required properdin. It has been designated the nephritic factor of the terminal pathway (NF_t). It is assumed that the nephritic factor-stabilized convertase has the structure $C3b,Bb,P,NF_t$ or $C3b_n,Bb,P,NF_t$ since two or more C3b molecules in close proximity are necessary for activation of C5. Because the convertase targeted by NF_t is assembled from three or more molecules rather than two, as for NF_a, its spontaneous formation in serum may be less frequent, accounting for the long incubation period required for its demonstration. When present in amounts sufficient to depress markedly the C3 level, the complement profile produced by NF_t is characterized by a severe depression of C5 and of one or more of the terminal components, C6, C7 and C9 (27). Depression of C8 may also be found but levels of this component may, for unknown reasons, be depressed in other hypocomplementemic nephritides. It should be noted that whereas NF_t appears solely responsible for the hypocomplementemia in all patients with MPGN type III, it may also be found in about one-third of the patients with MPGN type I (27).

3.   Nephritic Factor of the Classical Pathway

Also described is a nephritic factor of the classical pathway, designated variously as NF_c, C4NeF, and $F_{4,2}$. This nephritic factor was first described in a patient with acute postinfectious glomerulonephritis (34) and subsequently in patients with SLE (35) and MPGN (36). It stabilizes the classical pathway convertase, C4b2a. Because C4b2a, as compared to C3b,Bb, is not being constantly formed, this nephritic factor does not in vivo or in vitro cause C3 conversion and hypocomplementemia (34). In vivo it would augment, however, the extent of C3 conversion produced by classical pathway activation (37).

4. Nephritogenicity of Nephritic Factors

Although Ohi and Yasugi (38) have associated the presence of NF_c with more severe disease in patients with MPGN, there has been until recently little evidence that NF_a and NF_t are nephritogenic. Nephritic factors have been considered to be epiphenomena and not involved in pathogenesis. Thus, renal function was reported to deteriorate in patients with MPGN II in the absence of nephritic factor (39). In converse fashion, nephritic factor could be present for long periods in patients with partial lipodystrophy (40) and also in otherwise normal subjects without renal disease developing (41–43). On the other hand, two observers have found the nephritis to be more severe in those with circulating nephritic factor (39,44). In addition, in patients with MPGN type II who have renal transplants, hypocomplementemia and recurrence of proteinuria and hematuria indicating recurrence of the nephritis seem to be associated (45).

It has recently been pointed out that nephritis is often present in several conditions in which, as a result of dysfunction of factor H, the C3b-dependent convertase circulates over long periods, (45). Thus, nephritis can be present in humans (45) and swine (46) homozygous deficient in factor H and in patients with Marder disease (47,48). Glomerulonephritis was also present in a patient with a circulating factor H inhibitor (49). The glomerular disease in humans with these forms of factor H dysfunction has been described generically as MPGN (50) or as atypical dense deposit disease (49,51). The disease in swine has a number of features in common with human MPGN type II (52). Since widely differing abnormalities produce the H dysfunction in these conditions and factor H may be absent or normal in concentration, it has been postulated that circulating convertase, common to all, is the nephritogenic agent (45). As a corollary, it was postulated that nephritic factors, also producing factor H dysfunction, and allowing active C3b,Bb to circulate, are nephritogenic (45). It is possible that the nephritis is more severe in patients with nephritic factor than in those with other forms of H dysfunction because the convertase stabilized by nephritic factor has a half life more than 15-fold greater than that present in, for instance, homozygous factor H deficiency.

To gain evidence that nephritic factor can alter the glomerulus, renal biopsies of hypocomplementemic patients with MPGN type II and, hence, presumably obtained when NF_a was circulating, were compared with those obtained during normocomplementemia (53). In biopsies obtained during hypocomplementemia, subepithelial deposits were present on the paramesangial portion of the GBM that were not found in biopsies obtained from normocomplementemic patients. These paramesangial deposits had strong concordance with mesangial granules fluorescing with anti-C3, a glomerular abnormality found by others in about 75% of the patients with MPGN type II (54). These deposits, or granules, contain no IgG, making it doubtful that they are composed of nephritic factor stabilized convertase. That deposits in the same location were found in the glomerular ultrastructure in Marder disease (47,48), and have been found by us in two patients with homozygous factor H deficiency, supports the concept that they are in some way the product of circulating convertase. There is, however, no direct evidence that they are nephritogenic.

In retrospect, two factors may mask a nephritogenic effect of nephritic factor. First, not all individuals with circulating convertase will develop nephritis, as attested to by the absence of nephritis in about one-half of the subjects with homozygous factor H deficiency and with Marder disease (45). Second, it is possible that a lag between the appearance of nephritic factor and the development of or worsening of the glomerular lesion obscures a cause and effect relationship.

C. Complement-Reactive Immunoglobulins

When the material in the circulation activating complement is an immunoglobulin but not aggregated as part of a complex, levels of the three classical pathway components may be reduced and that of C3 in the normal range. When such a molecule activates the classical pathway, the paucity of sites on which C4b can bind prevents formation of C4b,2a and C4b decays in the fluid phase with little C3b formation. This complement profile is usually not accompanied by nephritis in patients with lymphoproliferative disorders and paraproteinemia (55) but nephritis is seen with essential cryoglobulinemia (56). This profile is also seen early in patients acutely ill with the nephritis of Henoch-Schoenlein purpura (57), but the nature of the circulating complement-reactive material is not known.

III. CIRCULATING PRODUCTS OF COMPLEMENT ACTIVATION

The complement reactions occurring in the circulation, and perhaps to a minor extent in the glomerulus, in nephritis are a source of circulating complement activation products. These have been used, especially in SLE, to gauge disease activity and some may contribute to pathogenesis.

A. $(C1INH)_2$, C1r-C1s (INC)

In SLE, elevated levels of complexes of the composition $(C1INH)_2C1r,C1s$, indicating classical pathway activation, have been found during relapse (58). The levels increased as C1q levels fell, except that at very low levels of C1q the INC levels were less than predicted and could be normal when C1q was virtually absent from the serum. This was attributed to a rate of INC removal from the circulation greater than the rate of synthesis of the C1 from which it was generated. In SLE, INC levels were of little value in gauging activity of the disease. Although there was evidence of classical pathway activation in patients with MPGN type I, serum INC levels were rarely elevated. Also, with rare exceptions, they were normal in MPGN type III as would be expected (58). Elevations were uncommon also in early specimens from patients with AGN (58) but were more frequently observed in another study (59). The observations suggest that in a minority of patients with AGN, classical pathway activation is an initial event.

B. C4d

Circulating C4d, indicating classical pathway activation, has been demonstrated in SLE. The ratio of C4d/C4 increases markedly with relapse and may accurately reflect the fractional catabolic rate of C4 (60). In AGN, the ratio is elevated in some patients in the first 10 days after onset and shows a negative correlation with the C4 level (61).

C. C3d and C3c

It has long been recognized that with hypercatabolism of C3, C3d appears in the circulation (62,63). This has been observed in SLE, MPGN, and AGN. The C3d level, in general, is inversely related to the level of C3. The ratio of C3d to native C3 has been considered a catabolic index of C3 (63). C3d, however, can be found in abnormal amounts in patients with SLE and MPGN who have low-normal levels of C3 (63). Also, in patients with IgA nephropathy who have no hypocomplementemia, levels of C3d may be greater than in normal plasma (reviewed in 64). The elevation was significantly greater in those patients with severe disease. We presume that C3d can be generated in sufficient quantity by the complement reaction in situ in the glomerulus to elevate the serum level. C3c has also been present with severe hypocomplementemia but is less abundant than C3d (62). The elevated C3d levels in the hypocomplementemic nephritides indicate that even though metabolic studies indicate that C3 synthesis is diminished (1,65), hypercatabolism is still occurring. It should be pointed out that with a constant C3 level, C3d accumulates in the plasma of the hypocomplementemic patient with MPGN, for example, but not in that of the normal subject. Thus, when C3 synthesis and catabolism are equal, C3d accumulates when there is hypocomplementemia and diminished C3 synthesis, presumably because catabolism is by C3 activation while in the normal subject it is by another route.

D. C3a desARG and C5a desARG

The removal by carboxypolypeptidase of the terminal arginine residues from the C3a and C5a generated by complement activation alters and in some cases abrogates their anaphylatoxin activity. The level of C3a desARG has been shown to be elevated with active SLE, with the extent of the elevation correlating with the severity of the relapse; the levels are said to more closely reflect SLE activity than do those of C3 (66). C5a desARG is less reflective of activity than C3a desARG. These split products may have a role in pathogenesis. C5a desARG is chemotactic for neutrophils, although to a lesser extent than C5a and can promote neutrophil degranulation. More important is that the split products induce neutrophils to increase their surface expression of CR-3, which could in turn cause them to aggregate, leading to both neutropenia and occlusive vasculopathy (66).

E. Ba and Bb

Complement activation also results in increased levels of breakdown products of factor B. Although with complement activation in nephritis, serum factor B levels are not greatly depressed, levels of Ba are often elevated, especially in MPGN (63). Ba levels will also occasionally be elevated in normocomplementemic patients, but in general the levels increase as levels of C3d increase and those of native C3 diminish (63). Others have shown that the Ba levels correlate better with disease activity than the levels of Bb (67). Ba levels were found to be more sensitive than a fall in C3 or C4, in indicating SLE relapse. However, the actual levels of Ba with active disease may overlap the normal range (67). Both Ba and Bb have biological activity. Consistent results have not been obtained with Ba but Bb augments the spreading of peritoneal macrophages, activates plasminogen, and inhibits the chemotactic activity of C5a desARG (reviewed in 67).

F. SC5b-9

C5b-9 stabilized by the S protein, assayed with a monoclonal antibody to the neoantigen expressed on polymeric C9, may be found in low concentration in normal plasma (68). The levels were found to be elevated at some time during a relapse in 13 of 14 patients with SLE but they correlated poorly with levels of C1q, C3, and C4. They were occasionally elevated in patients with acute infections and in patients with IgA nephropathy, MPGN, and membranous glomerulopathy. Mollnes et al. (69) also showed elevated levels in a few patients clinically suspected of having complement activation. They subsequently showed that the levels were elevated in patients with the "slow" nephritic factor and in a patient with AGN but, as would be expected, not in a patient with partial lipodystrophy (31). In general, the data would suggest that the measurement as a diagnostic tool would give a number of false-positives results.

IV. CHARACTERISTICS OF THE COMPLEMENT ACTIVATION IN SPECIFIC GLOMERULONEPHRITIDES

A. Systemic Lupus Erythematosus

In overt lupus nephritis (WHO classes II-V), IgG is always present in mesangial and capillary wall deposits. Although in our series (Table 1) C3 was always present in the glomerular deposits, others have often found it to be absent, especially in WHO class II, in which deposits are confined to the mesangium and mesangial proliferation may not be present (70). C4 can be absent when proliferation is low grade and deposits infrequent (class II and III). It is most often present when the glomerulus is diffusely proliferative and there are abundant capillary wall and mesangial deposits.

When lupus nephritis is active and the disease is severe, the complement profile indicates classical pathway activation, as would be expected from the presence of circulating immune complexes (9). As shown in Figure 1, the C3 level is usually only moderately depressed compared to other hypocomplementemic nephritides. In our experience, all patients with active lupus nephritis will have one or more of the three classical pathway components depressed, and in 90% two will be depressed. Most consistently depressed is C4 and most variable is C1q. Among the terminal components, C5 and C8 may be in normal concentration or moderately depressed and levels of C6, C7, and C9 are normal. A depressed C8 level may be seen in several hypocomplementemic nephritides and its significance is not clear. This complement profile is very similar to that seen in the nephritis of chronic bacteremia (11) and in about one-third of the hypocomplementemic patients with membranoproliferative glomerulonephritis (MPGN) type I (Fig. 2A).

Whereas, as noted above, the levels of a number of circulating activation products of complement are elevated with active lupus, activity of the disease is most commonly assessed by levels of complement components. There is confusion in the literature, however, as to the measurements of greatest value in predicting incipient relapses and gauging the response to treatment. We, as well as others (71–73), have found C4 levels of value in this assessment. A progressive fall in serial specimens, even though the level remains in the normal range, and with the C3 level in some patients remaining normal, presages a relapse. Only in patients with consistently low C4 levels as a result of a multiplicity of null genes for C4, not uncommon in lupus (18), have the levels not correlated with disease activity. On the contrary, others have reported that C4 levels may often be normal with relapse (74–76) and have found the measurement of C3 to be of greater value (74). In assessing these observations, a number of factors must be considered. First, the reductions in C3 and C4 levels with nephritis would be blunted if the assessment included data from relapses of extrarenal lupus since, in this situation, complement perturbation is less severe

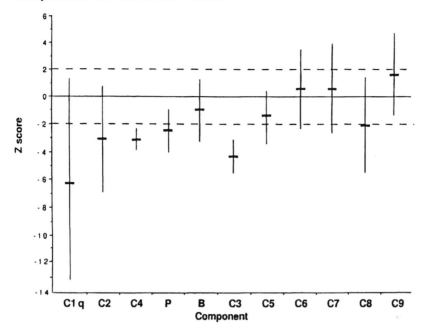

Figure 1 Systemic lupus erythematosus. Each vertical line represents the range of concentration (±2SD) of the complement component indicated on the ordinate. Data are from serum specimens from 29 patients obtained at the time of onset or relapse. The mean concentration is indicated by the heavy bar. The area between the dashed horizontal lines, indicating the normal range (Z = ±2), was derived from measurements on 163 normal subjects.

(71). Second, C3 levels may not be responsive in patients who have, when the disease is active, a circulating inhibitor of C3 conversion (77). In these patients, C3 levels may be in the normal range or even elevated but C4 levels still fall and mirror disease activity. Third, Milgrom et al. (60) found levels of C4d to be very high and C4 levels very low with relapse, so that an antiserum highly reactive with C4d used for C4 measurement by radial immunodiffusion or nephelometry would give spuriously normal levels of C4. Animals immunized with C4 may form large amounts of antibody reacting with C4d (60, 78). Taken together, the observations suggest that, if we assume C4d is not measured concurrently, the C4 level should provide the best index of lupus activity.

B. Membranoproliferative Glomerulonephritis Type I

This form of MPGN is characterized by subendothelial and mesangial glomerular deposits that always contain C3, often IgG, and, in about 75% of the cases, C4 (Table 1). In our experience (27), the complement profile in 23% of the patients gives evidence of only classical pathway activation (Fig. 2A). In another 23% terminal components are depressed together with, in some patients, depression of classical components (Fig. 2B). In another 23%, C3 is the only component in low concentration. The remaining 31% were normocomplementemic on presentation and remained normocomplementemic. This frequency of normocomplementemia agrees with the frequency of 36% for all types of MPGN observed by Cameron et al. (79). The heterogeneity of the profiles indicates that immune complexes,

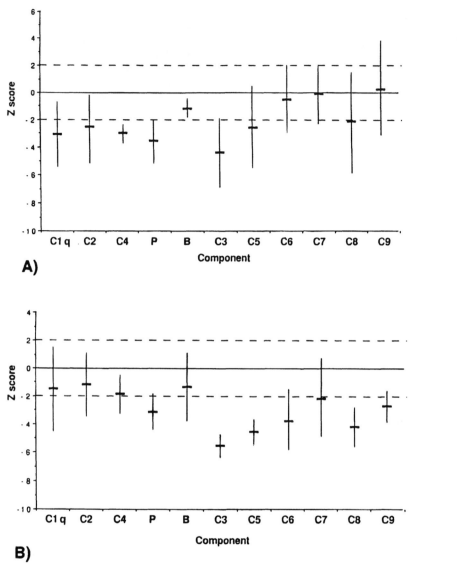

Figure 2 (A) MPGN type I. Mean and range of complement component concentrations in eight patients with signs of classic pathway activation predominating. Data are graphed as in Figure 1. (B) MPGN type I. Mean and range of complement component concentrations in seven patients with signs of terminal pathway activation predominating. Data are graphed as in Figure 1.

NF_t, and perhaps NF_a may circulate in these patients. Circulating immune complexes would appear basic to pathogenesis, however, in that with all profiles glomerular morphology of MPGN type I is identical to that found in patients with circulating immune complexes as the result of chronic bacteremia (10, 80). However, the nature and origin of the antigen component of the circulating immune complexes in MPGN type I are unknown. The patients are often systemically ill on presentation. Of those not presenting with signs and symptoms of nephritis, over half had fatigue, pallor, or weight loss for an extended period before diagnosis (81). The disease might be thought of as "slow" lupus with the kidney being the only target organ.

C. MPGN Type II

Dense deposit disease, as MPGN type II is also known, is a systemic disease. Not only are there so-called dense deposits in the glomerular basement membrane but also there are abnormalities in the basement membranes of the eye (82), spleen (83), Bowman's capsule, and renal tubules (84). The increased density of the GBM is the result of a structural change rather than a deposit. Its development in normal kidneys transplanted to these patients is further evidence that the disease is systemic (85). The main complement component in the glomeruli is C3 and it is possible that nonspecific glomerular protein trapping is responsible for the occasional finding of C4 and IgG (Table 1). With fluorescein-labeled antibody to C3, the margins of the GBM fluoresce, rings are seen in the mesangium that are probably remnants of shed basement membrane containing dense deposit, and paramesangial deposits, designated mesangial granules, may be present (54). The latter, as noted above, correspond to subepithelial deposits on the paramesangial portion of the glomerular basement membrane and are seen when the nephritic factor of the amplification loop is present (53).

The complement profile is unique in that the only component consistently in low concentration is C3. In some specimens, there may be mild depression of factor B and C5 (Fig 3). Hypocomplementemia, and presumably nephritic factor, was present in 54% of the adults and 73% of the children in the series by Cameron et al. (79). In our series, the incidence in children was 82% (27). The densification of the basement membrane is not produced by either nephritic factor or hypocomplementemia. It also appears to bear little relationship to the development of the glomerulonephritis since, within a few months, the dense deposits can develop in the renal transplant in the absence of both hypocomplementemia and of recurrence of the glomerulonephritis (86).

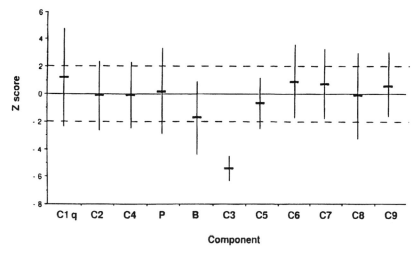

Figure 3 MPGN type II. Mean and range of complement component concentrations in seven patients at time of presentation or of relapse. Data are graphed as in Figure 1.

D. MPGN Type III

This disease differs from MPGN type I by the position of the deposits in the ultrastructure of the glomerular capillary wall and by apparent splitting and fraying of the GBM as seen in silver stains (87). It differs also in that, in the absence of renal insufficiency, the patients are usually in good health and hematuria and proteinuria are found by chance (81). The glomerular deposits contain C3 and, in some patients, IgG albeit the amount is less than seen in MPGN type I or in SLE (81). C4 is rarely present. The complement profile is distinctive; even with marked C3 depression there is no sign of classical pathway activation but there is marked depression of C5 and moderate depression of C7 and/or C9, and less commonly C6. As with other hypocomplementemias, C8 levels are also depressed (Fig. 4). This profile is produced by NF_t, the "slow" nephritic factor, which is properdin dependent and has been demonstrated to activate C5 and C9 in vitro (32). Hypocomplementemia was present or subsequently developed in 84% of the children in our series (88). An association between the glomerular abnormality and the presence of nephritic factor has not yet been demonstrated for MPGN type III as it has for MPGN type II (53).

E. Acute Poststreptococcal Glomerulonephritis

Since the observations by Schick early in this century, acute poststreptococcal glomerulonephritis (AGN) has been considered a disease of immune complex origin. In the average 10 day interval between the streptococcal infection and the development of nephritis, this concept assumes that antibody is made to products of a nephritogenic streptococcus and the resulting immune complexes are deposited in the glomeruli producing the disease. Support for this pathogenesis is the similar interval between the administration of a foreign protein and the development of serum sickness nephritis, the morphological similarities with the glomerular lesion produced after certain regimens of foreign protein injection

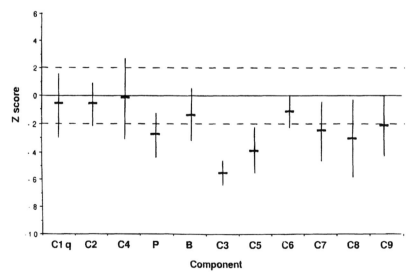

Figure 4 MPGN type III. Mean and range of complement component concentrations in eight patients at time of presentation. Data are graphed as in Figure 1.

(89,90), and the evidence for classical pathway activation early in the disease as manifested by the occasional depression of the C4 level and the occasional presence of classical pathway activation products as discussed above. However, deposits in the glomeruli are mainly subepithelial. In contrast to the nephritides of known immune complex origin (nephritis of chronic bacteremia, lupus nephritis and MPGN type I), subendothelial deposits are rare. Furthermore, C4 is rarely present in the glomerular deposits, suggesting that in their formation classical pathway activation did not occur. Finally, a small percentage of patients have no IgG in their glomerular deposits (91–93). It is possible that further studies of the nephritis strain-associated protein (NSAP), considered the nephritogenic extracellular product of certain strains of streptococci (94), will result in revision of the immune complex concept. NSAP has been shown to be a constituent of the glomerular deposits both in the human disease (95) and in rabbits infected with nephritogenic streptococci (96). More important is that NSAP has been found to activate the complement system both by itself and as an NSAP–anti-NSAP complex (97). It seems possible that basic to the pathogenesis of AGN is the deposition of NSAP in the glomerulus, alone or combined with antibody.

The cause of the perturbation of the complement system, often profound, found in the circulation in this disease, is not known. As shown in Figure 5, the complement profile is characterized by reduced levels of C3, properdin, and C5, with normal levels of other terminal components. Occasional patients will have slightly depressed C2 and C4 levels in very early specimens (61). It should be emphasized that this evidence of classical pathway activation is very transient whereas the C3 level may remain low for as long as 6 weeks. Most patients have low C3 levels from the onset but, in our experience, only the properdin level will be depressed in some and in 10% all components are in normal concentration throughout the disease course (98). In view of the low level of C5 in AGN and the requirement for C3b deposition on the solid phase for the activation of C5, Endre et al. (1) have proposed that the hypocomplementemia results from the deposition of C3b on the glomerular capillary wall. However, C5 levels are depressed in MPGN types I and

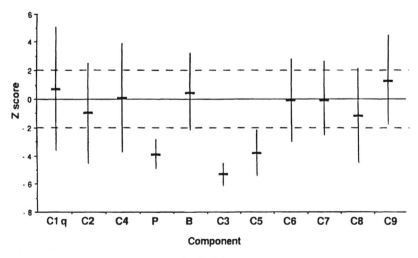

Figure 5 Acute poststreptococcal glomerulonephritis. Mean and range of complement component concentrations in 40 patients at time of presentation. Data are graphed as in Figure 1.

III and in SLE, in which diseases circulating complement-reactive material is thought to produce the hypocomplementemia. A circulating factor producing hypocomplementemia in AGN has not been recognized. Limited C3 conversion has been reported in mixtures containing AGN serum, but the results are inconsistent and the extent of the conversion variable (99,100).

Whatever the condition's cause, there is no evidence that the hypocomplementemia is related to the pathogenesis of the nephritis. Many patients with mild, subclinical disease have a severe hypocomplementemia (101,102). Also, there is no data to show that normo-complementemic patients have a disease different from those with hypocomplementemia. For diagnostic purposes, in a patient with recent advent of nephritis, hypocomplementemia is highly suggestive of AGN but the diagnosis cannot be ruled out in its absence.

F. Nephritis of Henoch-Schonlein Purpura

Henoch-Schoelein purpura HSP appears to be a biphasic disease in which a vasculitis of variable severity is often followed by chronic, usually asymptomatic, mesangial IgA deposition that may eventually lead to renal failure (57). The IgA deposition is indistinguishable from that of IgA nephropathy. By inhibition assays (103,104), complexes have been found in the initial vasculitic phase and may be responsible for the large glomerular subendothelial deposits found in this phase (57,105) that are often accompanied by a monocytic infiltrate (57). The subendothelial deposits contain IgG, IgA, and C3 but no C4. During this acute phase there may be evidence of classical pathway activation with reduced levels of C2, C4, and properdin but normal levels of C3. What is activating the classical pathway at this stage is not clear. The circulating complexes noted above, described as large, should produce reduced C3 levels. The profile resembles that seen in essential cryoglobulinemia (56) and it is possible that a protein with similar complement reactive properties but that does not precipitate in the cold is present. How this protein would relate to the glomerular deposits is not clear.

During the second phase of the disease, characterized by mesangial deposition of IgA, the mix of complement proteins present in the glomerulus probably depends on the severity of the mesangial inflammatory process. If severe, C3 and terminal components (106) will be present and often IgG and IgM as well as with IgA. That complement activation is continuing in the glomerulus, is, as noted above, suggested by the elevated serum C3d levels (64). By analogy to IgA nephropathy, however, C5b-9 may have no role in producing the glomerulitis (see below).

G. IgA Nephropathy

Commensurate with its importance as a cause of renal failure, the pathogenesis of IgA nephropathy has been the subject of considerable investigation. The disease is characterized in the young by a predisposition to recurrent episodes of gross hematuria concurrent with an infection and in the older patient by constant microhematuria and proteinuria. Usually renal function deteriorates slowly during a period when the disease is largely silent. Initially, renal biopsy shows only slight mesangial proliferation, without significant infiltration of circulating cells, and deposits containing IgA and C3 in a submesangial position. In many cases, IgG and IgM are also present but less abundant and in a different distribution than IgA. Also, by immunofluorescence, J chain is detectable in the deposits in the absence of IgM (107), which is evidence that the deposits are rich in polymerized IgA (pIgA). Whether the pIgA is part of an immune complex or whether a predisposition to form pIgA is basic to the disease is not known.

Much attention has been paid to the ability of the mesangial IgA to activate complement. There is no evidence from in vitro studies that IgA in any form activates the classical pathway. In consonance with this, C4 and C1q are usually absent from the glomerular deposits in IgA nephropathy (106). A number of studies have, on the other hand, shown that IgA can activate the alternative pathway. Human IgA_1, IgA_2, and secretory IgA coated on microwell plates activated the alternative pathway (108), but immune complexes made with IgA antibody did not (109). Aggregated IgA deposited on erythrocytes activated the alternative pathway depending on their abundance, size, and method of aggregation (110). An immune complex formed with a mouse myeloma IgA reactive with a specific antigen activated the alternative pathway in both mouse and guinea pig serum. C3, however, did not bind and C5 cleavage did not occur, probably because there was no solid-phase site for C3b attachment (111). That C5b-9 can be produced by alternative pathway activation by IgA was evidenced by the lysis in rat serum of TMP-conjugated rat red cells coated with dimeric or polymeric but not monomeric IgA (112). Also, immune precipitates made with monomeric, dimeric, or polymeric IgA of rat origin activated the alternative pathway of rat serum. Polymeric IgA was four times as effective in activating the pathway as its monomeric form (112). Thus, there is considerable evidence that mesangial IgA, by virtue of its high content of polymeric IgA, activates exclusively the alternative pathway. The presence in the deposits of terminal pathway components as well as C5b-9 in the same distribution as IgA and C3 suggests that the terminal pathway is activated as well (106). There is evidence, however, that the C5b-9 is not essential for the induction of the disease. First, C3 may be absent from the glomeruli, as noted in Table 1. Second, IgA nephropathy has been observed in four patients who are homozygous C9 deficient (113). All four were older children or young adults and, conforming to the course in that age group, the disease had not progressed during periods of observation of up to 9 years. Although C5b-9 appears unnecessary for initiation of the disease, a role in its progression cannot be ruled out.

H. Membranous Nephropathy

Membranous nephropathy is characterized ultrastructurally by beadlike subepithelial deposits separated by projections of lamina densa. The deposits contain IgG, C3, terminal components, and in less than half the patients, C4. The disease is characterized clinically by proteinuria that may be massive and is the most common cause of nephrotic syndrome in adults. Study of the disease has been facilitated by the availability of an experimental nephritis, known as Heymann, or autologous immune complex, nephritis, which models the disease almost perfectly. The experimental disease is produced by antibody to an epithelial cell antigen known in the rat as GP330 or Fx1A, located in the clathrin-coated pits. The antibody penetrates the GBM to form complexes in situ that are patched and capped by the epithelial cells to form the beadlike deposits. Complement, also penetrating the GBM, reacts, presumably via the alternative pathway (114), with the complexes to form C5b-9 (4). Whereas some of the C5b-9 must be inactivated by S protein, a fraction inserts in the epithelial cell membrane (115). It has been shown that when the animals are depleted of C3 (4) or C6 (116) prior to receiving antibody in the passive Heymann nephritis model, proteinuria does not develop. In the depleted animals, the amount of antibody in the deposits was the same as in the controls, giving evidence that the proteinuria is C5b-9 dependent. The C5b-9 inserted in the epithelial cell is endocytosed and undergoes transcellular transport and exocytosis into the urinary space and can be detected in the final urine (117). It is of interest that in other experimental nephritides C5b-9 is not excreted even though present in the glomerular deposits. These experimental nephritides include nephrotoxic nephritis, subendothelial immune complex nephritis and nephritis produced by antibody to mesangial cell membranes and by cationized IgG. Absence of urinary C5b-9 in the latter disease is of greatest interest because it is characterized by subepithelial deposits containing C5b-9 and by massive proteinuria, thus closely resembling membranous nephropathy and Heymann nephritis (117).

Although in the Heymann model the assembly of C5b-9 on the epithelial cell is essential for the development of proteinuria, the excretion of C5b-9 does not parallel the extent of the proteinuria. In the passive Heymann model, C5b-9 appears in the urine before proteinuria is detectable and the severity of the proteinuria that develops subsequently is independent of the rate of C5b-9 excretion (118).

Possible mechanisms by which proteinuria might be produced by the insertion in the epithelial cell of C5b-9 have been discussed by Couser et al. (119). Most likely is activation of the epithelial cell with release of toxic mediators, although denuding of the lamina rara externa by detachment of the epithelial cell podocyte may contribute. Whatever the mechanism, the rate of protein excretion appears not to be a measure of activity of the disease as judged by excretion of C5b-9.

These observations, by analogy to human idiopathic membranous nephropathy, have not only revealed intimate details of pathogenesis but also have the potential to provide a measure of activity of the human disease, allowing treatment to be applied with greater effect. Although the antigen responsible for the subepithelial deposits in human membranous nephropathy has not been identified, observations from several centers suggest that high rates of C5b-9 excretion are an indicator of immunologically active disease. Thus, in one study, C5b-9 excretion was high in patients with disease of recent onset with high rates of protein excretion (120) and in another it was high mainly in those deemed to have an unstable clinical course (121). In a third more longitudinal study, those in whom C5b-9 excretion became normal had a better clinical outcome than those with continuing excretion (122). This is an example of the direct applicability to human disease of detailed study of a disease model.

V. COMPLEMENT ACTIVATION IN THE GLOMERULUS AND ITS CONTROL

A. Nephritides Dependent on Complement Activation

To date, the complement system has been found to be central to the pathogenesis of three forms of experimental nephritis and there is evidence for its involvement in a human nephritis for which there is no experimental counterpart. A very early study (123) demonstrated that the attraction of neutrophils into the glomerulus by complement breakdown products could be a cause of nephritis. This mechanism is, in all likelihood, operative in exudative nephritides in humans. The role of complement in a second form of experimental nephritis arose from the studies by Couser and his group of Heymann nephritis in the rat. As noted above, they demonstrated that insertion of C5b-9 in the glomerular epithelial cell is basic to this lesion and there is strong evidence that the mechanism is similar in human membranous nephropathy. The third experimental glomerulonephritis is the mesangial proliferation produced by antithymocyte serum reacting with mesangial cells. This disease has recently been shown to depend on insertion of C5b-9 in the mesangial cells (5). Whereas no human nephritis is known to be produced by antibody to mesangial cells, the observation suggests that mesangial proliferation, as seen in human disease, could be the result of complement activation in the mesangium. Finally, as noted above (45), there is circumstantial evidence that, by some mechanism, circulating convertase, particularly that stabilized by nephritic factor, is nephritogenic. Certainly other complement dependent nephritogenic mechanisms await elucidation.

B. Membrane-Associated Control Proteins and C3b Deposition in the Glomerulus

Basic to the generation of C5a or C5b-9 is the glomerular deposition of C3b. C3b deposition can occur as a result of activation of C3 by the classical pathway convertase, C4b,2a, or as a bystander event dependent on the constant formation of $C3(H_2O)$ and the constant "tickover" of the amplification loop. Bystander deposition of C3b is prevented in the normal glomerulus by membrane-associated control proteins. These include membrane cofactor protein (MCP,CD46) and decay-accelerating factor (DAF,CD55). In the normal glomerulus, MCP is found in the mesangium and on glomerular capillary walls but it is most abundant at the juxto-glomerular apparatus (124,125). DAF, on the other hand, is virtually confined to the juxtoglomerular apparatus (126). Human mesangial cells in culture upregulate their production of DAF in response to insertion of C5b-9 in the cell membrane (127). MCP production in vitro is much less responsive to this stimulus (122,128). In vivo, membrane-associated DAF was found to increase with glomerular disease, particularly in HUS and MPGN, whereas that in the juxtoglomerular apparatus often disappeared (126). MCP, differing from its behavior in vitro, is more abundantly expressed in vivo with disease. In immunohistochemical terms, the increase occurs on the glomerular capillary walls or in the mesangium, or both. The increase in glomerular MCP is most consistent in MPGN and acute poststreptococcal glomerulonephritis and less consistent in IgA nephropathy, lupus, and membranous nephropathy (124). Staining for MCP was most intense in areas in which C3b/iC3b was most abundant, but the intensity of staining for C3dg, deposited alone, did not correlate with MCP staining (124).

There is a third membrane control protein in the glomerulus, CR-1, located on epithelial cells. It was reported in 1975 that C3b-coated erythrocytes and bacteria adhere to the podocytes of the normal glomerulus. Using this method of detection, many investigators found diseases and conditions in which CR-1 was absent from epithelial cells but the results were not uniform. Some found absence of CR-1 with deposits of C3 in the capillary wall and others with deposits in the mesangium. It would appear that in disease the receptors are to a variable extent blocked by C3b, since they were found to be normally present in most diseases when visualized with labeled polyclonal monospecific antibody to CR-1. This antibody bound equally in the presence and absence of C3b. CR-1 was absent diffusely or focally with hyalinosis, in many forms of rapidly progressive glomerulo-nephritis, in diabetic nephropathy, and in amyloidosis. In the diseases of immune origin such as MPGN and particularly proliferative lupus nephritis, CR-1 was absent (129,130). The reason for its absence in those proliferative nephritides as well as its role in the function of the glomerular epithelial cell is not clear.

Although deposition of C3b in the normal glomerulus is prevented largely by MCP and, with nephritis, this protection, as well as that afforded by DAF, is augmented, C3b deposition still occurs. It has been shown that in SLE, IgA nephropathy, AGN and MPGN types I and III, 8–70% of the C3 deposited in the glomerulus, as detected by a monoclonal antibody to C3c, is C3b with the remainder being iC3b (131). We presume that the C3b is deposited on C3b acceptors that restrict the inactivation of C3b by factors H and I and are distant from membrane-bound DAF and MCP. Restrictive C3b acceptors would include IgG when aggregated as part of an immune complex (132), IgA as found in the mesangium in IgA nephropathy (108,110–112), and the C3 convertase derived from C4, which is designated C4b,2a,3b (133,134). One or more of these acceptors can be found in most nephritides. They are, however, lacking in approximately 25% of the cases of AGN in which glomerular IgG is not present and in most cases of MPGN types II and III. In AGN, as noted above, it is possible that NSAP itself, located in subepithelial deposits and in the mesangium (95), provides a restricted site. In MPGN type III, the glomeruli are usually devoid of all immunoglobulins and of C4 (81) and the sites restricting inactivation of C3b, which was found to make up 8–25% of the deposited C3 (131), are not known. The fraction of glomerular C3 that is C3b in MPGN type II has not been determined.

C. Control of C5b-9

Whatever the site of C3b deposition, it is apparently sufficient in all the nephritides to activate C5, the first step in the formation of C5b-9 (135). For this activation, two or more C3b molecules must be in close proximity on a solid phase. The end product of C5 activation, C5b-9, has been found immunohistochemically, usually by monoclonal antibody to a neoantigen on the polymerized C9, in nearly all nephritides (136).

It is well known that whereas a single C5b-9 can cause hemolysis of a red cell, a multiplicity of hits is needed for lysis of a nucleated cell. A sublytic attack on a nucleated cell, however, serves to activate it and, for mesangial cells in culture, results in the extracellular release of autocoids, matrix components, and various cytokines and enzymes (reviewed in 137). C5b-9 was found codeposited with C3 in the glomerulus in a number of diseases (136,138). Although this observation could be taken as positive evidence for a role of C5b-9 in glomerular injury, the subsequent observation that the S protein was codeposited with C3 and C5b-9 made conclusions difficult (139,140). The S protein, also known as vitronectin, can bind to C5b-7 in the course of C5b-9 assembly. This does not interfere with the addition of C8 and C9 to the complex but the C9 does not polymerize. As a result SC5b-9 will not insert into cell membranes and remains in the fluid phase. It may be detected in the circulation in a number of glomerulonephritides. The codeposition of the S protein with the neoantigen of C5b-9 makes inconclusive the role of C5b-9 in producing the glomerular lesion, since only SC5b-9 deposited from the circulation may be present. That SC5b-9 can deposit in tissue from the circulation is indicated by its demonstration in sclerotic tissue, hyaline deposits, and the glomerular mesangium in diabetic nephropathy, all in the absence of immunoglobulin or C3 (139,140). The problem is further compounded by the observation that C5b-9, after insertion in the membrane and in the form C5b-9m, can also bind S protein. Although the amount bound is small, it can be detected immunohistochemically (141).

Although in human disease direct evidence that C5b-9 activates mesangial cells is lacking, there is, as described above, strong experimental evidence that C5b-9 insertion in glomerular epithelial cells is responsible for the proteinuria of Heymann nephritis and, by analogy, human membranous nephropathy.

More recently it has been shown that clusterin (SP-40,40) also binds to both C5b-9 and to SC5b-9 and renders C5b-9 cytolytically inactive (142). Clusterin can be found in association with C5b-9 and S protein in the glomerulus. It is more frequently found colocalized with C5b-9 in deposits containing immunoglobulins (143). The ability of clusterin to inactivate C5b-9 and the role of C5b-9 in Heymann nephritis was elegantly demonstrated by perfusion of an isolated kidney in which passive Heymann nephritis had been induced with blood depleted of clusterin. Proteinuria was significantly increased compared with control perfusion with unmodified blood. The subepithelial deposits and C3 deposition were similar (144).

Protection is also afforded glomerular cells from C5b-9 attack by two membrane-associated control proteins. The C8-binding protein (homologous restriction factor, membrane attack inhibiting factor) and CD59 (HRF20,p-18) both act on C8 and C9 and inhibit formation of poly-C9, thus preventing penetration of the cell membrane (145,146). The C8-binding protein is found on glomerular mesangial and epithelial cells in culture and its expression is transiently enhanced by treatment of the cells with interleukin 1β, C5b-9, or endotoxin (147). CD59 is present immunohistochemically on mesangial cells and on the capillary walls of normal glomeruli (148,149). In nephritis, there is little increase in capillary wall CD59 but in diffuse lupus nephritis there is a marked increase in the amount in the mesangium (149).

Thus, the regulatory proteins by which glomerular cells are protected from C5b-9 attack are present in both cell membranes and plasma. The membrane-associated proteins are DAF, MCP, the C8 binding protein, and CD59. There are data suggesting that these proteins become more abundant in the face of an inflammatory reaction. The plasma proteins are S protein, clusterin, factors H and I, and, controlling the classic pathway, C4-binding protein. Proteins in both categories either prevent the formation of C5b-9 or bind and render ineffective that formed to protect bystander cells. No data have implicated C5b-9 as basic to the pathogenesis of any of the human nephritides, except membranous nephropathy, by analogy from the studies of Heymann nephritis.

REFERENCES

1. Endre ZH, Pussell BA, Charlesworth JA, Coovadia HM, Seedat YK. C3 metabolism in acute glomerulonephritis: implications for sites of complement activation. Kidney Int 1984; 22:937–941.
2. Unanue, ER, Dixon FJ. Experimental glomerulonephritis. IV. Participation of complement in nephrotoxic nephritis. J Exp Med 1964; 119:965–982.
3. Brady HR. Leukocyte adhesion molecules and kidney diseases. Kidney Int 1994; 45:1285–1300.
4. Salant DJ, Belok S, Madiao MP, Couser WG. A new role for complement in experimental membranous nephropathy in rats. J Clin Invest 1980; 66:1339–1350.
5. Brandt J, Pippin J, Schulze M, Hämsch GM, Alpers CE, Johnson RJ, Gordon K, Couser WG. Role of the complement membrane attack complex (C5b-9) in mediating experimental mesangioproliferative glomerulonephritis. Kidney Int 1996; 49:335–343.
6. Silva FG, Hogg RJ. IgA nephropathy. In: Tisher CC, Brenner BM, eds. Renal Pathology with Clinical and Functional Correlations. Philadelphia: Lippincott, 1989; 440.
7. Levy M, Broyer M, Arsan A, Levy-Bentolila D, Habib R. Anaphylactoid purpura nephritis in childhood: natural history and immunopathology. Advances in Nephrology 1976; 6:183–228.

8. Noel LH, Zanatti M, Droz D, Barbanel C. Long-term prognosis of idiopathic membranous glomerulonephritis. Study of 116 untreated patients. Am J Med 1979; 66:82–90.

9. Edberg JC, Tosic L, Wright EL, Sutherland WM, Taylor RP. Quantitative analysis of the relationship between C3 consumption, C3b capture, and immune adherence of complement-fixing antibody/DNA immune complexes. J Immunol 1988; 141:4258–4265.

10. Strife CF, McDonald BM, Ruley EJ, McAdams AJ, West CD. Shunt nephritis: the nature of the serum cryoglobulins and their relation to the complement profile. J Pediatr 1976; 88:403–413.

11. West CD. The complement profile in clinical medicine. Complement Inflamm 1989; 6:49–64.

12. Miller GW, Nussenzweig V. A new complement function: solubilization of antigen–antibody aggregates. Proc Natl Acad Sci USA 1975; 72:418–422.

13. Takahashi M, Tack BF, Nussenzweig V. Requirements for the solubilization of immune aggregates by complement. J Exp Med 1977; 145:86–100.

14. Hebert LA, Cosio FG. The erythrocyte–immune complex–glomerulonephritis connection in man. Kidney Int 1987; 31:877–885.

15. Medof ME, Iida K, Mold C, Nussenzweig V. Unique role of the complement receptor CR-1 in the degradation of C3b associated with immune complexes. J Exp Med 1982; 156:1739–1754.

16. Ross GD, Yount WJ, Walport MJ, Windfield JB, Parker CJ, Fuller CR, Taylor RP, Myones BL, Lachmann PJ. Disease-associated loss of erythrocyte complement receptors (CR-1, C3b receptors) in patients with systemic lupus erythematosus and other diseases involving autoantibodies and/or complement activation. J Immunol 1985; 135:2005–2014.

17. Atkinson JP. Complement activation and complement receptors in systemic lupus erythematosus. Semin Immunol Pathol 1986; 9:179–194.

18. Fielder AHL, Walport MJ, Batchelor JR, Rynes RI, Black CM, Dodi IA, Hughes GRV. Family study of the major histocompatibility complex in patients with systemic lupus erythematosus: importance of null alleles of C4A and C4B in determining disease susceptibility. Br Med J 1983; 286:425–428.

19. Ross SC, Densen P. Complement deficiency states and infection: epidemiology, pathogenesis and consequences of neisserial and other infections in an immune deficiency. Medicine (Baltimore) 1984; 63:243–273.

20. Minota S, Terai C, Nojima Y, Takano K, Takai E, Miyakawa Y, Takaku F. Low C3b receptor reactivity on erythrocytes from patients with systemic lupus erythematosus detected by immune adherence hemagglutination and radio immunoassays with monoclonal antibody. Arthritis Rheum 1984; 27:1329–1335.

21. Spitzer RE, Vallota EH, Forristal J, Sudora E, Stitzel A, Davis NC, West CD. Serum C3 lytic system in patients with glomerulonephritis. Science 1969; 164:436–437.

22. Davis AE, Ziegler JB, Gelfand EW, Rosen FS, Alper CA. Heterogeneity of nephritic factor and its identification as an immunoglobulin. Proc Natl Acad Sci 1977; 74:3980–3983.

23. Daha MR, Van Es LA. Further evidence for the antibody nature of C3 nephritic factor (C3NeF). J Immunol 1979; 123:755–758.

24. Daha MR, Fearon DT, Austen KF. C3 nephritic factor (C3NeF): stabilization of fluid phase and cell-bound alternative pathway convertase. J Immunol 1976; 116:1–7.

25. Weiler JM, Daha MR, Austen KF, Fearon DT. Control of the amplification convertase of complement by the plasma protein β1H. Proc Natl Acad Sci USA 1976; 73:3268–3272.

26. Sissons JGP, Leibowitch J, Amos W, Peters DK. Metabolism of the fifth component of complement and its relation to the metabolism of the third component in patients with complement activation. J Clin Invest 1977; 59:704–715.

27. Varade WS, Forristal J and West CD. Patterns of complement activation in idiopathic membranoproliferative glomerulonephritis, types I, II and III. Am J Kidney Dis 1990; 16:196–206.

28. Peters DK, Martin A, Weinstein A, Cameron JS, Barratt TM, Ogg CS, Lachmann PJ. Complement studies in membranoproliferative glomerulonephritis. Clin Exp Immunol 1972; 11:311–320.

29. Vallota EH, Forristal J, Spitzer RE, Davis NC, West CD. Characteristics of a non-complement-dependent C3-reactive complex formed from factors in nephritic and normal serum. J Exp Med 1970; 131:1306–1334.

30. Ohi H, Watanabe S, Fujita T, Seki M, Hatano M. Detection of C3bBb-stabilizing activity (C3 nephritic factor) in the serum from patients with membranoproliferative glomerulonephritis. J Immunol Methods 1990; 131:71–76.

31. Mollnes TE, Ng WC, Peters DK, Lea T, Tschopp J, Harboe M. Effect of nephritic factor on C3 and on the terminal pathway of complement in vivo and in vitro. Clin Exp Immunol 1986; 65:73–79.

32. Clardy CW, Forristal J, Strife CF, West CD. A properdin dependent nephritic factor slowly activating C3, C5, and C9 in membranoproliferative glomerulonephritis, types I and III. Clin Immunol Immunopathol 1989; 50:333–347.

33. Tanuma Y, Ohi H, Hatano M. Two types of C3 nephritic factor: properdin-dependent C3NeF and properdin-independent C3NeF. Clin Immunol Immunopathol 1990; 56:226–238.

34. Halbwachs L, Leveille M, Lesabre P, Wattell S, Leibowitch J. Nephritic factor of the classical pathway of complement. Immunoglobulin G autoantibody directed against the classical pathway C3 convertase enzyme. J Clin Invest 1980; 65:1249–1256.

35. Daha MR, Hazevoet HM, Van Es LA, Cats A. Stabilization of the classical pathway C3 convertase C42, by a factor F42, isolated from serum of patients with systemic lupus erythematosus. Immunology 1980; 40:417–424.

36. Tanuma Y, Ohi, H. Watanabe S, Seki M, Hatano M. C3 nephritic factor and C4 nephritic factor in the serum of two patients with hypocomplementemic membranoproliferative glomerulonephritis. Clin Exp Immunol 1989; 76:82–85.

37. Gigli I, Sorvillo J, Mecarelli-Halbwachs L, Leibowitch J. Mechanism of action of the C4 nephritic factor. Deregulation of the classical pathway C3 convertase. J Exp Med 1981; 154:1–12.

38. Ohi H, Yasugi T. Occurrence of C3 nephritic factor and C4 nephritic factor in membranoproliferative glomerulonephritis (MPGN). Clin Exp Immunol 1994; 95:316–321.

39. Schena FP, Pertosa G, Stanziale P, Vox E, Pecoraro C, Andreucci VE. Biological significance of the C3 nephritic factor in membranoproliferative glomerulonephritis. Clin Nephrol 1982; 18:240–246.

40. Sissons JGP, West RJ, Fallows J, Williams DG, Boucher BJ, Amos N, Peters DK. The complement abnormalities of lipodystrophy. N Engl J Med 1976; 294:461–465.

41. Alper CA, Bloch KJ, Rosen FS. Increased susceptibility to infection in a patient with type II essential hypercatabolism of C3. N Engl J Med 1973; 288:601–606.

42. Edwards KM, Alford R, Gewurz H, Mold C. Recurrent bacterial infections associated with C3 nephritic factor and hypocomplementemia. N Engl J Med 1983; 308:1138–1141.

43. Gewurz AT, Imherr SM, Struss S, Gewurz H, Mold C. C3 nephritic factor and hypocomplementemia in a clinically healthy individual. Clin Exp Immunol 1983; 54:253–258.

44. Klein M, Poucell S, Arbus GS, McGraw M, Rance CP, Yoon S-J, Baumal R. Characteristics of a benign subtype of dense deposit disease: comparison with the progressive form of this disease. Clin Nephrol 1983; 20:163–171.

45. West CD. Occasional hypothesis. Nephritic factors predispose to chronic glomerulonephritis. Am J Kidney Dis 1994; 24:956–963.

46. Høgåsen K, Jansen JH, Mollnes TE, Hovdenes J, Harboe M. Hereditary porcine membranoproliferative glomerulonephritis type II is caused by factor H deficiency. J Clin Invest 1995; 95:1054–1061.

47. Marder HK, Coleman TH, Forristal J, Beischel L, West CD. An inherited defect in the C3 convertase, C3b,Bb, associated with glomerulonephritis. Kidney Int 1983; 23:749–758.

48. Linshaw MA, Stapleton FB, Cuppage FE, Forristal J, West CD, Schreiber RD, Wilson CB. Hypocomplementemic glomerulonephritis in an infant and mother. Evidence for an abnormal form of C3. Am J Nephrol 1987; 7:470–477.

49. Meri S, Koisteinen V, Meittinen A, Tornroth T, Seppala IJT. Activation of the alternative pathway of complement by monoclonal γ light chains in membranoproliferative glomerulonephritis. J Exp Med 1992; 175:939–950.

50. Lopez-Larrea C, Dieguez MA, Enguix A, Dominguez O, Marin B, Gomez E. A familial deficiency of complement factor H. Biochem Soc Trans 1987; 15:648–649.

51. Levy M, Halbwachs-Mecarelli L, Gubler N-C, Kohout G, Bensenouci A, Hiaudet P, Hauptmann G, Lesavre P. H deficiency in two brothers with atypical dense intramembranous deposit disease. Kidney Int 1986, 30:949–956.

52. Jansen JH. Porcine membranoproliferative glomerulonephritis with intramembranous dense deposits (porcine dense deposit disease). APMIS 1993; 101:281–289.

53. West CD, McAdams AJ. Paramesangial glomerular deposits in membranoproliferative glomerulonephritis type II correlate with hypocomplementemia. Am J Kidney Dis 1995; 25:853–861.

54. Kim Y, Vernier RL, Fish AJ, Michael AF. Immunofluorescent studies of dense deposit disease. The presence of railroad tracks and mesangial rings. Lab Invest 1979; 474–480.

55. Gelfand JA, Boss GR, Conley CL, Reinhart R, Frank MM. Acquired C1 esterase inhibitor deficiency and angioedema: a review. Medicine 1979; 58:321–328.

56. Tarantino A, Anelli A, Costantino A, De Vecchi A, Monte G, Massaro L. Serum complement pattern in essential mixed cryoglobulinemia. Clin Exp Immunol 1978; 32:77–85.

57. West CD, McAdams AJ, Welch TR. Glomerulonephritis in Henoch-Schoenlein purpura without mesangial IgA deposition. Pediatr Nephrol 1994; 8:677–683.

58. Waldo FB, West CD, Quantitation of $(C1INH)_2C1rC1s$ complexes in glomerulonephritis as an indicator of C1 activation. Clin Immunol and Immunopathol 1987; 42:239–249.

59. Hack CE, Hannema AJ, Erenberg-Belmer AJM, Out TA, Aaberse RC. A C1-inhibitor-complex assay (INCA): a method to detect C1 activation in vitro and in vivo. J Immunol 1981; 127:1450–1453.

60. Milgrom H, Curd JG, Kaplan RA, Muller-Eberhard HJ, Vaughan JH. Activation of the fourth component of complement (C4) asessment by rocket immunoelectrophoresis and correlation with the metabolism of C4. J Immunol 1980; 124:2780–2785.

61. Wyatt RJ, Forristal J, West CD, Sugimoto S, Curd JG. Complement profiles in acute post-streptococcal glomerulonephritis. Pediatr Nephrol 1988; 2:219–223.

62. West CD, Winter S, Forristal J, McConville JM, Davis AC. Evidence for in vivo breakdown of β1C-globulin in hypocomplementemic glomerulonephritis. J Clin Invest 1967; 26:539–548.

63. Perrin LH, Lambert PH, Miescher PA. Complement breakdown products in plasma from patients with systemic lupus erythematosus and patients with membranoproliferative or other glomerulonephritides. J Clin Invest 1975; 56:165–176.

64. Wyatt RJ, Julian BA. Activation of complement in IgA nephropathy. Am J Kidney Dis 1988; 12:437–442.

65. Alper CA, Rosen FS. Studies of the in vivo behavior of human C'3 in normal subjects and patients. J Clin Invest 1967; 46:2021–2034.

66. Abramson SB, Weissmann G. Complement split products and the pathogenesis of SLE. Hosp Pract 1988; December 15:45–56.

67. Kolb WP, Morrow PR, Tamerius JD. Ba and Bb fragments of factor B activation: fragment production, biological activities, neoepitope expression and quantitation in clinical samples. Complement Inflamm 1989; 6:175–204.

68. Falk RJ, Dalmasso AP, Kim Y, Lam S, Michael A. Radioimmunoassay of the attack complex of complement in serum from patients with systemic lupus erythematosus. N Engl Med 1985; 312:1594–1599.

69. Mollnes TE, Lea T, Frøland SS, Harboe M. Quantification of the terminal complement complex in human plasma by an enzyme-linked immunosorbent assay based on monoclonal antibodies against a neo-antigen of the complex. Scand J Immunol 1985; 22:197–202.

70. Hill GS, Hinglais N, Tron F, Bach J-F. Systemic lupus erythematosus. Morphologic correlations with immunologic and clinical data at the time of biopsy. Am J Med 1978; 64:61–79.

71. Lloyd W, Schur PH. Immune complexes, complement, and anti-DNA in exacerbations of systemic lupus erythematosus (SLE). Medicine (Baltimore) 1981; 60:208–217.

72. Cameron JS, Lessof MH, Ogg CS, Williams BD, Williams DG. Disease activity in the nephritis of systemic lupus erythematosus in relation to serum complement concentrations, DNA-binding capacity and precipitating anti-DNA antibody. Clin Exp Immunol 1976; 25:418–427.

73. Swaak AJG, Groenwold J, Bronsveld W. Predictive value of complement profiles and anti-dsDNA in systemic lupus erythematosus. Ann Rheum Dis 1986; 45:359–366.

74. Ricker DM, Hebert LA, Rohde R, Sedmak DD, Lewis EJ, Clough JD, The Lupus Collaborative Study Group. Serum C3 levels are diagnostically more sensitive and specific for systemic lupus erythematosus activity than are serum C4 levels. Am J Kidney Dis 1991; 18:678–685.

75. Morrow WJW, Isenberg DA, Todd-Pokropek A, Parry HF, Snaith ML. Useful laboratory measurements in the management of systemic lupus erythematosus. Q J Med 1982; 51:125–138.

76. Valentijn RM, van Overhagen H, Hazevoet HM, Hermans J, Cats A, Daha MR, van Es LA. The value of complement and immune complex determinations in monitoring disease activity in patients with systemic lupus erythematosus. Arthritis Rheum 1985; 28:904–913.

77. Waldo FB, Forristal J, Beischel L, West CD. A circulating inhibitor of fluid phase amplification C3 convertase formation in systemic lupus erythematosus. Clin Invest 1985; 75:1786–1795.

78. Nitsche JF, Tucker SE III, Sugimoto S, Vaughn JH, Curd JG. Rocket immunoelectrophoresis of C4 and C4d. A simple sensitive method for detecting complement activation in plasma. Am J Clin Pathol 1981; 76:679–684.

79. Cameron JS, Turner DR, Heaton J, Gwyn Williams D, Ogg CS, Chantler C, Haycock GB, Hicks J. Idiopathic mesangiocapillary glomerulonephritis. Comparison of types I and II in children and adults and long-term prognosis. Am J Med 1983; 74:175–192.

80. Michael AF, Herdman RC, Fish AJ, Pickering RJ, Vernier RL. Chronic membranoproliferative glomerulonephritis with hypocomplementemia. Transplant Proc 1969; 1:925–932.

81. Jackson EC, McAdams AJ, Strife CF, Forristal J, Welch TR, West CD. Differences between membranoproliferative glomerulonephritis types I and III in clinical presentation, glomerular morphology, and complement perturbation. Am J Kidney Dis 1987; 9:115–120.

82. Leys A, Prosmans W, Van Damme-Lombaerts R, Van Damme B. Specific eye fundus lesions in type II membranoproliferative glomerulonephritis. Pediatr Nephrol 1991; 5:189–192.

83. Thorner P, Baumal R. Extra-glomerular dense deposits in dense deposit disease. Arch Pathol Lab Med 1982; 106:628–631.

84. Churg J, Duffy JL, Bernstein J. Identification of dense deposit disease. A report for the International Study of Kidney Diseases in Children. Arch Pathol Lab Med 1979; 103:67–72.

85. Cameron JS. Glomerulonephritis in renal transplants. Transplantation 1982; 34:237–245.

86. Liebowitch J, Halbwachs L, Wattel S, Gaillard M-H, Droz D. Recurrence of dense deposits in transplanted kidney. II Serum complement and nephritic factor profiles. Kidney Int 1979; 15:396–403.

87. Strife CF, McEnery PT, McAdams AJ, West CD. Membranoproliferative glomerulonephritis with disruption of the glomerular basement membrane. Clin Nephrol 1977; 7:65–72.

88. West CD. Idiopathic membranoproliferative glomerulonephritis in childhood. Pediatr Nephrol 1992; 6:96–103.

89. Fish AJ, Michael AJ, Vernier RL, Good RA. Acute serum sickness nephritis in the rabbit: an immune deposit disease. Am J Pathol 1966; 49:997–1022.

90. Germuth FG, Rodriguez E: Immunopathology of the Renal Glomerulus. Boston: Little Brown, 1973: 20.

91. Fish AJ, Herdman RC, Michael AF, Pickering RJ, Good RA. Epidemic acute glomerulonephritis associated with type 49 streptococcal pyoderma. II. Correlative study of light, immunofluorescent and electron microscopic findings. Am J Med 1970; 48:28–39.

92. Michael AF, Drummond KN, Good RA, Vernier RL. Acute poststreptococcal glomerulonephritis: immune deposit disease. J Clin Invest 1966; 45:237–248.

93. Berger J, Yaneva H, Hinglais N. Immunohistochemistry of glomerulonephritis. Adv Nephrol Necker Hosp 1971; 1:11–30.

94. Johnston KH, Zabriskie JB. Purification and partial characterization of the nephritis strain-associated protein from streptococcus pyogenes, group A. J Exp Med 1986; 163:697–712.

95. Villarreal H Jr, Fischetti VA, Van De Rijn I, Zabriskie JB. The occurrence of a protein in the extracellular products of streptococci isolated from patients with acute glomerulonephritis. J Exp Med 1979; 149:459–472.

96. Holm SE, Bergholm A-M, Johnston KH. A streptococcal plasminogen activator in the focus of infection and in the kidneys during the initial phase of experimental streptococcal glomerulonephritis. APMIS 1988; 96:1097–1108.

97. Peake PW, Pussell BA, Karplus TE, Riley EH, Charlesworth JA. Post-streptococcal glomerulonephritis: studies on the interaction between nephritis strain-associated protein (NSAP), complement and the glomerulus. APMIS 1991; 99:460–466.

98. Strife CF, McAdams AJ, McEnery PT, Bove KE, West CD. Hypocomplementemic and normocomplementemic acute nephritis in children; a comparison with respect to etiology, clinical manifestations, and glomerular morphology. J Pediatr 1974; 84:29–38.

99. Sjoholm AG. Complement components and complement activation in acute post-streptococcal glomerulonephritis. Int Arch Allergy Immunol 1979; 58:274–284.

100. Gwyn Williams D, Peters DK, Fallows J, Petrie A, Kourilsky O, Morel-Maroger L, Cameron JS. Studies of serum complement in the hypocomplementaemic nephritides. Clin Exp Immunol 1974; 18:391–405.

101. Derrick CW, Reeves MS, Dillon HC Jr. Complement in overt and asymptomatic nephritis after skin infection. J Clin Invest 1970; 49:1178–1187.

102. Sagal I, Treser G, Ty A, Yoshizawa N, Kleinberger H, Yuceoglua M, Wasserman E, Lange K. Occurrence and nature of glomerular lesions after group A streptococci infections in children. Ann Intern Med 1973; 79:492–499.

103. Levinsky RJ, Barratt TM. IgA immune complexes in Henoch-Schoenlein purpura. Lancet 1979; 2:1100–1103.

104. Kauffmann RH, Herrmann WA, Meyer CJLM, Daha MR, Van Es LA. Circulating IgA-immune complexes in Henoch-Schoenlein purpura. A longitudinal study of their relationship to disease activity and vascular deposition of IgA. Am J Med 1980; 69:859–865.

105. Heaton JM, Turner DR, Cameron JS. Location of glomerular "deposits" in Henoch-Schoenlein nephritis. Histopathology 1977; 1:93–104.

106. Rauterberg EW, Lieberknecht H-M, Wingen A-M, Ritz E. Complement membrane attack (MAC) in idiopathic IgA-glomerulonephritis. Kidney Int 1987; 31:820–829.

107. Komatsu N, Nagura H, Watanabe K, Nomoto Y, Kobayashi K. Mesangial deposition of J chain linked polymeric IgA in IgA nephropathy. Nephron 1983; 33:61–64.

108. Hiemstra PS, Biewenga J, Gorter A, Stuurman ME, Faber A, van Es LA, Daha MR. Activation of complement by human serum IgA, secretory IgA and IgA-1 fragments. Mol Immunol 1988; 25:527–533.

109. Russell MW, Mansa B. Complement-fixing properties of human IgA antibodies. Alternative pathway complement activation by plastic-bound, but not specific antigen-bound, IgA. Scand J Immunol 1989; 30:175–183.

110. Hiemstra PS, Gorter A, Stuurman ME, van Es LA, Daha MR. Activation of the alternative pathway of complement by human serum IgA. Eur J Immunol 1987; 17:321–326.

111. Pfaffenbach G, Lamm ME, Gigli I. Activation of the guinea pig alternative complement pathway by mouse IgA immune complexes. J Exp Med 1982; 155:231–247.

112. Reits M, Hiemstra PS, Bazin H, van Es LA, Vaerman JP, Daha. MR. Activation of rat complement by soluble and insoluble rat IgA immune complexes. Eur J Immunol 1988; 18:1873–1880.

113. Yoshioka K, Takemora T, Akano N, Okada M, Yagi K, Maki S, Inai S, Akita H, Koitabashi Y, Takekoshi Y. IgA nephropathy in patients with congenital C9 deficiency. Kidney Int 1992; 42:1253–1258.

114. Quigg RJ, Cybulsky AV, Salant DJ. Effect of nephritogenic antibody on complement regulation in cultured rat glomerular epithelial cells. J Immunol 1991; 147:838–845.

115. Kerjaschki D, Schulze M, Binder S, Kain R, Ojha PP, Susani M, Horvat R, Baker PJ, Couser WG. Transcellular transport and membrane insertion of the C5b-9 membrane attack complex of complement by glomerular epithelial cells in experimental membranous nephropathy. J Immunol 1989; 143:546–552.

116. Baker PJ, Ochi RF, Schulze M, Johnson RJ, Campbell C, Couser WG. Depletion of C6 prevents development of proteinuria in experimental membranous nephropathy in rats. Am J Pathol 1989; 135:185–194.

117. Schulze M, Baker PJ, Perkinson DT, Johnson RJ, Ochi RF, Stahl RAK, Couser WG. Increased urinary excretion of C5b-9 distinguishes passive Heymann nephritis in the rat. Kidney Int 1989; 35:60–68.

118. Pruchno CJ, Burns MM, Schulze M, Johnson RJ, Baker PJ, Alpers CE, Couser WG. Urinary excretion of the C5b-9 membrane attack complex of complement as a marker of immune disease activity in autologous immune complex nephritis. Am J Pathol 1991; 138:203–211.

119. Couser WG, Pruchno CJ, Schulze M. The role of C5b-9 in experimental membranous nephropathy. Nephrol Dial Transplant 1992; 7(Suppl 1):25–31.

120. Schulze M, Donadio JV, Pruchno CJ, Baker P, Johnson RJ, Stahl RAK, Watkins S, Martin DC, Wurzner R, Gotze O, Couser WG. Elevated urinary excretion of the C5b-9 complex in membranous nephropathy. Kidney Int 1991; 40:533–538.

121. Brenchley PEC, Coups BC, Short CD, O'Donoghue DJ, Ballardie FW, Mallick MP. Urinary C3dg and C5b-9 indicate active immune disease in human membranous nephropathy. Kidney Int 1992; 41:933–937.

122. Kon SP, Coupes B, Short CD, Solomon LR, Raftery MJ, Mallick NP, Brenchley PE. Urinary C5b-9 excretion and clinical course in idiopathic human membranous nephropathy. Kidney Int 1995; 48:1953–1958.

123. Cochrane CG, Unanue ER, Dixon FJ. A role of polymorphonuclear leukocytes and complement in nephrotoxic nephritis. J Exp Med 1965; 122:99–116.

124. Endoh M, Yamashina M, Ohi H, Funahashi K, Ikuno T, Yasugi T, Atkinson JP, Okada H. Immunohistochemical demonstration of membrane cofactor protein (MCP) of complement in normal and diseased kidney tissues. Clin Exp Immunol 1993; 94:182–188.

125. Nakanishi I, Moutabarrik A, Hara T, Hatanak M, Hayashi T, Syouji T, Okada N, Kitamura E, Tsubakihara Y, Matsumoto M, Seya T. Identification and characterization of the membrane cofactor protein (CD46) in human kidneys. Eur J Immunol 1994; 24:1529–1535.

126. Cosio FG, Sedmak DD, Mahan JD, Nahman MS Jr. Localization of decay-accelerating factor in normal and diseased kidneys. Kidney Int 1989; 36:100–107.

127. Shibata T, Cosio FG, Birmingham DJ. Complement activation induces the expression of decay-accelerating factor on human mesangial cells. J Immunol 1991; 147:3901–3908.

128. Cosio FG, Shibata T, Rovin BH, Birmingham DJ. Effects of complement activation products on the synthesis of decay accelerating factor and membrane cofactor protein by human mesangial cells. Kidney Int 1994; 46:986–992.

129. Kazatchkine MD, Fearon DT, Appay MD, Mandet C, Bariety J. Immunohistochemical study of the human glomerular C3b receptor in normal kidney and in seventy-five cases of renal diseases. Loss of C3b receptor antigen in focal hyalinosis and in proliferative nephritis of systemic lupus erythematosus. J Clin Invest 1982; 69:900–912.

130. Emmancipator SN, Iida K, Nussenzweig V, Gallo GR. Monoclonal antibodies to human complement receptor (CR1) detect defects in glomerular diseases. Clin Immunol and Immunopathol 1983; 27:170–175.

131. Pan C, Strife CF, McAdams AJ, West CD. Activated C3(C3b) in the nephritic glomerulus. Pediat Nephrol 1993; 7:379–386.

132. Fries LF, Gaither TA, Hammer CH, Frank MN. C3b covariantly bound to IgG demonstrates a reduced rate of inactivation by factors H and I. J Exp Med 1984; 160:1640–1655.

133. Meri S, Pangborn NK. The mechanism of activation of the alternative pathway by the classical pathway (abstract). Compl Inflamm 1989; 6:367.

134. Takata Y, Kineshita T, Kozono H, Takeda J, Tanake E, Hong K, Inoue K. Covalent association of C3b with C4b within the C5 convertase of the classical complement pathway. J Exp Med 1987; 165:1494–1507.

135. Daha MR, Fearon DT, Austin KF. C3 requirements for formation of alternative pathway C5 convertase. J Immunol 1976; 117:630–634.

136. Falk RJ, Dalmasso AP, Kim Y, Tsai CH, Scheinman JI, Gewurz H, Michael AF. Neoantigen of the polymerized ninth component of complement. Characterization of a monoclonal antibody and immunohistochemical localization in renal disease. J Clin Invest 1983; 72:560–573.

137. Sterzel RB, Schulze-Lohoff E, Marx M. Cytokines and mesangial cells. Kidney Int 1993; 43:S26–31.

138. Hinglais N, Kazatchkine MD, Bhakdi S, Appay M-D, Mandet C, Grossetete J, Bariety J. Immunohistochemical study of the C5b-9 complex of complement in human kidneys. Kidney Int 1986; 30:399–410.

139. Bariety J, Hinglais N, Bhakdi S, Mandet C, Rouchon M, Kazatchkine MD. Immunohistochemical study of complement S protein (vitronectin) in normal and diseased human kidneys: relationship to neoantigens of the C5b-9 terminal complex. Clin Exp Immunol 1989; 75:76–81.

140. Falk RJ, Podack E, Dalmasso AP, Jennette JC. Localization of S protein and its relationship to the membrane attack complex of complement in renal tissue. Am J Pathol 1987; 127:182–190.

141. Bhakdi S, Cäflein R, Halstensen TS, Hugo F, Preissner KT, Mollnes TE. Complement S-protein (vitronectin) is associated with cytolytic membrane bound C5b-9 complexes. Clin Exp Immunol 1988; 74:459–464.

142. Choi NH, Mazda T, Tomita M. A serum protein SP-40,40 modulates the formation of the membrane attack complex of complement on erythrocytes. Mol Immunol 1989; 26:835–840.

143. French LE, Tschopp J, Schifferli JA. Clusterin in renal tissue: Preferential localization with the terminal complement complex and immunoglobulin deposits in the glomeruli. Clin Exp Immunol 1992; 88:389–393.

144. Saunders JR, Aminian A, McRae JL, O'Farrell KA, Adam WR, Murphy BF. Clusterin depletion enhances immune glomerular injury in the isolated perfused kidney. Kidney Int 1994; 45:817–827.

145. Rollins SA, Zhao J, Ninomiya H, Sims PJ. Inhibition of homologous complement by CD59 is mediated by a species-selective recognition conferred through binding to C8 within C5b-8 or C9 within C5b-9. J Immunol 1991; 146:2345–2351.

146. Schönermark S, Rauterberg EW, Shin ML, Löke S, Roelcke D, Hänsch GM. Homologous species restriction in lysis of human erythrocytes: a membrane derived protein with C8-binding capacity functions as an inhibitor. J Immunol 1986; 136:1772–1776.

147. Schieren G, Schönermark M, Barunger M, Hänsch GM. Expression of the complement regulator factor C8 binding protein on human glomerular cells protects them from complement-mediated killing. Exp Nephrol 1994; 2:299–305.

148. Nose M, Katoh M, Okada N, Kyogoku M, Okada H. Tissue distribution of HRF20, a novel factor preventing the membrane attack of homologous complement, and its predominant expression on endothelial cells in vivo. Immunology 1990; 70:145–149.

149. Tanai H, Matsuo S, Fukatsu A, Nishikawa K, Sakamoto N, Yoshika K, Okada N, Okada H. Localization of 20-kD homologous restriction factor (HRF20) in diseased human glomeruli. An immunofluorescent study. Clin Exp Immunol 1991; 84:256–262.

27

Role of Complement in Diseased and Normal Human Skin

KIM B. YANCEY

National Cancer Institute, National Institutes of Health,
Bethesda, Maryland

THOMAS J. LAWLEY

School of Medicine, Emory University, Atlanta, Georgia

Complement has long been regarded as a potent effector mechanism in a variety of inflammatory and autoimmune skin diseases. Foremost examples of these disorders are leukocytoclastic vasculitis and autoimmune blistering diseases, respectively. Recent investigations have substantiated the traditional view that lesion formation in some of these disorders is complement-dependent, but other experimental studies have indicated that complement is not required for the development of other immune skin diseases. This chapter will provide an overview of the role that complement plays in skin diseases and review recent experimental studies regarding the association of C3dg with normal human epidermal basement membrane as well as the production of complement components by human keratinocytes.

I. PATHOPHYSIOLOGY OF BLISTERING DISEASES

There are two major categories of blistering skin diseases: one represents a group of autoimmune disorders, the other a group of genetic diseases. Patients with the former have acquired diseases that are characterized by the presence of specific autoantibodies directed against antigens in normal human skin. In fact, autoantibodies from such patients have been used to isolate these antigens and demonstrate that they represent important structural proteins in human skin. Recent studies have shown that the genes encoding some of these structural proteins are mutated in patients with various genetic skin diseases. Hence, acquired or inherited abnormalities in key structural proteins in human skin result in disease phenotypes characterized by blister formation.

A number of recent studies have shown that autoantibodies play a key effector role in the pathophysiology of many blistering diseases. However, the basis for the initiation of autoimmune responses in these patients is largely unknown. Studies aimed at characterizing T-cell antigen receptors and major histocompatibility complex haplotypes in these patients will, it is hoped, elucidate further the pathophysiological basis of these autoimmune diseases. The role of complement in the pathophysiology of autoimmune diseases characterized by inflammation and blister formation in human skin is detailed below.

A. Pemphigus

Pemphigus is a blistering disease characterized by a loss of cohesion between epidermal cells (a process termed acantholysis) that results in intraepithelial blisters (1,2). The most common form of the disease, pemphigus vulgaris (PV), is characterized by blister formation just above the basal layer of keratinocytes in epidermis and mucous membranes. In another form of the disease, pemphigus foliaceus (PF), blisters form in a more superficial layer of the epidermis (specifically, usually just beneath the stratum corneun) and rarely involve mucous membranes.

In PV, clinical lesions typically consist of flaccid blisters situated on either normal-appearing or erythematous skin. Such lesions rupture easily, enlarge peripherally, and may result in denuded areas that cover large portions of the body surface. Lesions in patients with PV often involve the oral mucosa as well as the skin of the scalp, face, neck, axillae, trunk, and groin. Some patients experience pruritus in association with early or healing lesions as well as severe skin pain if lesions become extensive. Because the plane of blister formation is above the lamina densa (i.e., the basement membrane proper), lesions heal without scarring unless complicated by secondary infection or mechanically induced dermal wounds. Prior to the availability of systemic glucocorticoids and other immunosuppressives, PV was almost always uniformly fatal within several years of onset. Even today, PV is a life-threatening disease.

As mentioned earlier, light microscopic studies of lesional skin from patients with PV demonstrate acantholytic, intraepithelial blisters in which basal keratinocytes remain attached to epidermal basement membrane. Focal collections of eosinophils and other leukocytes in blister cavities and the adjacent epidermis and dermis are also commonly observed. Direct immunofluorescence microscopic examination of lesional or normal skin from patients with PV reveals deposits of IgG on the surface of keratinocytes (3,4). These deposits are derived from circulating IgG autoantibodies directed against a 130 kD cadherin molecule (i.e., desmoglein 3, the PV antigen) that is localized to desmosomes of keratinocytes in epidermis and mucous membranes (5). (Fig. 1). These IgG autoantibodies are specific to patients with PV and have been shown to be pathogenic (i.e., directly responsible for blister formation in this disease; see below).

In addition to deposits of IgG, keratinocytes in lesional skin from patients with PV demonstrate cell surface deposits of C3 and other classical pathway components (6). Additional evidence of complement activation at sites of PV lesions was derived from studies indicating that complement levels in blister fluid are markedly decreased in comparison to those in serum (7). Moreover, although PV IgG autoantibodies were originally thought to be unable to fix complement, a number of more recent studies indicate that some, if not most, of these autoantibodies fix complement in vitro (8–10). These findings are in concert with the presence of component complements on the surface of keratinocytes in these patients' lesional skin.

The immunopathological features of PV suggest that IgG autoantibodies in these patients play a central role in disease pathophysiology. Clinical features of PV that support this hypothesis include the following: autoantibody titers generally correlate with disease activity in patients with PV; neonatal PV can develop as a consequence of transplacental passage of maternal IgG autoantibodies (moreover, this rare form of pemphigus resolves

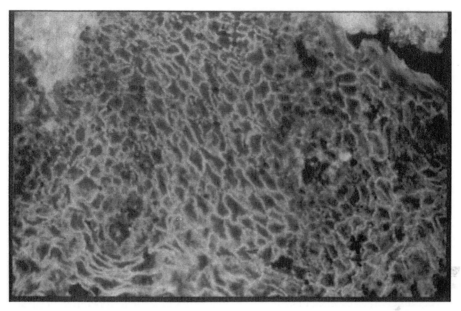

Figure 1 On indirect immunofluorescence microscopic examination IgG autoantibodies from patients with pemphigus vulgaris bind the surface of epithelial cells in cryosections of monkey esophagus. Deposits of IgG are found in the same pattern in these patients' epidermis; deposits of C3 are similarly found in their lesional skin.

as maternal IgG is catabolized); and removal of PV IgG autoantibodies by plasmapheresis (coupled with the use of immunosuppressives) is an effective therapy for the disease. Despite this strong evidence, many years of research were required to demonstrate convincingly that PV IgG can directly cause acantholysis and blister formation. In the mid-1970s, Michel and co-workers developed a skin organ culture model in which acantholysis occurred in the presence of PV serum or PV IgG, but not in the presence of normal human serum or IgG (11,12). Several groups have shown that PV IgG-induced acantholysis in such organ culture models is not dependent upon complement activation. Instead, it is thought that PV IgG binds to the surface of keratinocytes and elicits the production of urokinase-type plasminogen activator that alters the surface of these cells and results in acantholysis.

Additional, and very convincing, evidence regarding the pathogenic activity of PV IgG has been developed in passive transfer animal models of this disease (13,14). In these models, passive transfer of PV IgG to newborn BALB/c mice has been shown to produce intraepidermal acantholytic blisters. Lesions develop in a dose-dependent manner and show deposits of IgG on the surface of lesional keratinocytes. Passive transfer studies conducted in complement-depleted newborn mice or with Fab fragments of PV IgG have confirmed that blisters develop in vivo independently of complement activation (15). Nonetheless, these studies have suggested that complement may enhance the pathogenic activity of PV IgG in vivo since less blister formation was observed in complement-depleted mice challenged with PV IgG. Moreover, in vitro studies have shown that PV IgG plus complement can induce the assembly of the membrane attack complex on the surface of human keratinocytes and produce altered plasma membrane integrity and cytotoxicity (10,16–18). Hence, while complement is not thought to play a central role in the initiation of lesion formation in PV, it is considered a relevant amplifying mechanism of disease. Experimental studies have shown that these same conclusions hold true for PF as well, although the autoantigen in this form of pemphigus is a 160 kD desmosomal cadherin called desmoglein 1. Finally, it should be noted that the dominant subclass of IgG autoantibodies in patients with PV and PF is IgG_4, a subclass that activates the classical pathway of complement very poorly, if at all (19,20).

B. Bullous Pemphigoid

Bullous pemphigoid (BP) is a chronic, subepidermal blistering disease usually seen in the elderly (1,2). Lesions typically consist of tense blisters situated on either normal-appearing or erythematous skin. Lesions are usually distributed over the flexor surfaces, axillae, groin, and lower abdomen; oral mucosal lesions are present in 10–40% of patients. Pruritus may be nonexistent or severe. Nontraumatized lesions heal without scarring. Biopsies of lesional skin demonstrate subepidermal blisters and accumulations of eosinophils and neutrophils along the epidermal basement membrane. The extent of the leukocytic infiltrate is greatest in patients with lesions based on inflamed skin.

Direct immunofluorescence microscopic examination of normal-appearing, perilesional skin from patients with BP shows linear deposits of IgG and/or C3 in epidermal basement membrane (21,22). Moreover, sera from approximately 85% of these patients contain circulating IgG autoantibodies that bind normal epidermal basement membrane as shown by indirect immunofluorescence microscopic examination (22,23). (Fig. 2). Autoantibodies in patients with BP recognize 230 and (in approximately 50% of patients with BP) 180 kD hemidesmosome-associated proteins in basal keratinocytes (24–28). These proteins are also termed bullous pemphigoid antigens 1 and 2 (BPAG1 and BPAG2), respectively. IgG autoantibodies against these antigens are thought to deposit in situ, form immune complexes, activate complement, and yield cleavage fragments (e.g., C3a, C5a) that subsequently produce dermal mast cell degranulation, granulocyte-rich leukocytic infiltrates, tissue damage, and blister formation (29–32).

A variety of immunopathological findings support the hypothesis that complement plays a key role in the pathophysiology of BP. As mentioned previously, C3 (and other classical and terminal pathway components) are found in association with IgG in these patients' epidermal basement membranes. At times, C3 is present even in the absence of detectable IgG; relatedly, BP IgG is typically capable of fixing complement in vitro. As in PV, complement levels in BP blister fluid are markedly decreased, whereas serum complement levels in these patients are normal (7). Additional experimental evidence supporting a key role for complement in the pathophysiology of BP was gathered by Gammon and co-workers in a series of studies employing an in vitro skin chamber leukocyte attachment assay (33–36). In this system, skin sections are incubated with aliquots of serum from a patient with BP (i.e., a source of BP IgG autoantibodies), washed, and then exposed to fresh normal human serum (i.e., a source of complement) and purified peripheral blood neutrophils. In this assay, neutrophils selectively adhere to epidermal basement membrane and provide a relative estimate of in vitro complement activation. These investigators obtained similar results using sections of skin from patients with BP that had preexisting deposits of IgG (34). Notable was that heat inactivation of the complement source or the use of C5-deficient serum has been shown to block the specific attachment of leukocytes in this experimental model (36). Hence, complement activation

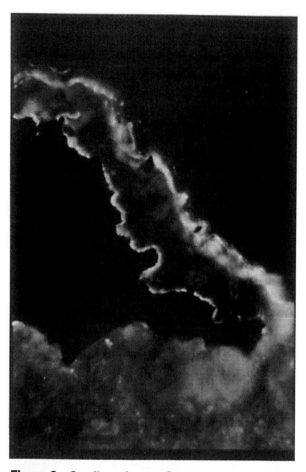

Figure 2 On direct immunofluorescence microscopic examination IgG autoantibodies from patients with bullous pemphigoid bind the epidermal side of 1 M NaCl split normal human skin, a sensitive test substrate that allows the regional localization of autoantigens in epidermal basement membrane. Autoantibodies from patients with this subepidermal blistering disease recognize bullous pemphigoid antigens 1 and 2, which are hemidesmosome-associated proteins in basal keratinocytes.

by immune complexes in the skin of patients with BP is thought to generate sufficient amounts of C5a to promote neutrophil adhesion to epidermal basement membrane (and presumably neutrophil degranulation that eventuates in tissue damage and blister formation).

While the results of the previously described in vitro studies offer very compelling evidence in support of an active role for complement in mediating lesion formation in BP, recent in vivo passive transfer experiments have been even more conclusive. These studies have been conducted in newborn BALB/c mice and have employed purified rabbit IgG directed against the murine homologue of the immunodominant epitope of BPAG2 (i.e., the region of the molecule bound by autoantibodies from most patients with BP) (37,38). In this passive transfer model of disease, rabbit anti-BPAG2 IgG induces subepidermal blisters in newborn BALB/c mice in a dose-dependent manner. Moreover, on histological and immunopathological examination these lesions resemble those seen in patients with BP (37). Passive transfer of pathogenic rabbit IgG to mice deficient in complement fails to induce lesion formation in vivo and further supports the hypotheses that this effector mechanism plays a central role in the pathogenesis of this human autoimmune disease (38).

C. Pemphigoid Gestationis

Pemphigoid gestationis (PG) is a rare, nonviral, subepidermal blistering disease of pregnancy and the puerperium (39). Lesions are usually distributed over the abdomen, trunk, and extremities; mucous membrane lesions are rare. Skin lesions in these patients consist of erythematous urticarial papules and plaques, vesiculopapules, and/or frank bullae. Lesions are almost always very pruritic. Severe exacerbations of PG frequently occur after delivery. In addition, this disease tends to recur in subsequent pregnancies, often beginning earlier during such gestations. Brief flares of disease may occur with resumption of menses or upon exposure to oral contraceptives. Occasionally, infants of affected mothers demonstrate transient skin lesions.

Biopsies of early lesional skin show teardrop-shaped subepidermal vesicles forming in dermal papillae in association with an eosinophil-rich leukocytic infiltrate. Differentiation of PG from other subepidermal bullous diseases by light microscopic examination is often difficult. However, direct immunofluorescence microscopic evaluation of normal perilesional skin from PG patients reveals the immunopathological hallmark of this disorder: linear deposits of C3 in the epidermal basement membrane. These deposits develop as a consequence of complement activation produced by low-titer IgG antibasement membrane autoantibodies (40,41) (Fig. 3). Recent studies have shown that the majority of PG sera contain autoantibodies that recognize BPAG2, the same 180 kD hemidesmosome-associated protein targeted by autoantibodies in patients with BP (27). The recognition of this common autoantigen by patients with BP and PG is thought to account for their resemblance clinically, histologically, immunopathologically, and pathophysiologically.

The development of specific IgG autoantibodies against BPAG2 is held to be key to the pathogenesis of PG. Once formed, such autoantibodies are thought to deposit in epidermal BM, activate complement, and generate inflammatory mediators (e.g., C4a, C3a, and C5a) that induce leukocytic infiltrates and dermal mast cell degranulation. Studies in animal models suggest that this inflammatory reaction accounts for the histological and immunopathological alterations in these patients' skin (37,38). Transplacental passage of maternal autoantibodies is held responsible for the development of similar lesions in affected neonates. Infant catabolism of maternal IgG results in resolution of their skin lesions. It is not currently known why anti-BPAG2 autoantibodies develop in patients with PG (39). Their formation is in some unknown way linked to pregnancy, parturition, and exposure to oral contraceptives, all of which are characterized by dynamic hormonal alterations. BPAG2 is present in human amnion and may represent an important antigen source for the initiation of the immunological processes that result in this autoimmune disease. Moreover, rare cases of PG have been reported in association with choriocarcinoma and hydatiform mole, which are selected neoplasms that may provide similar antigenic and hormonal stimuli. Unlike patients with BP, patients with PG show a high incidence of HLA-B8 and HLA-DR3 as well as the paired haplotype HLA-DR3, -DR4. However, these haplotypes are neither requisite nor sufficient for the development of this disease.

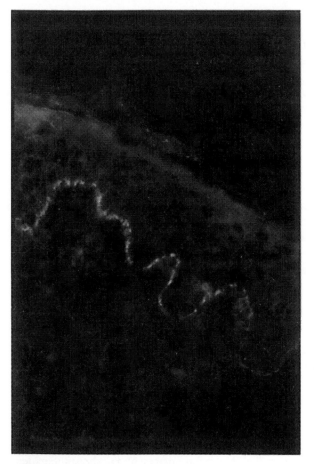

Figure 3 In complement fixation indirect immunofluorescence microscopic study of serum from a patient with pemphigoid gestationis, a cryosection of normal human skin was exposed to the patient's serum, washed, treated with an aliquot of fresh normal human serum as a complement source, washed, and then stained with a fluorescein isothiocyanate-conjugated antibody against human C3. The continuous deposits of C3 signify the presence of complement-fixing, IgG antiepidermal basement membrane autoantibodies in the patient's serum.

Additional study is required to elucidate the exact pathophysiological basis of this autoimmune subepidermal blistering disease.

D. Cicatricial Pemphigoid

Cicatricial pemphigoid (CP) is an autoimmune subepithelial blistering disease characterized by erosive lesions of mucous membranes and skin that result in scarring of at least some sites of involvement (42). Common sites of involvement include the oral mucosa and conjunctiva; other sites that may be affected include the nasopharyngeal, laryngeal, esophageal, genital, and rectal mucosae. Skin lesions (present in approximately one-third of patients) tend to predominate on the scalp, face, and upper trunk. Serious complications may arise in patients with CP as a consequence of ocular, oral, laryngeal, or esophageal lesions. Biopsies of lesional tissue generally demonstrate subepithelial bullae and a mono-nuclear-predominant leukocytic infiltrate; granulocytes may be seen in biopsies of early lesions. Direct immunofluorescence microscopic examination of perilesional tissue typically demonstrates deposits of IgG, IgA, and/or C3 in these patients' epithelial basement membranes. Although CP was once thought to be a single nosological entity, it is now largely regarded as a disease phenotype that may develop as a consequence of an autoimmune reaction against a variety of different molecules in epithelial basement membranes (43,44). Patients with CP have been shown to have anti-basement membrane autoantibodies directed against BPAG2, laminin 5, or other antigens yet to be completely defined (45,46). Lesions in these various forms of CP are thought to be autoantibody mediated. It has recently been demonstrated that passive transfer of antilaminin 5 IgG to newborn BALB/c mice produces subepithelial blisters that are clinically, histologically, and immunopathologically similar to those seen in patients with CP (47). Antilaminin 5 IgG induces identical lesions in C5- or mast cell-deficient mice. These experimental findings indicate that antibodies directed against laminin 5 are directly pathogenic in vivo (and that this protein plays an important role in epithelial adhesion to basement membranes).

E. Epidermolysis Bullosa Acquisita

Epidermal bullosa acquisita (EBA) is an acquired, polymorphic, subepidermal blistering disease (48,49). Since lesions generally occur in sites prone to minor trauma (e.g., dorsum of the hands, elbows, knees, etc.), EBA is regarded as a mechanobullous disease. Patients with classical or noninflammatory EBA have blisters on noninflamed skin, atrophic scars, milia, nail dystrophy, and oral lesions. Other patients with EBA have widespread inflammatory lesions that resemble severe BP. Some patients present with an inflammatory blistering disease that subsequently evolves into the classical noninflammatory form of this disorder.

The histological appearance of lesional skin from patients with EBA varies depending on the type or character of lesion being studied. Noninflammatory bullae show subepidermal blisters with a sparse leukocytic infiltrate and resemble those in patients with porphyria cutanea tarda. Inflammatory vesiculobullous lesions consist of a subepidermal blister and neutrophil-rich leukocytic infiltrates in the superficial dermis. Patients with EBA have continuous deposits of IgG (and frequently C3 as well as other complement components) in a linear pattern within the epidermal basement membrane zone (48,49). On ultrastructural examination these immunoreactants are found in the sublamina densa region in association with anchoring fibrils. Approximately 25–50% of patients with EBA have circulating IgG antibasement membrane autoantibodies directed against type VII collagen, which makes up anchoring fibrils (50,51) (Fig. 4).

Immunopathological evidence again strongly suggests that EBA is an autoimmune disease in which lesions form as a consequence of immune complex-mediated complement activation. In fact, Gammon et al. have shown that immune complexes formed in vivo in the skin of patients with EBA or in vitro by treating normal human skin with these patients' anti-type VII collagen autoantibodies are capable of mediating complement activation, leukocyte attachment, and dermal–epidermal separation (35). However, these findings do not explain lesion formation in noninflammatory forms of the disease in which there are also immunoreactants present in situ. Moreover, passive transfer of these patients' autoantibodies to mice results in epidermal basement membrane deposits of human IgG, murine C3, and the murine membrane attack complex along with edema and granulocyte-

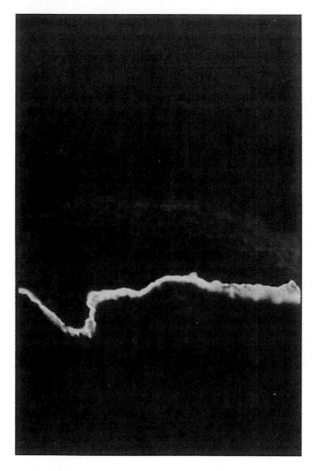

Figure 4 On indirect immunofluorescence microscopic examination IgG autoantibodies from patients with epidermolysis bullosa acquisita bind the dermal side of 1 M NaCl split normal human skin. This reactivity signifies the binding of anti-type VII collagen autoantibodies to anchoring fibrils located in the sublamina densa region of epidermal basement membrane.

rich infiltrates in the papillary dermis, but no frank subepidermal blisters (52). Hence, factors other than complement-binding autoantibodies are currently thought to be important in the development of lesions in patients with EBA.

F. Dermatitis Herpetiformis

Dermatitis herpetiformis (DH) is an intensely pruritic, chronic papulovesicular skin disease characterized by lesions symmetrically distributed over extensor surfaces (i.e., elbows, knees, buttocks, back, scalp, and posterior neck) (53,54). Because pruritus is prominent, patients may present with excoriations and crusted papules but no observable primary lesions. Almost all patients with DH have an associated, usually subclinical, gluten-sensitive enteropathy, and more than 90% express the HLA-B8/DRw3 and HLA-DQw2 haplotypes. DH is typically chronic.

Light microscopic studies of early lesional skin from patients with DH reveal neutrophil-rich infiltrates, edema, and microvesicles within dermal papillae. Older lesions may demonstrate nonspecific features of a subepidermal bulla or an excoriated papule. Direct immunofluorescence microscopic examination of normal-appearing perilesional skin demonstrates granular deposits of IgA in the papillary dermis and along the epidermal basement membrane (53,55,56) (Fig. 5). IgA deposits in the skin are unaffected by control of disease with medication. However, these immunoreactants may diminish in intensity or disappear in patients maintained for long periods on a strict gluten-free diet and hence attest to the central role that dietary gluten plays in the pathogenesis of this disease (57).

Unlike patients with pemphigus, BP, PG, or EBA, patients with DH do not have circulating antiepidermal basement membrane autoantibodies that account for the presence of immunoreactants in their skin. Nonetheless, the regular finding of IgA deposits in the skin of virtually all DH patients has led to the hypothesis that the bound IgA somehow leads to lesion formation. In brief, the bound IgA is thought to activate complement,

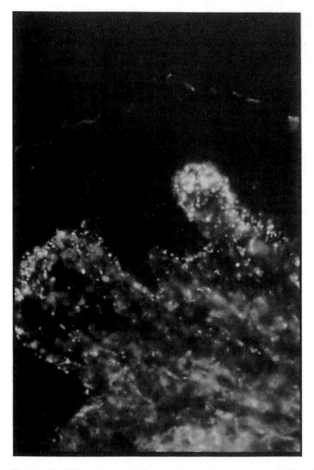

Figure 5   Direct immunofluorescence microscopic examination of normal-appearing perilesional skin from a patient with dermatitis herpetiformis shows granular deposits of IgA in dermal papillae and along the epidermal basement membrane. Deposits of C3 are typically found in the same distribution in these patients' skin.

generate chemotactic factors, and result in an influx of neutrophils that produce subepidermal blisters. In support of this, various investigators have demonstrated that C3 is often found in these patients' skin at the same location as IgA (58–60). The sequence by which IgA activates complement is thought to be through the alternative pathway (since the classical pathway is not activated by IgA). When early complement components are detected in the skin of patients with DH, they are those of the alternative complement pathway (e.g., properdin and factor B) (60). Often the fifth component of complement is also detected in areas of skin corresponding to the IgA deposits. To determine the origin of IgA found in the skin of patients with DH, the IgA subclass composition has been studied. Although IgA_2 is present to a greater extent than IgA_1 in secretory IgA (suggesting its importance in the mucosal immune response), IgA_1 is the only subclass that has been identified in the skin of DH patients (61).

The lack of IgA antibasement membrane autoantibodies in patients with DH has led to the hypothesis that these patients may have circulating immune complexes that originate in the gut, enter the circulation, eventually deposit in skin, and initiate lesions. Although IgG-containing circulating immune complexes have been detected in only a small percentage of patients with DH, several groups have identified IgA-containing circulating immune complexes in 25–30% of random serum samples from these patients (62,63). However, the presence or level of IgA-containing circulating immune complexes does not correlate with disease activity, mode of medical treatment, or dietary gluten challenge (54,64). Moreover, IgA-containing circulating immune complexes are present in an even higher percentage of patients with celiac disease despite the fact such patients lack deposits of IgA in their skin.

At present, it is thought that intestinal gluten sensitivity plays a central role in the pathophysiology of DH, since strict adherence to a gluten-free diet typically reduces these patients' medication requirements and, in some cases, provides complete control of skin lesions. Moreover, the resolution of cutaneous IgA deposits in patients maintained for long periods on strict gluten-free diets (as well as their reappearance following gluten challenge) further substantiates the important role of gluten in this disease (57). It is currently not known whether the IgA produced in the gut has specificity for unique skin proteins, or whether the IgA binds to antigens in the gut and somehow forms immune complexes which then circulate and deposit in skin. To date, attempts to identify gluten or gliadin peptides in the skin of patients with DH have been unsuccessful. However, in spite of these negative findings, the possibility that the IgA in the skin of patients with DH is directed against gluten proteins or cross-reacting antigens remains compelling because of the gastrointestinal and immunological findings related to the gluten-sensitive enteropathy in these patients. Once IgA deposits in skin, the cascade of events that mediate tissue injury seems straightforward. However, the finding of IgA and complement in all skin sites (i.e., nonlesional as well as lesional skin from patients with DH), makes it necessary to postulate that additional factors are required to explain the initiation of lesions. With these additional factors, IgA is thought to activate the alternative pathway of complement, produce anaphylatoxins, and generate neutrophil-rich infiltrates and tissue damage (i.e., microabscesses and microvesicles in the papillary dermis) characteristic of early DH lesions.

II. PATHOPHYSIOLOGY OF PORPHYRIA

The role of complement activation in porphyria has been investigated in depth. Lim and Gigli have conducted a series of studies indicating that the photosensitivity associated with porphyria cutanea tarda, porphyria variegata, and erythropoietic photoporphyria is mediated, at least in part, by complement activation (65,66). In this regard, it is known that many patients with these diseases have deposits of C3 in superficial dermal blood vessel walls as well as their epidermal basement membrane. Studies have shown that the addition of porphyrins to guinea pig sera in vitro, followed by irradiation with 405 nm light, causes dose-dependent decreases in CH_{50} and titers of C3 and C5. Further studies have documented the activation of complement and the generation of complement cleavage fragments with neutrophil chemotactic activity (i.e., C5a) in the sera of patients with erythropoietic protoporphyria or porphyria cutanea tarda following its exposure to ultraviolet light. Blister fluid from patients with erythropoietic protoporphyria has also been shown to contain C5a.

III. PATHOPHYSIOLOGY OF CUTANEOUS LEUKOCYTOCLASTIC VASCULITIS

The pathophysiology of cutaneous leukocytoclastic vasculitis is intimately related to activation of the complement system. Moreover, the Arthus reaction, an experimental animal model of leukocytoclastic vasculitis, requires an intact complement system. In this reaction, an animal is immunized with a protein antigen and then skin tested with the same antigen approximately 2 weeks later (67). An Arthus reaction develops rapidly and reaches peak intensity within 4–10 h following intradermal administration of antigen. On clinical examination one sees erythema and swelling followed by purpura and in some instances cutaneous necrosis. On histopathological examination there is massive infiltration of polymorphonuclear neutrophils, leukocytoclasis, and endothelial cell damage. Immuno-fluorescence studies have shown that antigen–antibody complexes and complement components deposit in vessel walls of lesional skin of Arthus reactions.

In humans, evidence for the importance of complement activation in the pathophysiology of necrotizing vasculitis emerged from studies that showed depressed levels of C1q, C4, C2, and C3 in serum samples from some of these patients (68). Moreover, deposits of C3 could be demonstrated in affected vessel walls. It is now known that activation of complement, generation of the chemotactic agent C5a, and assembly of the membrane attack complex are important events that eventuate in local tissue damage in this disorder. A key element in the pathogenesis of this series of events is the subendothelial deposition of circulating immune complexes in postcapillary venules (69). If these immune complexes contain IgM or IgG, they activate complement via the classical pathway. If they contain mainly IgA (e.g., Henoch-Schönlein purpura), complement may be activated via the alternative pathway. In either case, C3a and C5a are generated. These anaphylatoxins are thought to diffuse out of blood vessels, cause degranulation of perivascular dermal mast cells, and result in the release of histamine and other proinflammatory mediators (29,30). Histamine causes further dilatation of postcapillary venules and endothelial cell separation that in turn results in further deposition of circulating immune complexes. In addition, C5a is an extremely potent chemoattractant that causes the rapid influx of neutrophils and monocytes. C5a also causes these leukocytes to aggregate, release lysosomal enzymes, and undergo an oxidative burst (31). These proteolytic enzymes, reactive oxygen metabolites, and the associated ischemia cause the tissue damage seen in sites of leukocytoclastic vasculitis. Studies have also implicated assembly of the membrane attack complex on the surface of endothelial cells in areas of tissue damage in patients with leukocytoclastic vasculitis. Boom et al. have demonstrated deposits of poly(C9) on endothelial cell membranes in skin biopsies from patients with vasculitis using both direct immunofluorescence and immunoelectron microscopic examination (70). These investigators believe that assembly of the membrane attack complex on endothelial cells begins with insertion of the C5b67 complex into the membrane phospholipid bilayer, with endothelial cells acting as innocent bystanders. The subsequent binding of C8 and C9 is thought to result in lysis of these cells.

IV. STUDIES OF C3dg IN NORMAL HUMAN EPIDERMAL BASEMENT MEMBRANE

Early immunopathological studies that examined normal human skin for the presence of immunoreactants found that polyclonal antibodies directed against human C3d bound epidermal basement membrane in a continuous pattern (71,72) (Fig. 6). Original impressions of this finding were that it signified passive incorporation of C3 cleavage fragments or the presence of a cross-reacting C3 analog at this site in normal human skin. More recent studies have confirmed these original findings, demonstrated that this reactivity signifies the presence of C3dg rather than a cross-reacting C3 analog, and suggested that this C3 cleavage fragment is constitutively incorporated rather than passively adsorbed within normal human epidermal basement membrane (73). These studies have employed various antibodies reactive with C3dg or closely related C3 cleavage fragments. Because antibodies against intact C3 usually do not recognize C3dg or C3d, it is apparent why the former do not bind normal human epidermal basement membrane in routine immunopathological studies. Polyclonal or monoclonal antibodies directed against human C3d as well as clone 9, a monoclonal antibody specific for C3g, bind normal adult epidermal basement membrane in a continuous, somewhat stitched pattern (73–75). Antihuman C3dg reactivity has also been observed in the basement membranes of cutaneous appendages such as hair follicles, although not in dermal microvascular basement membranes. Moreover, 3F3, a murine monoclonal antibody raised against a homogenate of human placental basement membranes and shown to be reactive with the C3d portion of human C3, binds normal epidermal basement membrane in the same continuous pattern (73,76). Again, 3F3 reactivity is present within epidermal adnexal basement membranes yet absent in dermal microvascular basement membranes.

The localization of C3dg in human epidermal basement membrane has been defined in several different ways (73). Antihuman C3dg antibodies have been shown to bind the base of the cleavage plane in 1 M NaCl split adult and neonatal human skin. Moreover, by immunoelectron microscopic examination these reagents have been shown to bind the base of the lamina densa and the sublamina densa region of normal human epidermal basement membrane. In these studies, the most intense staining has been noted in the sublamina densa region where association of anti-human C3dg reactivity with anchoring fibrils has been suggested. Although the exact relationship between C3dg and anchoring fibrils is currently unknown, the precise ultrastructural localization of anti-human C3dg reactivity within epidermal basement membrane suggests that this finding is not secondary to random reactivity of the C3 thioester.

As mentioned above, it was not originally known if anti-human C3dg reactivity within normal human epidermal basement membrane signified the presence of a specific C3 cleavage fragment or a cross-reacting C3 analog at this site in skin. To examine this

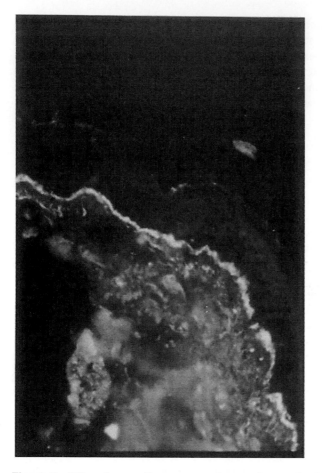

Figure 6   Direct immunofluorescence microscopic examination of a cryosection of normal skin stained with a monoclonal antibody specific for C3d shows a continuous, stitched pattern of staining in epidermal basement membrane. No staining is evident in dermal microvascular basement membranes. Antibodies directed against C3 or C3c show no evidence of reactivity to sequential sections of this same substrate.

question, a variety of specificity studies have been performed. Direct immunofluorescence microscopic studies utilizing antibodies directed against C3, C3c, C5, IgG, IgA, or IgM show no reactivity to normal human skin. These findings confirm that C3dg is the relevant C3 epitope present in normal epidermal basement membrane and demonstrate that deposits of immune complexes or subclinical inflammatory reactions are not responsible for the observed anti-human C3dg reactivity. Other specificity studies have shown that the binding of monoclonal or polyclonal antihuman C3dg antibodies to normal human epidermal basement membrane is blocked by pretreating these agents with aged human serum containing large amounts of C3dg or purified human C3d. In contrast, preadsorption of antitype IV collagen antibodies with aged serum does not interfere with this reagent's staining of epidermal or microvascular basement membranes. Moreover, treatment of skin sections with antibodies directed against C3, C3c, C5, laminin 1, types IV or VII collagen, or antibodies against BPAGs or KF-1 antigen does not block antihuman C3dg reactivity with normal human epidermal basement membrane.

Specificity studies regarding the presence of C3dg in normal human epidermal basement membrane have been confirmed and extended by examination of skin from a patient with congenital C3 deficiency. Congenital C3 deficiency is a rare condition typically characterized by an autosomal recessive pattern of inheritance, recurrent bacterial infections, and selected autoimmune syndromes. In studies of multiple samples of skin from a patient with documented C3 deficiency, monoclonal as well as polyclonal antibodies directed against human C3dg have found no evidence of epidermal BM reactivity. Multiple experiments, including those utilizing high concentrations of polyclonal antihuman C3dg antibodies (i.e., 10 mg/ml), have found no evidence of C3dg within this patient's epidermal basement membrane. Control direct immunofluorescence microscopic studies found that this patient's skin contains normal relative amounts and distribution of laminin 1, types IV and VII collagen, BPAGs, and other relevant adhesion proteins. In vitro treatment of this patient's skin sections with normal serum, aged serum containing C3dg, purified hemolytically active C3, or zymosan–serum reaction mixtures did not result in incorporation of C3dg (or other C3 fragments) within epidermal or dermal microvascular basement membranes. These studies indicate that C3/C3dg binding sites are not accessible within assembled matrices of the epidermal basement membrane and raise the possibility that C3 or C3 fragments are not passively adsorbed at this site in normal human skin.

While the exact manner of C3dg incorporation within epidermal basement membrane is unknown, recent studies have shown that hydrolyzed C3 and C3d bind laminin 1 in vitro. This finding has been proposed to account for the presence of C3d within human renal and placental basement membranes. However, an alternative hypothesis seems likely for epidermal basement membrane because laminin and C3dg display different regional and ultrastructural distributions in normal human skin. Specifically, C3dg is absent from laminin 1-rich microvascular basement membranes and does not reside within the laminin 1-rich lamina dense of epidermal basement membrane. Studies of papulonodular basal cell carcinoma tumor-nest basement membranes have further supported the idea that C3dg binding to epidermal basement membrane is not mediated via attachment to laminin 1 (77). Specifically, these tumor-nest basement membranes are rich in laminin 1 yet entirely devoid or very deficient in C3dg. Types IV and VII collagen are also present in these tumor-nest basement membranes and thus are also unlikely sites for passive incorporation of C3dg. Additional studies are needed to define the basis of C3dg incorporation and binding within epidermal basement membrane. These studies are important to define the biological significance of this protein within normal epithelial basement membranes as well as to gain insights regarding the binding of C3 (or C3 containing immune complexes) in diseased epithelial basement membranes.

V. KERATINOCYTE COMPLEMENT COMPONENT BIOSYNTHESIS

A. C3

C3, the third component of complement, plays a pivotal role in both the classical and alternative activation pathways. C3 is the most abundant serum complement component (normal concentration 1.2–1.5 mg/ml) and is a 195 kD glycoprotein that consists of disulfide-linked 120- and 75-kD alpha and beta chains, respectively. The C3 alpha chain contains an internal thioester bond that becomes exposed and highly reactive upon cleavage of the native molecule. Although the liver is considered the main source of circulating C3, various cell types have been shown to produce this complement protein and are considered potentially important local sources.

Biosynthetic radiolabeling studies have demonstrated that A-431 cells, a human epidermoid carcinoma cell line, and human keratinocytes synthesize and secrete C3 as two disulfide-linked polypeptide chains of 120 and 75-kD (78). Moreover, epithelial cell-derived C3 comigrates in sodium dodecyl sulfate polyacrylamide gel electrophoresis (SDS-PAGE) with that produced by HepG2 cells, a human hepatoma cell line previously used to elucidate complement component biosynthesis. Pulse-chase studies in A-431 cells demonstrate that epithelial cell-derived C3 is produced as a 195kD precursor molecule, pro-C3, which is processed intracellularly by limited proteolysis into 120- and 75-kD C3 alpha and beta chains. Comparative studies demonstrate that A-431 cell-derived C3 is synthesized, processed, and secreted in parallel but in lower quantity than that produced by HepG2 cells. Treatment of biosynthetically labeled A-431 cell culture supernatants with normal human serum and zymosan produces C3 alpha chain cleavage and specific C3 fragments not present in control culture supernatants treated with heat-inactivated human serum and zymosan. Northern blot analysis of total cellular RNA extracted from A-431 cells, human keratinocytes, and HepG2 cells reveals qualitative identify of a 5.1-kb C3 mRNA species in these three cell types. Thus, epithelial cells should be viewed as a potential source of the acute phase reactant, biologically active C3, as well as a local source of important C3 cleavage fragments such as C3a, a vasoactive anaphylatoxin; C3b, an opsonin; C3d,k, a known inhibitor of T-cell proliferation; and C3d, a B-lymphocyte growth factor. Constitutive and/or induced C3 synthesis in epithelial cells may play an important role in local inflammatory and immunological reactions. Moreover, epithelial cell C3 synthesis may have direct relevance to the presence of C3dg within selected normal primate epithelial basement membranes, including epidermal basement membrane (79).

B. Factor B

Factor B, the major zymogen protease of the alternative complement pathway, is a single-chain beta-globulin with a normal serum concentration of 225 μg/ml. Factor B is encoded by a single gene positioned on the short arm of human chromosome six in the region of the class III major histocompatibility complex. During complement activation, factor B binds C3b and is subsequently cleaved by factor D into two fragments, Ba and Bb. The smaller Ba fragment is released into the circulation whereas the carboxy terminal segment, Bb, remains associated with C3b. Together the latter function as the catalytically active component of the complex proteases of the alternative complement pathway (i.e., C3bBb, the alternative pathway C3 convertase; and C3bBbC3b, the alternative pathway C5 convertase). Factor Bb serine protease activity within these complexes serves as a major complement activation and amplification mechanism.

Biosynthetic radiolabeling studies have demonstrated that human keratinocytes and A-431 cells synthesize and secrete factor B as a monomeric 105-kD protein (80). Epithelial cell-derived factor B comigrates in SDS-PAGE with that produced by HepG2 cells. Comparative pulse-chase studies in A-431 and HepG2 cells have shown that this alternative pathway complement component is produced as comigrating 100-kD intracellular proteins that are processed in both cell types to 105 kD extracellular factor B. Treatment of biosynthetically radiolabeled A-431 cell culture media with cobra venom factor and factor

D for 60 min at 37°C produces the specific factor B cleavage products Ba and Bb. These fragments are not identifiable in control culture media subjected to similar treatment in the absence of alternative pathway activators. Northern blot analysis of total cellular RNA from human keratinocytes, A-431 cells, and HepG2 cells has revealed qualitative identity of a 2.8-kb factor B mRNA species in these three cell types. The relative level of factor B mRNA expression in these cells parallels their level of factor B protein synthesis (i.e., HepG2 cells>A-431 cells>human keratinocytes).

Epithelial cells should be viewed as a potential source of Bb, a novel serine protease and immunomodulatory complement cleavage fragment. Although Bb is generally recognized for its ability to cleave C3 and C5 when bound to C3b, the free form of this protease retains some ability to cleave these "downstream" complement components and may in fact activate other zymogens such as plasminogen activator. It is also likely that other proteases such as trypsin, plasmin, and kallikrein can convert epithelial cell-derived factor B to Bb, just as these enzymes can activate circulating factor B in humans. The potential immunomodulatory activities of Bb in human skin are also of significance. In addition to its traditional role as a migration inhibition factor that induces monocyte and macrophage spreading, Bb also stimulates monocyte cytotoxicity, lymphocyte blastogenesis, and clonal expansion of antigen-activated B cells.

In summary, epithelial cells are potential sources of both C3 and factor B. The fact that human keratinocytes make both of these complement components reduces cellular and plasma requirements for pathway activation in skin. Moreover, various proteases present in human skin may also cleave these components to produce cleavage fragments with a broad array of biological activities. It is of great biological interest that epithelial cells in direct contact with the environment and various bacterial, viral, parasitic, and chemical offenders have retained the ability to produce protective complement pathway components that are more highly conserved than specific antibody itself.

REFERENCES

1. Stanley JR. Pemphigus and pemphigoid as paradigms of organ-specific, autoantibody-mediated diseases. J Clin Invest 1989; 83:1443–1448.
2. Stanley JR. Cell adhesion molecules as targets of autoantibodies in pemphigus and pemphigoid, bullous diseases due to defective epidermal cell adhesion. Adv Immunol 1992; 53:291–325.
3. Beutner EH, Jordon RE. Demonstration of skin antibodies in sera of pemphigus vulgaris patients by indirect immunofluorescent staining. Proc Soc Exp Biol Med 1964; 117:505–510.
4. Chorzelski TP, von Weiss JR, Lever WF. Clinical significance of autoantibodies in pemphigus. Arch Dermatol 1966; 93:570–576.
5. Amagai M, Klaus-Kovtun V, Stanley JR. Autoantibodies against a novel epithelial cadherin in pemphigus vulgaris, a disease of cell adhesion. Cell 1991; 67:869–877.
6. van Joost T, Cormane RH, Podman, KW. Direct immunofluorescent study of the skin on occurrence of complement in pemphigus. Br J Dermatol 1972; 87:466–474.
7. Jordon RE, Day NK, Luckasan JR, Good RA. Complement activation in pemphigus vulgaris blister fluid. Clin Exp Immunol 1973; 15:53–63.
8. Nishikawa T, Kurihara S, Harada T, Sugawara M, Hatano H. Capability of complement fixation of pemphigus antibodies in vitro. Arch Dermatol Res 1977; 260:1–6.
9. Hashimoto T, Sugiura M, Kurikara S, Nishikawa T. In vitro complement activation by intercellular antibodies. J Invest Dermatol 1982; 78:316–318.
10. Kawana S, Janson M, Jordon RE. Complement fixation by pemphigus antibody. I. In vitro fixation to organ and tissue culture skin. J Invest Dermatol 1984; 82:506–510.

11. Michel B, Ko C. An organ culture model for the study of pemphigus acantholysis. Br J Dermatol 1977; 96:295–302.

12. Scaletta LJ, Occhino JC, MacCallum DK, Lillie JH. Isolation and immunologic identification of basement membrane zone antigens from human skin. Lab Invest 1978; 39:1–9.

13. Anhalt GJ, Labib RS, Voorhees JJ, Beals TF, Diaz LA. Induction of pemphigus in neonatal mice by passive transfer of IgG from patients with the disease. N Engl J Med 1982; 306:1189–1196.

14. Roscoe JT, Diaz L, Sampaio SA, Castro RM, Labib RS, Takahaski Y, Patel H, Anhalt GJ. Brazilian pemphigus foliaceus autoantibodies are pathogenic to BALB/c mice by passive transfer. J Invest Dermatol 1985; 85:538–541.

15. Anhalt GJ, Till GO, Diaz LA, Labib RS, Patel HP, Eaglstein NE. Defining the role of complement in experimental pemphigus vulgaris in mice. J Immunol 1986; 137:2835–2840.

16. Kawana S, Geoghegan WD, Jordon RE. Complement fixation by pemphigus antibody. II. Complement enhanced detachment of epidermal cells. Clin Exp Immunol 1985; 61:517–525.

17. Kawana S, Geoghegan WE, Jordon RE. Complement activation by pemphigus antibody. III. Altered epidermal cell membrane integrity mediated by pemphigus antibody and complement. J Invest Dermatol 1986; 86:29–33.

18. Xia P, Jordon RE, Geoghegan WD. Complement fixation by pemphigus antibody. V. Assembly of the membrane attack complex on cultured human keratinocytes. J Clin Invest 1988; 82:1939–1947.

19. Jones CC, Hamilton RG, Jordon RE. Subclass distribution of human IgG autoantibodies in pemphigus. J Clin Immunol 1988; 8:43–49.

20. Rock B, Martins CR, Theofilopoulos AN, Balderas RS, Anhalt GJ, Labib RS, Futamura S, Rivitti EA, Diaz LA. The pathogenic effect of IgG4 autoantibodies in endemic pemphigus foliaceus (fogo selvagem). N Engl J Med 1989; 320:1463–1469.

21. Jordon RE, Beutner EH, Witebsky E, Blumenthal G, Hale WH, Lever WF. Basement zone antibodies in bullous pemphigoid. JAMA 1967; 200:751–756.

22. Jordon RE, Bushkell LL. The complement system in pemphigus, bullous pemphigoid, and herpes gestationis. Int J Dermatol 1979; 18:271–281.

23. Sams WM, Schur P. Studies of the antibodies in pemphigoid and pemphigus. J Lab Clin Med 1973; 82:249–255.

24. Stanley JR, Hawley-Nelson P, Yuspa SH, Shevach EF, Katz SI. Characterization of bullous pemphigoid antigen: a unique basement membrane protein of stratified squamous epithelia. Cell 1981; 24:897–903.

25. Stanley JR, Tanaka T, Mueller S, Klaus-Kovtun V, Roop D. Isolation of complementary DNA for bullous pemphigoid antigen by use of patients' autoantibodies. J Clin Invest 1988; 82:1864–1870.

26. Mueller S, Klaus-Kovtun V, Stanley JR. A 230-kD basic protein is the major bullous pemphigoid antigen. J Invest Dermatol 1989; 92:33–38.

27. Morrison LH, Labib RS, Zone JJ, Diaz LA, Anhalt GJ. Herpes gestationis autoantibodies recognize a 180-kD human epidermal antigen. J Clin Invest 1988; 81:2023–2026.

28. Diaz LA, Ratrie H, Saunders WS, Futamura S, Squiquera HL, Anhalt GJ, Giudice GJ. Isolation of a human epidermal cDNA corresponding to the 180-kD autoantigen recognized by bullous pemphigoid and herpes gestationis sera. J Clin Invest 1990; 86:1088–1094.

29. Hugli TE. Human anaphylatoxin (C3a) from the third component of complement: primary structure. J Biol Chem 1975; 250:8293–8301.

30. Yancey KS, Hammer CH, Harvath L, Renfer L, Frank MM, Lawley TJ. Studies of human C5a as a mediator of inflammation in normal human skin. J Clin Invest 1985; 75:486–495.

31. Yancey KB. Biological properties of human C5a: selected in vitro and in vivo studies. Clin Exp Immunol 1988; 71:207–210.

32. Swerlick RA, Yancey KB, Lawley TJ. A direct in vivo comparison of the inflammatory properties of human C5a and C5a des Arg in human skin. J Immunol 1988; 140:2376–2381.

33. Gammon WR, Lewis DM, Carlo JR, Sams WM, Wheeler CE. Pemphigoid antibody mediated attachment of peripheral blood leukocytes at the dermal-epidermal junction of human skin. J Invest Dermatol 1980; 75:334–339.

34. Gammon WR, Merritt CC, Lewis DM, Sams WM, Carlo JR, Wheeler CE. An in vitro model of immune complex-mediated basement membrane zone separation caused by pemphigoid antibodies, leukocytes, and complement. J Invest Dermatol 1982; 78:285–290.

35. Gammon WR, Inman AO, Wheeler CE. Differences in complement-dependent chemotactic activity generated by bullous pemphigoid and epidermolysis bullosa acquisita immune complexes: demonstration by leukocyte attachment and organ culture methods. J Invest Dermatol 1984; 83:57–61.

36. Gammon WR, Yancey KB, Mangum K, Hendrix JD, Hammer CH. Generation of C5-dependent bioactivity by tissue-bound anti-BMZ autoantibodies. J Invest Dermatol 1989; 93:195–200.

37. Liu Z, Diaz LA, Troy JL, Taylor AF, Emery DJ, Fairley JA, Giudice GJ. A passive transfer model of the organ-specific autoimmune disease, bullous pemphigoid, using antibodies generated against the hemidesmosomal antigen, BP180. J Clin Invest 1993; 92:2480–2488.

38. Liu Z, Giudice GJ, Swartz SJ, Fairley JA, Till GO, Troy JL, Diaz LA. The role of complement in experimental bullous pemphigoid. J Clin Invest 1995; 95:1539–1544.

39. Yancey KB. Herpes gestationis. Dermatol Clin 1990; 8:727–735.

40. Katz SI, Hertz KC, Yaoita H. Herpes gestationis: immunopathology and characterization of the HG factor. J Clin Invest 1976; 57:1434–1438.

41. Jordon RE, Heine KG, Tappeiner G, Bushkell LL, Provost TT. The immunopathology of herpes gestationis: immunofluorescence studies and characterization of the "HG factor." J Clin Invest 1976; 57:1426–1433.

42. Fine JD, Neises GR, Katz SI. Immunofluorescence and immunoelectron microscopic studies in cicatricial pemphigoid. J Invest Dermatol 1984; 82:39.

43. Domloge-Hultsch N, Gammon WR, Briggaman RA, Gil SG, Carter WG, Yancey KB. Epiligrin, the major human keratinocyte integrin ligand, is a target in both an acquired autoimmune and an inherited subepidermal blistering skin disease. J Clin Invest 1992; 90:1628–1633.

44. Domloge-Hultsch N, Anhalt GJ, Gammon WR, Lazarova Z, Briggaman RA, Welch M, Jabs DA, Huff C, Yancey KB. Anti-epiligrin cicatricial pemphigoid: a subepithelial bullous disorder. Arch Dermatol 1994; 130:1521–1529.

45. Kirtschig G, Marinkovich MP, Burgeson RA, Yancey KB. Anti-basement membrane autoantibodies in patients with anti-epiligrin cicatricial pemphigoid bind the α subunit of laminin 5. J Invest Dermatol 1995; 105:543–548.

46. Balding SD, Prost C, Diaz LA, Bernard P, Bedane C, Aberdam D, Giudice GJ. Cicatricial pemphigoid autoantibodies react with multiple sites on the BP180 extracellular domain. J Invest Dermatol 1996; 106:141–146.

47. Lazarova Z, Yee C, Darling T, Briggaman RA, Yancey KB. Passive transfer of anti-laminin 5 antibodies induces subepidermal blisters in neonatal mice. J Clin Invest 1996; 98:1509–1518.

48. Gammon WR, Briggaman RA, Wheeler CE. Epidermolysis bullosa acquisita presenting as an inflammatory disease. J Am Acad Dermatol 1982; 7:382–387.

49. Briggaman RA, Gammon WR, Woodley DT. Epidermolysis bullosa acquisita of the immuno-pathological type (dermolytic pemphigoid). J Invest Dermatol 1985; 85:79–84.

50. Woodley DT, Briggaman RA, O'Keefe EJ, Inman AO, Queen LL, Gammon WR. Identification of the skin basement membrane autoantigen in epidermolysis bullosa acquisita. N Engl J Med 1984; 310:1007–1013.

51. Woodley DT, Burgeson RE, Lunstrum GP, Bruckner-Tuderman L, Reese MJ, Briggaman RA. The epidermolysis bullosa acquisita antigen is the globular carboxyl terminus of type VII collagen. J Clin Invest 1988; 81:683–687.

52. Borradori L, Caldwell JB, Briggaman RA, Burr CE, Gammon WR, James WD, Yancey KB. Passive transfer of autoantibodies from a patient with mutilating epidermolysis bullosa acquisita induces specific alterations in the skin of neonatal mice. Arch Dermatol 1995; 131:590–595.

53. Katz SI, Hall RP, Lawley TJ, Strober W. Dermatitis herpetiformis: the skin and the gut. Ann Intern Med 1980; 93:857–874.

54. Hall RP. The pathogenesis of dermatitis herpetiformis: recent advances. J Am Acad Dermatol 1987; 16:1129–1144.

55. Cormane RH. Immunofluorescent studies of the skin in lupus erythematosus and other diseases. Pathol Eur 1967; 2:170–180.

56. van der Meer J. Granular deposits of immunoglobulins in the skin of patients with dermatitis herpetiformis. Br J Dermatol 1969; 81:49–53.

57. Leonard J, Haffenden G, Tucker W, Fry L. Gluten challenge in dermatitis herpetiformis. N Engl J Med 1983; 308:816–819.

58. Seah PP, Mazaheri MR, Fry L. Complement in the skin of patients with dermatitis herpetiformis. Br J Dermatol 1973; 89:12.

59. Provost TT, Tomasi TB. Evidence for the activation of complement via the alternate pathway in skin diseases. II. Dermatitis herpetiformis. Clin Immunol Immunopathol 1974; 3:178–186.

60. Katz SI, Hertz KC, Crawford PS, Grazze L, Frank MM, Lawley TJ. Effects of sulfones on complement deposition in dermatitis herpetiformis and on complement-mediated guinea pig reactions. J Invest Dermatol 1976; 67:688–690.

61. Hall RP, Lawley TJ. Characterization of circulating and cutaneous IgA immune complexes in patients with dermatitis herpetiformis. J Immunol 1985; 135:1760–1765.

62. Zone JJ, Provost TT. IgA immune complexes in dermatitis herpetiformis. J Invest Dermatol 1980; 75:152–155.

63. Hall RP, Lawley TJ, Heck JA, Katz SI. IgA containing immune complexes in dermatitis herpetiformis, Henoch-Schonlein purpura, systemic lupus erythematosus, and other diseases. Clin Exp Immunol 1980; 40:431–437.

64. Yancey KB, Cason JC, Hall RP, Lawley TJ. Dietary gluten challenge does not influence the levels of circulating immune complexes in patients with dermatitis herpetiformis. J Invest Dermatol 1983; 80:468–471.

65. Lim HW, Gigli I. Role of complement in porphyrin-induced phototoxicity. J Invest Dermatol 1981; 76:4–9.

66. Lim HW, Poh-Fitzpatrick MB, Gigli I. Activation of the complement system in patients with porphyrias after irradiation in vivo. J Clin Invest 1984; 74:1961–1965.

67. Yancey KB, Lawley TJ. Circulating immune complexes: their immunochemistry, biology, and detection in selected dermatologic and systemic diseases. J Am Acad Dermatol 1984; 10:711–731.

68. McDuffie FC, Sams WM, Maldonado JE, Andreini PH, Conn DL, Sarnayoa EA. Hypocomplementemia with cutaneous vasculitis and arthritis. Possible immune complex syndrome. Mayo Clin Proc 1973; 48:340–348.

69. Braverman IM, Yen A. Demonstration of immune complexes in spontaneous and histamine-induced lesions and in normal skin of patients with leukocytoclastic vasculitis. J Invest Dermatol 1975; 64:105–112.

70. Boom BW, Out-Luiting CJ, Baldwin WM, Daha MR, Vermeer BJ. The role of membrane attack complex (MAC) in the manifestation of leukocytoclastic vasculitis of the skin. J Invest Dermatol 1986; 87:130.

71. Baart de la Faille-Kuyper EH, van der Meer JG, Baart de la Faille HB. An immunohistochemical study of the skin of healthy individuals. Acta Dermatol Venereol (Stockh) 1974; 54:271–274.

72. Nieboer C. Immunofluorescence patterns in sun-exposed and non-exposed skin of healthy individuals. Acta Dermatol Venereol (Stockh) 1980; 61:471–479.

73. Basset-Seguin N, Dersookian M, Cehrs K, Yancey KB. C3d,g is present in normal human epidermal basement membrane. J Immunol 1988; 141:1273–1280.

74. Lachmann PJ, Oldroyd RG, Milstein C, Wright BW. Three rat monoclonal antibodies to human C3. Immunol 1980; 41:503–515.

75. Lachmann PJ, Pangburn MK, Oldroyd RG. Breakdown of C3 after complement activation. Identification of a new fragment, C3g, using monoclonal antibodies. J Exp Med 1982; 156:205–216.

76. Leivo I, Engvall E. C3d fragment of complement interacts with laminin and binds to basement membranes of glomerulus and trophoblast. J Cell Biol 1986; 103:1091–1100.

77. Basset-Seguin N, Uhle P, Emanuel D, Henry P, Yancey KB. Defective expression of basement membrane-associated C3d,g in papulonodular basal cell carcinomas. J Invest Dermatol 1989; 92:734–738.

78. Basset-Seguin N, Caughman SW, Yancey KB. A-431 cells and human keratinocytes synthesize and secrete the third component of complement. J Invest Dermatol 1990; 95:621–625.

79. Basset-Seguin N, Porneuf M, Dereure O, Mils V, Tesnieres A, Yancey KB, Guilhou JJ. C3d,g deposits in inflammatory skin diseases: use of psoriatic skin as a model of cutaneous inflammation. J Invest Dermatol 1993; 101:827–831.

80. Yancey KB, Overholser O, Domloge-Hultsch N, Li LJ, Caughman SW, Bisalbutra P. Human keratinocytes and A-431 cells synthesize and secrete factor B, the major zymogen protease of the alternative complement pathway. J Invest Dermatol 1992; 98:379–383.

28

Complement and Neuromuscular Diseases

MILAN BASTA and MARINOS C. DALAKAS

National Institute of Neurological Disorders and Stroke,
National Institutes of Health, Bethesda, Maryland

I. INTRODUCTION

Neuromuscular diseases (NMD) encompass a heterogeneous group of disorders affecting peripheral nerve, neuromuscular junction, and muscle, causing muscle weakness and long-term disability. Their cause is often unclear, but degenerative, hereditary, infectious, metabolic, toxic, or autoimmune factors have been implicated. In a subset of NMD reviewed in this chapter (Table 1), disturbed immunoregulation leading to production of autoantibodies and activation of the complement system appears to play a major role in the disease pathogenesis. In many of these disorders, however, the autoimmunity is complex, because cellular factors such as macrophages, activated T cells, or cytokines appear to be intertwined with the effector arm of the humoral immune response.

Even in those neuromuscular diseases in which autoantibodies have been demonstrated, the role of complement, for the most part, has been incompletely studied. For example, in Guillain-Barré syndrome and other demyelinating polyneuropathies, various IgG and IgM autoantibodies against peripheral nerve glycolipids or glycoproteins, such as gangliosides GM1, GQ1b, GD1a, GD2, GD3, or GT1b, have been described. Information on the requirement of complement in the disease process is emerging only recently. In myasthenia gravis, the prototypic autoimmune disease, the pathogenic antibodies against the acetylcholine receptors (AChR) fix complement, but when antigenic modulation via cross-linking takes place, complement may not be required. In other diseases such as dermatomyositis or peripheral nerve vasculitis, the antibodies that fix complement remain uncharacterized. In a recently defined X-linked, nonimmune vacuolated myopathy, the complement system appears to be activated through the alternative pathway, leading to MAC deposits on muscle fibers. In spite of these uncertainties, the complement and its activation products seem to play key roles in certain autoimmune neuromuscular disorders. In this chapter we will review the evidence of complement involvement in these diseases, discuss its significance in their pathogenesis, and address how certain immunomodulating therapies suppress disease activity by intercepting complement fragments.

II. PERIPHERAL NEUROPATHIES

A. Guillain-Barré Syndrome

Guillain-Barré syndrome (GBS) is an acute inflammatory demyelinating polyneuropathy, characterized by symmetrical weakness of skeletal muscles, areflexia, and mild sensory

Table 1 Autoimmune Neuromuscular Disorders in Which
Complement Plays a Role in Pathogenesis

Peripheral neuropathies
   Guillain-Barré syndrome
   Chronic inflammatory demyelinating polyneuropathy
   Vasculitic polyneuropathy
   IgM monoclonal gammopathy with polyneuropathy
   Diabetic polyneuropathy

Diseases of the neuromuscular junction
   Myasthenia gravis
   Lambert-Eaton myasthenic syndrome

Myopathies
   Dermatomyositis
   Necrotizing myopathy with pipestem capillaries
   X-linked vacuolated myopathy

changes that develop over a period of 1–4 weeks (1). Although the cause of the disease
has not been clarified, there is strong evidence supporting an immune pathogenesis.
Segmental loss of myelin in large-diameter peripheral nerve fibers, preceded by a functional
blockade in the roots and peripheral nerve, probably by circulating factors against antigens
at the nodes of Ranvier, appears to be the major cause for the acute lesion that leads to
severe muscle weakness (2). Complement, fixed by the putative antibodies directed against
myelin or nodal antigens, may play a role in the pathogenesis of GBS, as suggested by
the following observations.

1. In-Situ Complement Deposition

Demonstration of deposition of complement components on myelinated fibers in peripheral
nerve biopsies represents direct evidence for complement involvement in the disease
process. Deposits of complement components C3 and C4 along with IgM have been
demonstrated by immunofluorescence on the myelin sheaths in the peripheral nerve biopsies from four of eight patients with GBS (3). The C3 deposition had a linear pattern and
in two biopsies colocalized with IgM and IgG. Furthermore, destruction of peripheral
nerve myelin appeared to correlate with positive staining for immune complexes. In
another immunofluorescent study, C3d and IgM were also found on the surface of the
myelin sheaths in two patients with GBS. In this study, C1q colocalized with C3d and
IgM, indicating activation of the classical pathway (4).

      A recent study combining light and electron microscopic evaluations has shown
C3d and C5b-9 deposition along the outer surface of the Schwann cells, but not on the
myelin sheath, in the nerve roots from three patients with GBS who died 3–9 days after
disease onset (5). The C3d-positive fibers, when subjected to ultrastructural analysis by
electron microscopic examination, contained vesicular changes in the outermost myelin
lamellae (Fig. 1). These changes were noted only within the first 3 days of disease, but
not 9 days later, suggesting that the putative antibodies bind to epitopes on the outer
surface of the Schwann cell very early in the disease process and activate complement,
leading to formation of the membranolytic attack complex that initiates the vesicular

degeneration of the myelin. Membrane-bound C5b-9 attack complex has been also detected by immunohistochemical evaluation using rabbit IgG antibody against C9 neoantigen in the autopsied peripheral nerves of another patient with GBS. The staining for C9 neoantigen was focal, segmental, and colocalized with IgM (6).

2. Complement Levels in the Serum and Cerebrospinal Fluid

Further support for the role of complement in the pathogenesis of GBS is based on finding increased concentration of various complement fragments in the sera and cerebrospinal fluid (CSF) of these patients.

The presence of terminal complement membrane complex in its inactive form (SC5b-9) was examined and quantitated by enzyme-linked immunosorbent assay (ELISA) in the serum of patients with GBS (6). The SC5b-9 was detected in the acute phase of GBS, but not after recovery or in healthy individuals. The levels of SC5b-9 correlated with the rapid fall of complement-fixing antiperipheral nerve myelin antibody and disappeared as the patients improved, suggesting that components of peripheral nerve myelin may be target of antibody-mediated complement attack. SC5b-9 complexes were likewise detected in the cerebrospinal fluid of 13 of 14 patients with GBS with a mean concentration of 3.08 µg/ml, compared to a mean concentration of 0.8 µg/ml found in only 3 of 11 disease controls (7).

Plasma and CSF levels of activated complement fragments C3a and C5a have been measured by radioimmunoassay (RIA) in patients with GBS and other noninflammatory neurological diseases (8). C3a and C5a levels are significantly higher in the CSF of patients with GBS than in disease controls; the plasma values, however, are not different between the two groups. Whether intrathecal increase of these potent mediators of inflammation represents a marker of a complement-mediated demyelinating process restricted to the root-segments enbathed into the CSF can only be speculated.

Our own study employed an in-vitro quantitative complement uptake assay to examine the role of complement in GBS and other autoimmune neuromuscular diseases (Table 2). The assay measures the capacity of a patient's serum, as a source of complement, to provide activated complement fragments generated during the incubation with corpuscular immune complexes for deposition onto the surface of sensitized cells (9). The C3 uptake, expressed as geometric and log means of triplicate counts per minute measurements, was high in patients with GBS compared to disease controls or healthy individuals. Among other diseases studied, only two complement-mediated autoimmune neuromuscular disorders, dermatomyositis and myasthenia gravis, had high C3 uptake, as discussed later. The results support the role of complement not only in the pathogenesis of GBS but also in the other two aforementioned neuromuscular diseases with complement activation, as described later. Continued activation of complement and accelerated production of fragments either fixed by the immunoglobulin onto the target tissue (myelinated nerve fibers) or present in the circulation in an inactive form appears to take place in these conditions. We have proposed that the complement uptake assay is not only a useful in vitro system for detection of complement activation but may also be used for monitoring disease activity and response to therapies.

3. Passive Transfer Studies

The in vivo effect of complement and complement-activating antibodies in the pathogenesis of GBS has been also assessed by passive transfer studies.

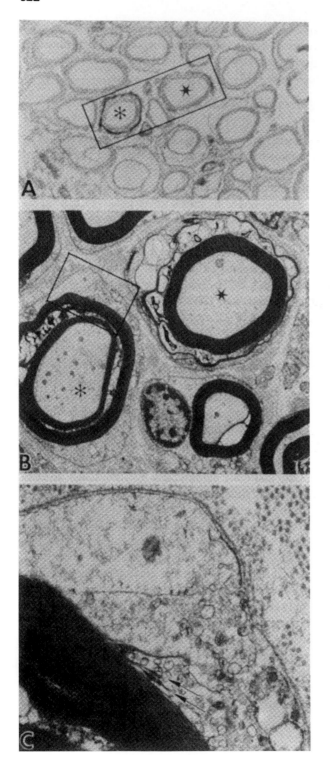

Table 2 Geometric Means and Mean Logs of Baseline C3 Uptake Values in Dermatomyositis (DM), Gullian-Barré Syndrome (GB), Myasthenia Gravis (MG), Inclusion Body of Myositis (IBM), and Normal Controls

Condition	N	Geometric mean[a]	Mean log
Active DM	10	11,640	4.066
Guillain-Barré	9	11,590	4.064
Myasthenia gravis	10	10,570	4.024
IBM	10	3,491	3.543
Normals	10	3,459	3.539

[a] All values calculated and expressed based on triplicate measurements of C3 uptake in counts per minute.

When injected into rat sciatic nerves, the GBS serum caused a complement-dependent demyelination and conduction block (10). The serum of patients with GBS in which antigalactocerbroside antibody activity was found likewise caused conduction blockade when injected with human complement into the rat sciatic nerve (11). However, other studies failed to demonstrate demyelination or conduction block following intraneural injections of GBS sera, despite the addition of complement (12). Sera from rabbits immunized with various gangliosides also produced demyelination after intraneural injections in a complement-dependent fashion (13). In spite of these inconsistent findings, it appears that sera from some patients with GBS contain high titers of antibodies that have a demyelinating effect in vivo in the presence of complement.

4. In Vitro Studies

Complement-dependent demyelination was also demonstrated in vitro, using cultured myelinated cells or myelin-producing Schwann cells and oligodendrocytes.

Myelin swelling is observed in spinal ganglionic cultures following prolonged exposure to GBS sera. The effect was noticed with five of the six tested GBS sera but only when fresh guinea pig serum as a source of complement was added (14). In addition, sera from patients with GBS had a demyelinatig effect on cultured dorsal root ganglionic cells in the presence of human complement (15). The sera from patients with GBS containing high titers of antiperipheral nerve myelin antibodies also causes demyelination, which is dependent on the generation of C5b-9 complexes on disassociated dorsal root ganglionic cultures (16). In this system, the C7-depleted human serum loses its demyelinating activity.

Figure 1 Thick and thin sections in this 8-day case demonstrate the deposition of C3d on the outer surface of two fibers (A). The boxed region in A is seen at higher power in B. The more darkly staining fiber (identified by the asterisk in A) is seen at increasing magnification in (B) and (C). At the ultrastructural level (B), the myelin disruption in fibers with C3d immunostaining consisted of vesicular changes in the sheath (B) and was usually seen in the outermost myelin lamellae (as illustrated by the fiber with the asterisk in B). The boxed region in B is seen at higher power in C. (C) The outermost lamellae of this fiber were amputated (arrows), with moderate numbers of vesicles present nearby. (A: $\times$ 1,500; B: $\times$ 4,830; C: $\times$ 27,600 before 20% reduction.) (Reprinted with permission by Lippincott-Raven Publishers, New York, NY.)

5. Comments

In general, none of the aforementioned studies provides by itself sufficient and overwhelming evidence for the role of complement in the pathogenesis of GBS. However, taken together, the data from the various in vivo and in vitro studies strongly suggest that complement is activated in the disease and participates in the acute demyelinating process. A number of issues, however, remain still unresolved. First, the in-situ deposition of complement has not always been accompanied by immunoglobulin deposits and vice versa. Second, time-course studies have been limited or fragmented. This is of fundamental concern, since the presence of complement or immune complex deposits is closely related to the age of the lesion. Furthermore, activation fragments are seen early in the disease and their correlation with disease activity or severity needs to be determined serially in a systematic fashion in a large number of samples. Finally, it remains to be determined if complement activation is uniformly present in all forms of GBS (axonal, demyelinating, pure motor) or is specific for certain disease subsets. Careful studies on the role of some specific autoantibodies associated with certain forms of GBS (i.e., anti-GQ1b in the Miller-Fisher variant) and their dependence on complement fixation to produce immune injury need to be performed.

B. Chronic Inflammatory Demyelinating Polyneuropathy

Chronic inflammatory demyelinating polyneuropathy (CIDP) represents a disease similar to GBS except for its course. In contrast to GBS, where the maximum deficit is reached within 4 weeks, the muscular weakness in CIDP progresses over a period of 2 or more months (17). CIDP is a chronic disease with remissions, exacerbations, or spontaneous improvement. Patients experience proximal and distal weakness, loss of tendon reflexes, and distal sensory loss.

The immunological events underlying CIDP have not been elucidated, and the role of complement in the initiation of the disease has not been examined as well as in patients with GBS. There is, however, evidence that the complement might be activated during the disease process.

Deposits of C3 on the outer portion of the myelin sheath have been demonstrated by immunofluorescence in two of four patients with CIDP. In one patient, immunoglobulin deposits were also found on the same site (4). Granular patterns of IgM and C3, by immunofluorescence staining, have also been demonstrated on the myelinated fibers and the intraneural blood vessels of sural nerve biopsies from patients with CIDP (18). It has been proposed that intravascular IgM-complement complexes might damage the blood–nerve barrier and facilitate passage of the putative anti-myelin-specific antibodies. Antiganglioside and anti-peripheral-nerve myelin antibodies recognizing neutral glycolipids are seen in the sera of some patients with CIDP (19), but their complement-fixing properties have not been studied. Most CIDP sera injected intraneurally in experimental animals failed to cause demyelination and passive transfer of patients' sera to monkeys had only mild effects (19). Because demyelination occurs in the presence of macrophages invading intact myelin, it is believed that in CIDP an antibody-dependent cellular cytotoxic reaction mediated by activated complement fragments attract macrophages to the myelin sheaths, which in turn become activated through CR1 receptor ligation (20). This hypothesis needs to be tested in various in vivo and in vitro systems.

As with other immunopathological parameters, the evidence for the role of humoral immunity and complement in the pathogenesis of CIDP is either indirect and circumstantial or limited and based on extrapolation and parallel with its acute counterpart, GBS. More data need to be gathered before complement can be established as a pathogenetic factor in CIDP.

C. Peripheral Vasculitic Neuropathy

Peripheral neuropathy is a common manifestation of vasculitides due to involvement of the intraneural blood vessels. Vasculitides make up a heterogeneous group of disorders characterized by inflammation and necrosis of blood vessels resulting in infarctions and ischemia of affected tissues. The precise incidence of vasculitic neuropathy is not known. Neuropathy occurs in all principal groups of vasculitides, which, according to modified Scott's classification (21), include systemic necrotizing vasculitis (polyarteritis nodosa, Wegener's granulomatosis, allergic angiitis, Churg Strauss syndrome, vasculitis with connective tissue diseases); hypersensitivity vasculitis (Henoch-Schonlein purpura, serum sickness, drug-induced vasculitis, vasculitis associated with infections, vasculitis associated with malignancy, vasculitis with connective tissue disease); giant cell arteritis (temporal arteritis, Takayasu's arteritis); isolated peripheral nerve vasculitis.

The classical clinical presentation of peripheral nerve vasculitis is a multiple mononeuropathy with acute onset of motor and sensory deficits, restricted to the distribution of individual peripheral nerves. Burning (dysesthetic) pain along the distribution of involved nerves is found in 70–80% of the patients. Nonspecific constitutional symptoms such as fever, malaise, and weight loss are common, according to the underlying disease. In isolated peripheral nerve vasculitis, the disease is entirely limited to the peripheral nerves.

Although most, if not all, vasculitides are thought to have an autoimmune pathogenesis, the mechanisms that trigger the putative autoimmune reaction, the targeted antigens, and the sequence of events that result in immune injury remain unknown. Passive deposition of immune complexes is probably the best understood mechanism of vasculitis. In this scenario, antibodies recognize and interact with circulating antigen(s) to form complexes that are deposited in the blood vessel walls and activate complement. This is followed by the release of complement-inflammatory mediators and chemotactic factors, leading to recruitment of lymphoid cells that infiltrate the vessel wall. In addition, formation of MAC causes direct injury to the blood vessels. Apart from the blood vessel injury related to deposits of circulating immune complexes, antibodies directed against endothelial cell antigens (AECA) may be involved in organ-specific vasculitis.

Studies of sural nerve biopsies from patients with peripheral nerve vasculitis demonstrate vascular and perivascular mononuclear cell infiltrates and necrosis of epineurial blood vessel wall (Fig. 2). Immunoglobulin and complement deposits are found, although the frequency may vary from 0 to 100% according to the site and the chronicity of the lesion (22). The pattern of immunostaining for immune complexes is often granular, similar to the pattern observed in other immune complex diseases (23). Immunoglobulin and C3 reactivity may be seen in biopsies of vasculitic as well as nonvasculitic and normal nerves, whereas epineurial C5 and C9 deposits are seen only in vasclutic lesions, suggesting that their presence may be more specific (24). In one study of 22 biopsy specimens from patients with systemic vasculitis and patients with isolated vasculitis of peripheral nerve, deposits of IgG, IgM, C3, and MAC were seen in all 14 biopsies from patients with systemic vasculitis, while deposits of MAC alone were seen in 4 of 8 nerve biopsies from

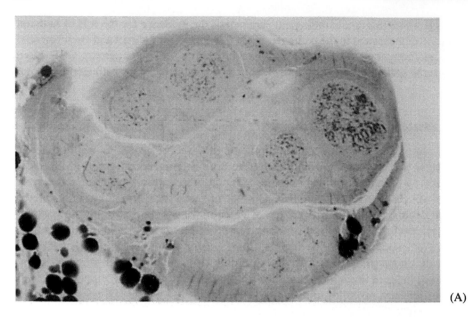

(A)

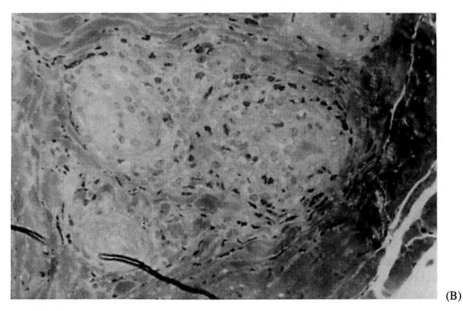

(B)

Figure 2 Cross-section of a nerve biopsy from a patient with vasculitis shows infarct within the nerve with obliteration of entire fascicles (A). High-power view of the endoneurial vessel from the same patient shows obliteration of the blood vessel wall with endothelial necrosis and inflammatory cells (B). These areas contain complement deposits (not shown).

patients with isolated peripheral nerve vasculitis (25). We have also demonstrated the presence of MAC on endoneurial blood vessels in patients with vasculitis (Dalakas et al., unpublished observation).

Although it appears that immune complexes play a prominent role in the pathogenesis of vasculitic neuropathies, it is argued that immunoglobulin and complement deposits may not be the only mechanism. Because these deposits are always associated with cellular infiltrates, they may represent secondary phenomena. It is possible that different mechanisms may be operative in different times during the evolution of the disease process. Epineurial vascular complexes composed of immunoglobulin and C3 can be also seen in nonvasculitic as well as normal nerves, suggesting that their presence may be related to a nonspecific disturbance of the blood–nerve barrier. In contrast, the presence of MAC, alone or concurrently with immunoglobulins, appears to be a more specific complement marker for the etiopathogenesis of vasculitis. The heterogeneity of peripheral vasculitic neuropathies, as a group, poses additional problems in exploring their pathogenesis. Studying well-defined subgroups of vasculitic patients will be necessary to estimate the prevalence and composition of complement fragments within the immune complex deposits.

D. Polyneuropathies with IgM Monoclonal Gammopathies

Acquired polyneuropathies associated with paraproteinemic diseases are characterized by the presence in serum of a monoclonal immunoglobulin produced by either malignant or normal plasma cells. Among paraproteinemic polyneuropathies, the one associated with a monoclonal IgM appears to be mediated by antibodies of the IgM isotype that recognize specific antigenic determinants on the myelin sheaths (26). More than half of those patients have antibodies against either myelin-associated glycoprotein (MAG) or the glycosphingolipid (SGPG). Other antigenic targets of monoclonal IgM include ganglioside GM1, GM2, GD1b, GD1a, LM1, and sulfatides. In up to two-thirds of these patients the monoclonal IgM recognizes an antigenic component in the peripheral nerve myelin (27).

The clinical picture of IgM anti-MAG neuropathy patients encompasses a mixed sensorimotor demyelinating polyneuropathy, or a sensory ataxic neuropathy (28). Immuno-histochemical studies of peripheral nerve biopsies show deposition of IgM and the complement fragment, C3d, on the myelin sheaths (29). C1q is also deposited at the same sites, suggesting activation of complement through the classical pathway. By electron microscopic examination, widening of the myelin lamellae, presumably due to deposition of IgM, is noted. Furthermore, the monoclonal IgM colocalizes along the myelin sheaths with C1q, C3d, and MAC (29). Terminal complex may contribute to myelin damage since there is a correlation between the number of fibers with abnormally spaced myelin and the extent of the deposition of the terminal complement complex. The abnormally spaced myelin could be a consequence of the influx of intracellular water following damage by MAC, thus representing a form of intramyelin edema. Additional evidence for the role of complement-fixing anti-IgM antibody is provided by passive transfer experiments. Injection of anti-MAG IgM monoclonal antibodies from patients with this neuropathy into the sciatic nerve of cats results in segmental demyelination (30). The effect is achieved only in the presence of fresh, non-heat-inactivated patients' sera supplemented with guinea pig complement. One hour after injection, immunofluorescencent staining detects IgM and C3 deposits along the injected nerve fascicle, while 4 h later the injected nerve fibers demonstrate extensive vesiculation of the myelin sheath (30).

Although the body of literature on the role of complement in inducing demyelination in IgM monoclonal gammopathy is not extensive, there is suggestive evidence for a complement-dependent process. Some earlier studies failed to detect complement at the sites of immunoglobulin deposits, but this could be due to the differences in the affinity of anticomplement antibodies used. The utilization of anti-C3d antibodies with increased specificity and sensitivity might have been an additional factor for the in-situ complement detection. Because paraproteinemic neuropathies are heterogeneous and the IgM recognizes various antigens including GM1, GD1b, MAG, and sulfatides, the role of the complement needs to be examined separately for each neuropathy subset.

E. Diabetic Polyneuropathy

Peripheral neuropathy is one of the major manifestations of diabetes mellitus; it has been estimated to occur in as many as 60% of patients. Neuropathy manifested by sensory loss and weakness can occur in several forms, such as distal symmetrical sensory, painful polyneuropathy, proximal diabetic neuropathy, and multifocal asymmetrical neuropathy.

The role of immunological mechanisms in the pathogenesis of a subset of patients with sensorimotor diabetic neuropathy has been suggested based on perineurial deposition of IgM, IgG, C3, and C4 in 6 of 16 nerve biopsies (31) and localization of C3d and C5b-9 within endoneurial and epineurial blood vessel walls in another 20 patients (32).

No definitive conclusion about the role of complement in the development of diabetic neuropathy can be made based on these two limited studies. However, research now underway is exploring whether a complement-mediated microangiopathy underlies the cause in a subset of patients with proximal motor diabetic polyneuropathy. The information is relevant because a major beneficial effect has been observed in some of these patients after treatment with intravenous immunoglobulin (IVIG). As discussed later, this suggests that complement activation may contribute to the development of peripheral nerve pathology in some patients with diabetic neuropathy.

III. DISEASES OF THE NEUROMUSCULAR JUNCTION

A. Myasthenia Gravis

Myasthenia gravis (MG) is the prototypic autoimmune disease that presents with easy fatigability, skeletal muscle weakness, ptosis, or diplopia. It may lead to life-threatening weakness of respiratory and swallowing muscles. The incidence has two age- and gender-related peaks: women are affected in the second and third decades, and men are affected after the fifth decade. In MG, the neuromuscular transmission is impaired due to antibody-mediated destruction of the nicotinic acetylcholine receptor (AChR) at the postsynaptic region of the end plate. Autoantibodies against the AChR are demonstrated by radioimmunoassay (RIA) in the sera of at least 90% of all patients with MG. These antibodies do not directly block neuromuscular transmission, but bind to the receptors causing their internalization and degradation either through cross-linking and antigenic modulation or through a complement-dependent process.

Several lines of evidence suggest that lysis of AChRs at the neuromuscular junction is complement-mediated in MG. Ultrastructural and light microscopic studies have localized IgG and C3 immune complexes as well as C9 and MAC at the motor end-plate (33). Due to MAC-mediated destruction, AChR-enriched membrane fragments of junctional folds are shed into the synaptic gap. As a consequence, there is a decreased number of postsynaptic folds and simplification of the end plate. The levels of the terminal complement components SC5b-9, assayed in the plasma of patients with MG by ELISA, are abnormally high in as many as 58% of patients (34). No clear correlation, however, exists between plasma SC5b-9 values, AchR antibody levels, and disease severity.

A more direct evidence for the role of complement in the pathogenesis of muscle weakness in MG was based on the observation that heat-inactivated serum causes lysis of cultured rat myotubes in the presence of guinea pig complement. This effect is prevented by heat-inactivation and C3-immunoabsorption of the guinea pig serum. An immunoglobulin fraction of MG sera also contains complement-dependent lytic activity against myotubes in culture (35). In vitro electrophysiological analysis has shown that heat-inactivated MG sera in conjunction with normal human serum as a source of complement causes contraction of the endplate areas of freshly dissociated rat muscle fibers, preceded by progressive depolarization of the muscle membrane. When MG sera alone and heat-inactivated normal human serum were used, these phenomena were not observed (36).

Additional evidence that the IgG antibody in MG is complement fixed was derived from passive transfer experiments using IgG fractions from patients with MG. The animals developed typical myasthenic features characterized by muscle weakness, reduction of miniature end-plate potentials, and a more than 50% decrease in the number of AChRs at the neuromuscular junction. Injection of the same IgG in mice depleted of C3 by cobra venom factor enhanced the degradation process (37).

Our study contributed to the body of evidence showing the role of complement in MG by demonstrating that sera of patients with active disease contain an increased number of activated complement components, measured by an in vitro C3 uptake assay (9). (Table 2).

The role of complement in the immunopathogenesis of MG seems to be unequivocally established. One unanswered question is whether complement is also activated in antibody-negative MG.

B. Lambert-Eaton Myasthenic Syndrome

Lambert-Eaton mysthenic syndrome (LEMS) is an autoimmune neuromuscular disorder often associated with small cell lung carcinoma and a high prevalence of autoantibodies. It is characterized by proximal muscle weakness and autonomic dysfunction that encompasses dry mouth, sexual impotence, and constipation. Ptosis and bulbar and respiratory symptoms may also occur. Clinical signs and symptoms are thought to be caused by an underlying impairment of neuromuscular transmission caused by antibodies that alter the presynaptic release of acetylcholine. The release of acetylcholine from storage vesicles in the nerve endings requires influx of calcium through voltage-gated channels in nerve terminals. In LEMS these channels are the target of pathogenic antibodies. The autoimmune neurological manifestations may reflect cross-reactivity against antigens of the tumor cells also found in synapses of the peripheral nervous system. The P/Q subtype of Ca^{2+} channels is the predominant mediator of neuromuscular transmission. Antibodies against P/Q type calcium channels are found in almost all patients with LEMS and cancer and in more than 90% of patients without cancer (38).

Passive transfer of sera or IgG fractions from patients with LEMS generally failed to produce convincing clinical weakness in recipient rodents, but resulted in a significant reduction in stimulus-dependent quantal release of acetylcholine, as measured microelectrophysiologically at the diaphragmatic endplates in vitro. This effect appears to be complement-independent, since the most potent patient's serum was effective in complement-deficient and complement-depleted mice (39). C3 could not be demonstrated electron microscopically on nerve terminals in biopsied muscle of patients with LEMS (40).

When applied to bovine adrenal chromaffin cells, IgG antibodies from patients with LEMS reduce the voltage-dependent Ca^{2+} channel currents by 40% (41). When the IgG samples are heat-inactivated, however, there is a significant (more than 50%) loss of their calcium current-suppressive activity, suggesting that residual complement proteins may accelerate the pathological effect of IgG.

There seems to be a consensus that LEMS is not a complement-dependent disorder, based primarily on the fact that complement was not required to induce characteristic changes in passive transfer studies. Only 1 (the most potent) of 26 LEMS sera, however, was tested in complement-deficient/depleted animals. On the other hand, there are some indications that complement may contribute to the involvement of antibodies in the pathogenesis of LEMS. Furthermore, the striking similarity of this disease to MG may justify the reexamination of the role of complement in the development of LEMS. Time course, in situ immunohistochemistry, and in vitro electrophysiological studies may be needed to assess the effectiveness of LEMS autoantibodies in the presence or absence of complement.

IV. MYOPATHIES

A. Dermatomyositis

Dermatomyositis (DM), along with polymyositis (PM) and inclusion body myositis (IBM), belongs to the group of acquired muscle diseases collectively called inflammatory myopathies because they have in common the presence of endomysial inflammation as a characteristic histological finding. Varying degrees of muscle weakness are present in all three conditions. DM differs from the other two because of additional distinct clinical features that include a characteristic rash and dilated capillaries at the base of the fingernails that occur even if the degree of muscle weakness is mild. An additional histological finding characteristic of DM is the presence of endomysial microangiopathy with capillary depletion that appears to be complement mediated (42).

The presence of immune complexes consisting of IgM, IgG, and C3 was initially observed in endomysial blood venules (43). Subsequent studies established that the endomysial capillaries are the primary site of immune injury in DM (44). The MAC was localized to the intramuscular capillaries by use of an antibody against the neoantigen exposed upon C5b-9 complex deposition (45). Further confirmation of complement-mediated injury to the capillaries was established using a lectin *Ulex europeus* (as a specific marker for endothelial cells) and antibodies to MAC in a double-localization method (Fig. 3). The deposition of MAC in muscle capillaries occurs in the perifascicular area early in the disease and precedes the consequences of endothelial cell destruction, such as microinfarcts and muscle fiber destruction. Complement fragments in the sera of patients with DM were quantitated by an in vitro C3 uptake assay, as described earlier for patients with GBS and MG. An increased C3 uptake is seen in DM patients and

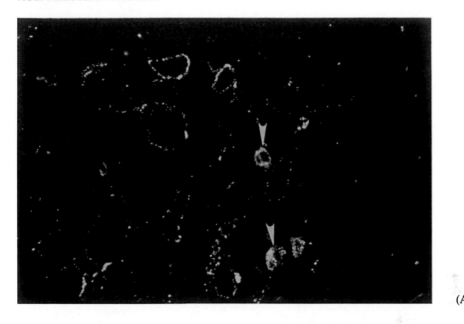

(A)

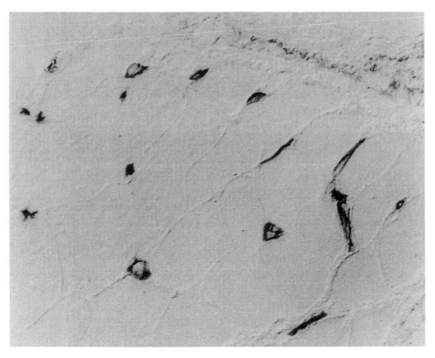

(B)

Figure 3 (A) Cross-section of a muscle biopsy from a patient with dermatomyositis immuno-stained with antibodies against MAC shows deposition of MAC on dilated capillaries (arrowheads) and on certain necrotic muscle fibers. The deposition of MAC leads to destruction of capillaries. The remaining capillaries are fewer in number and have a dilated lumen (B), as shown with immunostaining using a lectin that binds to endothelial cells. Normally, one or two capillaries surround each muscle fiber.

correlates with disease activity (9). In addition to MAC, C3bNEO antigen is also found deposited on the muscle capillaries, (Fig. 4); signifying deposition of C3b into immune complexes (46).

The mechanism of complement activation in DM is still unclear. Circulating antibodies against endothelial cells (AECA) have been demonstrated in the sera of patients with

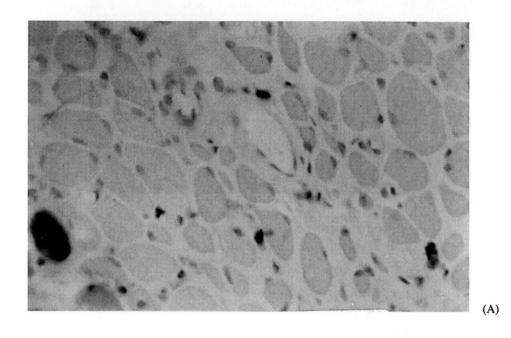

(A)

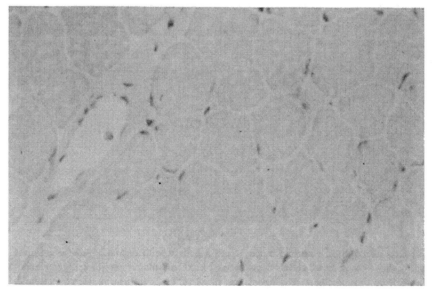

(B)

Figure 4 Cross-section of a muscle biopsy from a patient with dermatomyositis stained with antibodies to C3bNEO demonstrates C3bNEO deposits on the capillaries and occasional muscle fibers (A). After successful treatment with IVIg, the C3BNEO deposits disappear (B).

DM and could potentially trigger the classical complement pathway. We have preliminary evidence (Basta and Dalakas, unpublished observation) that IgG purified from DM sera binds to human umbilical vein endothelial cells (HUVEC) and recognizes endothelial cell proteins in Western blot assays. Purified IgG from the patients' sera in the presence of complement from fresh guinea pig serum appears to cause lysis of HUVEC (Basta and Dalakas, unpublished results).

Complement-mediated microangiopathy has been unquestionably established as a pathological event that precedes development of clinical signs and symptoms in DM. It remains to be elucidated what triggers complement activation and subsequent deposition of MAC in the endomyseal capillaries. The incidence of antiendothelial cell antibodies, their target antigens, and their complement-fixing properties need to be studied. Our preliminary data suggest that patients' IgG that exerted the cytotoxic effect in cultured HUVEC may represent specific, complement-dependent antiendothelial cell antibodies.

B. Necrotizing Myopathy with Pipestem Capillaries

Four patients with a unique microanagiopathy characterized by microvascular MAC deposition, capillary depletion, and necrotizing myopathy have been recognized (47). The disorder presents clinically with muscle pain and moderate proximal muscle weakness. The most prominent pathological finding in muscle biopsies is heavy hyalinization and thickening of capillary walls, giving them a "pipestem" appearance, similar to those seen in diabetes. In this myopathy, the number of capillaries is diminished and there are widespread intracapillary MAC deposits, resembling the findings in patients with DM as described earlier. However, these patients do not have the clinical picture of DM.

This disease appears to add to the growing list of neuromuscular diseases in which complement-dependent microangiopathy is the pathogenic hallmark. Whether these patients represent a distinct entity or a subset of dermatomyositis is unclear. It is interesting that hyalinized and thickened blood vessels with MAC deposition can be also found in the peripheral nerves of patients with diabetes. Whether these similarities point to an underlying immune process in certain subsets of diabetic neuropathy remains to be established.

C. X-Linked Vacuolated Myopathy

This is an X-linked recessive disorder with early childhood onset, and is characterized by very slow progression of proximal limb muscle weakness, elevation of serum creatine kinase, and normal life expectancy. Muscle biopsies show excessive autophagic activity and exocytosis of electron-dense membranous bodies. In later stages of the disease, the incidence of vacuolated muscle fibers may reach almost 50%. MAC is deposited on the sarcolemma and within vacuoles in a large number of muscle fibers. Granular MAC deposits are also present in the vessel walls. No immunostaining for immunoglobulins is seen, suggesting activation of the alternative pathway or an antibody-independent activation of the classical pathway (48). This disease is an example of nonlethal assembly of MAC, in which shedding of membrane fragments containing terminal complement complex appears to be protective against complement attack. Levels of C5 and C9 are elevated in the serum of patients with this disorder, supporting the role of complement in the disease pathogenesis (49).

The role of complement activation in this rare hereditary disease is interesting but provocative. The pathway of activation is unknown. It is intriguing that there appears to be a protective mechanism against MAC damage through shedding of membrane fragments containing MAC. It should be noted, however, that this mechanism is not absolutely protective because enough MAC complexes remain on muscle fibers that may be responsible for the pathological changes and the manifestations of clinical muscle weakness.

V. AUTOIMMUNE CHANNELOPATHIES

An increasing body of evidence supports the view that different ionic channels represent targets of an immune attack, with the subsequent functional blockade leading to abnormalities of peripheral nerve conduction and neuromuscular transmission.

Demyelination and associated conduction block are usually blamed for the clinical manifestations of Guillain-Barré syndrome, CIDP, and other neuropathies associated with antibodies to gangliosides including GM1 and GQ1b. However, after successful therapy conduction block can recover before the remyelination process is completed, suggesting a more complex pathophysiology or reversible functional blockade preceding myelin or axonal damage (2).

Rabbit polyclonal antibodies against GM1 ganglioside were found to suppress voltage-sensitive sodium currents in isolated rat nerve fibers. The effect was complement dependent and accompanied by an increase in K^+ and nonspecific leakage currents (50). In the absence of complement, however, anti-GM1 antibodies increased the rise and the amplitude of K^+ currents. These observations suggest that anti-GM1 antibodies react with antigenic determinants, probably sialic acid residues, of sodium channels in the axonal membrane and form antibody–complement complexes that block Na^+ channels, resulting in axonal damage, as reflected by an increase in leakage currents. In the absence of complement, anti-GM1 antibodies have a different effect, manifested as an increase in K^+ currents. The degree of complement involvement at the site of nodal membrane seems to correlate with the variety of clinical manifestations associated with anti-GM1 antibodies (50).

IgG isolated from patients with amyotrophic lateral sclerosis (ALS) is reported to bind to purified L-type voltage-gated calcium channels (VGCCs) from skeletal muscle cells and reduce calcium current amplitudes (51). Passive transfer of the patients' serum may also cause alteration of presynaptic voltage-dependent calcium currents and calcium-dependent release of neurotransmitters in recipient animals (52). Whether this effect is reproducible or complement dependent remains to be established. As previously discussed, LEMS is mediated by anti-P/Q-type calcium channel antibodies, but the role of complement remains to be clarified.

Complement and its fragments may not only exert a functional or even anatomical blockade of nerve conduction along with complement-fixing autoantibodies against the channels but may also have an effect directly or through their receptors linked to ion channels by second messenger system. For instance, C5a has been shown to cause hyperpolarization of the plasma membrane of inflammatory cells due to increased K^+ permeability. This electrophysiological event represents an early response of these cells to C5a and precedes physical signs of macrophage activation such as membrane spreading, ruffling, and pseudopod formation (53). The nature of ion channels that mediate C5a-induced hyperpolarization of macrophages remains unknown, but it is postulated that Ca^{2+}-activated

K^+ channels are involved. The hypothesis is that ligation of C5a receptor via pertussis-toxin sensitive G proteins activates K^+ channels. One pathway may engage rapid signaling by the release of intracellular Ca^{2+} close to a K^+ channel, similar to the neurotransmitter release at the presynaptic plasma membrane. At least one more pathway must exist, since even when Ca is clamped, further ligation of C5a receptor leads to further increases of outward K^+ currents (54).

Autoimmune channelopathies represent a new concept in the pathophysiology of neuromuscular diseases and an emerging field of the neuropathology and electrophysiology of demyelination or membrane disruption. Although more work is needed, the present evidence suggests that complement alone or in conjunction with immunoglobulin can directly or indirectly, transiently or permanently, affect ionic channels and their function, leading to various clinical manifestations.

VI. THERAPY OF NEUROMUSCULAR DISEASES

In general, the treatment of autoimmune neuromusclar diseases is based on the use of immunosuppressive or immunomodulatory therapies. Oral prednisone represents the first line of drugs for the immunotherapy of these diseases, with a notable exception of the GBS in which steroids are contraindicated. Cytostatic drugs, such as cyclophosphamide, cyclosporin, and azathioprine, are widely used as second-line therapeutic agents. Combination therapy is common in vasculitic neuropathies and the neuropathies associated with IgM monoclonal gammopathy. Plasmapheresis has been also effective in GBS and in short-term management of patients with MG (55).

High-dose intravenous immunoglobulin (IVIG) therapy deserves special mention as an immunomodulatory therapy because it exerts a beneficial effect in most of the diseases listed in Table 1. IVIG is equally effective if not superior to plasmapheresis in GBS, dramatically improves signs and symptoms of patients with active DM, can produce rapid reversal of myasthenic weakness, and has been shown to be reasonably effective in CIDP, and in occasional patients with diabetic polyneuropathy and polyneuropathy associated with IgM gammopathy (55).

While the positive effect can be ascribed to a variety of different mechanisms of action of IVIG (56), the complement scavenger action of intravenous immunoglobulin could play a predominant role in the treatment of the diseases discussed in this chapter, because complement involvement plays a role in their pathogenesis. This issue has been formally addressed in the study designed to examine if the beneficial effect of IVIG, previously noted in the Forssman shock model, and in clinical trials with patients with DM, could be exerted through the same mechanism of preventing the deposition of activated complement fragments on target cells. Repeat muscle biopsies from patients whose condition improved after IVIG therapy, showed disappearance of C3bNEO and MAC deposits from the endomysial capillaries (Fig. 4). This could mean that infused immunoglobulin intercepts the incorporation of C3b into the C5 convertase through formation of covalent or noncovalent complexes between specific acceptor sites within the immunoglobulin molecule and C3b. The resulting unavailability of C3b for incorporation into the C5 convertase can result in the prevention of MAC formation, as supported by the absence of MAC in post-IVIG muscle biopsies. Furthermore, the in vitro uptake of C3 in the sera of patients before IVIG (baseline C3 uptake) was high, correlated with the disease activity, and was significantly suppressed in the post-IVIG samples. These in vitro findings support the role of complement in DM and suggest that the high rate of complement activation may be responsible for the formation of a large number of activated early components (46). The C3 uptake was also increased in two other neuromuscular diseases, CBS and MG, in which IVIG is effective (9).

More clinical trials and careful in situ and in vitro studies in patients with autoimmune neuromuscular disorders may clarify further the role of complement-immunoglobulin complex formation in suppressing the deposition of activated complement fragments into target tissues.

REFERENCES

1. Asbury AK, Cornblath DR. Assessment of current diagnostic criteria for Guillain-Barre syndrome. Ann Neurol 1990; 27(Suppl):21–24.
2. Waxman SG. Sodium channel blockade by antibodies: a new mechanism of neurological disease? Ann Neurol 1995; 37:421–423.
3. Luijten, JAFM, Faille-Kuyper, EHB. The occurrence of IgM and complement factors along myelin sheaths of peripheral nerves. An immunohistochemical study of the Guillain-Barre syndrome. J Neurol Sci 1972; 15:219–224.
4. Hays, AP, Lee, SSI, Latov, N. Immune reactive C3d on the surface of myelin sheaths in neuropathy. J Neuroimmunol 1988; 18:231–244.
5. Hafer-Macko, CE, Sheikh, KA, Li, CY, Ho, TW, Cornblath, DR, McKhann, GM, Asbury, AK, Griffin, JW. Immune attack on the Schwann cell surface in acute inflammatory demyelinating polyneuropathy. Ann Neurol 1996; 39:625–635.
6. Koski, CL, Sanders, ME, Swoveland, PT, Lawley, TJ, Shin, ML, Frank, MM, Joiner, KA. Activation of terminal components of complement in patients with Guillain-Barre syndrome and other demyelinating neuropathies. J Clin Invest 1987; 80:1492–1497.
7. Sanders, M, Koski, CL, Robbins, D, Shin, ML, Frank, MM, Joiner, KA. Activated terminal complement in cerebrospinal fluid in Guillain-Barre syndrome and multiple sclerosis. J Immunol 1986; 136:4456–4459.
8. Hartung, HP, Schwenke, C, Bitter-Suermann, D, Toyka, KV. Guillain-Barre syndrome: activated complement components C3a and C5a in CSF. Neurology 1987; 37:1006–1009.
9. Basta, M, Dalakas, MC. Increased in vitro uptake of the complement C3b in the serum of patients with Guillain-Barre syndrome, myasthenia gravis and dermatomyositis. J Neuroimmunol 1996; 70:227–229.
10. Saida, T, Saida, K, Lisak, RP, Brown, M, Silberberg, DH, Asbury, AK. In-vivo demyelinating activity of sera from patients with Guillain-Barre syndrome. Ann Neurol 1982; 11:69–75.
11. Santoro, M,, Uncini, A, Corbo, M, Staugaitis, SM, Thomas, FP, Hays, AP, Latov, N. Experimental conduction block induced by serum from a patient with anti-GM1 antibodies. Ann Neurol 1992; 31:385–390.
12. Oomes, PG, van der Meche, FGA, Markus-Silvis, L. In-vivo effects of sera from Guillain-Barre subgroups: an elctrophysiological and histological study on rat nerves. Muscle Nerve 1991; 14:1013–1020.
13. Summer, AJ, Saida, K, Saida, T, Silberberg, D, Asbury, AK. Acute conduction block associated with experimental antiserum-mediated demyelination of peripheral nerve. Ann Neurol 1982; 11:469–477.
14. Dubois-Dalco, M, Buyse, M, Buyse, G, Gorce, F. The action of Guillain-Barre syndrome serum on myelin. A tissue culture and electron microscopic analysis. J Neurol Sci 1970; 13:67–83.
15. Cook, SD, Dowling, PC, Murray, MR, Whitaker, JN. Circulating demyelinating factors in acute idiopathic polyneuropathy. Arch Neurol 1971; 24:136–144.

16. Sawant-Mane, S, Clark, MB, Koski, CL. In-vitro demylination by serum antibody from patients with Guillain-Barre syndrome requires terminal complement complexes. Ann Neurol 1991; 29:397–404.

17. Dalakas, MC, Engel, WK. Chronic relapsing (dysimmune) polyneuropathy: pathogenesis and treatment. Ann Neurol 1981; 10(suppl):134–145.

18. Dalakas, MC, Engel, WK. Immunoglobulin and complement deposits in nerves of patients with chronic relapsing polyneuropathy. Arch Neurol 1980; 37:637–640.

19. Hartung, HP, Reiners, K, Toyka, KV, Pollard, JD. Guillain-Barre syndrome and CIDP. In: Hohlfeld R, ed. Immunology of Neuromuscular Disease. Dordrecht/Boston/London: Kluwer Academic Publishers, 1994:84–85

20. Toyka, KV, Hartung, HP. Chronic inflammatory polyneuritis and related neuropathies. Curr Opin Neurol 1996; 9:240–250.

21. Kissel, JT, Mendell, JR. Peripheral neuropathy due to vasculitis: immunopathogenesis, clinical features and treatment. In: Hohlfeld R, ed. Immunology of Neuromuscular Disease. Dordrecht/Boston/London: Kluwer Academic Publishers, 1994:114.

22. Midroni G, Bilbao JUM. Biopsy Diagnosis of Peripheral Neuropathy. Boston: Butterworth-Heinemann, 1995.

23. Pangyres, PK, Blumbergs, PC, Leong ASY, Bourne, AJ. Vasculitis of peripheral nerve and skeletal muscle: clinicopathological correlation and immunopathic mechanisms. J Neurol Sci 1990; 100:193–202.

24. Engelhardt, A, Lorler, H, Neundorfer, B. Immunohistochemical findings in vasculitic neuropathies. Acta Neurol Scand 1993; 87:318–321.

25. Kissel, JT, Reithman, JL, Omerza, J, Rammohan, KW, Mendell, JR. Peripheral nerve vasculitis: immune characterization of the vascular lesions. Ann Neurol 1989; 25:291–297.

26. Dalakas, MC, Engel, WK. Polyneuropathy with monoclonal gammopathy. studies of 11 patients. Ann Neurol 1981; 10:45–52.

27. Dalakas, MC. Autoimmune Neuropathies. In: Rich RR, ed. Clinical Immunology. St. Louis: Mosby Year Book, 1995:1384–1387.

28. Dalakas, MC, Quarles, RH. Autoimmune ataxic neuropathies (sensory ganglionopathies): are glycolipids the responsible autoantigens? Ann Neurol 1996; 39:419–422.

29. Monaco, S, Bonetti, B, Ferrari, S, et al. Complement-mediated demyelination in patients with IgM monoclonal gammopathy and polyneuropathy. N Engl J Med 1990; 322:649–652.

30. Hays, AP, Latov, N, Takatsu, M, Sherman, WH. Experimental demyelination of nerve induced by serum of patients with neuropathy and an anti-MAG IgM M-protein. Neurology 1987; 242–256.

31. Graham, AR, Johnson, PC. Direct immunofluorescence findings in peripheral nerve from patients with diabetic neuropathy. Ann Neurol 1985; 17:450–454.

32. Younger, DS, Rosoklija, G, Hays, AP, Trojaborg, W, Latov, N. Diabetic peripheral neuropathy: a clinicopathologic and immmunohistochemical analysis of sural nerve biopsies. Muscle Nerve 1996; 19:722–727.

33. Nakano, S, Engel, AG. Myasthenia gravis: quantitative immunocytochemical analysis of inflammatory cells and detection of complement membrane attack complex at the end-plate in 30 patients. Neurology 1993; 43:1167–1172.

34. Barohn, RJ, Brey, RL. Soluble terminal complement components in human myasthenia gravis. Clin Neurol Neurosurg 1993; 95:285–290.

35. Ashizawa, T, Appel, SH. Complement-dependent lysis of cultured rat myotubes by myasthenic immunoglobulins. Neurology 1985; 35:1748–1753.

36. Mzrzymas, JW, Lorenzon, P, Riviera, AP et al. An electrophysiological study of the effects of myasthenia gravis sera and complement on rat isolated muscle fibers. J Neuroimmunol 1993; 45:155–162.

37. Toyka, KV, Drachman, DB, Griffin, D. et al. Myasthenia gravis. Study of humoral immune mechanisms by passive transfer to mice. N Engl J Med 1977; 296:125–131.

38. Lennon, VA, Kryzer, TJ, Griesmann, MS et al. Calcium-channel antibodies in the Lambert-Eaton syndrome and other paraneoplastic syndromes. N Engl J Med 1995; 332:1467–1474.
39. Lambert, EH, Lennon, VA. Selected IgG rapidly induces Lambert-Eaton myasthenic syndrome in mice: complement independence and EMG abnormalities. Muscle Nerve 1988; 11:1133–1145.
40. Engel, AG, Lambert, EH, Howard JRFM. Immune complexes (IgG and C3) at the motor end-plate in myasthenia gravis. Ultrastructural and light microscopic localization and electrophysiologic correlations. Mayo Clin Proc 1977; 267–280.
41. Kim, YI, Neher, E. IgG from patients with Lambert-Eaton syndrome blocks voltage-dependent calcium channels. Science 1988; 239:405–408.
42. Dalakas, MC. Polymiositis, dermatomyositis, and inclusion-body myositis. N Engl J Med 1991; 325:1487–1498.
43. Whitaker, JN, Engel, WK. Vascular deposits of immunoglobulin and complement in idiopathic inflammatory myopathy. N Engl J Med 1972; 286:33–338.
44. Emslie-Smith, AM, Engel, AG. Microvascular changes in early and advanced dermatomyositis: a quantitative study. Ann Neurol 1990; 27:343–356.
45. Kissel, JT, Mendell, JR, Rammohan, KW. Microvascular deposition of complement membrane attack complex in dermatomyositis. N Engl J Med 1986; 314:329–334.
46. Basta, M, Dalakas, MC. High dose intravenous immunoglobulin exerts its beneficial effect in patients with dermatomyositis by blocking endomysial deposition of activated complement fragments. J Clin Invest 1994; 94:1729–1735.
47. Emslie-Smith, AM, Engel, AG. Necrotizing myopathy with pipestem capillaries, microvascular deposition of the complement membrane attack complex (MAC), and minimal cellular infiltration. Neurology 1991; 41:936–939.
48. Kalimo, H, Savontaus, ML, Lang, H, et al. X-linked myopathy with excessive autophagy: a new hereditary muscle disease. Ann Neurol 1988; 23:258–265.
49. Louboutin, JP, Villanova, M, Ulrich, G. Elevated levels of complement components C5 and C9 and decreased antitrypsin activity in the serum of patients with X-linked vacuolated myopathy. Muscle Nerve 1996; 19:1144–1147.
50. Takigawa, T, Yasuda, H, Kikkawa, R. et al. Antibodies against GM1 ganglioside affect K^+ and Na^+ currents in isolated rat myelinated nerve fibers. Ann Neurol 1995; 37:436–442.
51. Delbono, O, Garcia, J, Appel, S. et al. IgG from amyotrophic lateral sclerosis affects tubular calcium channels of skeletal muscle. Am J Physiol 1991; 260:C1347–C1351.
52. Appel, SH, Engelhardt, JI, Garcia J, et al. Imunoglobulins from animal models of motor neuron disease and from human amyotrophic lateral sclerosis patients passively transfer physiological abnormalities to the neuromuscular junction. Proc Natl Acad Sci USA 1991; 88:647–651.
53. Gallin, EK, Gallin, JI. Interaction of chemotactic factors with human macrophages. Induction of transmembrane potential changes. J Cell Biol 1977; 75:277–289.
54. Fan, Y, McCloskey, MA. Dual pathway for GTP-dependent regulation of chemoattractant-activated K^+ conductance in murine J774 monocytes. J Biol Chem 1994; 269:31533–31543.
55. Hohlfeld, R. Immunology of Neuromuscular Disease, 1st ed. Dordrecht/Boston/London: Kluwer Academic Publishers, 1994.
56. Dwyer, JM. Manipulating the immune system with immune globulin. N Engl J Med 1992; 326:107–116.

Index

Page numbers in *italic* indicate figures; page numbers followed by "t" indicate tables.

T - #1070 - 101024 - C0 - 254/178/31 [33] - CB - 9780824798987 - Gloss Lamination